Abdomen and Thoracic

Ayman S. El-Baz • Luca Saba • Jasjit Suri

Editors

Abdomen and Thoracic Imaging

An Engineering & Clinical Perspective

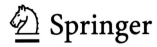

Springer

Editors
Ayman S. El-Baz
Department of Bioengineering
University of Louisville
Louisville, KY, USA

Luca Saba
University of Cagliari
Cagliari, Italy

Jasjit Suri
Biomedical Technologies, Inc
    Idaho State University (Affiliated)
Roseville, CA, USA

ISBN 978-1-4899-7958-2   ISBN 978-1-4614-8498-1 (eBook)
DOI 10.1007/978-1-4614-8498-1
Springer New York Heidelberg Dordrecht London

Springer is part of Springer Science+Business Media (www.springer.com)

Ayman S. El-Baz would like to dedicate this book to his wife, daughter, son, mother, and father.

Luca Saba would like to dedicate this book to his parents Giovanni Saba and Raffaela Polla for their love.

Jasjit Suri would like to dedicate this book to his children Harman Suri and Neha Suri, and his loving wife Malvika.

Contents

Computer-Aided Diagnosis Systems for Acute Renal Transplant Rejection: Challenges and Methodologies

Mahmoud Mostapha, Fahmi Khalifa, Amir Alansary, Ahmed Soliman, Jasjit Suri, and Ayman S. El-Baz

Abstract This chapter overviews one of the most critical problems in urology, namely detection of acute renal transplant rejection. Developing an effective, fast, and accurate computer-aided diagnosis (CAD) system for early detection of acute renal rejection is of great clinical importance for the management of these patients. For this reason, CAD systems for early detection of renal transplant rejection have been investigated in a huge number of research studies using different image modalities, such as ultrasound (US), magnetic resonance imaging (MRI), computed tomography (CT), and radionuclide imaging. A typical CAD system for kidney diagnosis consists of a set of processing steps including, but not limited to, image registration to account for kidney motion, segmentation of the kidney and/or its compartments (e.g., cortex, medulla), construction of agent kinetic curves, functional parameters estimation, and diagnosis and assessment of the kidney status. Due to the widespread popularity of US and MRI, this chapter overviews the current state-of-the-art CAD systems that have been developed for kidney diagnosis using these two image modalities. In addition, the chapter addresses several challenges that researchers face in developing efficient, fast, and reliable CAD systems for early detection of kidney diseases.

M. Mostapha • F. Khalifa • A. Alansary • A. Soliman
BioImaging laboratory, Bioengineering Department and with the Electrical and Computer Engineering Department, University of Louisville, Louisville, KY 40292, USA

J. Suri
Biomedical Technologies, Inc., Roseville CA, USA

A.S. El-Baz (✉)
BioImaging laboratory, Bioengineering Department, University of Louisville, Louisville, KY 40292, USA
e-mail: aselba01@exchange.louisville.edu

A.S. El-Baz et al. (eds.), *Abdomen and Thoracic Imaging: An Engineering & Clinical Perspective*, DOI 10.1007/978-1-4614-8498-1_1,
© Springer Science+Business Media New York 2014

1

Introduction

Early detection of kidney rejection is important for clinical management in patients with transplanted kidneys [1]. In the USA, approximately 17,736 renal transplants are performed annually [2], and given the limited number of donors, transplanted kidney salvage is an important goal. Renal transplantation complications could be divided into 6 classes: urologic complications, fluid collections, vascular complications, neoplasms, recurrent native renal disease, and graft dysfunction [3]. Urologic complications include urine leaks associated with discharged urinomas, which have different sizes and occurs within 2 weeks from transplantation. Also, transplant patients face the high risk of developing calculous disease and urinary obstruction. Around transplantation fluid collections have been usually recorded in up to 50 % of renal transplantations and include urinomas, hematomas, lymphoceles, and abscesses. The size, location, and the growth possibility of these collections greatly influence their clinical relevance [4]. vascular complications include transplanted artery stenosis, infarction, arteriovenous fistulas [AVFs] and pseudoaneurysms, and renal vein thrombosis. Although these complications are found in only 10 % of transplantation cases, they represent significant reasons for serous graft dysfunction that has high mortality rates [5]. Cancer development highly increases after kidney transplantation, especially when immunosuppression period is extended. Neoplasms risks include renal cell carcinomas and lymphomas [6]. Recurrent disease is rare in the early stage posttransplantation and is usually detected in long-term renal transplant recipients with diabetes, amyloidosis, and cystinosis [7]. Renal graft dysfunction causes are acute tubular necrosis (ATN), rejection (hyperacute, acute, and chronic), and drug nephrotoxicity [8]. ATN is found initially in most cadaveric grafts and usually diminishes within 2 weeks depending on ischemic insult. ATN is usually related to the donor kidney and is commonly observed in patients whose transplants are from living relatives [9]. Acute rejection is found in up to 40 % of patients within 3 weeks after transplantation and it is typically reversible through high-dose steroids or antibody therapy [10]. Chronic rejection manifested itself as a gradual deterioration in graft function starting at 3 months posttransplantation [11]. The recurrent previous episodes of acute rejection is the main cause for chronic rejection [10]. Since finding an effective treatment of chronic rejection is still an ongoing research, avoiding episodes of acute rejection is the ideal way of preventing chronic rejection [9]. Drug toxicity also contributes in degrading the grafted kidney functions. Cyclosporine imposes a high nephrotoxic potential as it can afferent glomerular arterioles [11].

Acute rejection, i.e., the immunological response of the human immune system to the foreign kidney, is the most important cause of renal dysfunction among other diagnostic possibilities. Acute rejection is still a risk for grafts, regardless of the progresses made within the last decades. The incidence of rejection episodes depends on several factors, e.g., the organ (status), comorbidities, medication, and compliance [12]. Chronic allograft deterioration and worsening long-term risk increases significantly with each acute rejection episode [13, 14]. Consequently, early detection and effective-fast treatment of acute rejection are crucial to preserve a graft's function. At present, the initial evaluation of renal dysfunction after transplantation is based on multiple blood tests and urine sampling (e.g., plasma creatinine, creatinine clearance). Creatinine clearance is a clinical measurement used to estimate renal function, specifically the filtration rate of the glomeruli, and its value is determined by measuring the concentration of endogenous creatinine (which is produced by the body) in both plasma and urine. Creatinine clearance is a slightly less accurate measure of the glomerular filtration rate than inulin clearance because, unlike inulin, a small amount of creatinine is reabsorbed by the kidney and is not excreted in the urine, thereby being lost to measurement. Difficulties involved in carrying out the inulin clearance procedure, however, render creatinine clearance the more practical clinical measurement with which to assess renal function [15]. However, the fact that creatinine clearance provides information on both kidneys together, but not unilateral information [16], and that significant change in creatinine level is only detectable after the loss of 60 % of the kidney function [17], limits the efficiency of such index in detecting renal rejection. Therefore, an obligating need for highly sensitive and specific detection of early acute detection still exists, with biopsy remaining the gold standard diagnostic procedure. However, biopsy as an invasive procedure imposes the risk of bleeding and infection to the patients, may cause injury to the graft, and is limited to patients who are not taking any anticoagulant drugs. Moreover, this procedure relies on few small samples from limited areas to determine the status of the entire organ. Therefore, this may lead to a wrong estimation of the extent of inflammation in the whole graft [18]. So, diagnostics with noninvasive image-based techniques to investigate the entire graft would yield much better results.

Several noninvasive imaging modalities have been used clinically used to asses transplanted kidneys. Radionuclide imaging (also called scintigraphy), the traditional method in renal imaging, is an excellent modality for evaluating graft function, both qualitatively and quantitatively, while screening for common complications [8]. However, this technique fails in showing accurate anatomical details due to its limited spatial resolution, so functional abnormalities inside different parts of the kidney (such as cortex and medulla) cannot be discriminated precisely [19]. Furthermore, radionuclide imaging includes radiation exposure [20], thus limiting the range of its applications, especially in monitoring such diseases as ATN or cyclosporin [21]. Ultrasound imaging (US) is usually used to evaluate the transplanted kidney early in the postoperative period, and it can also be used for long-term follow-up assessment of the transplanted kidney. US is a relatively cheap and non-nephrotoxic modality; however, sensitivity and reliability of this method mainly depend on the investigator's experience [22]. During an episode of rejection, both two-dimensional and Doppler ultrasound show unspecific features. Doppler may give high pulsatility index (PI) and resistivity index (RI) values (>0.8), which is an indication similar to those of ATN [23, 24]. However, by knowing the course of the finding, discrimination between these two complications could be achieved, as acute rejection usually needs more than few weeks to develop [3]. Computed tomography (CT) is a commonly available technology that uses contrast agents that allows accurate evaluation of various diseases in renal transplantation and with lower costs than magnetic resonance (MR) imaging [25]. However, information gathered by CT to detect renal acute rejection is unspecific and the contrast agents used still are nephrotoxic. Therefore, currently CT has a limited role in diagnosing acute renal rejection [12]. Magnetic resonance imaging (MRI) provides excellent morphological information. Excellent temporal and spatial resolution were possible, thanks to the use of multichannel coils and parallel imaging, which allowed advanced analysis of different aspects of renal function which might be useful to distinguish acute rejection from ATN [26, 27]. More recently, dynamic contrast-enhanced magnetic resonance imaging (DCE-MRI) has gained considerable attention in detecting acute renal rejection due its ability to provide both functional and anatomical information, and the use of the FDA approved contrast agent Gd-DTPA is harmless since it is freely filtered and not reabsorbed by the kidney [28]. However, even with an imaging technique like DCE-MRI, there are several problems because the abdomen is scanned repeatedly and rapidly after the injection of the contrast agent. Therefore, developing a noninvasive CAD system from DCE-MRI is still a challenging problem due to the following reasons: (1) the spatial resolution of the dynamic MR images is low due to fast scanning, (2) the images suffer from the motion induced by the breathing patient which necessitates advanced registration techniques, and (3) the intensity of the kidney changes nonuniformly as the contrast agent perfuses into the cortex which complicates the segmentation procedures [29].

In literature, the development of computer-aided diagnosis (CAD) systems for detecting acute renal rejection using different image modalities is an ongoing area of increased research. The success of the CAD systems can be measured based on the diagnostic accuracy, speed, and automation level [30]. The most popular image modalities used for the diagnosis of kidney diseases are ultrasound (US) and magnetic resonance imaging (MRI). In the following sections, we will first review quickly the anatomy and the functions of the kidney, then we will overview different CAD systems for diagnosis of acute renal rejection using these two imaging modalities.

Anatomy and Functions of the Kidney

Kidneys are bean-shaped organs, located at the back of the abdominal cavity, one on each side of the spinal column, just below the rib cage [31] as shown in Fig. 1. Each kidney is about the size of a fist, but every day, they process about 200 quarts of blood to make the 2 quarts of waste products and extra water which becomes urine [32]. It is the urine production that keeps the blood clean and chemically balanced, making the kidneys vital organs for the body. A cross section of a kidney, as shown in Fig. 2, consists of three regions: the pelvis, the cortex, and the medulla. The pelvis region is only an extension of the ureter into the kidney, while the cortex (outer portion) and the medulla (inner portion) are the main two structural regions.

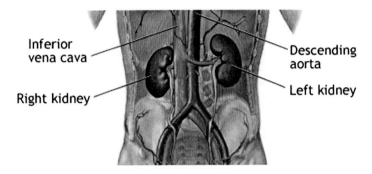

Fig. 1 Schematic of the abdominal area of the human body showing the location of a the kidney

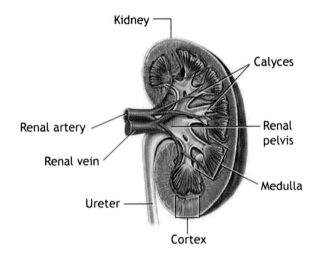

Fig. 2 A schematic showing the anatomy of the human kidney

The cortex and medulla consist of nearly 1 million functional units called nephrons, which are 45–65 mm in length and 0.05 mm in width [33]. Nephrons in the cortex and the medulla process the blood that enters the kidney in several steps to form the urine. The urine then escapes into the pelvis to be transported via ureter tubes to the urinary bladder and with the urethra to the outside environment [31].

The actual process of creating the urine from the blood takes place in the nephrons. Each nephron consists of a glomerulus, its tubule and its blood supply as seen in Fig. 3. The tubule is also divided into four parts: Bowman's capsule, proximal tubule, loop of Henle, and distal tubule. The blood meets the glomerulus structure and the urine starts to formulate through three main processes. These processes include filtration by the glomerulus, as well as reabsorption and secretion by the tubular cells. By means of these processes, the important products such as the amino acids and water in the body are conserved, whereas the metabolic wastes (urea, uric acid, creatinine, ammonia) are excreted out of the body.

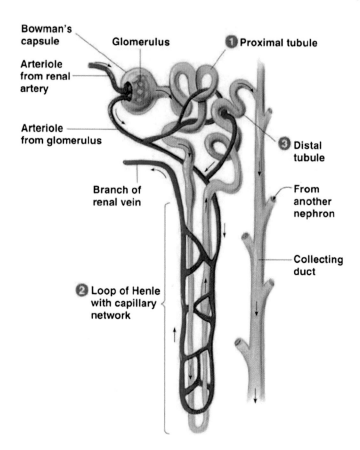

Fig. 3 Structure of a nephron

The first process, the filtration, occurs in the glomerulus. The differences in the blood pressure and the protein osmotic (oncotic) pressure allow the glomerulus to act as an ultra-filter and allow only small particles to enter the fluid that goes into the Bowman's capsule. As a result, the fluid enters the Bowman's capsule lacks the blood cells and the proteins. From the Bowman's capsule, this filtrated fluid goes into the tubular cells which actively transport the necessary materials such as glucose back into the body. This active transportation is called reabsorption, and it helps to retain normal blood levels of necessary materials. On the other hand, a process called secretion is responsible for removing some substances from the blood and adding to the tubular [33]. By the end of these three steps, the urine of a healthy kidney should be free of protein, glucose, and any blood cells.

In ultrasound, ultrasonic sound waves are transferred at high frequency by a transducer, and transfer through the skin and other body tissues to the kidney. The sound waves reflect from the kidney like an echo and come back to the transducer. The transducer collects the reflected waves, which are then altered into an electronic image of the kidney. The speed at which the waves travel is highly affected by various types of body tissues. By introducing additional mode to the ultrasound, the blood flow could be estimated. A Doppler probe inside the transducer gauges the velocity and direction of blood flow in the vessel by allowing sound waves to be audible. The loudness degree of the sound waves shows the level of blood flow in a blood vessel. Also, obstruction of blood flow could be determined by the absence of these sounds. In DCE-MRI, as the contrast agent Gd-DTPA passes through the cortex, the signal intensity is expected to increase before it decreases slightly due to water reabsorption. Constant signal intensity is then expected followed by a decrease due to the washout of the contrast agent. In a healthy kidney, the signal intensity increases instantly after the contrast agent is introduced in around 40 s and peaks within 100 s and starts to drop slowly to its initial value while the urine is formed [34].

Ultrasound

Ultrasound is currently still the first choice in the early assessment of the transplanted kidney or in the long-term follow-up. After 24–48 h posttransplantation, a baseline US evaluation is performed with a detailed examination of renal size, echogenicity, collecting system, ureter condition, and evaluation of any postoperative collections. Graft enlargement (swelling, more globular shape), reduction of corticomedullary differentiation, increased echogenicity, prominent medullary pyramids, or irregularities in the graft perfusion are all typical US findings in case of acute renal rejection [12]. Color Doppler (CD) and power Doppler (PD) are used to investigate blood flow in the renal and iliac vessels, and "flow quantification" can be measured using resistivity index (RI), pulsatility index (PI), and systolic/diastolic ratio [22]. The Doppler resistive index (RI) developed by Leandre Pourcelot is a measure of pulsatile blood flow that mirrors the resistance to blood flow caused by microvascular bed distal to the site of measurement. RI is usually determined as a standard practice in clinical monitoring, and it can depend on the recipient's vessels and their elasticity beside the graft vessels [35]. RI was found to be a useful parameter in quantifying the variations in renal blood flow that might be associated with renal disease. RI is defined as $\dfrac{PSV - EDV}{PSV}$, where PSV: peak systolic velocity and EDV: end diastolic velocity [36]. Figure 4 shows how RI is calculated from a CD sonogram. Contrast-enhanced Ultrasound (CEUS) is used to evaluate cortical perfusion since CD and PD can only estimate perfusion in large arteries [37], see Fig. 5.

Recently, the are several studies that evaluate the performance of the conventional ultrasound parameters such as the resistance index (RI) in the diagnosis of early allograft dysfunction. According to [38, 39], RI is not an exact indicator of renal graft dysfunction, and it could only provide a prognostic marker of the graft. Saracino et al. [40] concluded that RI measurements taken early after kidney

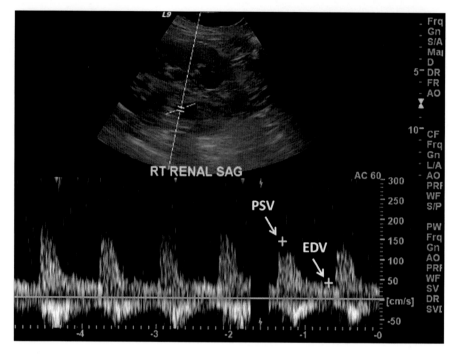

Fig. 4 The process of calculating renal resistance index from CD sonogram

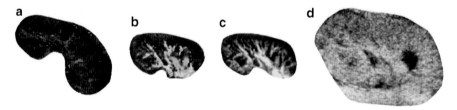

Fig. 5 Illustration of gray-scale sonography (**a**), color Doppler (**b**), power Doppler (**c**), and CEUS (**d**). Note that CD or PD cannot evaluate the cortical perfusion; however, CEUS can explore this area

transplant could predict long-term renal function. However, Kramann et al. [23] focused in their research on evaluating the ability of RI measurements to predict renal allograft survival on the time point of RI measurement. They found that RI measurements should be taken 12–18 months posttranplantation in order to be able to predict long-term allograft survival. Also, Khosroshahi et al. [41] compared Doppler US images of the donor's kidney before and 6–12 months after transplantation and showed that a significant increase in the RI couldn't be related to the graft enlargement. Krejčí et al. [42] examined the potential of US evaluation in the detection of subclinical acute rejection using a composite gray-scale, CD, and PD imaging, and it was proven that a significant differentiation between different groups could be achieved. Damasio et al. [43] investigated the use of Doppler US in the case of dual kidney transplantation (DKT), and it was concluded that DKT patients had higher RI and lower kidney volumes than single kidney transplantation (SKT) patients. Chudek et al. [44] tried to characterize factors that influence PI and RI in patients with immediate (IGF), slow (SGF), or delayed (DGF) kidney graft function, and found that ischemic injury which occurred mainly prior to organ harvesting played a dominant role determining intrarenal resistance in the early posttransplant period. Fischer et al. [45] proved the superiority of ultrasound contrast media (USCM) to conventional US that uses the RI indicator in the diagnosis of early allograft dysfunction. In addition, Benozzi et al. [46] found that both US and CEUS could identify grafts with early dysfunction, but only some CEUS-derived parameters could differentiate between ATN and acute renal rejection. A summary of recent studies relating to acute renal rejection with different US findings is given in Table 1.

Magnetic Resonance Imaging

Magnetic resonance imaging (MRI) has become the most powerful and central noninvasive tool for clinical diagnosis of diseases [47]. The main advantage of MRI is that it offers the best soft tissue contrast among all imaging modalities (e.g., US and CT). However, structural MRI lacks functional information. Dynamic contrast-enhanced magnetic resonance imaging (DCE-MRI) is a special MR technique that has emerged as a new noninvasive technique to provide superior information of the anatomy, function, and metabolism of tissue [26, 48]. The technique involves the acquisition of serial MR images with high temporal resolution before, during, and several times after the administration of a contrast agent (e.g., gadolinium) into the blood stream. In DCE-MRI, the signal intensity in target tissue changes in proportion to the contrast agent concentration in the volume element of measurement, or voxel. DCE-MRI is commonly used to enhance the contrast between different tissues, particularly normal and pathological. A typical example of a dynamic MRI time series data of the kidney is shown in Fig. 6.

DCE-MRI has been extensively used in many clinical applications, including the study of the hemodynamic (i.e., perfusion) and properties of tissues (blood flow, blood volume, mean transit time), microvascular permeability and extracellular leakage space, detection of renal transplant diseases, and MR angiography [49]. Advantages of DCE-MRI techniques over other imaging modalities include the lack of ionizing radiation, increased spatial resolution, the ability to provide superior anatomical and functional information, and the feasibility to be used as early as possible (even one day posttransplantation) for the assessment and follow-up of the transplanted kidney. Unlike the brain where the widely used clinical agent gadolinium is confined by the blood–brain barrier and behaves essentially like an intravascular agent, in the kidney tissue the contrast agent gadolinium behaves as a

Table 1 Summary of studies on acute renal rejection with different US findings

Study	Objective	Methods	Conclusions
Fischer et al. [45]	Compare the ability of USCM in diagnosing early allograft dysfunction with the traditional US modalities that relies on the RI parameter.	An overall of 48 successive kidney recipients undertook US examination after USCM administration 4–10 days after transplantation.	Conventional US that rely on RI measurements are inferior to USCM when it comes to diagnosing early kidney allograft dysfunction.
Kirkpantur et al. [38]	Investigate the correlation relationship between RI and renal histopathologic characteristics in grafted kidneys.	The intrarenal RI was retrospectively compared with biopsy results in 28 kidney recipients.	RI appeared to offer a predictive indicator for the graft rather than yielding a precise diagnosis of renal graft dysfunction.
Kramann et al. [23]	Evaluate the ability of RI measurements to predict renal allograft survival through a retrospective single-center analysis, but with special focus on the time point of RI measurement.	In total, 88 patients with an RI measurement 0–3, 3–6, and 12–18 months after transplantation were involved and separated into two groups according to RI threshold of 0.75.	RI obtained 12–18 months after transplantation was found to be able to help in predicting long-term allograft results, while RI acquired during the first 6 months after transplantation failed to predict renal allograft dysfunction.
Seiler et al. [39]	Test the hypothesis that renal RI represents a sign of systemic vascular damage rather than an organ-specific indicator.	Renal and splenic RIs besides common carotid intima-media thickness (IMT) were measured in 87 stable transplant recipients.	Results backed the belief that renal RI is not a specific marker of allograft dysfunction.
Benozzi et al. [46]	Compare the results of CEUS and PD in renal transplanted kidneys within 30 days after transplantation.	Altogether, 39 kidney recipients experienced CEUS and US examinations at 5, 15, and 30 days after transplantation. The outcomes were correlated with clinical findings and functional evolution.	Although US and CEUS both could recognize grafts with early dysfunction, only some CEUS-derived factors could separate ATN from acute renal rejection.
Krejčí et al. [42]	Assess the prospect of ultrasound evaluation in the recognition of subclinical acute rejection that are diagnosed in stable	Gray-scale assessment, CD imaging, and PD imaging were performed before each of 184 protocol graft biopsies in 77 patients in the third week, third month, and	Groups with borderline changes and subclinical acute rejection and groups with normal histological finding and clinically manifested acute

(continued)

Table 1 (continued)

Study	Objective	Methods	Conclusions
	grafts by protocol biopsy.	first year after transplantation.	rejection could be successfully divided using a combined gray-scale, PD and CD assessment.
Damasio et al. [43]	Analyze CD results in patients with dual kidney transplanta- tion (DKT) and com- pare renal volume and resistive index (RI) values between DKT and single kid- ney transplantation (SKT).	Reviewing the clinical and imaging findings [30 CDUS, five mag- netic resonance (MR) and one computed tomography (CT) examination] in 30 patients with DKT. Renal volumes and RI were compared with 14 SKT patients and comparable levels of renal function.	CD provided beneficial information in patients with DKT, and DKT patients had higher RI and lower volumes than SKT patients.
Khosroshahi et al. [41]	Compare the Doppler US variations in the donor's kidney before transplanta- tion with the recipient's kidney at 6 to 12 months after transplantation.	Before transplantation, the size, cortical thickness, echogenicity, anastomo- sis, mean pulsatility index (MPI), and RI of the 20 kidney donors were documented. In addition, the same parameters were measured in the recipient's kidney at 6 to 12 months after transplantation	Findings showed a sig- nificant enlargement of the kidney size accompanied with an insignificant increase in MPI and RI of the transplanted kidney.
Saracino et al. [40]	Evaluate the potential for RI measured early after kidney trans- plant to also predict long-term renal function.	RI measurements of 79 transplant patients within 1 month after the transplant were divided into two groups based on RI median value of 0.635.	Early determination of RI can help predict long-term graft func- tion in kidney trans- plant recipients.
Chudek et al. [44]	Describe factors that affect PI and RI in patients with imme- diate (IGF), slow (SGF), or delayed (DGF) kidney graft function.	PI and RI were measured in 200 transplanted patients at 2 to 4 days after transplantation. Patients with acute rejection episodes within the first month were discarded. IGF, SGF, and DGF were defined based on different creatinine levels.	A central role in the determination of intrarenal resistance in the early period after transplantation is played by ischemic injury, which tran- spired primarily prior to organ harvesting.

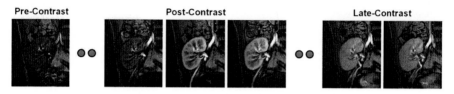

Fig. 6 DCE-MRI images taken at different time points post the adminstration of the contrast agent showing the change of the contrast as the contrast agent perfuses into the tissue beds for kidney

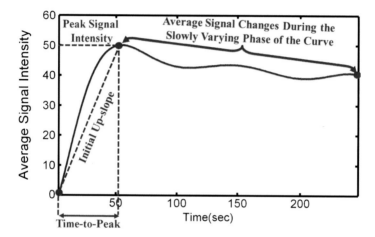

Fig. 7 Typical DCE-MRI TIC representing the average intensity of the kidney measured before and after the adminstration of the contrast agent into the blood stream. The figure illustrates typical transient phase (peak value, time to the first peak, and the initial up-slope) and the tissue distribution phase parameters that can be estimated and used for diagnosis

leakage agent, namely it distributes in the extra cellular extra vascular space, and at short times (up to about 2 min) after administration at DCE-MRI, time-intensity curves (TIC) that represent the average intensity of the kidney can be constructed. Importantly, from these TICs empirical parameters (indexes) that reflect the delivery of agent to the tissue bed can be estimated (see Fig. 7). Other clinically important functional parameters, such as fractional plasma volume (FPV), renal blood flow (RBF), glomerular filtration rate (GFR), renal plasma flow (RPF), and cortical and medullary blood volumes, can also be estimated from the perfusion curves [50]. Whereas these TICs represent global information about the kidney condition, it is conceivable that a vascular insult can be confined to a local territory. Thus for visual local assessment it is helpful for the radiologists that the perfusion indexes can be displayed as pixel-by-pixel parametric maps (see Fig. 8) overlayed on an anatomic image. This is of great importance, in case of kidney dysfunction, the radiologist can investigate which kidney regions need attention during follow-up of the treatment and thus determine the appropriate therapy.

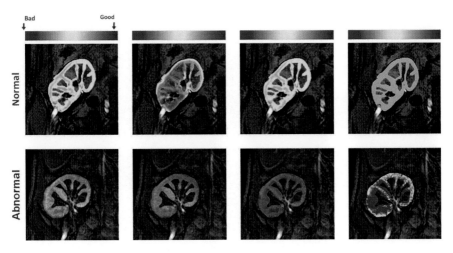

Fig. 8 Perfusion maps for the four perfusion indexes estimated from the normalized TICs: peak signal intensity (*first column*), initial up-slope (*third column*), average plateau (*second column*), and time-to-peak (*last column*); for a normal subject (*upper row*) and acute rejection subject (*lower row*). The *red* and *blue* hues of each color scale correspond to respective highest and lowest values, respectively. Note all indexes show worsening of perfusion with pathology

Developing a CAD for early and noninvasive diagnosis of the kidney is an ongoing area for research interest. However, DCE-MRI exhibits multiple challenges stemming from (1) the need to image very quickly, to capture the transient first-pass transit effects, while maintaining adequate spatial resolution (2) varying signal intensities over the time course of agent transit, and (3) nonrigid deformations, or shape changes, may occur related to pulsatile or transmitted effects from adjacent structures, such as bowel. A schematic diagram of a typical CAD system for detection of acute rejection is shown in Fig. 9. The motion correction step of the kidney on DCE-MRI time series is a preprocessing step in developing the CAD system to compensate for the global and/or local motion of the kidney. Next, the kidney objects are segmented and the functional unit (i.e., renal cortex) is extracted in order to determine dynamic agent delivery. In the final step, perfusion is estimated from contrast agent kinetics using empiric indexes (see Fig. 7) and classification is performed based on the extracted features to distinguish between acute rejection and non-rejection. Below, we will overview the related work on renal image segmentation and registration as well as the todays' CAD systems for kidney diagnosis.

Related Work on Renal Image Segmentation and Registration

Dynamic MR images are subject to relatively low signal-to-noise, nonuniform intensity distribution over the time series images, and geometric kidney deformations caused by gross patient motion, transmitted respiratory effects, and intrinsic

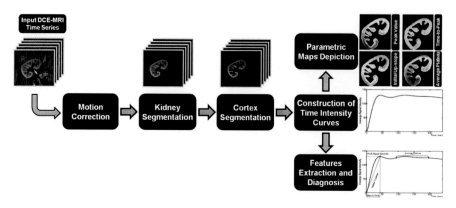

Fig. 9 Typical computer-aided diagnosis (CAD) system for diagnosis of acute renal rejection. The input of a CAD system is the DCE-MRI medical images. The motion correction step is used to handle global and/or local motion during data acquisition. The renal cortex is segmented after kidney object segmentation since it is the cortex that is primarily affected by the perfusion deficits that underlie the pathophysiology of acute rejection. Then, the time intensity curves are constructed and perfusion features are extracted and used for diagnosis

and transmitted pulsatile effects. Therefore, accurate segmentation and registration of dynamic MR renal images is a challenge. These two basic steps are commanding the major attention in this research area for automated analysis of dynamic perfusion MRI. Particularly, kidney motion effects can be compensated for by specific use of global and local registration techniques. On the other hand, kidney segmentation techniques can be classified into three main categories: threshold-based, deformable boundary-based, and probabilistic or energy minimization-based methods. Below we review the related work on kidney segmentation and registration techniques addressing the above-mentioned challenges.

Threshold-based techniques segment the kidney and its internal structures (i.e., cortex and medulla) by analyzing an empirical probability distribution, or histogram of pixel intensities in a region-of-interest (ROI). Earlier computerized renal image analysis (e.g., [51–54]) was usually carried out either manually or semiautomatically. Typically, the user defines an ROI in one image and for the rest of the images, image edges were detected and the model curve was matched to these edges. However, the manual ROI placements are based on the users' knowledge of anatomy and thus are subject to inter- and intra-observer variability. Also, valuable information, being inherent in the DCE-MRI signal intensity time series (sequences), is not used. Additionally, these approaches are very slow, even though semiautomated techniques (e.g., [51, 54]) do reduce the processing time. Giele et al. [55] introduced an approach for the segmentation and registration and of the kidney on DCE-MRI. First, the kidney contour is drawn manually by the user in a single high-contrast image. Then, the phase difference movement detection (PDMD) method is employed to correct kidney displacements. Their method demonstrated better performance than direct image intensity matching and cross-correlation. However, when compared with the radiologist results, the PDMD method accuracy was about 68 % and a manual mask to register the time frames was still required. Additionally, only translational motion was handled, while rotational motion was not mentioned, although the existence of the latter has been discussed in a number of studies [51, 56, 57]. De Priester et al. [54] subtracted the average of pre-contrasted images (10 frames) from the average of early enhanced images (30 frames) and thresholded the resulting difference image to obtain a kidney mask. Objects smaller than a certain size (700 pixels) were removed, and the remaining kidney object was closed using morphological erosion and manual processing. This approach was further expanded by Giele [58] by applying an erosion filter to the mask image in order to obtain a contour at a second subtraction stage. Koh et al.[59] segmented kidneys with the morphological 3D H-maxima transform. Rectangular masks and edge information are used to exclude training data or prior knowledge. Simple thresholding is too inaccurate to segment human organs in DCE-MRI, because these specific regions have similar gray level (intensity) distributions.

Evolving deformable boundary methods have been explored as a more accurate means of kidney segmentation. A series of studies on both rats and human subjects [57, 60–65] has been conducted for the registration and segmentation of kidneys from DCE-MRI. A multi-step segmentation and registration in the study on humans by Sun et al. [57, 62] initially corrects the large-scale motion by using an image gradient-based similarity rigid registration (only translational). Once roughly aligned, a high-contrast image is subtracted from a pre-contrast image and a level set approach was used to extract the kidney border from the difference image. Then, the segmented kidney contour is propagated over the other frames to search for the rigid (rotation and translation) registration parameters. For rat studies, Sun et al. [60, 61, 63] used a variational level set approach to find the kidney borders. Their framework integrated a subpixel motion model and temporal smoothness constraints. For segmenting the cortex and medulla, the level set approach by Chan and Vese [66] was used. The deformable model-based segmentation has been improved by hybrid edge- and region-based models in a number of studies [67, 68]. Some works have focused on segmenting multiple objects with multiphase level set methods [69, 70]. Abdelmunim et al. [71] incorporated both image and shape prior information into a variational level set framework for kidney segmentation. However, their model did not adequately account for spatial dependencies between the pixels and therefore are quite sensitive to imperfect kidney contours and image noise. Yuksel et al. [72, 73] proposed a parametric deformable model approach for the segmentation of the kidney where the deformable contour evolution was constrained using two density functions. The first describes the kidney shape prior and is constructed using the average signed distance maps of the training samples. The second functional describes the pixel-wise image intensity distribution of the kidney and its background, estimated using an adaptive linear combinations of discrete Gaussians (LCDG) [74–81]. El-Baz et al. [82–84] proposed a parametric deformable model-based approach for the segmentation of the kidney using shape and visual appearance priors. The shape model is constructed from a linear combination of vectors of distances between the training boundaries and their common centroid. The appearance prior is modeled with a spatially homogeneous second-order Markov-Gibbs random field (MGRF) of gray levels with analytically estimated pairwise potentials. The current appearance model is described with the LCDG model [74–81]. Khalifa et al. [29, 85] proposed an automated level set-based framework for the segmentation of kidney from dynamic MRI. They proposed a stochastic force that accounts for a shape prior and features of image intensity and pairwise MGRF spatial interactions [75, 86–88]. These features are integrated into a joint MGRF image model of the kidney and its background to constrain the evolution of the deformable contour [89–92]. They employed a two-stage registration methodology using first an affine transformation to account for the global motion, followed by a partial differential equation (PDE)-based approach for local motion correction [90, 92]. The segmentation approach in [29, 89] was later extended to deal with 3D data in [93, 94]. Gloger et al. [95] presented a level set-based approach using the shape prior information and Bayesian statistical concepts for generating the shape probability maps. However, the shape prior model in [29, 89, 93–95] did not impose temporal constraints on kidney segmentation.

The graph cut-based segmentation algorithm by Boykov et al. [96, 97] minimizes the energy of a temporal MGRF model of intensity curves. Each voxel is described with a vector of intensity values over time. Initially, several seed points are placed on the objects and on the background to give user-defined constraints as well as expert samples of intensity curves. These samples are used to compute a two-dimensional histogram further acting as a data penalty function in minimizing the energy. Although the results looked promising, manual interaction was still required. Rusinek et al. [98] proposed a graph cut-based segmentation formwork to assess cortical and medullary functional parameters. Their method employed a rigid registration step to account for the kidney displacements and the approach has been tested on simulated and in-vivo data. Ali et al. [99] used the graph cut-based minimization of an energy functional combining a shape constraint with boundary properties. The constraint was built using a Poisson probability distribution and distance maps. Chevaillier et al. [100, 101] proposed a semiautomated method to segment internal structures (i.e., cortex, medulla, and pelvis) from DCE-MRI time series by using k-means-based partitioning to classify pixels according to contrast evolution using vector quantization algorithm. However, it was only tested on eight data sets for normal kidneys, and user interaction was still required. A similar segmentation by Song et al. [102] has only been tested on two MRI data sets, with simulated rotation and translation rigid motion, for one normal and one abnormal kidney. An automated framework proposed by Zöllner et al. [103] assesses renal function by deriving voxel-based functional information from DCE-MRI, the nonrigid image registration compensating for the motion and deformation of the kidney during DCE-MRI acquisitions. The k-means clustering method [104] was used for extracting functional information about different regions of the kidney according to their dynamic contrast enhancement patterns. An automated wavelet-based k-means clustering framework for segmenting the kidneys was proposed by Li et al. [105]. The images were co-aligned using B-splines registration and cross-correlation (CC) cost function and their framework was tested on seven subjects (four volunteers and three patients). Yang et al. [106] proposed a framework for the classification of kidney tissue using fuzzy c-mean clustering. In order to reduce the motion artifacts, their framework employed a nonrigid registration step using the demons algorithm [107] and the squared pixel distance as a similarity metric and the squared gradient of the transformation field as the smoothness regularization term. To summarize, the reviewed methodologies for kidney segmentation and registration are presented in Table 2.

Renal CAD Systems

The integration of accurate kidney segmentation and motion correction into a complete computer-aided diagnostic (CAD) system for renal assessment is still a challenge. In recent years, several CAD systems have been proposed to analyze kidney function using DCE-MRI. The DCE-MRI of the kidney has the ability to characterize tissue-specific functional changes, and the potential to measure both total and cortical volume, and other functional parameters such as renal blood flow (RBF) and glomerular filtration rate (GFR). Farag et al. [108] and El-Baz et al.[109–112] proposed an automated framework for early diagnosis of acute renal transplant rejection. Their CAD system included parametric deformable model segmentation, nonrigid alignment, and classification of the kidney status using empirical parameters estimated from the perfusion curves. They proposed a new external energy to control the evolution of the deformable boundary using the density estimations one for a shape model and the other for gray level distribution estimated using linear combination of Gaussian (LCG) [75, 86–88, 113–120]. They proposed a geometric-based nonrigid registration approach that deforms the kidney objects over a set of closed equi-spaced contours) iso-contours. The evolution of the iso-contours is guided by an exponential speed function by minimizing the distances between the corresponding pixel pairs on the reference and target iso-contours. Correspondence between the target and reference iso-contours is evaluated by their normalized cross-correlation (NCC). Their frameworks were tested on 30 data sets and the evaluation of the kidney status was based on four empirical parameters (peak signal intensity, time-to peak, the slope between the peak and the first minimum (wash-in slope), and the slope between the peak and the signal measured from the last image in the sequence (wash-out slope)). Similar CAD systems were proposed in [121, 122]. They employed a global alignment step based on maximizing a special Gibbs energy function, the perfusion curves were estimated from the whole kidney rather than the cortex, and the system was tested on a larger cohort of 100 patients.

A semiautomated approach by Rusinek et al. [98] assessed cortical and medullary functional parameters (RPF, GFR, vascular volumes of the cortex and medulla, and rate of water absorption) using simulated and in-vivo data. Their framework employed an initial rigid alignment (translation only) step followed by a graph cut-based segmentation approach. Zikic et al. [123] evaluated kidney kinetic parameters after motion correction using template-matching-based registration

Table 2 Summary of kidney segmentation and registration techniques using MRI

Study	Database	Dim	AL	Approach	Performance
De Priester et al. [54]	18 data sets (9 subjects)	2D	UI	• Thresholding, • Morphological erosion and manual processing.	N/A
Giele et al. [55, 58]	5 data sets	2D	UI	• Manual segmentation of the kidney, • PDMD registration.	ACC: 68 %
Sun et al. [62]	5 subjects	2D	UI	• Multi-step rigid registration, • level set segmentation for the kidney and the cortex.	Error is at most one pixel size (for one sequence of 150 image frames)
Sun et al. [60, 61, 63]	20 data sets	2D	A	• Variational level set.	Visual evaluation by an expert.
Abdelmunim et al. [71]	39 data sets to build shape prior (Testing data N/A)	2D	A	• Shape-based segmentation using level set.	N/A
Yuksel et al. [72, 73]	N/A	2D	UI	• Shape-based segmentation using parametric deformable model.	E: 0.382 % (for one image only)
El-Baz et al. [82–84]	2700 images	2D	A	• Scale invariant feature transform (SIFT)-based alignment, • Shape-based segmentation using parametric deformable model, • Second-order MGRF spatial interaction model of gray scale images.	E: 0.83±0.45 %
Khalifa et al. [29]	26 data sets	2D	A	• Affine registration, • Shape-based segmentation using level set, • Second-order MGRF spatial interaction model.	E: 1.29±0.60
Khalifa et al. [85]	50 data sets	2D	A	• Affine registration, • Shape-based segmentation using level set, • Higher-order MGRF spatial interaction model.	DSC: 0.982±0.016
Khalifa et al. [127]	50 data sets	2D	A	• Affine registration, • Shape-based segmentation using level set, • Second-order MGRF spatial interaction model.	DSC: 0.970±0.02
	18 data sets	3D+time	UI		N/A

(continued)

Table 2 (continued)

Study	Database	Dim	AL	Approach	Performance
Boykov et al. [96]				• Graph cut-based segmentation, • Temporal MGRF.	
Boykov et al. [97]	1 data set	3D	UI	• Graph cut-based segmentation, • Temporal MGRF.	N/A
Rusinek et al. [98]	40 data sets (18 simulated and 22 clinical data sets)	3D+time	UI	• Mutual Information (MI)-based rigid registration (translation only), • Graph cut-based segmentation.	AD cortex: 7.2±6.1, AD medulla: 6.5±4.6
Ali et al. [99]	N/A	2D	UI	• Mutual information (MI)-based affine registration, • Graph cut shape-based segmentation.	E: 5.7±0.9 % (tested on 33 slices)
Chevaillier et al. [100, 101]	8 data sets	2D	UI	• k-means based clustering based on contrast evolution using a vector quantization algorithm.	DSC cortex: 0.79, DSC cortex: 0.70, DSC cavities: 0.77
Song et al. [102]	4 subjects	3D+time	UI	• Fourier-based registration, • Template-based segmentation.	N/A
Zöllner et al. [103]	4 data sets	3D+time	A	• B-splines nonrigid registration, • k-means clustering.	Average similarity score of 0.96
Li et al. [105]	7 data sets	3D+time	A	• B-splines nonrigid registration, • wavelet-based k-means clustering.	ACC cortex: 88 %, ACC medulla: 91 %, ACC pelvis: 98 %
Yang et al. [106]	N/A	3D+time	UI	• Demons algorithm nonrigid registration, • Fuzzy c-mean clustering.	N/A

*AL denotes Automation Level (A: Automatic, UI: User Interactive). *N/A denotes not applicable.
*DSC denotes the Dice similarity coefficient; DSC = $2TP/(2TP+FP+FN)$ — TP: true positive, FP: false positive, FN: false negative.
*Dim denotes the approach dimension (2D or 3D).
*ACC denotes accuracy; ACC= $(TP+TN)/(TP+FP+FN+TN)$— TN: true negative.
*E denotes percentage error; E = $(FP+FN)/(TP+FN)$ %
*AD denotes the absolute disparity.

and normalized gradient field (NGF), as the contrast-invariant similarity measure. However, the kidney was segmented manually, only the translational motion was considered, and the evaluation of perfusion parameters (plasma volume and tubular flow) was performed visually by trained physicians for 10 data sets of healthy volunteers. Semiautomated evaluation of renal function was explored by De Senneville [124] using rigid-body registration to handle kidney motion inside a user-defined ROI. The renal cortex was segmented manually, and the GFR was estimated with Patlak-Rutland tracer kinetic model. Their method demonstrated a significant uncertainty reduction on the computed GFR for native kidneys, but not the transplanted ones. Anderlik et al. [125] proposed a framework for quantitative assessment of kidney function using a two-step motion correction and pharmacokinetic modeling. The GFR was estimated from the time-intensity curves using Sourbron et al. [126] compartment model. Their framework has been tested on 11 data sets. Zöllner et al. [103] employed a nonrigid registration using B-splines and mutual information (MI) as a similarity metric. Functional information was extracted regionally using k-means clustering [104]. This system was tested only on four DCE-MRI data sets and the evaluation of kidney regions was assessed qualitatively according to their mean signal intensity time courses.

An automated framework for the classification of kidney transplant status was proposed by Khalifa et al. [29, 85, 127]. In their framework, the kidney was segmented using a stochastic geometrical deformable model approach and the local motion of the kidney is corrected for by a Laplace partial differential equation-based nonrigid alignment method [90, 92]. The system was tested on 26 data sets and the kidney status was evaluated using K-nearest neighbor classifier based on empirical parameters estimated from the agent kidney kinetic curves. Their framework was later extended in [127] by using analytical function-based model to fit agent kinetic curves derived from the cortex rather than the whole kidney as in [29]. For the classification of kidney status, five features (three are derived from the gamma-variate functional model and two are from the perfusion data, namely the time-to-peak and average plateau, see Fig. 7) were chosen and the study included 50 transplant patients (27 non-rejection and 23 acute rejection). Semiautomated estimation of renal parameters was performed by Hodneland et al. [128]. A viscous fluid model combined with an NGF-based cost function was used for elastic kidney registration. However, the kidney was segmented interactively with the nearest neighbor approach, the framework was tested only on 4 data sets of two healthy volunteers, and the reported GFR measurements were slightly underestimated relative to the creatinine reference values. Positano et al. [129] proposed a CAD system for the estimation for renal parameters. Their system included a two-step rigid registration framework to compensate for kidney motion using MI and adaptive prediction of kidney position over the course of the respiratory cycle. The perfusion indices (peak signal intensity, mean transit time (MTT), initial up-slope, and time to peak) were estimated from the extracted perfusion curves from the automatically and manually registered datasets were similar as well. However, their registration method could address only the global motion, but not the local motion. A summary of current CAd system for kidney diagnosis is presented in Table 3.

Table 3 Summary of MRI CAD systems for diagnosis of kidney function

Study	Database	Dim	AL	Approach	Objective and System Evaluation
Farag et al. [108] and El-Baz et al. [109–112]	30 data sets	2D	A	• Parametric deformable model, • Iso-contours non-rigid registration, • Cortex segmentation, • Estimation of cortical parameters: peak-signal intensity, time-to-peak, wash-in and wash-out slopes.	• To classify acute rejection and non rejection transplant, • The classification accuracy was 86.67 % for training and 93.3 % for testing.
Rusinek et al. [98]	40 data sets	3D+time	UI	• Mutual Information (MI)-based rigid registration (translation only), • Graph cut-based segmentation, • Multicompartmental modeling, • Estimation of cortical and medullary parameters: RPF, GFR, vascular volumes, and rate of water absorption.	• The purpose of the study was to estimate the accuracy, precision, and efficiency to measure: cortical and medullary volumes, and functional parameters (RPF and GFR) from the multicompartmental model of perfusion curves. • The average estimation errors were 7.5 % for RPF 13.5 % for GFR.
El-Baz et al. [121, 122]	100 data sets	2D	A	• Global alignment using an MGRF similarity metric, • Parametric deformable model, • Iso-contours non-rigid registration, • Estimation of kidney parameters: peak-signal intensity, time-to-peak, wash-in and wash-out slopes.	• To classify acute rejection and non rejection transplant, • The classification accuracy was 100 % for training and 94 % for testing.
Zikic et al. [123]	10 data sets	2D	UI	• NGF-based template-matching registration, • Manual segmentation of the kidney, • Modeling of perfusion curves using two-compartment model to estimate Plasma volume and tubular flow.	• The goal of this study was to the of perfusion and filtration parameters, • Motion correction effect has been evaluated visually using frequency spectrum of the signal, • The perfusion parameter results have been evaluated by trained physicians.
De Senneville [124]	20 data sets	2D	UI	• Rigid-body registration, • Manual correction of kidney borders in the co-aligned images,	• The goal of this study was to quantify motion correction accuracy on tracer kinetic models,

(continued)

Table 3 (continued)

Study	Database	Dim	AL	Approach	Objective and System Evaluation
				• Modeling of perfusion curves using PatlakRutland model and estimation of the GFR.	• Significant uncertainty reduction on the computed GFR for native kidneys, but not the transplanted ones.
Anderlik et al. [125]	11 data sets	3D+time	UI	• Rigid-body registration followed by B-Splines nonrigid registration, • Semi-automated segmentation of the kidney, • Modeling of perfusion curves and estimation of the GFR.	• Quantitative assessment of kidney function using DCE-MRI, • No evaluation is performed.
Khalifa et al.[29]	26 data sets	2D	A	• Affine MI-based rigid alignment, • Shape-based segmentation using level set, • Laplace-based iso-contours non-rigid registration, • Estimation of kidney functional parameters: time-to-peak and wash-out slope.	• To classify acute rejection and non rejection transplant, • The classification accuracy was 100 % for training and 93 %testing.
Hodneland et al. [128]	4 data sets	3D+time	UI	• Viscous fluid model nonrigid registration, • Nearest neighbor segmentation, • Construction and modeling of perfusion curves using Patlak model to estimate GFR.	• To present an image processing pipeline for in vivo estimation of GFR using DCE-MRI, • GFR measurements were slightly underestimated relative to the creatinine reference values.
Zöllner et al. [103]	4 data sets	3D+time	A	• Rigid registration followed by B-Splines nonrigid registration, • k-means clustering, • Construction of regional perfusion curves.	• To evaluate the effect of motion correction and segmentation on the intensity time curves on kidney compartments (cortex, medulla, and pelvis), • Average similarity score of 0.96, • Evaluation of kidney regions was assessed qualitatively according to their intensity time courses.
Positano et al. [129]	20 data sets	2D	UI	• Two-steps MI-based rigid alignment and an adaptive predictor of kidney position over the course of the respiratory cycle, • Manual segmentation of the renal cortex,	• To evaluate perfusion parameters extracted from manually and automatically constructed perfusion curves, • The mean distance between the automatically and manually detected contours was 2.95 ± 0.81 mm

(continued)

Table 3 (continued)

Study	Database	Dim	AL	Approach	Objective and System Evaluation
				• Fitting of perfusion curve was to a bicompartmental model, • Estimation of perfusion parameters: peak signal intensity, mean transit time (MTT), initial up-slope, and time-to-peak.	• The perfusion parameters for automatically and manually registered data sets have good agreement.
Khalifa et al.[127]	50 data sets	2D	A	• Affine MI-based rigid alignment, • Shape-based segmentation using level set, • Laplace-based iso-contours nonrigid registration, • Cortex segmentation, • Gamma-variate modeling of perfusion curves, • Estimation of functional parameters: three gamma-variate functional parameters, time-to-peak, and average plateau.	• To classify acute rejection and non rejection transplant, • The classification accuracy was 100 % for both training and testing.

*AL denotes Automation Level (A: Automatic, UI: User Interactive) *Dim denotes the approach dimension (2D or 3D)

Discussion and Conclusions

Designing efficient and reliable CAD systems for early detection of renal transplant complications is very important, since early detection of renal transplant complications, specially renal rejection, can be potentially mitigated by the adminstration of anti-rejection medications. In this chapter, we overview recent CAD systems for the detection of kidney rejection using ultrasound and magnetic resonance imaging modalities. This chapter addresses current approaches and their strengths and limitations. In the final section, we summarize this work by outlining the research challenges that face each stage in kidney diagnosis CAD systems. In addition, the suggested trends to solve these challenges are presented.

Several challenges and aspects have been facing the development of accurate and fast CAD systems for early detection of renal transplant complications. These challenges can be summarized as follows.

- Most clinical and research studies focus on 2D time series analyses that are compatible with data acquisitions for real patient scenarios. However, the extension of the work to deal with 4D (3D + time) is one of the major challenges. The goal of DCE-MRI is to obtain the best feasible temporal resolution while maintaining good spatial resolution. Therefore, the acquisition of 3D data with higher spatial resolution greatly affects the temporal resolution and vice versa. Thus, a compromise in choosing the acquisition parameters for 3D time series (4D) is required to achieve a sufficiently high signal-to-noise ratio (SNR), since an ideal rapid isotropic 3D imaging of the moving kidneys is not achievable [124].
- Accurate delineation of kidney borders requires new segmentation models to account for the large inhomogeneities that exist in the kidney (i.e., cortex, medulla). This can be achieved by integrating into the segmentation techniques both the spatial interactions information between the kidney pixels and the intensity information. Most popular spatial interaction models are MGRF-based methods using binary maps and pairwise relationships for 2D and 3D images (see, e.g., [29, 75, 86, 90– 94, 130, 131]). A recent study by Khalifa et al. [85] demonstrated the advantage of higher-order MGRF spatial model over the second-order one for the segmentation of the kidney from DCE-MRI. Also, a new trend in medical image analysis is to learn the appearance of the kidney using MGRF from gray-scale images instead of binary maps [132–139].
- Motion artifacts present one of the major challenges for automated analysis of DCE-MRI. Both global and local kidney deformations affect accurate analysis of perfusion data. In literature, a tremendous number of image registration methods have been proposed to handel both global and local motion in medical images (please see [140] for more details). A new trend to provide more accurate registration is the use of higher-order similarity metrics [141–145]. Unlike other registration methods that are prone to image intensity variations over the time series, other sophisticated methods [29, 112, 127] explicitly depend

only on the geometric features to compensate for the kidney motion. These approaches can be extended to delay with 3D data.
- Fusion of information from different modalities (US, MRI, and CT) is also another major challenge. This is due to the fact that different modalities give different clinical information and have their own image resolutions.

References

1. Nankivell BJ, Alexander SI (2010) Rejection of the kidney allograft. North Eng J Med 363 (15):1451–1562
2. USRDS (2010) US Renal Data System Annual Data Report 2011: Atlas of Chronic Kidney Disease and End-Stage Renal Disease in the United States, National Institutes of Health, National Institute of Diabetes and Digestive and Kidney Diseases, Bethesda
3. Park SB, Kim JK, Cho K-S (2007) Complications of renal transplantation ultrasonographic evaluation. J Ultras Med 26(5):615–633
4. Akbar SA, Jafri SZH, Amendola MA, Madrazo BL, Salem R, Bis KG (2005) Complications of renal transplantation. Radiographics 25(5):1335–1356
5. Höhnke C, Abendroth D, Schleibner S, Land W (1987) Vascular complications in 1,200 kidney transplantations. Trans Proc 19(5):36–91
6. Scott M, Sells R (1988) Primary adenocarcinoma in a transplanted cadaveric kidney. Transplantation 46(1):157–158
7. Mathew T (1988) Recurrence of disease following renal transplantation. Am J Kidney Diseases: Official J Nat Kidney Found 12(2):85–96
8. Brown ED, Chen MY, Wolfman NT, Ott DJ, Watson NE (2000) Complications of renal transplantation: Evaluation with US and radionuclide imaging. Radiographics 20(3):607–622
9. Baxter G (2001) Ultrasound of renal transplantation. Clin Radiol 56(10):802–818
10. Pirsch JD, Ploeg RJ, Gange S, D'Alessandro AM, Knechtle SJ, Sollinger HW, Kalayoglu M, Belzer FO (1996) Determinants of graft survival after renal transplantation. Transplantation 61(11):1581–1586
11. Isoniemi HM, Krogerus L, von Willebrand E, Taskinen E, Ahonen J, Häyry P, et al. (1992) Histopathological findings in well-functioning, long-term renal allografts. Kidney Intern 41 (1):155–160
12. Grabner A, Kentrup D, Schnöckel U, Schäfers M, Reuter S (2013) Non-invasive diagnosis of acute renal allograft rejection- Special focus on gamma scintigraphy and positron emission tomography. In: Current issues and future direction in kidney transplantation, ch. 4. In Tech, New York
13. Matas AJ, Gillingham KJ, Payne WD, Najarían JS (1994) The impact of an acute rejection episode on long-term renal allograft survival (t1/2) 1, 2. Transplantation 57(6):857–859
14. Wu O, Levy AR, Briggs A, Lewis G, Jardine A (2009) Acute rejection and chronic nephropathy: A systematic review of the literature. Transplantation 87(9):1330–1339
15. "Creatinine clearance," http://www.britannica.com/EBchecked/topic/1346079/creatinine-clearance
16. Bennett H, Li D (1997) MR imaging of renal function. Magnet Reson Imag Clin North Am (1):5–18
17. Myers GL, Miller WG, Coresh J, Fleming J, Greenberg N, Greene T, Hostetter T, Levey AS, Panteghini M, Welch M, Eckfeldt JH (2006) Recommendations for improving serum creatinine measurement: A report from the laboratory working group of the national kidney disease education program. Clin Chem 52(1):5–18
18. Yang D, Ye Q, Williams M, Sun Y, Hu TC-C, Williams DS, Moura JM, Ho C (2001) USPIO-enhanced dynamic MRI: evaluation of normal and transplanted rat kidneys. Magnet Reson Med 46(6):1152–1163

19. Giele ELW (2002) Computer methods for semi-automatic MR renogram determination. Technische Universiteit Eindhoven
20. Taylor A, Nally JV (1995) Clinical applications of renal scintigraphy. Am J Roentgenol 164 (1):31–41
21. Heaf J, Iversen J (2000) Uses and limitations of renal scintigraphy in renal transplantation monitoring. Eur J Nucl Med 27(7):871–879
22. Kolofousi C, Stefanidis K, Cokkinos DD, Karakitsos D, Antypa E, Piperopoulos P (2012) Ultrasonographic features of kidney transplants and their complications: An imaging review. ISRN Radiol 2013
23. Kramann R, Frank D, Brandenburg VM, Heussen N, Takahama J, Krüger T, Riehl J, Floege J (2012) Prognostic impact of renal arterial resistance index upon renal allograft survival: The time point matters. Nephrol Dialys Transplant 27(10):3958–3963
24. Cosgrove DO, Chan KE (2008) Renal transplants: What ultrasound can and cannot do. Ultrasound Quart 24(2):77–87
25. Sebastià C, Quiroga S, Boyé R, Cantarell C, Fernandez-Planas M, Alvarez A (2001) Helical CT in renal transplantation: Normal findings and early and late complications. Radiographics 21(5):1103–1117
26. Michaely H, Herrmann K, Nael K, Oesingmann N, Reiser M, Schoenberg S (2007) Functional renal imaging: Nonvascular renal disease. Abdom Imag 32(1):1–16
27. Grenier N, Basseau F, Ries M, Tyndal B, Jones R, Moonen C (2003) Functional MRI of the kidney. Abdom Imag 28(2):164–175
28. Choyke P, Frank J, Girton M, Inscoe S, Carvlin M, Black J, Austin H, Dwyer A (1989) Dynamic Gd-DTPA-enhanced MR imaging of the kidney: Experimental results. Radiology 170(3):713–720
29. Khalifa F, El-Baz A, Gimel'farb G, El-Ghar MA (2010) Non-invasive image-based approach for early detection of acute renal rejection. In: Proceedings of international conference on medical image computing and computer-assisted intervention (MICCAI'10), Beijing, 20–24 September 2010, pp 10–18
30. El-Baz A, Beache GM, Gimel'farb G, Suzuki K, Okada K, Elnakib A, Soliman A, Abdollahi B (2013) Computer-aided diagnosis systems for lung cancer: Challenges and methodologies. Int J Biomed Imag 2013
31. Kimber DC, Gray CE, Stackpole CE, Miller MA, Drakontides AB, Leavell LC (1977) Kimber-Gray-Stackpole's anatomy and physiology. Macmillan, New York
32. "Your kidneys and how they work," http://kidney.niddk.nih.gov/kudiseases/pubs/yourkidneys/.
33. Kapit W, Macey R, Meisami E (1987) The physiology coloring book. 2nd edn. C. M. Wilson and Ed.HarperCollins Publishers, Benjamin Cummings, San Fransisco
34. Szolar DH, Preidler K, Ebner F, Kammerhuber F, Horn S, Ratschek M, Ranner G, Petritsch P, Horina JH (1997) Functional magnetic resonance imaging of human renal allografts during the post-transplant period: Preliminary observations. Magnet Reson Imag 15(7):727–735
35. Heine GH, Gerhart MK, Ulrich C, Köhler H, Girndt M (2005) Renal Doppler resistance indices are associated with systemic atherosclerosis in kidney transplant recipients. Kidney Int 68(2):878–885
36. Tublin ME, Bude RO, Platt JF (2003) The resistive index in renal Doppler sonography: Where do we stand? Am J Roentgenol 180(4):885–892
37. Jimenez C, Lopez MO, Gonzalez E, Selgas R (2009) Ultrasonography in kidney transplantation: Values and new developments. Transplant Rev 23(4):209–213
38. Kirkpantur A, Yilmaz R, Baydar DE, Aki T, Cil B, Arici M, Altun B, Erdem Y, Erkan I, Bakkaloglu M, Yasavul U, Turgan C (2008) Utility of the Doppler ultrasound parameter, resistive index, in renal transplant histopathology. Transplant Proc 40(1):104–106
39. Seiler S, Colbus SM, Lucisano G, Rogacev KS, Gerhart MK, Ziegler M, Fliser D, Heine GH (2012) Ultrasound renal resistive index is not an organ-specific predictor of allograft outcome. Nephrol Dialysis Transplant 27(8):3315–3320

40. Saracino A, Santarsia G, Latorraca A, Gaudiano V (2006) Early assessment of renal resistance index after kidney transplant can help predict long-term renal function. Nephrol Dialysis Transplant 21(10):2916–2920
41. Khosroshahi HT, Tarzamni M, Oskuii RA (2005) Doppler ultrasonography before and 6 to 12 months after kidney transplantation. Transplant Proc 37(7):2976–2981
42. Krejčí K, Zadražil J, Tichý T, Al-Jabry S, Horčička V, Štrebl P, Bachleda P (2009) Sonographic findings in borderline changes and subclinical acute renal allograft rejection. Eur J Radiol 71(2):288–295
43. Damasio M, Cittadini G, Rolla D, Massarino F, Stagnaro N, Gherzi M, Paoletti E, Derchi L (2013) Ultrasound findings in dual kidney transplantation. La Radiologia Medica 118 (1):14–22
44. Chudek J, Kolonko A, Krol R, Ziaja J, Cierpka L, Wicek A (2006) The intrarenal vascular resistance parameters measured by duplex Doppler ultrasound shortly after kidney transplantation in patients with immediate, slow, and delayed graft function. Transplant Proc 38 (1):42–45
45. Fischer T, Filimonow S, Dieckhöfer J, Slowinski T, Mühler M, Lembcke A, Budde K, Neumayer H-H, Ebeling V, Giessing M, Thomas A, Morgera S (2006) Improved diagnosis of early kidney allograft dysfunction by ultrasound with echo enhancer: A new method for the diagnosis of renal perfusion. Nephrol Dialys Transplant 21(10):2921–2929
46. Benozzi L, Cappelli G, Granito M, Davoli D, Favali D, Montecchi M, Grossi A, Torricelli P, Albertazzi A (2009) Contrast-enhanced sonography in early kidney graft dysfunction. Transplant Proc 41(4):1214–1215
47. Mansfield P (2004) Snapshot magnetic resonance imaging (nobel lecture). Angew Chem Int Ed 43(41):5456–5464
48. Prasad PV (2006) Functional MRI of the kidney: Tools for translational studies of pathophysiology of renal disease. Am J Physiol: Renal Physiol 290(5):958–974
49. Collins DJ, Padhani AR (2004) Dynamic magnetic resonance imaging of tumor perfusion. IEEE Eng Med Biol Mag 23(5):65–83
50. Bokacheva L, Rusinek H, Zhang JL, Lee VS (2008) Assessment of renal function with dynamic contrast-enhanced MR imaging. Mag Reson Imag Clin North Am 16(4):597–611
51. Von Schulthess GK, Kuoni W, Gerig G, Duewell S, Krestin G (1991) Semiautomated ROI analysis in dynamic MRI studies, Part II: Application to renal function examination. J Comput Assist Tomogr 15(5):733–741
52. Gerig G, Kikinis R, Kuon W, van Schulthess GK, Kübler O (1992) Semiautomated ROI analysis in dynamic MRI studies: Part I: Image analysis tools for automatic correction of organ displacements. IEEE Trans Image Process 11(2):221–232
53. Yim PJ, Marcos HB, Choyke PL, McAuliffe M, McGarry D, Heaton I (2001) Registration of time-series contrast enhanced magnetic resonance images for renography. In: Proceedings of the IEEE symposium on computer-based medical systems (CMBS'01), vol 1, Bethesda, 24–26 July 2001. IEEE, Piscataway, pp 516–520
54. de Priester JA, Kessels AG, Giele EL, Den Boer JA, Christiaans ML, Hasman A, Van Engelshoven JA (2001) MR renography by semiautomated image analysis: Performance in renal transplant recipients. J Mag Reson Imag 14(2):134–140
55. Giele EW, de Priester JA, Blom JA, den Boer JA, van Engelshoven JA, Hasman A, Geerlings M (2001) Movement correction of the kidney in dynamic MRI scans using FFT phase difference movement detection. J Mag Reson Imag 14(6):741–749
56. Krestin GP (1994) Magnetic resonance imaging of the kidneys: Current status. Magnet Resonan Quart 10(1):2–21
57. Sun Y (2004) Registration and segmentation in perfusion MRI: Kidneys and hearts. Ph.D. dissertation, Carnegie Mellon University, Pittsburg
58. Giele E (2002) Computer methods for semi-automatic MR renogram determination. Ph.D. dissertation, Eindhoven University of Technology, Eindhoven

59. Koh HK, Shen W, Shuter B, Kassim AA (2006) Segmentation of kidney cortex in MRI studies using a constrained morphological 3D H-maxima transform. In: Proceedings of international conference on control, automation, robotics and vision (ICARCV'06), Singapore, 26–29 December 2006. IEEE, Piscataway, pp 1–5

60. Sun Y, Moura JM, Yang D, Ye Q, Ho C (2002) Kidney segmentation in MRI sequences using temporal dynamics. In: Proceedings of IEEE international symposium on biomedical imaging: from Nano to Macro (ISBI'02), Washington, DC, 7–10 July 2002, pp. 98–101

61. Sun Y, Yang D, Ye Q, Williams M, Moura JMF, Boada F, Liang Z-P, Ho C (2003) Improving spatiotemporal resolution of USPIO-enhanced dynamic imaging of rat kidneys. Magnet Resonan Imag 21(6):593–598

62. Sun Y, Jolly MP, Moura JMF (2004) Integrated registration of dynamic renal perfusion MR images. In: Proceedings of IEEE international conference on image processing (ICIP'04), vol 3, Singapore, 24–27 October 2004, pp 1923–1926

63. Sun Y, Moura JMF, Ho C (2004) Subpixel registration in renal perfusion MR image sequence. In: Proceedings of IEEE international symposium on biomedical imaging: from nano to macro (ISBI'04), Arlington, 15–18 April 2004, pp 700–703

64. Song T, Lee VS, Rusinek H, Kaur M, Laine AF (2005a) Automatic 4-D registration in dynamic MR renography. In: Proceedings of IEEE conference on engineering in medicine and biology society (EMBS'05), Shanghai, 1–4 September 2005, pp 3067–3070

65. Song T, Lee VS, Rusinek H, Kaur M, Laine AF (2005b) Automatic 4-D registration in dynamic MR renography based on over-complete dyadic wavelet and Fourier transforms. In: Proceedings of international conference on medical image computing and computer-assisted intervention (MICCAI'05), Palm Springs, 26–29 October 2005, pp 205–213

66. Chan TF, Vese LA (2001) Active contours without edges. IEEE Trans Image Proces 10 (2):266–277

67. Kim S (2005) A hybrid level set approach for efficient and reliable image segmentation. In: Proceedings of IEEE international symposium on signal processing and information technolology, Athens, 21 December 2005, pp 743–748

68. Kim S, Lim H (2005) A hybrid level set segmentation for medical imagery. In: Proceedings of IEEE nuclear science symposium conference record, vol 3, Puerto Rico, 23–29 October 2005, pp 1790–1794

69. Lie J, Lysaker M, Tai X-C (2006) A binary level set model and some applications to Mumford-Shah image segmentation. IEEE Trans Image Process 15(5):1171–1181

70. Yan P, Kassim AA, Shen W, Shah M (2009) Modeling interaction for segmentation of neighboring structures. IEEE Trans Inform Technol Biomed 13(2):252–262

71. Abdelmunim HE, Farag AA, Miller W, AboelGhar M (2008) A kidney segmentation approach from DCE-MRI using level sets. In: Computer vision and pattern recognition workshops, (CVPRW'08), vol 1, Anchorage, 23–28 June 2008, pp 1–6

72. Yuksel SE, El-Baz A, Farag AA, El-Ghar M, Eldiasty T, Ghoneim MA (2007) A kidney segmentation framework for dynamic contrast enhanced magnetic resonance imaging. J Vibrat Contrl 13(9–10):1505–1516

73. Yuksel SE, El-Baz A, Farag AA (2006) A kidney segmentation framework for dynamic contrast enhanced magnetic resonance imaging. In: Proceedings of international symposium on mathematical methods in engineering, (MME'06), Ankara, 27–29 April 2006, pp 55–64

74. El-Baz A, Mohamed RM, Farag AA, Gimel'farb G (2005) Unsupervised segmentation of multi-modal images by a precise approximation of individual modes with linear combinations of discrete Gaussians. In: Computer vision and pattern recognition workshops (CVPRW'2005), San Diego, June 20–26. IEEE Computer Society, Piscataway, pp 54–54

75. El-Baz A (2006) Novel stochastic models for medical image analysis. Ph.D. dissertation, University of Louisville, Louisville, KY

76. El-Baz A, Gimel'farb G (2007) EM based approximation of empirical distributions with linear combinations of discrete Gaussians. In: Proceedings of IEEE international conference on image processing (ICIP'07), vol 4, San Antonio, 16–19 September 2007, pp 373–376

77. El-Baz A, Gimel'farb G, Kumar V, Falk R, El-Ghar MA (2009) 3D joint Markov-Gibbs model for segmenting the blood vessels from MRA. In: Proceedings of IEEE international symposium on biomedical imaging: from nano to macro (ISBI'09), pp 1366–1369

78. El-Baz A, Gimelfarb G, Falk R, El-Ghar MA, Kumar V, Heredia D (2009) A novel 3D joint Markov-Gibbs model for extracting blood vessels from PC–MRA images. In: Proceedings of international conference on medical image computing and computer-assisted intervention (MICCAI'09), London, 20–24 September 2009, pp 943–950

79. El-Baz A, Gimel'farb G (2011) Accurate modeling of marginal signal distributions in 2D/3D images. In: El-Baz A, Acharya R, Mirmedhdi M, Suri JS (eds) Handbook of multi modality state-of-the-art medical image segmentation and registration methodologies, vol 1, chap 7. Springer, New York, pp 189–213

80. El-Baz A, Gimelfarb G, Elnakib A, Falk R, El-Ghar MA (2011) Fast accurate unsupervised segmentation of 3D magnetic resonance angiography. In: Atherosclerosis disease management, chap 14. Springer, New York, pp 411–432

81. El-Baz A, Elnakib A, Khalifa F, El-Ghar MA, McClure P, Soliman A, Gimel'farb G (2012) Precise segmentation of 3-D magnetic resonance angiography. IEEE Trans Biomed Eng 59 (7):2019–2029

82. El-Baz A, Gimel'farb G (2008a) Robust image segmentation using learned priors. In: Proceedings of IEEE international conference on computer vision (ICCV'09), Kyoto, September 27–October 4, 2008. IEEE, Piscataway, pp 857–864

83. El-Baz A, Gimel'farb G (2008b) Image segmentation with a parametric deformable model using shape and appearance priors. In: Proceedings of IEEE international conference on computer vision and pattern recognition (CVPR'08), Anchorage, 24–26 June 2008, pp 1–8

84. El-Baz A, Gimel'farb G (2009) Robust medical images segmentation using learned shape and appearance models. In: Proceedings of international conference on medical image computing and computer-assisted intervention (MICCAI'09), London, September 20–24. Springer, Berlin, pp 281–288

85. Khalifa F, Beache GM, El-Ghar MA, El-Diasty T, Gimel'farb G, Kong M, El-Baz A (2013) Dynamic contrast-enhanced MRI-based early detection of acute renal transplant rejection. IEEE Trans Med Imag 32(10):1910–1927

86. Farag A, El-Baz A, Gimel'farb G (2006) Precise segmentation of multimodal images. IEEE Trans Image Proces 15(4):952–968

87. El-Baz A, Farag AA, Gimel'farb G (2005) Iterative approximation of empirical grey-level distributions for precise segmentation of multimodal images. EURASIP J Appl Signal Process 2005:1969–1983

88. El-Baz A, Farag A, Ali A, Gimelfarb G, Casanova M (2006) A framework for unsupervised segmentation of multi-modal medical images. In: Computer vision approaches to medical image analysis (CVAMIA'06). Springer, Berlin, pp 120–131

89. Khalifa F, Beache GM, El-Baz A, Gimel'farb G (2010) Shape-appearance guided level-set deformable model for image segmentation. In: Proceedings of IAPR international conference on pattern recognition (ICPR'10), Istanbul, 23–26 August 2010, pp 4581–4584

90. Khalifa F, Beache GM, Nitzken M, Gimel'farb G, Giridharan GA, El-Baz A (2011) Automatic analysis of left ventricle wall thickness using short-axis cine CMR images. In: Proceedings of IEEE international symposium on biomedical imaging: from nano to macro (ISBI'11), Chicago, 30 March–2 April 2011, pp 1306–1309

91. Khalifa F, Gimel'farb G, El-Ghar MA, Sokhadze G, Manning S, McClure P, Ouseph R, El-Baz A (2011) A new deformable model-based segmentation approach for accurate extraction of the kidney from abdominal CT images. In: Proceedings of IEEE international conference on image processing (ICIP'11), Brussels, 11–14 September 2011, pp 3393–3396

92. Khalifa F, Beache GM, Gimel'farb G, Giridharan GA, El-Baz A (2012) Accurate automatic analysis of cardiac cine images. IEEE Trans Biomed Eng 59(2):445–455

93. Khalifa F, Beache GM, Gimel'farb G, El-Baz A (2011) A novel approach for accurate estimation of left ventricle global indexes from short-axis cine MRI. In: Proceedings of IEEE international conference on image processing (ICIP'11), Brussels, 11–14 September 2011, pp 2697–2700

94. Khalifa F, Elnakib A, Beache GM, Gimel'farb G, El-Ghar MA, Sokhadze G, Manning S, McClure P, El-Baz A (2011) 3D kidney segmentation from CT images using a level set approach guided by a novel stochastic speed function. In: Proceedings of international conference on medical image computing and computer-assisted intervention (MICCAI'11), Toronto, 18–22 September 2011, pp 587–594

95. Gloger O, Tönnies KD, Liebscher V, Kugelmann B, Laqua R, Völzke H (2012) Prior shape level set segmentation on multistep generated probability maps of MR datasets for fully automatic kidney parenchyma volumetry. IEEE Trans Med Imag 31(2):312–325

96. Boykov Y, Lee VS, Rusinek H, Bansal R (2001) Segmentation of dynamic N-D data sets via graph cuts using Markov models. In: Proceedings of international conference on medical image computing and computer-assisted intervention (MICCAI'01), Utrecht, 14–17 October 2001, pp 1058–1066

97. Boykov Y, Funka-Lea G (2006) Graph cuts and efficient N-D image segmentation. Int J Comput Visison 70(2):109–131

98. Rusinek H, Boykov Y, Kaur M, Wong S, Bokacheva L, Sajous JB, Huang AJ, Heller S, Lee VS (2007) Performance of an automated segmentation algorithm for 3D MR renography. Magnet Resonance Med 57(6):1159–1167

99. Ali AM, Farag AA, El-Baz A (2007) Graph cuts framework for kidney segmentation with prior shape constraints. In: Proceedings of international conference on medical image computing and computer-assisted intervention (MICCAI'07), vol 1, Brisbane, October 29–November 2, pp 384–392

100. Chevaillier B, Ponvianne Y, Collette J-L, Mandry D, Claudon M, Pietquin O (2008) Functional semi-automated segmentation of renal DCE-MRI sequences. In: Proceedings of IEEE international conference acoustics, speech, and signal processing (ICASSP'08), Las Vegas, March 30–April 4, 2008, pp 525–528

101. Chevaillier B, Mandry D, Collette J-L, Claudon M, Galloy M-A, Pietquin O (2011) Functional segmentation of renal DCE-MRI sequences using vector quantization algorithms. Neural Process Lett 34(1):71–85

102. Song T, Lee VS, Rusinek H, Wong S, Laine AF (2006) Four dimensional MR image analysis of dynamic renography. In: Proceedings of IEEE conference on engineering in medicine and biology society (EMBS'06), New York, August 30–September 3, 2006, pp 3134–3137

103. Zöllner F, Sance R, Rogelj P, Ledesma-Carbayo MJ, Rørvik J, Santos A, Lundervold A (2009) Assessment of 3D DCE-MRI of the kidneys using non-rigid image registration and segmentation of voxel time courses. Comput Med Imag Graph 33(3):171–181

104. MacQueen JB (1967) Some methods for classification and analysis of multivariate observations. In: Proceedings of 5th Berkeley symposium on mathematical statistics and probability, University of California Press, California, pp 281–297

105. Li S, Zöllner FG, Merrem AD, Peng Y, Roervik J, Lundervold A, Schad LR (2012) Wavelet-based segmentation of renal compartments in DCE-MRI of human kidney: Initial results in patients and healthy volunteers. Computer Med Imag Graph 36(1):108–118

106. Yang X, Ghafourian P, Sharma P, Salman K, Martin D, Fei B (2012) Nonrigid registration and classification of the kidneys in 3D dynamic contrast enhanced (DCE) MR images. In: Proceedings of SPIE medical imaging 2012: image processing (SPIE'12), vol 8314. SPIE, The International Society for Optical Engineering, Bellingham, pp 1–9

107. Wang H, Dong L, O'Daniel J, Mohan R, Garden AS, Ang KK, Kuban DA, Bonnen M, Chang JY, Cheung R (2005) Validation of an accelerated demons algorithm for deformable image registration in radiation therapy. Phys Med Biol 50(12):2887–2905

108. Farag A, El-Baz A, Yuksel S, El-Ghar MA, Eldiasty T (2006) A framework for the detection of acute rejection with dynamic contrast enhanced magnetic resonance imaging. In: Proceedings of IEEE international symposium on biomedical imaging: from nano to macro (ISBI'06), Arlington, 6–9 April 2006, pp 418–421

109. El-Baz A, Farag A, Fahmi R, Yuksel S, El-Ghar MA, Eldiasty T (2006) Image analysis of renal DCE MRI for the detection of acute renal rejection. In: Proceedings of IAPR international conference on pattern recognition (ICPR'06), Hong Kong, 20–24 August 2006, pp 822–825

110. El-Baz A, Farag A, Fahmi R, Yuksel S, Miller W, El-Ghar MA, El-Diasty T, Ghoneim M (2006) A new CAD system for the evaluation of kidney diseases using DCE-MRI. In: Proceedings of international conference on medical image computing and computer-assisted intervention (MICCAI'06), Copenhagen, 1-6 October 2006, pp 446–453

111. El-Baz A, Farag AA, Yuksel SE, El-Ghar MEA, Eldiasty TA, Ghoneim MA (2007) Application of deformable models for the detection of acute renal rejection. In: Farag AA, Suri JS (eds) Deformable models, vol 1, chap 10, pp 293–333

112. El-Baz A, Gimel'farb G, El-Ghar MA (2007) New motion correction models for automatic identification of renal transplant rejection. In: Proceedings of international conference on medical image computing and computer-assisted intervention (MICCAI'07), Brisbane, October 29–November 2, 2007, pp 235–243

113. Farag AA, El-Baz A, Gimel'farb G (2004) Precise image segmentation by iterative EM-based approximation of empirical grey level distributions with linear combinations of Gaussians. In: Computer vision and pattern recognition workshops, (CVPRW'04), Washington, DC, 27 June–2 July. IEEE Computer Society, Piscataway, pp 109–109

114. Farag A, El-Baz A, Gimel'farb G (2004) Density estimation using modified expectation maximization for a linear combination of Gaussians. In: Proceedings of IEEE international conference on image processing (ICIP'04), vol 3, Singapore, 24–27 October 2004, pp 1871–1874

115. Gimel'farb G, Farag A, El-Baz A (2004) Expectation-maximization for a linear combination of Gaussians. In: Proceedings of IEEE international conference on pattern recognition (ICPR'04), vol 4, Cambridge, 23–26 August 2004, pp 422–425

116. El-Baz A, Farag A, Gimelfarb G (2005) Cerebrovascular segmentation by accurate probabilistic modeling of TOF-MRA images. In: Image analysis, Proceedings of the 14 Scandinavian Conference on Image analysis (SCIA'05), Joensuu, June 19–22. Springer, Heidelberg. pp 1128–1137

117. El-Baz A, Farag AA, Gimelfarb G, Hushek SG (2005) Automatic cerebrovascular segmentation by accurate probabilistic modeling of TOF-MRA images. In: Proceedings of international conference on medical image computing and computer-assisted intervention (MICCAI'05), Palm, Spring, October 26–29. Springer, Berlin, pp 34–42

118. El-Baz A, Farag AA, Gimelfarb G, El-Ghar MA, Eldiasty T (2006) A new adaptive probabilistic model of blood vessels for segmenting MRA images. In: Proceedings of international conference on medical image computing and computer-assisted intervention (MICCAI'06), Copenhagen, 1–6 October 2006, pp 799–806

119. El-Baz A, Farag A, Gimel'farb G, El-Ghar MA, Eldiasty T (2006a) Fast unsupervised segmentation of 3D magnetic resonance angiography. In: Proceedings of IEEE international conference on image processing (ICIP'06). IEEE, Piscataway, pp 93–96

120. El-Baz A, Farag A, Gimel'farb G, El-Ghar MA, Eldiasty T (2006b) Probabilistic modeling of blood vessels for segmenting MRA images. In: Proceedings of IAPR international conference on pattern recognition (ICPR'06), vol 3. IEEE, Piscataway, pp 917–920

121. El-Baz A, Gimel'farb G, El-Ghar MA (2008a) A novel image analysis approach for accurate identification of acute renal rejection. In: Proceedings of IEEE international conference on image processing (ICIP'08), San Diego, 12–15 October 2008, pp 1812–1815

122. El-Baz A, Gimel'farb G, El-Ghar MA (2008b) Image analysis approach for identification of renal transplant rejection. In: Proceedings of IAPR international conference on pattern recognition (ICPR'08), Tampa, 8–11 December 2008, pp 1–4

123. Zikic D, Sourbron S, Feng X, Michaely HJ, Khamene A, Navab N (2008) Automatic alignment of renal DCE-MRI image series for improvement of quantitative tracer kinetic studies. In: Proceedings of SPIE medical imaging 2008: image processing (SPIE'08), vol 6914. SPIE, Bellingham, pp 1–8

124. de Senneville BD, Mendichovszky IA, Roujol S, Gordon I, Moonen C, Grenier N (2008) Improvement of MRI-functional measurement with automatic movement correction in native and transplanted kidneys. J Magnet Resonan Imag 28(4):970–978

125. Anderlik A, Munthe-Kaas A, Oye O, Eikefjord E, Rorvik J, Ulvang D, Zollner F, Lundervold A (2009) Quantitative assessment of kidney function using dynamic contrast enhanced MRI-Steps towards an integrated software prototype. In: Proceedings of the 6th international symposium on image and signal processing and analysis (ISPA'09), Salzburg, 16–18 September 2009, pp 575–581

126. Sourbron SP, Michaely HJ, Reiser MF, Schoenberg SO (2008) MRI- measurement of perfusion and glomerular filtration in the human kidney with a separable compartment model. IEEE Eng Med Biol Mag 43(1):40–48

127. Khalifa F, El-Ghar MA, Abdollahi B, Frieboes H, El-Diasty T, El-Baz A (2013) A comprehensive non-invasive framework for automated evaluation of acute renal transplant rejection using DCE-MRI. NMR in Biomedicine 26(11):1460–1470

128. Hodneland E, Kjorstad A, Andersen E, Monssen J, Lundervold A, Rorvik J, Munthe-Kaas A (2011) In vivo estimation of glomerular filtration in the kidney using DCE-MRI. In: Proceedings of the 7th international symposium on image and signal processing analysis (ISPA'11), Dubrovnik, 4–6 September 2011, pp 755–761

129. Positano V, Bernardeschi I, Zampa V, Marinelli M, Landini L, Santarelli MF (2012) Automatic 2D registration of renal perfusion image sequences by mutual information and adaptive prediction. Mag Resonan Mater Phys Biol Med pp 1–11

130. El-Baz A, Farag A, Gimelfarb G (2005) MGRF controlled stochastic deformable model. In: Image analysis, Proceedings of the 14 Scandinavian conference on image analysis (SCIA'05), Joensuu, June 19–22. Springer, Heidelberg, pp 1138–1147

131. Khalifa F, Beache GM, Firjani A, Welch KC, Gimel'farb G, El-Baz A (2010) Deformable model guided by stochastic speed with application in cine images segmentation. In: Proceedings of IEEE international conference on image processing (ICIP'10), Hong Kong, 26–29 September 2010, pp 1725–128

132. El-Baz A, Gimelfarb G, Falk R, Abo El-Ghar M (2009) Automatic analysis of 3D low dose CT images for early diagnosis of lung cancer. Pattern Recogn 42(6):1041–1051

133. El-Baz A, Gimelfarb G, Falk R, El-Ghar MA (2011) 3D MGRF-based appearance modeling for robust segmentation of pulmonary nodules in 3D LDCT chest images. In: El-Baz A, Suri JS (eds) Lung imaging and computer aided diagnosis, chap. 3. CRC, Boca Raton, pp 51–63

134. El-Baz A, Gimelfarb G, Falk R, El-Ghar MA, Suri JA (2011) Appearance analysis for the early assessment of detected lung nodules. In: El-Baz A, Suri JS (eds) Lung imaging and computer aided diagnosis, chap. 17. IEEE, Piscataway, pp 395–404

135. El-Baz A, Khalifa F, Elnakib A, Nitzken M, Soliman A, McClure P, El-Ghar MA, Gimelfarb G (2012) A novel approach for global lung registration using 3D Markov-Gibbs appearance model. In: Proceedings of international conference on medical image computing and computer-assisted intervention (MICCAI'12), Nice, 1–5 October 2012. Springer, Berlin, pp 114–121

136. El-Baz A, Gimel'farb G, Abou El-Ghar M, Falk R (2012) Appearance-based diagnostic system for early assessment of malignant lung nodules. In: Proceedings of IEEE international conference on image processing (ICIP'12), Orlando, September 30–October 3, pp 533–536

137. El-Baz A, Soliman A, McClure P, Gimelfarb G, Abou El-Ghar M, Falk R (2012) Early assessment of malignant lung nodules based on the spatial analysis of detected lung nodules. In: Proceedings of IEEE international symposium on biomedical imaging: from nano to macro (ISBI'12), Barcelona, 2–5 May 2012, pp 1463–1466

138. El-Baz A, Gimel'farb G, Falk R, El-Ghar M (2010) Appearance analysis for diagnosing malignant lung nodules. In: Proceedings of IEEE international symposium on biomedical imaging: from nano to macro (ISBI'10), Rotterdam, 14–17 April 2010, pp 193–196

139. Farag AA, El-Baz A, Gimelfarb G, Falk R, El-Ghar MA, Eldiasty T, Elshazly S (2006) Appearance models for robust segmentation of pulmonary nodules in 3D LDCT chest images. In: Proceedings of international conference on medical image computing and computer-assisted intervention (MICCAI'06), Copenhagen, 1–6 October 2006, pp 734–741

140. Khalifa F, Beache GM, Gimel'farb G, Suri JS, El-Baz A (2011) State-of-the-art medical image registration methodologies: A survey. In: El-Baz A, Acharya UR, Mirmedhdi M, Suri JS (eds) Handbook of multi modality state-of-the-art medical image segmentation and registration methodologies, vol 1, chap 9. Springer, New York, pp 235–280

141. Rueckert D, Clarkson MJ, Hill DLG, Hawkes DJ (2000) Non-rigid registration using higher-order mutual information. In: Proceedings of SPIE medical imaging 2000: image processing (SPIE'00), vol 3979, pp 438–447

142. Khalifa F, Beache GM, Elnakib A, Sliman H, Gimel'farb G, Welch KC, El-Baz A (2012) A new nonrigid registration framework for improved visualization of transmural perfusion gradients on cardiac first-pass perfusion MRI. In: Proceedings of IEEE international symposium on biomedical imaging: from nano to macro (ISBI'12), Barcelona, 2–5 May 2012, pp 828–831

143. Khalifa F, Beache GM, Firjani A, Welch KC, Gimel'farb G, El-Baz A (2012) A new nonrigid registration approach for motion correction of cardiac first-pass perfusion MRI. In: Proceedings of IEEE international conference on image processing (ICIP'12), Lake Buena Vista, 30 September–3 October, 2012, pp 1665–1668

144. Khalifa F, Beache GM, Gimel'farb G, El-Baz A (2012) A novel CAD system for analyzing cardiac first-pass MRI images. In: Proceedings of IAPR international conference on pattern recognition (ICPR'12), Tsukuba Science City, 11–15 November 2012, pp 77–80

145. Khalifa F, Beache GM, Elnakib A, Sliman H, Gimel'farb G, Welch KC, El-Baz A (2013) A new shape-based framework for the left ventricle wall segmentation from cardiac first-pass perfusion MRI. In: IEEE international symposium on miomedical imaging: from nano to macro (ISBI'13), San Francisco, 7–11 April 2013. IEEE, Piscataway, pp 41–44

Biography

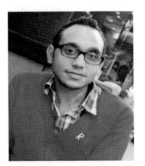

Mahmoud Mostapha received his B.Sc. degree in Electronics and Communications Engineering from Mansoura University, Mansoura, Egypt, in 2009. In January 2013 he joined the BioImaging Laboratory at University of Louisville, Louisville, KY, USA, as a research assistant. He is currently pursuing his M.S. in the ECE Department at the University of Louisville. His current research is focused on developing new computer assisted diagnostic (CAD) system for brain disorders from diffusion tensor MRI images.

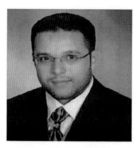

Fahmi Khalifa received his B.Sc. and M.S. degrees in Electrical Engineering from Mansoura University, Mansoura, Egypt, in 2003 and 2007, respectively. In May 2009 he joined the BioImaging Laboratory at University of Louisville, Louisville, KY, USA, as a graduate research assistant. His current research includes developing new computer aided diagnostic (CAD) systems, image modeling, shape analysis, and 2D and 3D image segmentation and registration.

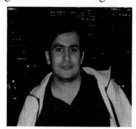

Amir Alansary received his B.Sc. Electrical Engineering from Mansoura University, Egypt, in 2009. Mr. Alansary was a part-time employee at the Middle East Technology company for 2 years, from February 2009 to February 2011. He joined the BioImaging Laboratory at University of Louisville, Louisville KY, as a research assistance in 2012. His general interests are in Digital Image Processing, Medical Imaging, and Computer Vision. Currently, Mr. Al Ansary is researching in Medical Image Analysis field and Autism Diagnostics.

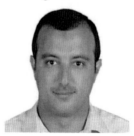

Ahmed Soliman received his B.Sc. and M.S. degrees in Computer Engineering from Mansoura University, Mansoura, Egypt. In December 2011 he joined the BioImaging Laboratory at University of Louisville, Louisville, KY, USA, as a research assistant. He has actively been working on Design of Computer Aided-Diagnostic Systems for Lung Segmentation and Early Detection of Lung Nodules.

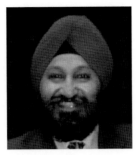

Jasjit Suri is an innovator, scientist, a visionary, an industrialist, and an internationally known world leader in Biomedical Engineering. Dr. Suri has spent over 20 years in the field of biomedical engineering/devices and its management. He received his Doctorate from University of Washington, Seattle and Business Management Sciences from Weatherhead, Case Western Reserve University, Cleveland, Ohio. Dr. Suri was crowned with President's Gold medal in 1980 and the Fellow of American Institute of Medical and Biological Engineering for his outstanding contributions.

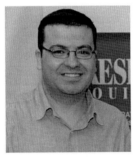

Ayman S. El-Baz, Ph.D., is an Associate Professor in the Department of Bioengineering at the University of Louisville, KY. Dr. El-Baz has 12 years of hands-on experience in the fields of bioimaging modeling and computer-assisted diagnostic systems. He has developed new techniques for analyzing 3D medical images. His work has been reported at several prestigious international conferences (e.g., CVPR, ICCV, and MICCAI) and in journals (e.g., IEEE TIP, IEEE TBME, IEEE TITB, and Brain). His work related to novel image analysis techniques for lung cancer and autism diagnosis has earned him multiple awards, including: first place at the annual Research Louisville 2002, 2005, 2006, 2007, 2008, 2010, 2011, and 2012 meetings, and the "Best Paper Award in Medical Image Processing" from the prestigious ICGST International Conference on Graphics, Vision and Image Processing (GVIP-2005). Dr. El-Baz has authored or coauthored more than 300 technical articles.

Kidney Detection and Segmentation in Contrast-Enhanced Ultrasound 3D Images

Raphael Prevost, Benoit Mory, Remi Cuingnet, Jean-Michel Correas, Laurent D. Cohen, and Roberto Ardon

Abstract Contrast-enhanced ultrasound (CEUS) imaging has lately benefited of an increasing interest for diagnosis and intervention planning, as it allows to visualize blood flow in real-time harmlessly for the patient. It complements thus the anatomical information provided by conventional ultrasound (US). This chapter is dedicated to kidney segmentation methods in 3D CEUS images. First we present a generic and fast two-step approach to locate (via a robust ellipsoid estimation algorithm) and segment (using a template deformation framework) the kidney automatically. Then we show how user interactions can be integrated within the algorithm to guide or correct the segmentation in real-time. Finally, we develop a co-segmentation framework that generalizes the aforementioned method and allows the simultaneous use of multiple images (here the CEUS and the US images) to improve the segmentation result. The different approaches are evaluated on a clinical database of 64 volumes.

Introduction

Ultrasound imaging (US) is a widely used modality due to its versatility, low cost, and real-time capabilities. Such acquisitions have been for a long time limited to 2D images but the recent development of 3D US allowed to consider new problems

R. Prevost (✉) • B. Mory • R. Cuingnet • R. Ardon
Philips Research Medisys, Suresnes, France
e-mail: prevost.raphael@gmail.com; benoit.mory@philips.com; remi.cuingnet@philips.com; roberto.ardon@philips.com

J.-M. Correas
Adult Radiology Department, Necker Hospital, Paris, France
e-mail: jean-michel.correas@nck.aphp.fr

L.D. Cohen
Paris Dauphine University, CEREMADE UMR 7534, Paris, France
e-mail: cohen@ceremade.dauphine.fr

A.S. El-Baz et al. (eds.), *Abdomen and Thoracic Imaging: An Engineering & Clinical Perspective*, DOI 10.1007/978-1-4614-8498-1_2,
© Springer Science+Business Media New York 2014

such as volumetric assessments of organs or image registration. In addition to conventional US, three-dimensional real-time visualization of vascularization can be achieved with contrast-enhanced ultrasound (CEUS) imaging. This rather new modality provides very useful information for lesions diagnosis or large vessels monitoring [1]. Gas-filled microbubbles, acting as amplifiers of the blood back-scattering signal, are used as a contrast agent. Because the bubbles are naturally eliminated by metabolism processes, this modality is considered as completely safe for the patients even with renal or liver failure (unlike contrast-enhanced CT, for example).

However the usually poor quality of CEUS images makes any computer-based analysis challenging: in addition to having powerful speckle noise, the image is very grainy and almost binary as a result of ultrasound interactions with individual bubbles. Unlike in conventional US [2], very few segmentation methods of 3D CEUS images have been reported. Among them, Gasnier et al. [3] introduced an interactive approach to segment and analyze tumors in this modality. However, their framework was specific to lesion segmentation, just as the automatic methods proposed in [4, 5]. In [6], Ma et al. developed an automatic algorithm to segment the heart left ventricle. This method, although applicable to other organs, does not provide any natural way to refine or correct the result interactively. Besides, it has been designed for images acquired with a particular transducer, producing sparse rotated slices instead of a whole 3D volume.

In this chapter, we address the problem of kidney segmentation in 3D CEUS images. This challenging issue is of great importance to assess quantitatively the volume of renal tissues. First, we present a generic and fast approach to automatically segment a kidney in CEUS volumes. Our method consists in detecting it in the image as an ellipsoid, and then deforming this ellipsoid to match precisely its boundary. Second, we extend this framework in order to take into account other kinds of information :

- *user interactions:* Because of the poor image quality or pathologies, image information may be sometimes unreliable and even misleading. In such cases, the clinician user should be able to guide or correct the segmentation easily and with a real-time feedback.
- *simultaneous use of another image:* Because of shadowing effects, pathologies, and limited field of view, parts of the kidney may be hardly visible in the image. In such cases even expert users may have difficulty delineating the true boundary of the organ by solely relying on one CEUS image. In clinical routine every CEUS acquisition is preceded by a conventional US acquisition to locate the kidney. Hence, the latter would be useful to complement the CEUS image and thus cope with missing and corrupted information.

Prior work on kidney segmentation in CEUS is limited to two of our conference papers [7, 8], of which this chapter is an extended version.

The remainder of the chapter is organized as follows. First of all, section "Material" is dedicated to the description of the material used throughout the chapter in validation experiments. In section "Kidney Detection via Robust Ellipsoid

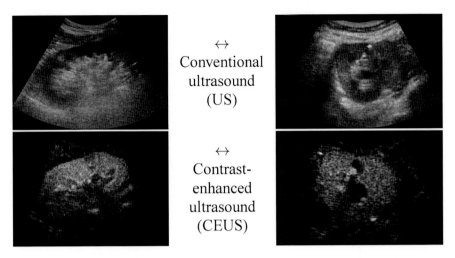

Fig. 1 Slices of conventional and contrast-enhanced ultrasound 3D images of the kidney for two different patients (*left* and *right*)

Estimation", we introduce a fast and robust method to estimate roughly the center, orientation, and sizes of the kidney. This is a done via an original variational framework for ellipsoid detection. The outcome of this step is then used as the prior model of a segmentation algorithm, based on template deformation, described in section "Kidney Segmentation via Implicit Template Deformation". Because of the inherent ambiguities in CEUS images, the obtained segmentation may be improved by using additional information. In section "Segmentation with User Interactions", we show how user interactions can be used inherently in our framework to correct the result in real-time. Then we extend our approach to multiple images, namely the CEUS and the US volumes (section "Joint Co-segmentation and Registration") which are not aligned. Thus a generic framework for joint co-segmentation and registration is introduced and applied to both the kidney detection and segmentation. We show that by taking additional information into account, the automatic kidney segmentation is more robust. Finally, we conclude the chapter by discussing potential improvements.

Material

This section describes the material used throughout the chapter. Our database is composed of 64 pairs of CEUS and US volumes acquired from 35 different patients, via an iU22 ultrasound system (Philips, The Netherlands). In order to have a clinically representative database, both healthy and diseased kidneys were considered. Images were acquired using different probes, namely V6-2 and X6-1 (Philips, The Netherlands) US probes, with various fields of view. The volumes size was

$512 \times 510 \times 256$ voxels with different spatial resolutions ($0.25 \times 0.25 \times 0.55$ mm in average). The acquisition protocol was as follows: first, the clinician scouted for the patient's kidney using conventional US and acquired a US volume. Then, 2.4 mL of Sonovue (Bracco, Italy) contrast agent was injected to the patient and a CEUS acquisition was performed after a few seconds. Indeed, dynamic CEUS images of a kidney show a cortical enhancement shortly followed by a medullary enhancement. Better visualization of kidney tissue is then available when the contrast agent has diffused as it is completely hyperechoic whereas its fatty surrounding produces no signal. Figure 1 shows a comparison of US and CEUS images for two patients of our database. Note that the US and CEUS images are not aligned as the clinician may have slightly moved the probe between the two acquisitions.

For each image, an expert was asked to segment the kidney with a semiautomatic tool. This segmentation was considered as the ground truth. The different approaches described in the chapter will be evaluated by computing the Dice coefficient between the segmentation result S and the ground truth $G\,T$, defined as

$$\text{Dice}(S, GT) = 2\;\frac{\text{Vol}(S \cap GT)}{\text{Vol}(S) + \text{Vol}(GT)}\;, \tag{1}$$

where $\text{Vol}(X)$ denotes the volume of a region X. Thus the higher the Dice coefficient, the better the segmentation is. In particular, this score is equal to 1 for a perfect segmentation and 0 for a completely non-overlapping segmentation.

All proposed methods were implemented in a C++ prototype and the computational times will be given for a standard computer (Intel Core i5 2.67 Ghz, 4GB RAM).

Kidney Detection via Robust Ellipsoid Estimation

Since kidney shape can be roughly approximated by an ellipsoid, the kidney automatic detection problem in CEUS images can be initially reduced to finding the smallest ellipsoid encompassing most of the hyperechoic voxels. A large number of methods (e.g., Hough transforms [9, 10]) have already been proposed to detect ellipses in images [11]. However their extension to 3D, though possible, is usually computationally expensive mainly because of the number of parameters to estimate (9 for a 3D ellipsoid). Furthermore, they do not explicitly use the fact that only one ellipsoid is present in the image. On the other hand, statistical approaches like robust Minimum Volume Ellipsoid (MVE) estimators [12] are better suited but require prior knowledge on the proportion of outliers (here the noise, artifacts, or neighboring structures), which may vary from one image to another and is thus not available. We therefore propose an original variational framework, which is robust and fast, to estimate the best ellipsoid in an image $I : \Omega \subset \mathbb{R}^3 \to \mathbb{R}^+$.

A Variational Framework for Robust Ellipsoid Estimation

In the considered framework, an ellipsoid is implicitly represented using an implicit function $\phi : \Omega \to \mathbb{R}$ that is positive inside the ellipsoid and negative elsewhere. ϕ can be parametrized by the center of the ellipsoid $\mathbf{c} \in \mathbb{R}^3$ and its sizes and orientations encoded by a 3×3 positive-definite matrix $\mathbf{M}$. We therefore define the implicit equation of an ellipsoid as

$$\phi_{\mathbf{c},\mathbf{M}}(\mathbf{x}) = 1 - (\mathbf{x} - \mathbf{c})^T \mathbf{M}(\mathbf{x} - \mathbf{c}) = 0 . \tag{2}$$

The detection method should be robust to outliers, i.e. bright voxels coming from noise, artifacts, or other neighboring structures. Excluding those outliers is done by estimating a weighting function w (defined over the image domain Ω into $[0,1]$) that provides a confidence score for any point $\mathbf{x}$ to be an inlier. The ellipsoid estimation is then formulated as an energy minimization problem with respect to $\mathbf{c}$, $\mathbf{M}$, and w:

$$\min_{\mathbf{c},\mathbf{M},w} \left\{ E_{\det}(\mathbf{c}, \mathbf{M}, w) = - \int_\Omega \phi_{\mathbf{c},\mathbf{M}}(\mathbf{x}) \, I(\mathbf{x}) \, w(\mathbf{x}) \, d\mathbf{x} \right.$$

$$\left. + \mu . \log\left(\frac{\mathrm{Vol}(\mathbf{M})}{|\Omega|}\right) . \left(\int_\Omega I(\mathbf{x}) \, w(\mathbf{x}) \, d\mathbf{x}\right) \right\} \tag{3}$$

$$\text{with} \quad \phi_{\mathbf{c},\mathbf{M}}(\mathbf{x}) = 1 - (\mathbf{x} - \mathbf{c})^T \mathbf{M}(\mathbf{x} - \mathbf{c})$$

$$\text{and} \quad \mathrm{Vol}(\mathbf{M}) = \frac{4\pi}{3} \sqrt{\det \mathbf{M}^{-1}} \quad \text{the ellipsoid volume.}$$

The ellipsoid detection energy $E_{\det}$ is composed of two terms:

- a *data-fidelity term*: The first term is an integral over the whole image domain Ω of the product $\phi_{\mathbf{c},\mathbf{M}}$ by $w\, I$. Note that $w\, I$ is highly positive at voxels that have a high intensity but are not outliers. To minimize the energy, such voxels must therefore be included inside the ellipsoid, i.e. where ϕ is positive.
- a *regularization term*: The second term penalizes the volume of the ellipsoid Vol (M) with respect to the domain volume $|\Omega|$. The logarithm provides a statistical interpretation of the problem and eases the minimization of the energy, as will be seen in the next subsection. It is normalized by $\int w\, I$ and weighted by a trade-off parameter $\mu > 0$.

Numerical Optimization

This ellipsoid estimation process can be viewed as fitting a Gaussian distribution to the bright pixels of the image by minimizing its negative log-likelihood. Therefore $E_{\det}$ has a statistical meaning and when w is fixed, the minimizers $(\mathbf{c}^*, \mathbf{M}^*)$ of $E_{\det}$

$(\cdot, \cdot, w)$ have a closed form. Indeed, $\mathbf{c}^*$ is the barycenter of all voxels $\mathbf{x}$ weighted by $I(\mathbf{x})w(\mathbf{x})$, while $\mathbf{M}^*$ is the inverse of the covariance matrix[1] of the same data. Besides, E_{det} is linear with respect to w which is by definition restricted to $[0,1]$. Therefore, at every voxel $\mathbf{x}$ the minimizer $w^*(\mathbf{x})$ is equal to 0 or 1, depending only on the sign of $\phi_{\mathbf{c},\mathbf{M}} - \mu \log\left(\frac{\text{Vol}(\mathbf{M})}{|\Omega|}\right)$. w^* is then the indicator of the current ellipsoid estimation which has been dilated proportionately to μ. Its purpose is to remove the contribution of the points which are far away from the current ellipsoid and may hinder its refinement.

The weighting function w is initialized to 1 everywhere. Minimization of E_{det} is then performed with an alternate iterative scheme that successively updates the variables $\mathbf{c}$, $\mathbf{M}$, and w, as summarized in Algorithm 1. As the energy E_{det} decreases at each step, the algorithm is guaranteed to converge. In practice, few iterations are required for convergence and total computational time is less than a second for a 3D image.

Algorithm 1: Robust ellipsoid detection algorithm

---

initialization $\forall\, \mathbf{x} \in \Omega,\ w(\mathbf{x}) \leftarrow 1$

repeat

> // Estimation of center $\mathbf{c}$ and matrix $\mathbf{M}$
>
> $\mathbf{c} \leftarrow \frac{1}{\int_{\Omega} Iw} \int_{\Omega} I(\mathbf{x})\, w(\mathbf{x})\, \mathbf{x}\, d\mathbf{x}$
>
> $\mathbf{M}^{-1} \leftarrow \frac{2}{\mu \int_{\Omega} Iw} \int_{\Omega} I(\mathbf{x})\, w(\mathbf{x})\, (\mathbf{x} - \mathbf{c})(\mathbf{x} - \mathbf{c})^T\, d\mathbf{x}$
>
> // Update of the weighting function w for each $\mathbf{x} \in \Omega$
>
> **if** $(\mathbf{x} - \mathbf{c})^T \mathbf{M}\, (\mathbf{x} - \mathbf{c}) \leq 1 - \mu \log\left(\frac{\text{Vol}(\mathbf{M})}{|\Omega|}\right)$ **then**
>
> > $\lfloor\ w(\mathbf{x}) \leftarrow 1$
>
> **else**
>
> > $\lfloor\ w(\mathbf{x}) \leftarrow 0$

until *convergence*;

The choice of μ is paramount as it controls the number of points that are taken into account for the ellipsoid matrix estimation. It should be set to values close to $\frac{2}{5}$ in 3D and $\frac{1}{2}$ in 2D (the proof is deferred in the appendix).

Figure 2 shows such a process for a synthetic 2D image. The first ellipse estimate is too large as all voxels are considered but far points are progressively eliminated via the weighting function w until the algorithm converges towards the good solution. We also present results on real CEUS data in Fig. 3. The estimated ellipsoids are not perfectly accurate but robust and close enough to be used as an initialization for a segmentation algorithm.

---

[1] Up to a constant multiplier.

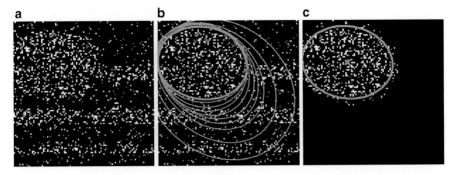

Fig. 2 (**a**) Original 2D synthetic image, corrupted by salt-and-pepper noise. (**b**) Evolution of the ellipse along the iterations (*orange*) and final result (*green*). (**c**) Ellipse contour and center superimposed on the product $w\,I$ at convergence

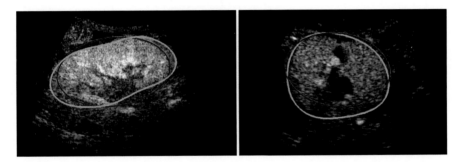

Fig. 3 Results of the ellipsoid detection (*red*) compared to the ground truth (*green*), on slices of the volumes shown in Fig. 1

Kidney Segmentation via Implicit Template Deformation

The previously detected ellipsoid will now be deformed to segment the kidney more precisely. We follow the template deformation framework described in [13, 14] and extended in [15], as it is a very efficient model-based algorithm and it has already been applied successfully to kidney segmentation in CT images [16].

Implicit Template Deformation Framework

Implicit template deformation is a framework where an implicit shape defined by a function $\phi_0 : \Omega \to \mathbb{R}$, called the *template*, is deformed so that its zero level set segments a given image $I : \Omega \to \mathbb{R}^+$. The segmenting implicit shape is the zero level set of a function $\phi : \Omega \to \mathbb{R}$, therefore defined with respect to this template and a transformation of the space $\psi : \Omega \to \Omega$ that becomes the unknown of the problem : $\phi = \phi_0 \circ \psi$. In our application, the template is the implicit function of the previously estimated ellipsoid $\phi_0 = \phi_c{}^*, M^*$ and ψ is sought such that the image gradient flux across the surface of the deformed ellipsoid $(\phi_0 \circ \psi)^{-1}(0)$ is maximum. The segmentation energy is then

$$E_{\text{seg}}(\psi) = \int_{\{\phi_0 \circ \psi = 0\}} -\left\langle \vec{\nabla} I(\mathbf{x}) , \vec{n}(\mathbf{x}) \right\rangle dS(\mathbf{x}) + \lambda \mathcal{R}(\psi), \tag{4}$$

where $\vec{n}(\mathbf{x})$ denotes the vector normal to the surface of the segmentation at point $\mathbf{x}$. $\mathcal{R}(\psi)$ is a regularization term which prevents large deviations from the original ellipsoid. Its choice will be detailed in section "Transformation Model" hereafter. λ is a positive scalar parameter that controls the strength of this shape constraint.

Using the divergence theorem, the first data-fidelity term can be rewritten as

$$\int_{\{\phi_0 \circ \psi = 0\}} -\left\langle \vec{\nabla} I(\mathbf{x}), \vec{n}(\mathbf{x}) \right\rangle dS(\mathbf{x}) = -\int_{\{\phi_0 \circ \psi \geq 0\}} div(\nabla I(\mathbf{x})) \, d\mathbf{x} = -\int_{\{\phi_0 \circ \psi \geq 0\}} \Delta I(\mathbf{x}) \, d\mathbf{x} \tag{5}$$

where Δ denotes the Laplacian operator. Introducing H the Heaviside function ($H(a) = 1$ if a is positive, 0 otherwise) yields a more convenient formulation of the segmentation energy :

$$E_{\text{seg}}(\psi) = -\int_{\Omega} H(\phi_0 \circ \psi(\mathbf{x})) \, \Delta I(\mathbf{x}) \, d\mathbf{x} + \lambda \mathcal{R}(\psi), \tag{6}$$

Transformation Model

The choice of the space of possible solutions ψ to Problem (6) is, in our case, intrinsically linked to the notion of *shape*. A *shape* can be considered as a set of objects sharing the same visual aspect. It should be invariant to geometric transforms such as translation, rotation, scaling, or shearing. We will refer to such a global transformation as the *pose*. To set up a clear distinction between the pose and the subsequent shape *deformation*, similarly to [17], we design our template transformation model ψ as a functional composition of a global transformation $\mathcal{G}$ and a nonrigid local transformation $\mathcal{L}$ (see Fig. 4):

$$\psi = \mathcal{L} \circ \mathcal{G} \tag{7}$$

Pose. $\mathcal{G} : \Omega \to \Omega$ is chosen as a parametric transform that coarsely aligns the template with the target surface in the image. It will basically correct or adjust the global position and scaling of the ellipsoid and can be chosen as a similarity. $\mathcal{G}$ is thus represented by a matrix in homogeneous coordinates defined by 7 parameters $\mathbf{p} = \{p_i\}_{i=1\ldots7}$ and noted $\mathcal{G}_{\mathbf{p}}$.

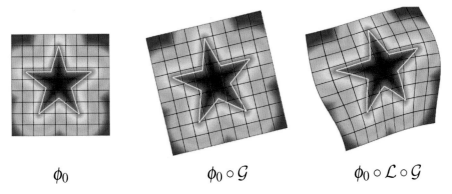

$$\phi_0 \qquad\qquad \phi_0 \circ \mathcal{G} \qquad\qquad \phi_0 \circ \mathcal{L} \circ \mathcal{G}$$

Fig. 4 Decomposition of the transformation ψ. The implicit template ϕ_0 undergoes a global transformation $\mathcal{G}$ and a local deformation $\mathcal{L}$

Deformation. $\mathcal{L} : \Omega \rightarrow \Omega$ is expressed using a displacement field $\mathbf{u}$ in the template referential $\mathcal{L} = Id + \mathbf{u}$. Similarly to problems in image registration and optical flow algorithms [18], $\mathbf{u}$ should be smoothly varying in space. While adding penalizations on differential terms of $\mathbf{u}$ to $\mathcal{R}(\psi)$ is a valid approach, efficient implementations are difficult to derive. Taking advantage of efficient linear filtering, smoothness of the displacement $\mathbf{u}$ is set as a built-in property defining it as a filtered version of an integrable unknown displacement field $\mathbf{v}$

$$\mathbf{u}(\mathbf{x}) = [K_\sigma * \mathbf{v}](\mathbf{x}) = \int_\Omega K_\sigma(\mathbf{x} - \mathbf{y}) \, \mathbf{v}(\mathbf{y}) \, d\mathbf{y} \tag{8}$$

where K_σ is a Gaussian kernel of scale σ. The overall transformation that can therefore be parametrized by $\mathbf{p}$ and $\mathbf{v}$ will be noted $\psi_{\mathbf{p},\mathbf{v}}$.

The proposed decomposition allows to define the shape prior term independently from the pose: $\mathcal{R}(\psi) = \mathcal{R}(\mathcal{L})$. $\mathcal{R}$ thus quantifies how much the segmenting implicit function ϕ deviates from the prior *shape* ϕ_0. Using the L_2 norm we choose to constraint $\mathcal{L}$ towards the identity :

$$\mathcal{R}(\mathcal{L}) = \frac{1}{2} \| \mathcal{L} - Id \|_2^2 = \frac{1}{2} \int_\Omega \| \mathbf{u}(\mathbf{x}) \|^2 \, d\mathbf{x} \tag{9}$$

The optimization problem to solve finally reads:

$$\min_{\mathbf{p},\mathbf{v}} \left\{ E_{\text{seg}}(\psi_{\mathbf{p},\mathbf{v}}) = - \int_\Omega H(\phi_0 \circ \psi_{\mathbf{p},\mathbf{v}}(\mathbf{x})) \, \Delta I(\mathbf{x}) \, d\mathbf{x} + \frac{\lambda}{2} \int_\Omega \| K_\sigma * \mathbf{v} \|^2 \right\} \tag{10}$$

with $\psi_{\mathbf{p},\mathbf{v}} = (Id + \mathbf{u}) \circ \mathcal{G}_{\mathbf{p}}$ and $\mathbf{u} = K_\sigma * \mathbf{v}$

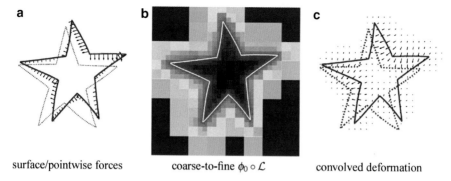

surface/pointwise forces   coarse-to-fine $\phi_0 \circ \mathcal{L}$ convolved deformation

Fig. 5 Fast template deformation with coarse-to-fine distance warp and convolutions. (**a**) Surface/pointwise forces. (**b**) Coarse-to-fine $\phi_0 \circ \mathcal{L}$. (**c**) Convolved deformation

Numerical Implementation

Problem (10) is minimized via a standard gradient descent simultaneously on the parameters of the pose $\mathcal{G}_p$ and the deformation field **v**. The descent evolution equations are obtained by applying calculus of variations to E_{seg}. We omit the tedious details but the final equations, after a variable substitution, read

$$\begin{cases} \dfrac{\partial \mathbf{p}}{\partial t} = - \displaystyle\int_{\Omega} \delta(\phi_0 \circ \mathcal{L}) \cdot \left\langle \nabla \phi_0 \circ \mathcal{L}, \ (Id + J_{\mathbf{u}}) \dfrac{\partial \mathcal{G}}{\partial \mathbf{p}} \mathcal{G}^{-1} \right\rangle \cdot \Delta I \circ \mathcal{G}^{-1} \\[3mm] \dfrac{\partial \mathbf{v}}{\partial t} = - \left[\delta(\phi_0 \circ \mathcal{L}) \cdot \nabla \phi_0 \circ \mathcal{L} \cdot \Delta I \circ \mathcal{G}^{-1} \ + \lambda \mathbf{v} \right] * K_{\sigma} \end{cases} \tag{11}$$

where δ denotes the Dirac distribution and $J_{\mathbf{u}}$ is the Jacobian matrix of the displacement field **u**.

A quick analysis of Eq. (11) reveals several key aspects for an efficient implementation. Interpolating $\phi_0 \circ \mathcal{L}$ and $\nabla \phi_0 \circ \mathcal{L}$ over the whole domain Ω would be extremely time-consuming. Nevertheless, since it is multiplied by $\delta(\phi_0 \circ \mathcal{L})$, the warped gradient field $\nabla \phi_0 \circ \mathcal{L}$ is only needed on the set $\{\phi_0 \circ \mathcal{L} = 0\}$ (Fig. 5a) which highly reduces the computational burden. Moreover, precise knowledge of the warped template $\phi_0 \circ \mathcal{L}$ is only necessary near its zero level set. We use a coarse-to-fine approach using octrees. At each level a decision is made to further refine the cell depending on the distance measure (Fig. 5b) drastically dropping complexity. Finally, stemming from the displacement model, extrapolating image and pointwise forces to the whole space boils down to a convolution with K_{σ} (Fig. 5c). In practice, our current 3D implementation supports up to 100 time steps per second for a discretization of the implicit function on a $64 \times 64 \times 64$ lattice.

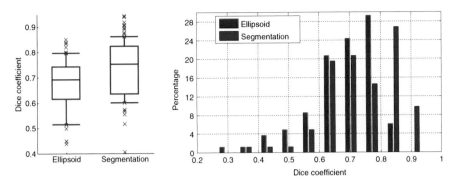

Fig. 6 Kidney detection (*red*) and segmentation (*blue*) results in terms of Dice coefficients shown as boxplots (*left*) and histograms (*right*). Boxplots show, respectively, the first decile, the first quartile, the median, the third quartile, and the ninth decile. Extreme points are shown separately

Results for Automatic Segmentation in CEUS Images

This validation has been performed on the CEUS images of the dataset presented in section "Material". The completely automatic pipeline had a computational time of around 5 s.

Quantitative results are reported in Fig. 6. The overall median Dice coefficient is 0.69 for the detection and 0.76 for the segmentation and 25 % of the database have a very satisfying segmentation (Dice coefficient higher than 0.85), given the very poor image quality and the presence of pathologies.

Figure 7 shows the obtained result for the two cases introduced in Fig. 1. The segmentations are very similar to the ground truth and can be considered as satisfying. Some cases are, however, more difficult (e.g., Fig. 10 in the next section) and will require additional information.

Segmentation with User Interactions

The previously described approach is fast and automatic, but fails in some difficult cases. Indeed ultrasound shadows or kidney pathologies make the image information unreliable and thus hinder the segmentation algorithm. It is therefore important to provide the clinician a way to guide or correct the segmentation easily and with a real-time feedback. As proposed in [15], this can be done easily within the implicit template deformation framework that was presented in section "Kidney Segmentation via Implicit Template Deformation".

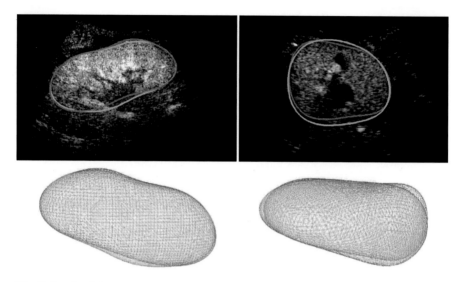

Fig. 7 Result of the automatic segmentation (*blue*) compared to the ground truth (*green*) on a particular slice (*top*) and in 3D (*bottom*)

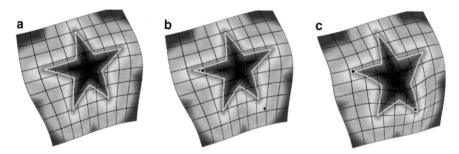

Fig. 8 User interactions as inside/outside points. (**a**) Template deformed without constraints. (**b**) User indicates points that should be inside (*blue*) and outside (*red*) the segmentation. (**c**) New segmentation that satisfies these constraints

User Interactions as Constraints

In this section, we show how the user can guide the segmentation by indicating points that should be inside or outside the segmentation (see Fig. 8).

Consider that the user provides N points $\{\mathbf{x}_k\}_k \subset \Omega^N$ in the image domain labeling each one as inside or outside of the surface to extract (which can be done via simple interactions such as a left click on an inside point, and a right click on an outside point). The implicit formulation allows to express this information merely as inequality constraints on the deformed implicit function, at points $\{\mathbf{x}_k\}_k$:

$$\forall k \in [|1,N|], \quad \gamma_k \cdot \phi_0 \circ \psi(\mathbf{x}_k) \geq 0 \tag{12}$$

where $\gamma_k = 1$ (resp. -1) for inside (resp. outside) points. Note that it is also possible to specify a point that should be exactly on the segmentation surface by labeling it as both inside and outside: the two inequality constraints are equivalent to an equality constraint. Then, putting together the initial formulation in Eq. (6) and the constraints of Eq. (12) yields a general formulation of implicit template deformation with user interactions, as the following minimization problem:

$$\min_{\psi} \left\{ E_{\mathrm{seg}}(\psi) = -\int_{\Omega} H(\phi_0 \circ \psi(\mathbf{x})) \, \Delta I(\mathbf{x}) \, d\mathbf{x} + \lambda R(\psi) \right\}$$
$$\text{subject to } \forall k \in [1,N], \quad \gamma_k \cdot \phi_0 \circ \psi(\mathbf{x}_k) \geq 0 \tag{13}$$

In the next subsection we propose a method to solve this problem efficiently. For the sake of genericity, no assumption is made on the representation of the deformation ψ and the model $\psi = \mathcal{L} \circ \mathcal{G}$ will be just a particular implementation of the approach described hereafter.

Optimization Scheme

Since $E_{\mathrm{seg}}(\psi)$ is a non-convex functional and has to be minimized under a set of nonlinear constraints, no specifically tailored algorithms are available. For this matter, we follow a general augmented Lagrangian methodology [19] and define an equivalent unconstrained problem that can be locally minimized by gradient descent. The constrained problem (13) can equivalently be written as an unconstrained minimization problem of the form

$$\min_{\psi} \left\{ \tilde{E}_{\mathrm{seg}}(\psi) = \max_{\alpha \geq 0} \left\{ E_{\mathrm{seg}}(\psi) - \sum_{k=1}^{N} \alpha_k c_k(\psi) \right\} \right\}$$
$$\text{with } c_k(\psi) = \gamma_k \cdot \phi_0 \circ \psi(\mathbf{x}_k) \tag{14}$$

where α_k is the Lagrange multiplier associated with the kth constraint. Equation (14) has the same set of solutions as the original problem in Eq. (13): if ψ satisfies all constraints c_k, then $\tilde{E}_{\mathrm{seg}}(\psi) = E_{\mathrm{seg}}(\psi)$; otherwise, $\tilde{E}_{\mathrm{seg}}(\psi)$ is infinite. Since $\tilde{E}_{\mathrm{seg}}$ jumps from finite to infinite values at the boundary of the feasible set, it is difficult to minimize it as such. A more practical approach is to introduce a smooth approximation $\tilde{E}_{\text{seg}}^{\nu}$ that depends on a quadratic penalty parameter ν. Parameter ν will be used to constrain the maximizers $(\alpha_k)_k$ to finite values. These multipliers are estimated iteratively and we introduce $(\alpha_k^j)_k$ the multipliers estimates at the jth iteration, in order to define the energy approximation

$$\tilde{E}_{\text{seg}}^{\nu}(\psi, \alpha^j) = \max_{\alpha \geq 0} \left\{ E_{\text{seg}}(\psi) - \sum_{k=1}^{N} \alpha_k c_k(\psi) - \frac{1}{2\nu} \sum_{k=1}^{N} \left(\alpha_k - \alpha_k^j \right)^2 \right\} \quad (15)$$

The maximizing Lagrange multipliers associated with each constraint $c_k(\psi)$ have a closed-form solution :

$$\alpha_k^{j+1} = \begin{cases} 0 & \text{if } \alpha_k^j - \nu c_k(\psi) \leq 0 \\ \alpha_k^j - \nu c_k(\psi) & \text{otherwise.} \end{cases} \quad (16)$$

Substituting (16) into (15) yields the following expression of the smooth approximation $\tilde{E}_{\text{seg}}^{\nu}$:

$$\tilde{E}_{\text{seg}}^{\nu}(\psi, \alpha^j) = E_{\text{seg}}(\psi) + \sum_{k=1}^{N} F_{\nu}\left(c_k(\psi), \alpha_k^j \right)$$

$$\text{with} \quad F_{\nu}(a, b) = \begin{cases} -ab + \dfrac{\nu}{2} a^2 & \text{if } \nu a \leq b \\ -\dfrac{1}{2\nu} b^2 & \text{otherwise.} \end{cases} \quad (17)$$

Finally, the alternate scheme described in Algorithm 2, in which the penalty parameter ν is gradually increased, will provide a local minimizer of E_{seg} that eventually satisfies the user constraints. Within this process, Step (1) is straightforward and Step (2) is very similar to the gradient descent proposed in section "Numerical Implementation":

$$\begin{cases} \dfrac{\partial \mathbf{p}}{\partial t} \leftarrow \dfrac{\partial \mathbf{p}}{\partial t} - \sum_{k=1}^{K} \gamma_k F(\alpha_k) \left\langle \nabla \phi_0 \circ \mathcal{L} \circ \mathcal{G}(\mathbf{x}_k), (Id + J_{\mathbf{u}}) \dfrac{\partial \mathcal{G}}{\partial \mathbf{p}}(\mathbf{x}_k) \right\rangle \\[3mm] \dfrac{\partial \mathbf{v}}{\partial t} \leftarrow \dfrac{\partial \mathbf{v}}{\partial t} - \left[\sum_{k=1}^{K} \gamma_k \delta_{\mathcal{G}(\mathbf{x}_k)} F_{\nu}(\alpha_k) \nabla \phi_0 \circ \mathcal{L} \right] * K_{\sigma} \end{cases} \quad (18)$$

Note that the additional terms in Eq. (18) are just pointwise contributions that do not influence the overall computational time.

Algorithm 2: Augmented Lagrangian Scheme For Inequality Constraints

---

initialization choose $v^0 > 0$ and set $\forall k,\ \alpha_k^0 \leftarrow 0$,

repeat

> choose $v^t > v^{t-1}$,
> set $j \leftarrow 0$,
> **repeat**
>> (1) ψ being fixed, update the Lagrange multipliers α^j using Eq (16)
>> (2) α^j being fixed, update ψ by minimizing $\tilde{E}_{seg}^{v^t}(\psi, \alpha^j)$ with gradient descent on Eq (17)
>> (3) increment $j \leftarrow j+1$
>
> **until** *convergence*;
> increment $t \leftarrow t+1$

until *a local minimum of $E_{seg}(\psi)$ satisfying $\forall k,\ c_k(\psi) \geq 0$ is found;*

Influence of User Interactions on Kidney Segmentation in CEUS

Validation of the user interactions has been performed on a subset of 21 CEUS volumes from 21 different patients of our database. For each case, the automatic segmentation has been run and its result was refined with user interactions from an expert. Figure 9 reports the Dice coefficients obtained as a function of the number of clicks. The score gradually increases as the user interacts with the algorithm but rapidly converges: most of the time, less than 3 clicks are needed for a fairly precise result (Dice ≥ 0.9).[2] The results also show that even when the initialization produces a low score, very few interactions can improve a lot the segmentation. The influence of user interactions is illustrated in Fig. 10, where we show results on a difficult case. The patient has a lot of renal cysts that are anechogenic and hinders the automatic segmentations. With 3 clicks, the segmentation is much closer to the ground truth.

Nevertheless, in some applications user interactions are not possible and the segmentation has to be automatic. In the next section, we propose to improve the kidney segmentation by using simultaneously and automatically the conventional US image

---

[2] The ground truth may not exactly be reached because of the high intra-operator variability.

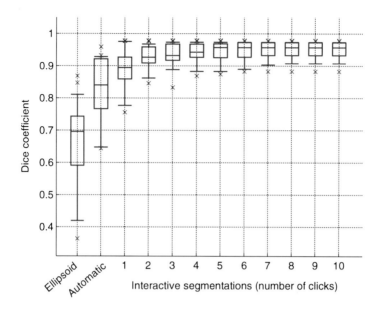

Fig. 9 Boxplots of the Dice coefficient between the ground truth and the segmentation at different steps of the proposed algorithm. Boxplots show, respectively, the first decile, the first quartile, the median, the third quartile, and the ninth decile. Extreme points are shown separately

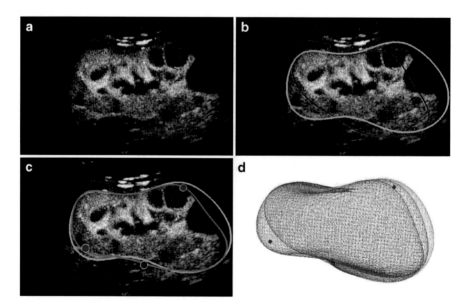

Fig. 10 Example of a segmentation with user interactions. (**a**) Slice of the original CEUS volume. (**b**) Comparison of the ground truth (*green*) and automatic segmentation (*red*). (**c**) Corrected segmentation (*blue*) with 2 inside points (*blue dots*) and one outside point (*red dot*). (**d**) 3D visualization of the ground truth (*green*), the automatic (*red*), and corrected (*blue*) segmentation, with constraint points

Joint Co-segmentation and Registration

Co-segmentation often denotes the task of finding an object in each image that shares the same appearance but not necessarily the same shape [20]. Here we look for the exactly same organ in two images but with a different appearance. As simultaneous acquisition of US and CEUS is not possible on current 3D imaging systems, the two images are in arbitrary referentials and need to be aligned. However, standard iconic registration methods are not adapted since visible structures, apart from the kidney itself, are completely different in US and CEUS. Co-segmentation shall therefore help registration, just as registration helps co-segmentation. This calls for a method that jointly performs these two tasks (see Fig. 11).

Although segmentation and registration are often seen as two separate problems, several approaches have already been proposed to perform them simultaneously. Most of them rely on an iconic registration guiding the segmentation (e.g., [21–23]). Yet they assume that the segmentation is known in one of the images, which is not the case in our application of co-segmentation. Moreover, as stated before, CEUS/ US intensity-based registration is bound to fail since visible structures do not correspond to each other. Instead of registering the images themselves, Wyatt et al. [24] developed a MAP formulation to perform registration on label maps resulting from a segmentation step. However no shape model is enforced and noise can degrade the results. In [25], Yezzi et al. introduced a variational framework that consists in a feature-based registration in which the features are actually the segmenting active contours.

In this section, we aim at extending both the previously described kidney detection and segmentation in a 3D CEUS image to a pair of 3D CEUS and US images. To that end, we develop a generic joint co-segmentation and registration framework inspired by [25]. This results in a fully automated pipeline to obtain both an improved kidney segmentation in CEUS and US images and a registration of them. But first of all, in order to use conventional US, we need to learn how the kidney looks like in such images.

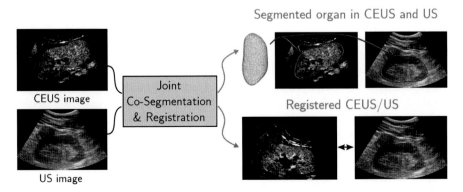

Fig. 11 Joint co-segmentation and registration. Given two different non-aligned images of the same object, the proposed method aims at segmenting this object in both images as well as estimating a rigid transformation between them

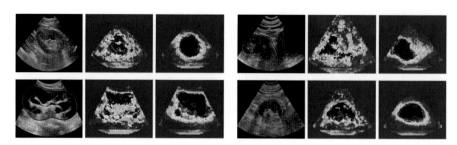

Fig. 12 Kidney appearance in US images (the kidney boundary is denoted in *red*). (*Left*) Original images showing the high variability of the database. (*Middle*) Kidney probability given by the first classifier. (*Right*) Final kidney probability p_{US}

Learning Appearance in Conventional Ultrasound

In CEUS images, bright areas indicate the presence of contrast agent which is mainly localized in the kidney. This is why we directly used the image intensity as a voxel probabilities to be inside the kidney. However in conventional US images, this does not hold and we need to transform the image into a more elaborate kidney probability map.

The kidney appearance has a much higher variability in US images, although their structure is consistent: kidneys are always composed of a bright sinus surrounded by a darker parenchyma (see Fig. 12). As intensity itself is not reliable enough, we chose to combine multiple image features using decision forests [26] to obtain a class posterior map p_{US}.

Recent work [27–31] demonstrated that adding contextual information allows to improve spatial consistency and thus classification performance. Here we propose to exploit the kidney structure in a simple yet efficient way. Similarly to the auto-context framework introduced by Tu et al. [32], contextual information is included by using two classifiers in cascade. A first classification (kidney vs background) is performed in each voxel using a decision forest. Then we use these class posterior probabilities as additional input of a second random forest that will give the final kidney probability p_{US}. In the remainder of the chapter, we will work on this map instead of the original US image.

The features used for the first decision forest were the intensity of the image and its Laplacian at the considered voxel as well as at its neighbors' within a $7 \times 7 \times 7$ local patch, at three different scales ($\sigma = 2,4,6$ mm). Intensities were normalized in each patch. For the second forest, we added the estimated class posterior as additional channels. Each forest was composed of 10 trees with maximum depth 15.

To validate this probability estimation, the patient database was split into two groups. Results on the whole dataset were then obtained using a two-fold cross-validation. Figure 13 shows the ROC and Precision-Recall curves computed (1) by

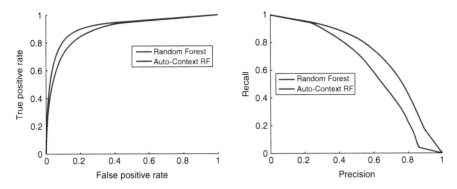

Fig. 13 Comparison of classification results for the single decision forest and the auto-context approach. (*Left*) ROC curve. (*Right*) Precision-Recall curve

the first decision forest and (2) using the auto-context approach with another forest in cascade. The latter provides better kidney probabilities with respect to all reported statistics. Indeed, taking into account structural information helps, for example, in distinguishing the kidney sinus from the background or the parenchyma from shadows and allows a more spatially coherent classification (see Fig. 12).

Generic Framework for Co-segmentation and Registration

In sections "Kidney Detection via Robust Ellipsoid Estimation" and "Kidney Segmentation via Implicit Template Deformation", we presented two variational methods to, respectively, detect and segment the kidney. They both consist in seeking ϕ as the minimizer of a functional of the following generic form

$$E_I(\phi) = \int_\Omega f(\phi(\mathbf{x})) \, r_I(\mathbf{x}) \, d\mathbf{x} + \mathcal{R}(\phi) \tag{19}$$

where f is a real-valued function and $r_I(\mathbf{x})$ denotes a pointwise score on whether $\mathbf{x}$ looks like an interior or exterior voxel in the image I. This is a standard setting in which the optimal implicit function ϕ must achieve a trade-off between an image-based term and a regularization term $\mathcal{R}$.[3]

---

[3] For example, the seminal method of Chan and Vese [33] falls in this framework with $f = H$ the Heaviside function and $r_I(\mathbf{x}) = (I(\mathbf{x}) - c_{\text{int}})^2 - (I(\mathbf{x}) - c_{\text{ext}})^2$ with c_{int} and c_{ext} denoting mean intensities inside and outside the target object.

We are interested in the case where a pair of images $I_1 : \Omega_1 \to \mathbb{R}$ and $I_2 : \Omega_2 \to \mathbb{R}$ of the same object are available. If those images were perfectly aligned, the energy in Eq. (19) can be straightforwardly generalized to perform co-segmentation :

$$E_{I_1,I_2}(\phi) = \int_{\Omega_1} f(\phi(\mathbf{x})) \, (r_{I_1}(\mathbf{x}) + r_{I_2}(\mathbf{x})) \, d\mathbf{x} + \mathcal{R}(\phi) \,. \tag{20}$$

Unfortunately, such an assumption rarely holds in medical applications unless the two images are acquired simultaneously. A more realistic hypothesis is to assume that the target object, segmented by ϕ, is not deformed between the two acquisitions, but only undergoes an unknown rigid transformation $\mathcal{G}_r$. The co-segmentation energy thus reads

$$E_{I_1,I_2}(\phi, \mathcal{G}_r) = \int_{\Omega_1} f(\phi(\mathbf{x})) \, r_{I_1}(\mathbf{x}) \, d\mathbf{x} + \int_{\Omega_2} f(\phi \circ \mathcal{G}_r(\mathbf{x})) \, r_{I_2}(\mathbf{x}) \, d\mathbf{x} + \mathcal{R}(\phi) \,. \tag{21}$$

Note that, after a variable substitution, it can be equivalently written

$$E_{I_1,I_2}(\phi, \mathcal{G}_r) = \int_{\Omega_1} f(\phi(\mathbf{x})) \, (r_{I_1}(\mathbf{x}) + r_{I_2} \circ \mathcal{G}_r^{-1}(\mathbf{x})) \, d\mathbf{x} + \mathcal{R}(\phi) \,. \tag{22}$$

Minimizing E_{I_1,I_2} with respect to ϕ and $\mathcal{G}_r$ simultaneously can be therefore interpreted as performing jointly segmentation (via ϕ) and rigid registration (via $\mathcal{G}_r$). This generalizes a more common co-segmentation approach (e.g., [34]) where the images are first aligned in a preprocessing step.

In the following, we apply this framework to the robust ellipsoid detection (section "Kidney Detection via Robust Ellipsoid Estimation") and implicit template deformation (section "Kidney Segmentation via Implicit Template Deformation") to build a completely automated workflow for kidney segmentation in CEUS and US images. Note that the kidney, which is surrounded by a tough fibrous renal capsule, is a rigid organ. The hypothesis of non-deformation is therefore justified.

Application to Kidney Detection

The robust ellipsoid detection setting of Eq. (3) falls into the framework described in Eq. (19) with :

- $f = I \, d$ and $r_I = -wI$;
- $\mathcal{R}(\phi_{\mathbf{c},\mathbf{M}}) = \mathcal{R}(\mathbf{M}) = \mu. \int_\Omega Iw. \log\left(\frac{\mathrm{Vol}(\mathbf{M})}{|\Omega|}\right).$

Expanding this algorithm to another image I_2 requires the introduction of another weighting function w_2. Following Eq. (21), we can now define the co-detection energy as

$$
\begin{aligned}
E_{\text{co-det}}(\mathbf{c}, \mathbf{M}, w_1, w_2, \mathcal{G}_r) = & -\int_{\Omega} \phi_{\mathbf{c},\mathbf{M}}(\mathbf{x}) \, w_1(\mathbf{x}) \, I_1(\mathbf{x}) \, d\mathbf{x} \\
& -\int_{\Omega} \phi_{\mathbf{c},\mathbf{M}} \circ \mathcal{G}_r(\mathbf{x}) \, w_2(\mathbf{x}) \, I_2(\mathbf{x}) \, d\mathbf{x} \\
& +\mu \left(\int_{\Omega} w_1 I_1 + w_2 I_2 \right) \log \left(\frac{\text{Vol}(\mathbf{M})}{|\Omega|} \right)
\end{aligned}
\tag{23}
$$

with $\text{Vol}(\mathbf{M}) = \dfrac{4\pi}{3} \sqrt{\det \mathbf{M}^{-1}}$ the ellipsoid volume.

To facilitate the resolution of such a problem, $\mathcal{G}_r$—as a rigid transformation—can be decomposed into a rotation and a translation. We can therefore equivalently write the energy as a function of the ellipsoid center $\mathbf{c}_2$ in the second image and the rotation matrix $\mathbf{R}$:

$$
\begin{aligned}
E_{\text{co-det}}(\mathbf{c}_i, w_i, \mathbf{R}, \mathbf{M}) = & -\int_{\Omega} \phi_{\mathbf{c}_1, \mathbf{M}}(\mathbf{x}) \, w_1(\mathbf{x}) \, I_1(\mathbf{x}) \, d\mathbf{x} \\
& -\int_{\Omega} \phi_{\mathbf{c}_2, \mathbf{R}^T \mathbf{M} \mathbf{R}}(\mathbf{x}) \, w_2(\mathbf{x}) \, I_2(\mathbf{x}) \, d\mathbf{x} \\
& +\mu \left(\int_{\Omega} w_1 I_1 + w_2 I_2 \right) \log \left(\frac{\text{Vol}(\mathbf{M})}{|\Omega|} \right)
\end{aligned}
\tag{24}
$$

Minimization of such functional is done in an alternate three-step process:

1. The statistical interpretation still holds for the ellipsoid centers and matrix: minimizers c_1^* and c_2^* are weighted centroids while minimizer $\mathbf{M}^*$ is related to the weighted covariance matrix of pixels coming from both images.
2. The unknown matrix $\mathbf{R}$ accounts for the possible rotation between the two images and can be parametrized by a vector of angles $\Theta \in \mathbb{R}^3$. A gradient descent is performed at each iteration to minimize the energy with respect to Θ.
3. The weights w_1 and w_2 are finally updated as indicator functions (up to a slight dilation) of the current ellipsoid estimates.

The complete minimization strategy is summarized in Algorithm 2. This algorithm is computationally efficient: closed-form solutions are available (except for $\mathbb{R}$) and the process, though iterative, usually converges in very few iterations.

Algorithm 3: Robust ellipsoid co-detection algorithm

---

initialization $\forall \mathbf{x} \in \Omega$, $w_1(\mathbf{x}) \leftarrow 1$, $w_2(\mathbf{x}) \leftarrow 1$

repeat

    // Estimation of centers $\mathbf{c}_1$ and $\mathbf{c}_2$ and matrix $\mathbf{M}$

$$\mathbf{c}_1 \leftarrow \frac{1}{\int_\Omega w_1 I_1} \int_\Omega w_1(\mathbf{x}) \, I_1(\mathbf{x}) \, \mathbf{x} \, d\mathbf{x}$$

$$\mathbf{c}_2 \leftarrow \frac{1}{\int_\Omega w_2 i_2} \int_\Omega w_2(\mathbf{x}) \, I_2(\mathbf{x}) \, \mathbf{x} \, d\mathbf{x}$$

$$\mathbf{M}^{-1} \leftarrow \frac{2}{\mu \int_\Omega w_1 I_1 + w_2 I_2} \left(\int_\Omega w_1(\mathbf{x}) \, I_1(\mathbf{x}) \, (\mathbf{x} - \mathbf{c}_1)(\mathbf{x} - \mathbf{c}_1)^T \, d\mathbf{x} \right.$$
$$\left. + \int_\Omega w_2(\mathbf{x}) \, I_2(\mathbf{x}) \, \mathbf{R}(\mathbf{x} - \mathbf{c}_2)(\mathbf{x} - \mathbf{c}_2)^T \, \mathbf{R}^T \, d\mathbf{x} \right)$$

    // Update of the rotation matrix by gradient descent with step Δt

    repeat

        | $\mathbf{R}(\Theta) \leftarrow \mathbf{R}(\Theta - \Delta t \, \nabla_\Theta E_{co-det}(\Theta))$

    until *convergence*;

    // Update of the weighting functions w_1 and w_2 for each $\mathbf{x} \in \Omega$

    if $(\mathbf{x} - \mathbf{c})^T \mathbf{M}(\mathbf{x} - \mathbf{c}) \leq 1 - \mu \log\left(\frac{Vol(\mathbf{M})}{|\Omega|}\right)$ **then**

        | $w_1(\mathbf{x}) \leftarrow 1$ **else** $w_1(\mathbf{x}) \leftarrow 0$

    if $(\mathbf{x} - \mathbf{c}_2)^T \mathbf{R}^T \mathbf{M} \mathbf{R}(\mathbf{x} - \mathbf{c}_2) \leq 1 - \mu \log\left(\frac{Vol(\mathbf{M})}{|\Omega|}\right)$ **then**

        | $w_2(\mathbf{x}) \leftarrow 1$ **else** $w_2(\mathbf{x}) \leftarrow 0$

until *convergence*;

Figure 14 shows an example of ellipse co-detection in synthetic images, where the probability of belonging to the target object is the image intensity. Despite the noise, the simulated shadow, and the reduced field-of-view effect, the co-detection algorithm provides a good estimate on the ellipse position, size, and orientation in both images.

Application to Kidney Segmentation

Implicit template deformation, as previously described in section "Kidney Segmentation via Implicit Template Deformation", is part of the framework defined in Eq. (19) with :

- $f = H$ and $r_l = -\Delta I$;
- $\mathcal{R}(\phi_0 \circ \psi) = \mathcal{R}(\mathcal{L}) = \frac{\lambda}{2} \, \|\mathcal{L} - Id\|_2^2$.

We can therefore extend it to co-segmentation using Eq. (21) by considering the following functional

$$
\begin{aligned}
E_{co-seg}(\phi_0 \circ \mathcal{L} \circ \mathcal{G}, \mathcal{G}_r) = \ & E_{co-seg}(\mathcal{L}, \mathcal{G}, \mathcal{G}_r) \\
= \ & - \int_\Omega H(\phi_0 \circ \mathcal{L} \circ \mathcal{G}) \, \Delta I_1(\mathbf{x}) \, d\mathbf{x} \\
& - \int_\Omega H(\phi_0 \circ \mathcal{L} \circ \mathcal{G} \circ \mathcal{G}_r) \, \Delta I_2(\mathbf{x}) \, d\mathbf{x} \\
& + \frac{\lambda}{2} \|\mathcal{L} - Id\|_2^2.
\end{aligned}
\tag{25}
$$

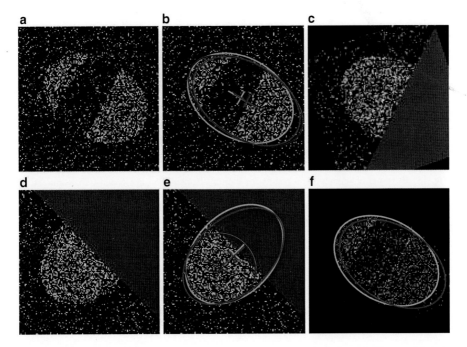

Fig. 14 Ellipse detection on two synthetic images I_1 (**a**) and I_2 (**d**). Detected ellipses with their center and main axes are shown in (**b**) and (**e**) for independent ellipse detection (*red*) and proposed method for co-detection (*blue*) compared to the ground truth (*green*). (**c**) Second image registered with the estimated transform $\mathcal{G}_r^{-1}$. (**f**) Combination of image terms $w_1 I_1 + (w_2 I_2) \circ \mathcal{G}_r^{-1}$ used for ellipse estimation at convergence

The energy $E_{\text{co-seg}}$ is then minimized with respect to the parameters of $\mathcal{G}$, $\mathcal{G}_r$ and each component of the vector field $\mathbf{u}$, through a gradient descent similar to section "Numerical Implementation".

Results for Kidney Co-segmentation in CEUS and US

The average overall computational time for kidney probability estimation in US, ellipsoid co-detection, and kidney co-segmentation was around 20 s with our implementation.

Validation was performed by comparing the co-segmentation approach to a segmentation from a single image (in both CEUS an US cases). Dice coefficients and relative error on the measured kidney volume are reported in Fig. 15. Using simultaneously the complementary information from US and CEUS images significantly improves the segmentation accuracy in both modalities. More specifically, the median Dice coefficient is increased from 0.74 to 0.81 in CEUS (p-value $<$ 10^{-4}) and 0.73 to 0.78 in US (p-value $< 10^{-4}$). Furthermore, the proposed approach

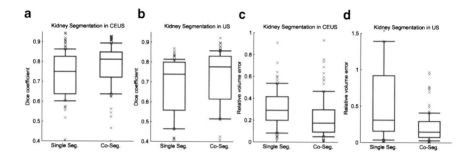

Fig. 15 Boxplots of segmentation results for kidney segmentation in US and CEUS images, in terms of Dice coefficients (**a**)–(**b**) and relative volume error (**c**)–(**d**). The proposed co-segmentation compares favorably to independent segmentation with a p-value $< 10^{-4}$. Boxplots show, respectively, the first decile, the first quartile, the median, the third quartile, and the ninth decile. Extreme points are shown separately

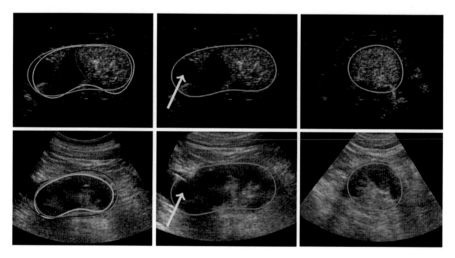

Fig. 16 Example of joint co-segmentation and registration for a CEUS (*top*) and a US (*bottom*) images. (*Left*) Comparison of independent segmentations (*red*) and the proposed co-segmentation (*blue*) with respect to the ground truths (*green*). (*Middle, Right*) Two views of the registered volumes that can be assessed by considering the position of the lesion (*yellow arrow*)

provides more reliable clinical information as the median error on the kidney volume is almost divided by two in CEUS (29 % versus 15 %) and in US (25 % versus 13 %). Figure 16 shows the joint co-segmentation and registration results for one case. Independent segmentation fails in both US and CEUS images because of the kidney lesion (indicated by the yellow arrow) that looks like the background in CEUS but like the kidney in US. Conversely, the proposed co-segmentation manages to overcome this difficulty by combining information from the two modalities. Furthermore, for this example, one can assess the estimated registration by comparing the location of the lesion in the two modalities. Results on another case were also displayed in Fig. 11.

Conclusion

This chapter addressed the problem of kidney segmentation in 3D CEUS images. Such a task is challenging because of the noise, the artifacts, and the partial occultation of the organ (due to the limited field of view).

A robust ellipsoid detector has been introduced to coarsely locate the kidney. The ellipsoid is then deformed to segment the kidney more precisely, by maximizing the image gradient flux through the segmentation boundary, using the template deformation framework. This method yields a fully automatic pipeline that provides a satisfying segmentation in a large number of cases but may fail when the image information is too ambiguous (shadows, pathologies, etc).

To overcome such difficulties, two extensions of this approach have been proposed to take into account additional information. First, we showed how user interactions can be exploited to guide the segmentation in real-time, by letting the user indicate points that should be inside/outside/on the segmentation. Then, we introduced a generic co-segmentation framework that generalizes any segmentation method to allow the simultaneous use of multiple images (here the CEUS and the US images). This results in both a better estimate of the organ shape and a registration of the images. The two aforementioned extensions are compatible and including user interactions in multiple images would be straightforward.

The kidney detection can still be improved by including more anatomical prior knowledge. A possible solution would be to constrain the ellipsoid's axis lengths or volume to be close to clinically meaningful values. Another way is the use of CT images of the same patient to extract a tailored model of the kidney and help both the CEUS detection and segmentation.

Appendix: Choice of the Parameter μ for Ellipsoid Detection

The choice of μ in Eq. (3) is paramount as it controls the number of points that are taken into account for the ellipsoid matrix estimation. To find a suitable value, let us consider an ideal case of an image I_0 in which there is one white ellipsoid ($I_0 = 1$) on a black background ($I_0 = 0$), whose implicit function is $\phi_{\mathbf{c}_0, \mathbf{M}_0}$. We also assume that the confidence weight is $w \equiv 1$ everywhere. Then the matrix estimated by our approach would be

$$\mathbf{M}^* = \mathrm{argmin}_{\mathbf{M}} \, E_{\det}(\mathbf{c}_0, \mathbf{M}, 1)$$

$$= \left[\frac{2}{\mu} \frac{1}{\int_\Omega I_0} \int_\Omega I_0(\mathbf{x}) \, (\mathbf{x} - \mathbf{c}_0)(\mathbf{x} - \mathbf{c}_0)^T d\mathbf{x} \right]^{-1} \qquad (26)$$

Using the fact that $I_0 = \mathbf{1}_{\{1 - (\mathbf{x} - \mathbf{c}_0)^T \mathbf{M}_0 (\mathbf{x} - \mathbf{c}_0) \geq 0\}}$ is the indicator of the ellipsoid yields

$$\mathbf{M}^* = \left[\frac{2}{\mu} \frac{1}{\mathrm{Vol}(\mathbf{M}_0)} \int_{\{1-(\mathbf{x}-\mathbf{c}_0)^T \mathbf{M}_0 (\mathbf{x}-\mathbf{c}_0) \geq 0\}} (\mathbf{x} - \mathbf{c}_0)(\mathbf{x} - \mathbf{c}_0)^T d\mathbf{x} \right]^{-1} \quad (27)$$

After a variable substitution $\mathbf{x} \leftarrow \mathbf{M}_0^{1/2}(\mathbf{x} - \mathbf{c}_0)$, this expression becomes

$$\mathbf{M}^* = \left[\frac{2}{\mu} \frac{\det(\mathbf{M}_0^{-1/2})}{\mathrm{Vol}(\mathbf{M}_0)} \mathbf{M}_0^{-1/2} \int_{\{\|\mathbf{x}\| \leq 1\}} \mathbf{x}\mathbf{x}^T d\mathbf{x} \ \mathbf{M}_0^{-1/2} \right]^{-1} \quad (28)$$

With $\mathrm{Vol}(\mathbf{M}_0) = \frac{4\pi}{3} \sqrt{\det(\mathbf{M}_0^{-1})} = \frac{4\pi}{3} \det(\mathbf{M}_0^{-1/2})$, we then obtain

$$\mathbf{M}^* = \left[\frac{2}{\mu} \frac{3}{4\pi} \mathbf{M}_0^{-1/2} \int_{\{\|\mathbf{x}\| \leq 1\}} \mathbf{x}\mathbf{x}^T d\mathbf{x} \ \mathbf{M}_0^{-1/2} \right]^{-1} \quad (29)$$

Note that the integral $\int_{\{\|\mathbf{x}\| \leq 1\}} \mathbf{x}\mathbf{x}^T d\mathbf{x}$ denotes the covariance matrix of a 3D unit ball, which is actually a scalar matrix that can be easily computed

$$\int_{\{\|\mathbf{x}\| \leq 1\}} \mathbf{x}\mathbf{x}^T d\mathbf{x} = \begin{pmatrix} 2\pi \frac{2}{3}\frac{1}{5} & 0 & 0 \\ 0 & 2\pi \frac{2}{3}\frac{1}{5} & 0 \\ 0 & 0 & 2\pi \frac{2}{3}\frac{1}{5} \end{pmatrix} = \frac{4\pi}{15} \begin{pmatrix} 1 & 0 & 0 \\ 0 & 1 & 0 \\ 0 & 0 & 1 \end{pmatrix} \quad (30)$$

Combining Eqs. (29) and (30) leads to

$$\mathbf{M}^* = \left[\frac{2}{\mu} \left(\frac{1}{5} \mathbf{M}_0^{-1} \right) \right]^{-1} \quad (31)$$

which yields the following relationship between $\mathbf{M}^*$ and $\mathbf{M}_0$:

$$\mathbf{M}^* = \frac{5}{2}\mu \mathbf{M}_0 \quad (32)$$

This shows that the exact solution $\mathbf{M}_0$ is retrieved for $\mu = \frac{2}{5}$. This value actually depends on the dimension of Ω. Here we assumed $\Omega \subset \mathbb{R}^3$ but for 2D images, the optimal value would rather be $\mu = \frac{1}{2}$.

References

1. Albrecht T et al (2004) Guidelines for the use of contrast agents in ultrasound. Ultraschall Med 25(4):249–256
2. Noble JA, Boukerroui D (2006) Ultrasound image segmentation: a survey. IEEE Trans Med Imag 25(8):987–1010
3. Gasnier A, Ardon R, Ciofolo-Veit C, Leen E, Correas J (2010) Assessing tumour vascularity with 3D contrast-enhanced ultrasound: a new semi-automated segmentation framework. In: Proceedings of IEEE ISBI 2010, pp 300–303. http://ieeexplore.ieee.org/xpls/abs_all.jsp?arnumber=5490351
4. Kissi A, Cormier S, Pourcelot L, Bleuzen A, Tranquart E (2004) Contrast enhanced ultrasound image segmentation based on fuzzy competitive clustering and anisotropic diffusion. In: IEEE IEMBS 2004, vol 1, pp 1613–1615. http://ieeexplore.ieee.org/xpl/login.jsp?tp=&arnumber=1403489
5. Prevost R, Cohen L, Correas J, Ardon R (2012) Automatic detection and segmentation of renal lesions in 3D contrast-enhanced ultrasound images. Proc. SPIE 8314:83141D–83141D1
6. Ma M, Stralen M, Reiber J, Bosch J, Lelieveldt B (2009) Left ventricle segmentation from contrast enhanced fast rotating ultrasound images using three dimensional active shape models. In: Proceedings of FIMH 2009, pp 295–302. http://ieeexplore.ieee.org/xpls/abs_all.jsp?arnumber=6235871
7. Prevost R, Mory B, Correas JM, Cohen LD, Ardon R (2012) Kidney detection and real-time segmentation in 3D contrast-enhanced ultrasound images. In: Proceedings of IEEE ISBI, pp 1559–62
8. Prevost R, Cuingnet R, Mory B, Correas JM, Cohen LD, Ardon R (2013) Joint co-segmentation and registration of 3D ultrasound images. In: To appear in Proceedings of IPMI, pp 268–279. Springer, Berlin, Heidelberg
9. Guil N, Zapata E (1997) Lower order circle and ellipse Hough transform. Pattern Recogn 30 (10):1729–1744
10. McLaughlin RA (1998) Randomized Hough transform: improved ellipse detection with comparison. Pattern Recogn Lett 19(3):299–305
11. Wong C, Lin S, Ren T, Kwok N (2012) A survey on ellipse detection methods. In: 2012 I.E. international symposium on industrial electronics (ISIE), pp 1105–1110. IEEE, New York
12. Van Aelst S, Rousseeuw P (2009) Minimum volume ellipsoid. Wiley Interdisciplin Rev: Comput Statist 1(1):71–82
13. Saddi K, Chefd'Hotel C, Rousson M, Cheriet F (2007) Region-based segmentation via non-rigid template matching. In: Proceedings of ICCV, pp 1–7. http://ieeexplore.ieee.org/xpls/abs_all.jsp?arnumber=4409152
14. Somphone O, Mory B, Makram-Ebeid S, Cohen LD (2008) Prior-based piecewise-smooth segmentation by template competitive deformation using partitions of unity. In: Proceedings of ECCV, pp 628–641. http://link.springer.com/chapter/10.1007/978-3-540-88690-7_47
15. Mory B, Somphone O, Prevost R, Ardon R (2012) Real-time 3D image segmentation by user-constrained template deformation. In: Proceedings of MICCAI. LNCS, vol 7510, pp 561–568. Springer, Berlin
16. Cuingnet R, Prevost R, Lesage D, Cohen LD, Mory B, Ardon R (2012) Automatic detection and segmentation of kidneys in 3D CT images using random forests. In: Proceedings of MICCAI. LNCS, vol 7512, pp 66–74. Springer, Berlin
17. Yezzi A, Soatto S (2003) Deformotion: deforming motion, shape average and the joint registration and approximation of structures in images. IJCV 53(2):153–167
18. Schunck B, Horn B (1981) Determining optical flow. In: Image understanding workshop, pp 144–156. http://www.sciencedirect.com/science/article/pii/0004370281900242
19. Nocedal J, Wright SJ (1999) Numerical optimization. Springer, Berlin
20. Vicente S, Kolmogorov V, Rother C (2010) Cosegmentation revisited: models and optimization. In: Proceedings of ECCV, vol 6312, pp 465–479

21. Wang F, Vemuri B (2005) Simultaneous registration and segmentation of anatomical structures from brain MRI. In: Proceedings of MICCAI. LNCS, vol 3749, pp 17–25. Springer, Berlin

22. Pohl K, Fisher J, Grimson W, Kikinis R, Wells W (2006) A Bayesian model for joint segmentation and registration. NeuroImage 31(1):228–239

23. Lu C, Duncan J (2012) A coupled segmentation and registration framework for medical image analysis using robust point matching and active shape model. In: IEEE Workshop on MMBIA, pp 129–136

24. Wyatt P, Noble JA (2002) MAP MRF joint segmentation and registration. In: Proceedings of MICCAI. LNCS, vol 2488, pp 580–587. Springer, Berlin

25. Yezzi A, Zöllei L, Kapur T (2003) A variational framework for integrating segmentation and registration through active contours. MedIA 7(2):171–185

26. Breiman L (2001) Random forests. Mach Learn 45(1):5–32

27. Payet N, Todorovic S (2010) 2-Random forest random field. In: Proceedings of NIPS 2010

28. Montillo A, Shotton J, Winn J, Iglesias J, Metaxas D, Criminisi A (2011) Entangled decision forests and their application for semantic segmentation of CT images. In: Proceedings of IPMI. LNCS, vol 6801, pp 184–196. Springer, Berlin

29. Kontschieder P, Bulò S, Criminisi A, Kohli P, Pelillo M, Bischof H (2012) Context-sensitive decision forests for object detection. In: Proceedings of NIPS, pp 440–448

30. Glocker B, Pauly O, Konukoglu E, Criminisi A (2012) Joint classification-regression forests for spatially structured multi-object segmentation. In: Proceedings of ECCV. LNCS, vol 7575, pp 870–881. Springer, Berlin

31. Zikic D, Glocker B, Konukoglu E, Criminisi A, Demiralp C, Shotton J, Thomas O, Das T, Jena R, Price S (2012) Decision Forests for Tissue-specific Segmentation of High-grade Gliomas in Multi-channel MR. In: Proceedings of MICCAI. LNCS, vol 7512, pp 369–376. Springer, Berlin

32. Tu Z, Bai X (2010) Auto-context and its application to high-level vision tasks and 3D brain image segmentation. IEEE TPAMI 32(10):1744–1757

33. Chan T, Vese L (2001) Active contours without edges. IEEE TIP 10(2):266–277

34. Han D, Bayouth J, Song Q, Taurani A, Sonka M, Buatti J, Wu X (2011) Globally optimal tumor segmentation in PET-CT images: A graph-based co-segmentation method. In: Proceedings of IPMI, pp 245–256. http://link.springer.com/chapter/10.1007/978-3-642-22092-0_21

Biography

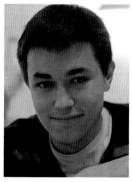

Raphael Prevost is currently working as a Ph.D. candidate at Philips Research

Medisys (Suresnes, France) in collaboration with Universite Paris Dauphine (Paris, France). Born in France in 1988, he received in 2010 the M.Sc. degree in Applied Mathematics from the engineering school ENSTA ParisTech (Paris, France), and the M.Sc. degree in Image Processing and Machine Learning from Ecole Normale Superieure (Cachan, France). His research interests lie in various fields of medical image processing such as segmentation, registration, and pattern recognition.

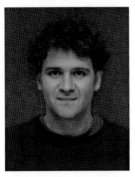

Benoit Mory born in Paris in 1976, received an engineer degree in signal and image processing in 1998 from Ecole Supérieure d'Electricité, France. After 10+ years of experience as a research scientist with Philips Research France in the area of multimedia indexing (MPEG-7) and medical image processing, he received a Ph.D. in Electrical Engineering in 2011 from Ecole Polytechnique Fédérale de Lausanne, Switzerland. He is currently a senior researcher at Medisys, Philips Research lab located in Suresnes, France. His latest research interests include 3D image segmentation with implicit surfaces and multi-modal image registration.

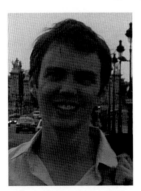

Rémi Cuingnet received the B.Sc. from Ecole Polytechnique in 2006, the M.Sc. in Electrical Engineering from Telecom ParisTech in 2007, and the Ph.D. in Physics from University Paris-Sud in 2011. From 2007 to 2011, he was a research assistant within the Research Center of the Brain and Spine Institute (CR-ICM) in Paris. He is now a research scientist at Philips Research (Suresnes, France). His research interests are in the area of statistical learning and medical image computing.

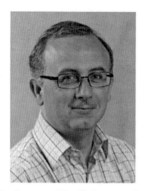

Jean-Michel Correas is a Professor of Radiology at the Paris-Descartes University and is a vice chairman of the Department of Adult Radiology in Necker University Hospital, Paris, France. He got an M.D. Ph.D. degree from the University of Tours under the supervision of Pr. Leandre Pourcelot. He spent almost 2 years in the USA as part of his Ph.D. participating in the preclinical and clinical research programs in a small company developing contrast agents for ultrasound. He was Visiting Professor of Radiology at the University of Toronto department of Imaging Research, where he was in charge of several research projects on Ultrasound Contrast Agents under Pr. PN Burns supervision, as part of his doctorate of science on Ultrasound Contrast Agents. He was deeply involved in the development of interventional uroradiology. After ablation of more than 80 hepatocellular carcinomas, he developed together with the Adult Urology department the minimally invasive treatment of renal tumors, starting in 2004. He performed more than 400 ablative procedures of renal masses.

Pr. Correas is a member of the French Society of Radiology, the French Society of Uroradiology, and the European Society of Radiology. He was elected as President of the French Society of Ultrasound in 2008.

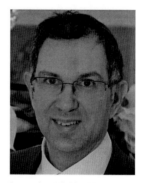

Laurent David Cohen was born in 1962. He was student at the Ecole Normale Superieure, rue d'Ulm in Paris, France from 1981 to 1985. He received the Master's and Ph.D. degrees in Applied Mathematics from University of Paris 6, France, in 1983 and 1986, respectively. He got the Habilitation à diriger des Recherches from University Paris 9 Dauphine in 1995.

From 1985 to 1987, he was member at the Computer Graphics and Image Processing group at Schlumberger Palo Alto Research, Palo Alto, California and Schlumberger Montrouge Research, Montrouge, France and remained consultant with Schlumberger afterwards. He began working with INRIA, France in 1988, mainly with the medical image understanding group EPIDAURE.

He obtained in 1990 a position of Research Scholar (Charge then Directeur de Recherche 1st class) with the French National Center for Scientific Research (CNRS) in the Applied Mathematics and Image Processing group at CEREMADE, Universite Paris Dauphine, Paris, France. His research interests and teaching at university are applications of Partial Differential Equations and variational methods to Image Processing and Computer Vision, like deformable models, minimal paths, geodesic curves, surface reconstruction, Image segmentation, registration, and restoration.

He is currently an editorial member of the *Journal of Mathematical Imaging and Vision*, the *International Journal for Computational Vision and Biomechanics*, and the journal *Computer Methods in Biomechanics and Biomedical Engineering: Imaging & Visualization*. He was also member of the program committee for about 40 international conferences. He authored about 200 publications in international Journals and conferences or book chapters, and 5 patents.

In 2002, he got the CS 2002 prize for Signal and Image Processing. In 2006, he got the Taylor & Francis Prize: "2006 prize for Outstanding innovation in computer methods in biomechanics & biomedical engineering."

He was 2009 laureate of Grand Prix EADS de l'Academie des Sciences.

He was promoted as IEEE Fellow 2010 for contributions to computer vision technology for medical imaging.

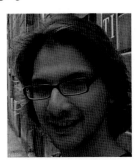

Roberto Ardon was born in Guatemala in 1977. He received an engineer degree in Applied Mathematics in 2001 from Ecole Centrale Paris, a master's degree in computer vision in the same year from Ecole Normale Supérieure de Cachan, and a Ph.D. with honors in Applied Mathematics from the Universite Paris Dauphine in 2005 within a collaboration with Philips Research Lab in Paris, Medisys. He is currently a senior researcher in Medisys, a team in which he joined as a permanent member in 2005. His research interests are in medical image analysis and computer vision.

Renal Cortex Segmentation on Computed Tomography

Xinjian Chen, Dehui Xiang, Wei Ju, Heming Zhao, and Jianhua Yao

Abstract The current procedure of renal cortex segmentation is subjective and tedious. This chapter introduces an automated framework for renal cortex segmentation on contrast-enhanced abdominal CT images. The framework consists of four parts: first, an active appearance model (AAM) is built using a set of training images; second, the AAM is refined by live wire (LW) method to initialize the shape and location of the kidney; third, an iterative graph cut-oriented active appearance model (IGC-OAAM) method is applied to segment the kidney; Finally, the identified kidney contour is used as shape constraints for renal cortex segmentation which is also based on IGC-OAAM. The chapter also discusses several other state-of-art techniques for segmentation and modeling of the kidneys.

Kidney Anatomy and Clinical Problem

The kidney consists of four anatomical structures, the renal cortex, renal column, renal medulla, and renal pelvis (shown in Fig. 1). The kidney acts as the body's garbage collection and disposal system. It helps to control water levels and eliminate wastes through urine as the body's filtering system. It also serves homeostatic functions such as the regulation of electrolytes, maintenance of acid–base balance, and regulation of blood pressure (via maintaining salt and water balance). However, its function may be disturbed by many kidney diseases, such as, kidney cancer,

X. Chen (✉) • D. Xiang • W. Ju • H. Zhao
School of Electronics and Information Engineering, Soochow University, Suzhou, China
e-mail: xjchen@suda.edu.cn; xiangdehui@suda.edu.cn; 287687047@qq.com

J. Yao
Department of Radiology and Imaging Sciences, National Institute of Health,
Bethesda, MD 20892, USA
e-mail: JYao@cc.nih.gov

A.S. El-Baz et al. (eds.), *Abdomen and Thoracic Imaging: An Engineering & Clinical Perspective*, DOI 10.1007/978-1-4614-8498-1_3,

69

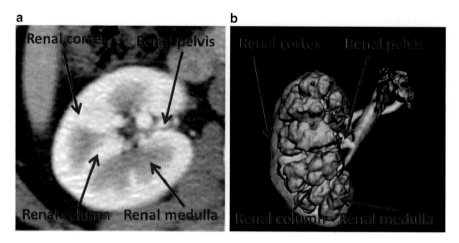

Fig. 1 Kidney. (**a**) The kidney in one CT slice. (**b**) Iso-surface rendering [7]

membranous nephropathy, nephritic syndrome, hypertensive renal disease, etc. Kidney cancer is one of the ten most common cancers in both men and women worldwide. Overall, the risk for developing kidney cancer is about 1 in 70 in lifetime [1]. Renal cell carcinoma which arises from the renal cortex is the most common type of kidney cancer in adults, responsible for approximately 80 % of cases [2]. Hence, the investigation of the renal cortex has great values for kidney cancer research. The renal cortex segmentation is of particular clinical importance. The renal cortical volume and thickness are effective biomarkers for renal function in many clinical situations, for instance, urological treatment decision-making [3], radiotherapy planning [4], and assessment of clinical outcomes of surgery [5, 6].

The renal cortex, medulla, and pelvis are three basic compartments of kidneys. Only out-layer of the kidney is strictly defined as a renal cortex because renal columns are anatomically and functionally different from the cortex. Several previous researches treated renal cortex and column as homogeneous structures though they are anatomically different. However, only the out-layer of the kidney (i.e., renal cortex) needs to be quantified with volume and thickness in most clinical applications. For certain clinical studies, it is advisable to measure the renal cortex precisely.

The renal cortex segmentation is one of fundamental steps for renal cortical volume and thickness measurement, since the quantification of renal cortical volume and thickness plays an important role in renal function analysis. However, kidney and renal cortex segmentation is a challenging task. As shown in Fig. 1, the location of kidney in abdomen and its specific internal anatomical structures in CT images are visualized in one slice (see Fig. 1a), and the surface of different internal anatomical structures is also rendered (see Fig. 1b). Surrounding anatomical structures or organs, such as liver, spine, and muscles, are located beside the kidney. In addition, the boundaries with adjacent anatomical structures are weak. Image artifacts, noise, and various pathologies, such as cancers and nephrolithiasis, pose more challenges. The renal cortex and renal column are fused as one connected component, since they have similar intensity distributions. The renal cortex is a non-fully closed structure due to the renal pelvis [7]. Currently, the renal cortex segmentations used in many clinical situations rely on manual methods, which are subjective, tedious, time-consuming, and prone to errors. Hence, there is a strong need to develop a fully automatic and accurate kidney and renal cortex segmentation.

Imaging Protocol

Computed tomography (CT) imaging, magnetic resonance imaging (MRI), and ultrasound (US) imaging are widely used for kidney examination and kidney diseases diagnosis because essential anatomical information, including kidney morphology and kidney ducts, can be readily obtained [8–11].

Computed tomography (CT) scan is a noninvasive diagnostic imaging modality that uses a combination of X-rays and computer technology to produce detailed cross-sectional images (often called slices) of the body. A beam of X-rays is aimed at one part of body, for instance, abdomen, which needs to be checked. Energy of beam attenuates as it passes through skin, bone, muscle, and other tissue. These variations can be detected by a two-dimensional monitor behind the body part. The X-ray beam moves in a circle around the body inside CT gantry. After the projection is accomplished in one direction, the X-ray signals are transmitted to a computer in order to reconstruct a series of slices.

CT imaging of the kidneys is useful in the examination of one or both of the kidneys to detect conditions obstructive conditions, such as kidney stones, congenital anomalies, polycystic kidney disease, accumulation of fluid around the kidneys, and the location of abscesses. The CT images can also present precise information about the size, shape, and position of a tumor. It is also useful in checking to see whether a cancer has spread to organs and tissues beyond the kidney and can help find enlarged lymph nodes that might contain cancer.

Although high resolution CT has taken the largest leap, MRI is also an imaging technique used primarily in medical settings to produce 3D high-quality morphologic images of the inside of the human body in the evaluation of renal abnormalities. MRI modality can be applicable to children and pregnant women since it does not lead to radiation exposure, compared to CT modality. MRI uses a powerful magnetic field, radio waves, and a computer to produce detailed pictures of organs, soft tissues, bone, and virtually all other internal body structures. The energy from the radio waves is absorbed and then released in a pattern formed by the type of body tissue and by certain diseases. A computer translates the pattern into a very detailed image of parts of the body. A contrast material called gadolinium is often injected into a vein before the scan to better see details. This contrast material cannot be used in people on dialysis, because in those people it could cause a severe side effect called nephrogenic systemic fibrosis. Additionally, dynamic contrast-enhanced MRI is often used for renal lesion characterization. The multiphase 3D volume interpolation is performed as multiple breath-hold sequences before and at timed intervals after intravenous bolus injection of a gadolinium-based contrast agent. It allows for more accurate computer-processed image subtraction and better degree of lesion enhancement with reproducible diaphragmatic excursion during breath-holds.

MRI still plays an important role in differentiating benign lesions versus malignant lesions of patients in renal imaging. MRI can achieve the similar accuracy as CT in detection and characterization of most renal lesions, including malignant renal lesions such as renal cell carcinomas, and benign renal lesions such as oncocytoma and angiomyolipoma. In addition, MRI has a high sensitivity in evaluating complicated cysts and early lymph node spread and can be used to analyze lesions with minimal amounts of fat or with intracellular fat. Functional MRI of the kidney has found broad clinical application. It can be used in the analyses of compromised renal function, severe contrast allergy. Attempts are being made to use MRI for imaging of renal function, including perfusion, glomerular filtration rate, and intra-renal oxygen measurement.

Ultrasound (US) imaging of kidney is also a noninvasive and painless modality used to obtain the size, shape, and location of the kidneys with no radiation exposure. This modality uses sound waves to create images of internal organs. A handheld transducer is utilized to send out ultrasonic sound waves at a frequency. The ultrasonic sound waves go through the skin and other body tissues to the organs and structures of the abdomen as the transducer is placed on the abdomen at certain locations and angles. The sound waves bounce off the tissues in the organs like an echo and return to the transducer. The transducer picks up the reflected waves, which are then converted into an image of the organs.

Ultrasound imaging can help determine if a kidney mass is solid or filled with fluid. Therefore, blood flow to the kidney can be assessed by using an additional mode of ultrasound technology during an ultrasound imaging. An ultrasound transducer with a Doppler probe is used to assess blood flow. By making the sound waves audible, the Doppler probe within the transducer evaluates the velocity and direction of blood flow in the vessel. The degree of loudness of the audible sound waves suggests the rate of blood flow within a blood vessel. Absence or faintness of these sounds may show an obstruction of blood flow. In addition, ultrasound imaging is suitable for detection and characterization of tumors, since the echo patterns produced by most kidney tumors are different from those of normal kidney tissue. Different echo patterns can distinguish some types of benign and malignant kidney tumors. This imaging modality can be used to guide a biopsy needle into the mass to obtain a sample if a kidney biopsy is needed.

General Frameworks

In computer vision and image analysis, image segmentation is a fundamental and challenging problem. In medical image processing, several challenges still remain in spite of several decades of research and many key technological advances. The medical image segmentation methods may be classified into three frameworks: image-based [12–23], model-based [24–32], and hybrid methods [33–40]. Image-based methods perform segmentation based only on information available in the image; these include thresholding, region growing [12], morphological operations [13], active contours [14, 15], level sets [16], live wire [17], watershed [18], fuzzy connectedness [19, 20], and graph cut [21, 22]. These methods perform well on high-quality images. However, the results are not as good when the image quality is inferior or boundary information is missing. In recent years, there has been an increasing interest in model-based segmentation methods. One advantage of these methods is that, even when some object information is missing, such gaps can be filled by drawing upon the prior information present in the model. The model-based methods employ object population shape and appearance priors such as atlases [24, 25, 29, 30, 41], statistical active shape models [26, 42, 43], and statistical active appearance models (AAMs) [27, 31, 32]. As such, hybrid methods that form a combination of two or more approaches are emerging as powerful segmentation tools, where their superior performances and robustness over each of the components are beginning to be well demonstrated [33–40].

Typically, image information, such as, the spatial information and intensity, were used for kidney and renal cortex segmentation with image-based methods. Boykov and colleagues [44] developed a temporal Markov model to describe the time intensity curves for each pixel and used the min-cut/max-flow algorithm for kidney segmentation [45]. Sun et al. [46] presented an integrated image registration algorithm to segment renal cortex in MR images. Zöllner et al. [47] applied automated image analysis methods in the assessment of human kidney perfusion based on 3D dynamic contrast-enhanced MRI data. Song et al. [48] combined spatial anatomical structures with temporal dynamics for dynamic MR images kidney segmentation.

Another type is model-based segmentation framework. Freiman et al. [49] proposed a nonparametric model constraint graph min-cut/max-flow approach for automatic kidney segmentation in CT images. Tsagaan et al. [50] integrated the gray level appearance of the target and statistical information of the shape into NURBS surface-based deformable model to automatically segment kidneys from abdominal 3D CT images. Touhami et al. [51] proposed a statistical method for fully automatic kidneys segmentation. They used spatial and gray-levels prior models by using a set of training images.

Several prior investigations have addressed the kidney and renal cortex segmentation on hybrid methods. In order to automatically segment kidney parenchyma in MR datasets, Gloger et al. [52] first applied a multistep refinement approach to improve the quality of the probability map, and then an extended prior shape level set segmentation method was used on the refined probability maps and combined

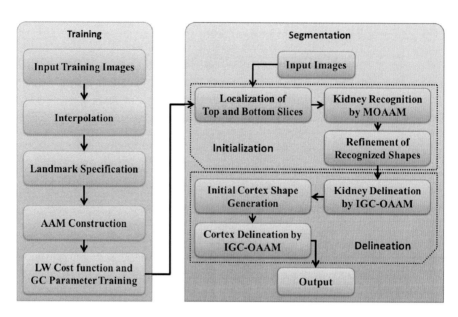

Fig. 2 The framework of the proposed method (*AAM* active appearance model, *LW* live wire, *GC* graph cuts, *MOAAM* multi-object active appearance model, *IGC-OAAM* iterative graph cut-oriented active appearance model)

several relevant kidney parenchyma features. Lin et al. [53] proposed a two-step fully automatic kidney parenchyma 3D segmentation technique in MR datasets to segment kidney in CT images. Xie et al. [54] introduced a texture and shape priors-based method in ultrasound images. Li et al. [55] presented a graph construction-based optimal graph search method for renal cortex segmentation on CT images. Li et al. [7] also presented an automatic renal cortex segmentation approach by the combination of the implicit shape registration and novel multiple surfaces graph search.

In Fig. 2, the kidney cortex framework is divided into two phases: training and segmentation. In the first phase, landmarking is used to annotate kidney' shape, an AAM is built, and then the live wire and graph cuts parameters are trained. The second phase consists of two main steps: initialization and delineation. In the initialization step, a pseudo 3D initialization strategy is applied such that the contour of the kidney is obtained slice by slice via a multi-object AAM method. A refinement operation may be done subsequently to correct improperly initialized slices. We employ the pseudo-3D initialization strategy motivated by its efficiency and ability to combine. The strategy is much faster while achieved a similar performance compared to a full 3D initialization method. Additionally, it is difficult to integrate AAM into live wire in 3D. In the delineation step, we compute the graph cuts cost based on the shape information generated from the oriented active appearance model (OAAM) initialization step. The kidney is delineated using the iterative graph cut OAAM method. After getting the kidney contour, we employ morphological operations to obtain the initial cortex shape. Finally, the shape constrained iterative graph cut OAAM method is applied once more to segment the renal cortex. The details of each step are described in the following sections.

Kidney Modeling

The literature is rich with kidney modeling approaches. To segment 3D kidneys in CT images, more detailed active shape models were generated and did not need to explicit or parametric formulations of the problem. The active shape model was quickly updated with additional prior knowledge. In addition, the crucial correspondence problem is solved by nonrigid image registration [56]. Tsagaan et al. [50] presented a deformable model-based approach for automated segmentation of kidneys from 3D abdominal CT images. Spatial and gray-levels kidney prior models were used according to a set of training images [51]. In the paper of Lin et al. [53] he presented a directional model-based approach for computer-aided kidney segmentation of CT images. Xie et al. [54] introduced a texture and shape priors-based method in ultrasound images. In the framework shown in Fig. 2, the top and bottom slices of each kidney are first manually selected before the AAM is constructed. Then linear interpolation is executed to generate the same number of slices for the kidney in every training image, in order to establish anatomical correspondences. 2D OAAMs are then built for each slice level from the images in the training set. The cost function of live wire and parameters of graph cuts are also obtained in this phase.

Landmark Specification

A 3D shape of kidney is represented as a stack of 2D contours and also manually annotated slice by slice. Because of its simplicity, generality, and efficiency, manual landmarking is still in use in clinical research, although semiautomatic or automatic methods are also available for annotating kidneys. Therefore, manual landmarking is applied to annotate kidney's shape. Prominent landmarks on each shape are identified by trained operators and also visualized on slices.

The equally spaced landmarking method [57] was assessed, in order to demonstrate that there is a strong correlation between the shapes annotated by the manual and semiautomated landmarking approaches. In practice, the shape of an object can be represented by a finite subset of a sufficient number of its points; hence the shape of a kidney is treated as an infinite point set. Then, different numbers of landmarks are used for different kidneys from different medical images based on their size. Numerous researches have been done for the analysis of effects of distribution of landmarks on model building and segmentation results; these experiments consequently were omitted while manual landmarking was validated by the equally spaced labeling method.

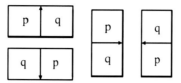

Fig. 3 The four possible situations that a boundary element is an oriented pixel edge. The inside of the boundary is to the left of the bel and the outside is to the right of the bel

Active Appearance Model Construction

The standard AAM [31, 32] method is applied to build the model after the landmarks are specified. Shape and texture information are integrated into the model. Suppose M_j denotes the AAM for slice level j and the number of slice levels is n, then the complete AAM M can be represented as $M = (M_1, M_2, \ldots, M_n)$.

Although a pseudo 3D initialization strategy is applied, the fully 3D AAM denoted M_{3D} is also constructed by using the method in [58]. This 3D model is used to only provide the delineation constraints as explained later.

Live Wire Cost Function and Graph Cuts Parameter Training

An oriented boundary cost function is designed for a kidney included in the model M as per the Live Wire method [16]. Following the original terminology and notation in [16], a *boundary element*, bel for short, is defined as an oriented edge between two pixels with values 1 and 0. A bel is represented as an ordered pair (p,q) of four-adjacent pixels where p is inside the kidney (pixel value is 1) and q is outside (pixel value is 0) for a given image slice I, as shown in Fig. 3. Every pixel edge of I is considered as constituting two potential bels(p,q) and (q,p) and possibly assign different cost values to them. The features assigned to each bel are used to represent the likelihood of the bel that belongs to the boundary of a particular object of interest.

The cost $c(l)$ associated with bel l is a linear combination of the costs assigned to its features,

$$c(l) = \frac{\sum_{i=1}^{nf} w_i c_f(f_i(l))}{\sum_{i=1}^{nf} w_i} \tag{1}$$

where, nf denotes the number of features, w_i denotes a positive constant indicating the emphasis given to feature f_i, and c_f denotes the function to convert feature values $f_i(l)$ at l to cost values $c_f(f_i(l))$. f_i may represent features such as intensity on the immediate interior of the boundary, intensity on the immediate exterior of the boundary, and gradient magnitude at the center of the bel in [16]. Different f_i may be combined, which depends on the intensity characteristics of the object of interest. As suggested in [16], c_f is chosen as an inverted Gaussian function, and all selected features are combined with uniform weights w_i. We employ the feature of live wire to define the best-oriented path between any two-landmark points (x_k and x_{k+1}) as a sequence of bels with minimal total cost:

$$\kappa(x_k, x_{k+1}) = \sum_{i=1}^{h} c(l_i) \tag{2}$$

where h is the number of bels in the best-oriented path ($l_1, l_2, \ldots, l_h$). The total cost structure $K(x)$ associated with all the landmarks may be formulated as

$$K(x) = \sum_{k=1}^{m} \kappa(x_k, x_{k+1}) \tag{3}$$

where m denotes the number of landmarks for the object of interest, and we assume that the contour is closed, i.e., $x_{m+1} = x_1$. In other words, $K(x)$ represents the sum of the costs associated with the best-oriented paths between all m pairs of successive landmarks of shape instance x. The parameters of $K(x)$ for each object shape x are obtained automatically as described in [16] by using the training images.

For the sake of continuity, the description of how the parameters of graph cuts are estimated is given in section "Kidney and Renal Cortex Segmentation" where the graph cuts algorithm is described.

Kidney Localization

The initialization step plays a critical role in the segmentation of kidney and renal cortex framework. The subsequent segmentation tends to have higher accuracy when initial model is localized in the region closer to kidney. To segment the kidneys in dynamic contrast-enhanced MRI, graph cut method was used based on min-cut/max-flow algorithm [45], where the localization was accomplished by painting foreground seed points and background seed points on some slices [44]. Tsagaan et al. [50] presented automated positioning method of an initial model for automated segmentation of kidneys from abdominal 3D CT images. The candidate kidney region was detected according to the statistical geometric location of kidney within the abdomen in [53]. This method can be applied to images of different sizes since they used the relative distance of the kidney region to the spine. In the work of Li et al. [55], the coarse pre-segmentation was firstly obtained by using Amira. Recently, the whole kidney was coarsely initialized using an implicit shape registration method in [7].

In this framework, the initialization method provides the shape constraints to the subsequent graph cuts delineation step and makes the delineation fully automatic.

The developed initialization method is divided into three main steps. First, a slice localization method is employed to identify the top and bottom slices of the kidneys. A linear interpolation is then utilized to generate the same number of slices for the given image of a subject as in the model. The kidneys are recognized slice by slice via the OAAM method. A multi-object strategy [59] is applied to help with kidney recognition. Even if just one kidney is to be segmented, other organs can also be included in the model to provide context and constraints. Finally, a refinement approach is used to adjust the initialization result.

Localization of Top and Bottom Slices

There are several recent researches related to slice localization. Haas et al. [40] created a navigation table with eight landmarks, which were identified in various ways. By using probabilistic boosting tree and Haar features, Seifert et al. [42] developed a method to detect invariant slices and single point landmarks in full body scans. Emrich et al. [60] introduced a CT slice localization approach by using k-nearest neighbor instance-based regression. The target of slice localization is to identify the top and bottom slices of the organ in our framework. The model can be utilized to locate slices, since the model is already trained for each kidney slice. The proposed approach is based on the similarity of the slice to the OAAM.

The top slice model is used for each slice in the image based on the recognition method described in section "Kidney and Renal Cortex Segmentation," in order to locate the top slice in a given image. Then the slice corresponding to maximal similarity or minimal distance is considered as the top slice of the kidney. Figure 4 shows the localization of the top slice in a CT image, where the distance value is computed from (5). The minimal value corresponds to the top slice of the left kidney. A similar method is applied to detect the bottom slice.

Kidney Recognition by Multi-object Active Appearance Model

The kidney recognition method is based on the AAM. The root mean square difference between the appearance model instance and the target image is achieved in traditional AAM matching method for object recognition. It is more suitable for matching appearances than for the detailed segmentation of target images in this procedure (shown in Fig. 5b). The reason is that the AAM is optimized on global appearance; therefore, it is less sensitive to local structures and boundary information in this procedure. In contrast, the live wire detects the boundary very well [16], but it needs good initialization of landmarks and user interaction. Therefore, live wire is integrated into AAM, in order to combine their complementary strengths. In the new procedure, the landmarks needed in the live wire are provided by the AAM; meanwhile, the shape model of the AAM can be improved by live wire.

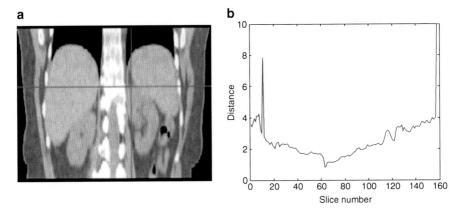

Fig. 4 Illustration of top slice recognition [61]. (**a**) A slice of the abdominal region. Cross point is the top slice of the left kidney. (**b**) The distance values of each slice to the top slice are plotted for the left kidney

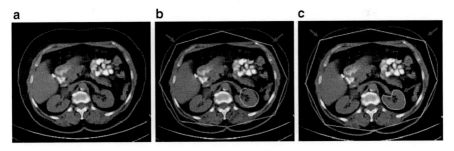

Fig. 5 Comparison of traditional active appearance model and oriented active appearance model segmentation [61]. (**a**) Original image. (**b**) Traditional active appearance model segmentation. (**c**) Oriented active appearance model segmentation

The live wire is fully integrated into AAM in two aspects: First, the shape model of the AAM is improved based on the live lire method; second, the live wire boundary cost is integrated into cost computation during the AAM optimization process. As shown in Fig. 5c, the boundary detection is much improved with the proposed OAAM segmentation, compared to traditional AAM method (see Fig. 5b).

Refinement of the Shape Model in Active Appearance Model by Live Wire

First, a rough placement of the model is achieved by using the conventional AAM searching method. The shape is obtained from the shape model of the AAM, and then live wire is applied to update the landmarks using only the shape model and the pose (i.e., translation, rotation, and scale) parameters in [33], as shown in Fig. 6. The refined shape model is subsequently transformed back into the AAM.

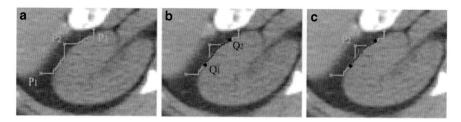

Fig. 6 The position of the landmarks [61]. (**a**) P_1, P_2, and P_3 are three landmarks from active appearance model. (**b**) The middle point Q_1 of the live wire segment between P_1 and P_2, and Q_2 for P_2 and P_3 are obtained. (**c**) Landmark P_2 is moved to the closest point P'_2 on the live wire segment from Q_1 to Q_2

Meanwhile, AAM refinement is utilized to yield its own set of coefficients for shape and pose.

Algorithm 1: Refine Active Appearance Model Shape Model Based on Live Wire

Input: The shape model x.
Output: Updated shape model x' and new affine transformation t'.
Begin

For each triple P_1, P_2, and P_3 of successive landmarks on x

1. Delineate from P_1 to P_2 and P_2 to P_3 via Live Wire.
2. Search the middle point Q_1 and Q_2 in the Live Wire segments obtained from P_1 to P_2 and from P_2 to P_3, respectively.
3. Delineate from Q_1 to Q_2 via Live Wire.
4. Search the point P'_2 on the Live Wire segment from Q_1 to Q_2 closest to P_2, and update P_2 to P'_2.

EndFor

5. Transform the obtained shape x_r into a new shape model instance x' by aligning x_r to the mean shape $\overline{x}$, in order to yield the new affine transformation t'.
6. Apply the model constraints to the new shape model x' so that the new shape is within the allowed shape-space.

End

Oriented Active Appearance Model Optimization

The boundary cost is not taken into consideration in the traditional AAM matching method, since the optimization is based only on the difference between the appearance model instance and the target image. Its performance can be considerably improved for AAM matching with the integration of the boundary cost. During the optimization process, the cost computation is performed with the combination of the live wire technique. Shape and texture information is represented as b, and it is the current estimate of the AAM parameters,

$$b = Q^T \begin{pmatrix} b_s \\ b_g \end{pmatrix} \tag{4}$$

where Q represents a matrix which specifies the modes of shape and appearance variation derived from the training set, b_s denotes the shape model parameters, and b_g denotes the appearance model parameters. Combined with the above shape model refinement approach, our optimization process is described as follows:

Algorithm 2: Oriented Active Appearance Model Optimization

Input: Model parameters vector b, pose vector t, texture vector u, weight parameters
$\quad \alpha_1 = \alpha_2 = 0.5$.
Output: Updated model parameters vector b, t and u.
Begin

1. Obtain shape parameters b_s from b, and refine b_s using *Algorithm 1* and get the
   updated shape model parameters b'_s and pose t', and update b by $b = Q^T \begin{pmatrix} b'_s \\ b_g \end{pmatrix}$.
2. Resample the image intensity as g'_{im} and compute the texture model frame using
   $g'_s = T_u^{-1}(g'_{im})$ based on the updated b and t'.
3. Evaluate the errors

   (a) Texture error $E_{aam} = |r(\phi)|^2$, where $\phi^T = (b^T|t'^T|u^T)$ and $r(\phi) = g'_s - g'_{im}$.
   (b) Total error by combining E_{aam} and live wire cost along the shape boundary E_{lw},

$$E_{total} = \alpha_1 \cdot E_{aam} + \alpha_2 \cdot E_{lw} \tag{5}$$

4. Compute the predicted displacements $\delta_\phi = - Rr(\phi)$, where

$$R = \left(\frac{\partial r^T}{\partial \phi} \frac{\partial r}{\partial \phi} \right)^{-1} \frac{\partial r^T}{\partial \phi}$$

5. Set $k = 1$,
6. Update the parameters $\phi \leftarrow \phi + k\delta_\phi$,
7. Repeat steps 1–3 based on the new parameters ϕ, and obtain the new error E'_{total}.
8. If $E'_{total} < E_{total}$, then accept the new parameters and go to step 9.
   Else try $k = 0.5, 0.25$, etc. and go to step 6.

9. Repeat starting with step 1 until no improvement is made to the total error.

End

In the process of initialization, a multiple resolution method is applied. It starts from the coarsest resolution and then iterated to convergence at each level before starting the next level. It is more efficient using this method than searching at a single resolution, and it can lead to a convergence to the correct solution using this method even when the model position is far away from the kidney. It may be necessary to get a discrepancy between these error functions because they run in shape-space and image-space, since the total error function is a linear combination of the nonlinear functions of live wire and AAM costs. Therefore, it may lead to $E' < E$ becoming false, because an increase in AAM costs may not be exactly overcome by the cost of the live wire. In addition, another important factor will affect this condition, since high variation of E_{aam} error stems from large texture nonuniformity even though the live wire cost becomes stable after several iterations. It is easily trapped in local minima during the process of conventional AAM optimization. Therefore, such difficulties may be overcome by changing the ratio of the contributing errors into the total cost, although it is difficult to solve this problem in a fail-safe manner.

Refinement of the 3D Recognized Shapes

The recognized shapes are stacked together to form 3D objects after kidneys are recognized in all slices. Sometimes the initialization result for one slice is far away from the results for its neighboring slices. This shows a failure of recognition for this slice. At most two slices failed in recognition in this sense in all of our tests. The new shape is interpolated from the shapes in neighboring slices once failure occurs. The following algorithm is applied to improve the recognized shape results.

Algorithm 3: Refinement of the 3D Recognized Shape

Input: Slices $1 \leq j \leq n$, weights $\eta_1 = 0.5$, $\eta_2 = 0.25$ and $\eta_3 = 0.25$, threshold of reliability T_j is estimated from training data.
Output: Refined 3D shape.
Begin
For $j = 1 : n$

1. Compute the distance between the centroids of the shapes in slices $j - 1$ and $j + 1$ as d_{j-1} and d_{j+1}
2. Compute the total reliability for slice j

$$rel_j = \eta_1 \cdot \left(\frac{e_{\max} - e}{e_{\max}} \right) + \eta_2 \cdot \exp \left(\frac{\left(d_{j-1} - \mu\left(d_{j-1}\right) \right)^2}{2 \cdot \mathrm{Var}\left(d_{j-1}\right)} \right)$$
$$+ \eta_3 \cdot \exp \left(-\frac{\left(d_{j+1} - \mu\left(d_{j+1}\right) \right)^2}{2 \cdot \mathrm{Var}\left(d_{j+1}\right)} \right)$$

3. If $rel_j < T_j$, then estimate the shape in slice j via interpolation from the neighboring slices.

   EndFor
   End

Here, $\mu(d_{j-1})$, $var(d_{j-1})$, $\mu(d_{j+1})$, and $var(d_{j+1})$ represent the mean and variance of d_{j-1} and d_{j+1}, respectively, which are estimated from training images during the model building process. e and $e_{\max}$ denote current and maximum slice localization errors, respectively. However, only one neighbor slice is applied to the above algorithm for the first and last slice.

Kidney and Renal Cortex Segmentation

Different approaches have been proposed to segment kidney and renal cortex. Many methods employ image information, such as, the spatial information and intensity. Sun et al. [46] presented an integrated image registration algorithm to segment renal cortex in MR images. Their method achieved temporal image registration by multiple steps. They first detected large-scale motion to register the images roughly, and then integrated region information and local gradient information with auxiliary image segmentation results to refine the registration results. Zöllner et al. [47] have applied automated image analysis methods in the assessment of human kidney perfusion based on 3D dynamic contrast-enhanced MRI data. This approach used a nonrigid 3D image registration method to reduce motion artifacts in the image time series. The subsequent k-means clustering method as used to segment the kidney compartments (cortex, medulla, and pelvis). Song et al. [48] developed a 4D level set approach for dynamic MR images kidney segmentation. Their method also combined spatial anatomical structures with temporal dynamics.

Spiegel et al. [56] proposed an active shape model generation method to segment 3D kidneys in CT images. Their approach method yielded more detailed active shape models and did not need explicit or parametric formulations of the problem. The active shape model was updated with additional prior knowledge quickly. Then they used nonrigid image registration to solve the crucial correspondence problem. Freiman et al. [49] proposed a nonparametric model constraint graph min-cut/max-flow approach for automatic kidney segmentation in CT images. The segmentation was considered as a maximum a-posteriori estimation problem in a model-driven Markov random field. Energy functional was built with a nonparametric hybrid shape and intensity model. The latent model and minimization of the energy functional were then computed with an expectation maximization algorithm. Tsagaan et al. [50] presented a deformable model-based approach for automated segmentation of kidneys from abdominal 3D CT images. They integrated the gray level appearance of the target and statistical information of the shape into NURBS surface-based deformable model. In addition, they proposed automated positioning method of an initial model. Touhami et al. [51] proposed a statistical method for fully automatic kidneys segmentation. They used spatial and gray-levels prior models by using a set of training images.

Gloger et al. [52] proposed fully automatic kidney parenchyma 3D segmentation technique in MR datasets by using Bayesian concepts for probability map generation. They first applied a multistep refinement approach to improve the probability map quality, and then an extended prior shape level set segmentation method was used on the refined probability maps and combined several relevant kidney parenchyma features. Lin et al. [53] presented a model-based approach for computer-aided kidney segmentation of CT images. Their approach was divided into two steps. First, the candidate kidney region was detected according to the statistical geometric location of kidney within the abdomen. This method can be applied to images of different sizes since they used the relative distance of the kidney region to the spine. In the second step, kidney region seed points were identified by using directional model, and then adaptive region growing was used by the properties of image homogeneity. Xie et al. [54] introduced a texture and shape priors-based method in ultrasound images. They applied a bank of Gabor filters on test images to extract texture features, and then constructed the texture model by estimating the parameters of a set of mixtures of half-planed Gaussians. Based on the texture model, the texture similarities of areas around the segmenting curve were computed respectively in the inside and outside regions. Finally, they combined the texture measures into the parametric shape model. Kidney segmentation was accomplished by calculating the parameters of the shape model to minimize a texture-based energy function. Li et al. [55] presented a graph construction-based optimal graph search method for renal cortex segmentation on CT images. The renal cortex segmentation problem was treated as a multiple surfaces extraction problem. More recently, Li et al. [7] developed an automatic renal cortex segmentation approach by the combination of the implicit shape registration and novel multiple surfaces graph search. The proposed approach consists of three steps. In the first step, the whole kidney was coarsely initialized using an implicit shape registration method, and the shapes built in the space of Euclidean distance functions. In the second step, the multiple surfaces graph searching algorithm was applied to obtain the outer and inner surfaces of renal cortex. In the end, a renal cortex refining scheme was utilized to detect and reduce incorrect segmentation pixels around the renal pelvis and to improve the segmentation accuracy.

In the cortex segmentation framework, the aim of this step is to finally precisely delineate the kidneys recognized in the previous step. An iterative algorithm is proposed by combining graph cuts and OAAM method for the kidney and renal cortex delineation. The iterative graph cut OAAM algorithm effectively integrates the shape information with the globally optimal 3D delineation ability of the Graph Cuts method.

Shape Integrated Graph Cuts

Graph Cuts segmentation can be considered as an energy minimization problem for a set of pixels P and a set of labels L, such that the goal is to find a labeling $f : P \rightarrow L$ that minimizes the energy function $\text{En}(f)$.

$$\text{En}(f) = \sum_{p \in P} R_p(f_p) + \sum_{p \in P, \ q \in N_p} B_{p,q}(f_p, f_q) \tag{6}$$

where N_p represents the set of pixels in the neighborhood of p, $R_p(f_p)$ represents the cost of assigning label $f_p \in L$ to p, and $B_{p,q}(f_p, f_q)$ represents the cost of assigning labels $f_p, f_q \in L$ to p and q. If $B_{p,q}$ in two-class labeling, $L = \{0,1\}$, is a sub-modular function, i.e., $B_{p,q}(0,0) + B_{p,q}(1,1) \le B_{p,q}(0,1) + B_{p,q}(1,0)$, the problem can be solved efficiently with graph cuts in polynomial time [22].

In this chapter, the unary cost $R_p(f_p)$ represents the sum of a data penalty $D_p(f_p)$ and a shape penalty $S_p(f_p)$ term. The data penalty term is defined according to image intensity and can be treated as a log likelihood of the image intensity for the target object. The shape prior term does not depend on image information, and the boundary term is defined according to the gradient of the image intensity.

Based on the shape prior, the proposed energy function is formulated as follows:

$$En(f) = \sum_{p \in P} \left(\alpha \cdot D_p(f_p) + \beta \cdot S_p(f_p) \right) + \sum_{p \in P, q \in N_p} \gamma \cdot B_{p,q}(f_p, f_q) \qquad (7)$$

where α, β, γ denote the weights for the data term, shape term S_p, and boundary term, respectively, satisfying $\alpha + \beta + \gamma = 1$. These terms are formulated as follows:

$$D_p(f_p) = \begin{cases} -\ln P(I_p|O) & \text{if } f_p = \text{object label} \\ -\ln P(I_p|B) & \text{if } f_p = \text{background label} \end{cases} \qquad (8)$$

$$B_{p,q}(f_p, f_q) = \exp\left(-\frac{(I_p - I_q)^2}{2\sigma^2} \right) \cdot \frac{1}{d(p,q)} \cdot \delta(f_p, f_q) \qquad (9)$$

$$\delta(f_p, f_q) = \begin{cases} 1 & \text{if } f_p \ne f_q \\ 0 & \text{otherwise} \end{cases} \qquad (10)$$

where I_p denotes the intensity of pixel p; *object label* denotes the label of the object (foreground); $P(I_p|O)$ and $P(I_p|B)$ denote the probability of intensity of pixel p belonging to object and background, respectively, which are estimated from object and background intensity histograms during the training phase; $d(p,q)$ denotes the Euclidian distance between pixels p and q; and σ denotes the standard deviation of the intensity differences of neighboring voxels along the boundary.

$$S_p(f_p) = 1 - \exp\left(-\frac{d(p, x_O)}{r_O} \right) \qquad (11)$$

where $d(p, x_O)$ denotes the distance from pixel p to the set of pixels which constitute the interior of the current shape x_O of object O (note that if p is in the interior of x_O, then $d(p, x_O) = 0$); r_O denotes the radius of a circle that just encloses x_O. The linear time method was applied to compute this distance [62].

The histograms of intensity are estimated for object and background from the training images in the training phase, in order to compute $P(I_p|O)$ and $P(I_p|B)$. α, β can be estimated by optimizing accuracy as a function of α, β and then compute $\gamma = 1 - \alpha - \beta$. The gradient descent method is used for the optimization. The true positive volume fraction [59] is used to represent the algorithm's accuracy $Accu(\alpha,\beta)$. After both α and β are initialized to 0.35, $Accu(\alpha,\beta)$ is computed optimally over the training data set to select the best α and β.

Minimizing En with Graph Cuts

The minimization of (7) can be achieved by graph cuts method. The graph is constructed as follows. $V = P \cup L$. V represents all the pixel nodes and terminals corresponding to the labels in L, which represent objects of interest and the background. $A = A_N \cup A_T$. A_N represents the n-links which connect pixels p and q ($p \in P$, $q \in N_p$), and $w_{p,q}$ represents its weight. A_T represents the set of t-links which connect pixel p and terminals $\ell \in L$, and $w_{p,l}$ represents its weight. The desired graph with cut cost $|C|$ is constructed using the following weight assignments:

$$w_{p,q} = \gamma \cdot B_{p,q} \tag{12}$$

$$w_{p,l} = K - \left(\alpha \cdot D_p(l) + \beta \cdot S_p(l) \right) \tag{13}$$

where K is a large constant in order to ensure the weights $w_{p,l}$ positive.

Iterative Graph Cut-Oriented Active Appearance Model

In this step, the location of recognized shapes is supposed to be close to the desirable boundaries in the given image. The proper position of the landmarks of the objects represented in the initialized shape x_{in} can be achieved when the graph cut cost is minimized in the iterative graph cut OAAM algorithm, described as follows.

Algorithm 4: Iterative Graph Cut-Oriented Active Appearance Model

Input: Initialized shapes x_{in}, shape distance $d = \infty$, $\varepsilon =$ a small value.
Output: Resulting shapes x_{out} and the associated kidney boundaries shape.
Begin
While $d > \varepsilon$ do

1. Perform graph cuts segmentation using (7) based on the OAAM initialized shapes x_{in};
2. Compute the new position of the landmarks by moving each landmark in x_{in} to the point closest on the graph cuts boundary; call the resulting shapes x_{in};
3. If no landmarks move, then set x_{new} as x_{out} and stop;
    Else, subject x_{new} to the constraints of model M_{3D}, and call the result x_{in}. And compute the shape distance d between the current shape and previous shape.

EndWhile

Perform one final Graph Cuts segmentation based on x_{out}, and obtain the associated shape boundaries.
End

In our implementation, $\varepsilon = 0.1$. The segmentation accuracies usually don't change much after two iterations in our test. The distance is constrained for a landmark to move within any iteration to six voxels, in order to make the change smoother.

Renal Cortex Segmentation

The renal cortex segmentation consists of three main steps: kidney delineation, cortex shape generation, and cortex delineation.

Kidney Delineation

The purpose of this step is to precisely delineate the kidney shapes recognized in the previous step. We propose an iterative graph cut OAAM method for the kidney's delineation, which effectively integrates the shape information from the OAAM initialization step with the globally optimal 3D delineation capability of the graph cuts method.

Renal Cortex Shape Construction

The initial cortex shape needs to be required after the kidney contour is obtained. A morphological operation (erosion) is applied to construct an initial renal cortex shape. The running times of erosion is estimated from the training data set which is actually related with the depth of the renal cortex.

Renal Cortex Delineation

Based on the former step, the initial cortex shape can be generated. The location of initialized cortex shapes is supposed to be close to the desirable boundaries in the given image. The iterative graph cut OAAM is applied again to refine the final renal cortex boundaries, and the obtained initial cortex shape is used as the shape constraint.

Experimental Results

The proposed method was tested on a clinical dataset which includes 27 patients (12 men and 15 women, age ranged from 19 to 63). The patients were injected with 130 mL of Isovue-300 contrast agent (Bracco Diagnostics, Milan, Italy) before image acquisition. These CT images were reviewed with a three-dimensional multi-planar reformatting interactive mode on an image-processing workstation (Advanced Workstation; GE Medical Systems). The pixel size varied from 0.55 to 1 mm, and slice thickness from 1 to 5 mm. All datasets were acquired from one of two different types of CT scanners (LightSpeed Ultra, GE Medical Systems, Milwaukee, WI; or Mx8000 IDT 16, Philips Medical Systems, Andover, MA). The leave-one-out strategy was adopted to evaluate the proposed method.

Table 1 Segmentation evaluation based on the "MICCAI 2007 grand challenge for liver segmentation" evaluation criteria

Method	OE (%)	VD (%)	AD (mm)	RMSD (mm)	MD (mm)
Kidney segmentation	3.6 ± 2.6	1.9 ± 2.1	0.9 ± 0.5	1.7 ± 1.1	16.9 ± 7.1
Cortex segmentation	12.7 ± 3.3	3.9 ± 5.2	1.5 ± 1.1	2.8 ± 2.6	19.5 ± 0.8

To quantitatively evaluate the proposed method, the MICCAI 2007 grand challenge for liver segmentation evaluation criteria: volumetric overlap error (OE), relative volume difference (VD), average symmetric surface distance (AD), root mean square symmetric surface distance (RMSD), and maximal symmetric surface distance (MD), were used to evaluate the proposed method.

Volumetric overlap error is defined as,

$$OE = 1 - \frac{|V_s \cap V_t|}{|V_s \cup V_t|} \tag{14}$$

where V_s and V_t are the manually segmented image and the computer segmentation result, respectively, while the intersection operation $\cap$ and union operation $\cup$ are the voxel wise *and* and *or* operation, respectively, and $|V|$ represents the number of voxels in region V.

To account for the extension of a result over-segmented or under-segmented, relative volume difference was calculated according to

$$SVD = \frac{|V_t| - |V_s|}{|V_s|} \tag{15}$$

To evaluate the global and local disagreement between the manually segmented image and the segmentation result image, average symmetric surface distance, root mean square symmetric surface distance, and maximal symmetric surface distance were calculated according to

$$AD = \frac{\sum_{p_s \in S_s} D(p_s, S_t) + \sum_{p_t \in S_t} D(p_t, S_s)}{|S_s| + |S_t|} \tag{16}$$

$$RMSD = \sqrt{\frac{\sum_{p_s \in S_s} D^2(p_s, S_t) + \sum_{p_t \in S_t} D^2(p_t, S_s)}{|S_s| + |S_t|}} \tag{17}$$

$$MD = max\left(\max_{p_s \in S_s} (D(p_s, S_t)), \max_{p_t \in S_t} (D(p_t, S_s)) \right) \tag{18}$$

where S_s and S_t are the surfaces of the manually segmented image and the segmentation result. $D(p,S)$ represents the minimum Euclidean distance between an arbitrary point p and surface S.

The Experimental results are summarized in Table 1. The average volumetric overlap error for kidney segmentation is about 3.6 %, while for cortex segmentation; the average overlap error is about 12.7 %.

The segmentation results are shown in Fig. 7c, d and g, h for the kidney and cortex by the proposed method, respectively. In addition, the error of cortex segmentation is higher than kidney segmentation, which may be due to the greater difficulty in cortex segmentation than kidney segmentation.

In terms of efficiency, the running time was tested for the kidney and cortex segmentation on an Intel Xeon E5440 workstation with 2.83 GHz CPU, 8 GB of RAM. For kidney segmentation, the time for the computation was reduced from 8 min for manual segmentation to about 1.3 min for automatic segmentation. For renal cortex segmentation, the time was reduced from 20 min for manual segmentation, to less than 2 min for automatic segmentation.

Conclusion and Discussion

In this chapter, we introduced a 3D automatic renal cortex segmentation method. This framework effectively integrates the AAM and live wire with graph cuts so that their complementary strengths can be fully exploited. It consists of two phases: training and segmentation. For the training part, we build an AAM and then trained the live wire and graph cuts parameters. In the second phase, we employed a pseudo-3D strategy and segmented the organs slice by slice via multi-object OAAM method which synergistically integrated the AAM with live wire methods. Subsequently, an iterative graph cut OAAM method is proposed which integrates the shape information. The approach was tested on a clinical abdominal CT dataset with 27 contrast-enhanced images. The experimental results showed that an overall renal cortex segmentation accuracy with overlap error ≤ 12.7 %, volume difference ≤ 3.9 %, average distance ≤ 1.5 mm, RMS distance ≤ 2.8 mm, and maximal distance ≤ 19.5 mm could be achieved.

For initialization, we applied a pseudo-3D strategy and integrated AAM with live wire methods to improve the performance. Besides, the multi-object strategy also helped initialization because of increased constraints. Compared to the real 3D AAM method, the pseudo 3D OAAM approach has comparable accuracy; meanwhile, it achieves roughly a 12-fold speed up. The aim of initialization is to provide rough object localization and shape constraints for a latter graph cuts method which will accomplish refined delineation. We suggest that it is better to employ a fast and robust method than a slow and more accurate technique for initialization.

For delineation, the shape constrained graph cuts method is the core part of the whole framework. Several similar researches were also done in the literatures [36–39]. However, they are mostly studied on 2D images, and it is difficult to compare with these methods since the testing data sets used are different.

So far, it has not received much attention to research on the localization of a CT slice within a human body, although it can greatly facilitate the workflow of a physician. It is an important part to localize the top and bottom slices of organs automatically in the whole framework. It can also be utilized to localize any slice by constructing the corresponding slice model.

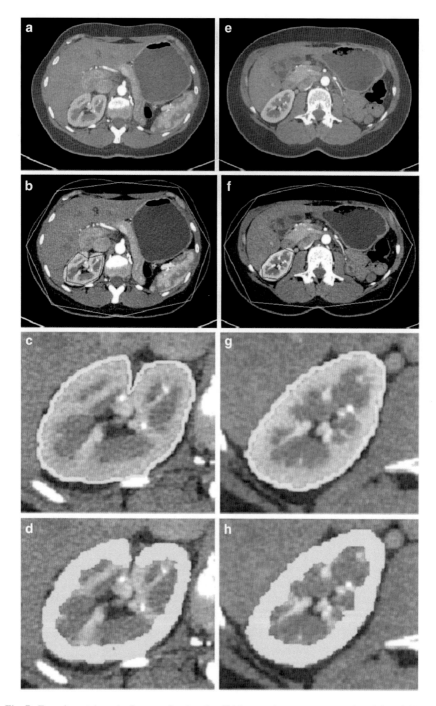

Fig. 7 Experimental results for two slice levels of kidney and cortex segmentation. (**a**) and (**e**) are the original slice images; (**b**) and (**f**) are multi-object active appearance model initialization result; (**c**) and (**g**) are the kidney segmentation results; (**d**) and (**h**) are the cortex segmentation results

In this chapter, only one object is delineated at a time. With the shape constraints of multiple organs, the proposed iterative graph cut OAAM method can be easily applied to segment multiple organs simultaneously. However, it is difficult to achieve a globally optimal min cut solution for simultaneously segmenting multiple objects for graph cuts. Global optimality is guaranteed for single object segmentation. The α-expansion method can accomplish segmentations only within a known factor of the global optimum for multiple objects [39].

The proposed method takes about 2 min for segmenting one organ. To make it more practical in clinical applications, the parallelization or multi-thread implementation of the algorithm may be a good choice. Anderson and Setubal [63] and Liu and Sun [64] proposed parallelization of the graph cuts methods and achieved good performance.

References

1. American Cancer Society (2010) http://wwwcancerorg/Cancer/KidneyCancer/DetailedGuide/kidney-cancer-adult-key-statistics
2. Rathmell WK, Martz CA, Rini BI (2007) Renal cell carcinoma. Curr Opin Oncol 19(3): 234–240
3. Beland MD, Walle NL, Machan JT, Cronan JJ (2010) Renal cortical thickness measured at ultrasound: is it better than renal length as an indicator of renal function in chronic kidney disease? Am J Roentgenol 195(2):W146–W149
4. Muto NS, Kamishima T, Harris AA, Kato F, Onodera Y, Terae S, Shirato H (2011) Renal cortical volume measured using automatic contouring software for computed tomography and its relationship with BMI, age and renal function. Eur J Radiol 78(1):151–156
5. Artunc F, Yildiz S, Rossi C, Boss A, Dittmann H, Schlemmer H, Risler T, Heyne N (2010) Simultaneous evaluation of renal morphology and function in live kidney donors using dynamic magnetic resonance imaging. Nephrol Dial Transplant 25(6):1986–1991
6. Stevens LA, Coresh J, Greene T, Levey AS (2006) Assessing kidney function—measured and estimated glomerular filtration rate. N Engl J Med 354(23):2473–2483
7. Li X, Chen X, Yao J, Zhang X, Yang F, Tian J (2012) Automatic renal cortex segmentation using implicit shape registration and novel multiple surfaces graph search. IEEE Trans Med Imaging 31(10):1849–1860
8. American Cancer Society (2013) How is kidney cancer diagnosed? http://wwwcancerorg/cancer/kidneycancer/detailedguide/kidney-cancer-adult-diagnosis
9. Medicine JH. Computed tomography (CT or CAT) scan of the kidney. http://wwwhopkinsmedicineorg/healthlibrary/test_procedures/urology/computed_tomography_ct_or_cat_scan_of_the_kidney_92,P07703/
10. Nikken J, Krestin G (2007) MRI of the kidney—state of the art. Eur Radiol 17(11):2780–2793
11. Cohen D, Brown JJ (2008) MR imaging of indeterminate renal lesions. Appl Radiol 37(11)
12. Rusko L, Bekes G, Nemeth G, Fidrich M (2007) Fully automatic liver segmentation for contrast-enhanced CT images. In: MICCAI workshop 3D segmentation in the clinic: a grand challenge, vol 2(7)
13. Fujimoto H, Gu L, Kaneko T (2002) Recognition of abdominal organs using 3D mathematical morphology. Syst Comput Japan 33(8):75–83
14. Kass M, Witkin A, Terzopoulos D (1988) Snakes: active contour models. Int J Comput Vis 1(4): 321–331

15. Liu F, Zhao B, Kijewski PK, Wang L, Schwartz LH (2005) Liver segmentation for CT images using GVF snake. Med Phys 32:3699
16. Malladi R, Sethian JA, Vemuri BC (1995) Shape modeling with front propagation: a level set approach. IEEE Trans Pattern Anal Mach Intell 17(2):158–175
17. Falcão AX, Udupa JK, Samarasekera S, Sharma S, Hirsch BE (1998) Lotufo RdA: user-steered image segmentation paradigms: live wire and live lane. Graph Mod Image Process 60(4): 233–260
18. Grau V, Mewes A, Alcaniz M, Kikinis R, Warfield SK (2004) Improved watershed transform for medical image segmentation using prior information. IEEE Trans Med Imaging 23(4): 447–458
19. Udupa JK, Samarasekera S (1996) Fuzzy connectedness and object definition: theory, algorithms, and applications in image segmentation. Graph Mod Image Process 58(3):246–261
20. Saha PK, Udupa JK (2001) Relative fuzzy connectedness among multiple objects: theory, algorithms, and applications in image segmentation. Comput Vis Image Underst 82(1):42–56
21. Boykov Y, Kolmogorov V (2004) An experimental comparison of min-cut/max-flow algorithms for energy minimization in vision. IEEE Trans Pattern Anal Mach Intell 26(9): 1124–1137
22. Kolmogorov V, Zabin R (2004) What energy functions can be minimized via graph cuts? IEEE Trans Pattern Anal Mach Intell 26(2):147–159
23. Besbes A, Komodakis N, Langs G, Paragios N (2009) Shape priors and discrete MRFs for knowledge-based segmentation. In: IEEE conference on computer vision and pattern recognition, 2009 (CVPR 2009), IEEE, pp 1295–1302
24. Cuadra MB, Pollo C, Bardera A, Cuisenaire O, Villemure J-G, Thiran J-P (2004) Atlas-based segmentation of pathological MR brain images using a model of lesion growth. IEEE Trans Med Imaging 23(10):1301–1314
25. Bazin P-L, Pham DL (2008) Homeomorphic brain image segmentation with topological and statistical atlases. Med Image Anal 12(5):616
26. Frangi AF, Rueckert D, Schnabel JA, Niessen WJ (2002) Automatic construction of multiple-object three-dimensional statistical shape models: application to cardiac modeling. IEEE Trans Med Imaging 21(9):1151–1166
27. Mitchell SC, Lelieveldt BPF, van der Geest RJ, Bosch HG, Reiver J, Sonka M (2001) Multistage hybrid active appearance model matching: segmentation of left and right ventricles in cardiac MR images. IEEE Trans Med Imaging 20(5):415–423
28. Bankman I (2000) Handbook of medical imaging: processing and analysis management. Academic, New York
29. Artaechevarria X, Munoz-Barrutia A, Ortiz-de-Solorzano C (2009) Combination strategies in multi-atlas image segmentation: application to brain MR data. IEEE Trans Med Imaging 28(8):1266–1277
30. Christensen GE, Rabbitt RD, Miller MI (1994) 3D brain mapping using a deformable neuro-anatomy. Phys Med Biol 39(3):609
31. Cootes TF, Edwards GJ, Taylor CJ (2001) Active appearance models. IEEE Trans Pattern Anal Mach Intell 23(6):681–685
32. Stegmann MB, Ersboll BK, Larsen R (2003) FAME-a flexible appearance modeling environment. IEEE Trans Med Imaging 22(10):1319–1331
33. Liu J, Udupa JK (2009) Oriented active shape models. IEEE Trans Med Imaging 28(4): 571–584
34. Haris K, Efstratiadis SN, Maglaveras N, Katsaggelos AK (1998) Hybrid image segmentation using watersheds and fast region merging. IEEE Trans Image Process 7(12):1684–1699
35. Yang J, Duncan JS (2004) 3D image segmentation of deformable objects with joint shape-intensity prior models using level sets. Med Image Anal 8(3):285
36. Freedman D, Zhang T (2005) Interactive graph cut based segmentation with shape priors. In: IEEE computer society conference on computer vision and pattern recognition, 2005 (CVPR 2005), IEEE, pp 755–762

37. Ayvaci A, Freedman D (2007) Joint segmentation-registration of organs using geometric models. In: 29th annual international conference of the IEEE engineering in medicine and biology society, 2007 (EMBS 2007), IEEE, pp 5251–5254

38. Malcolm J, Rathi Y, Tannenbaum A (2007) Graph cut segmentation with nonlinear shape priors. In: IEEE international conference on image processing, 2007 (ICIP 2007), IEEE, pp IV-365–IV-368

39. Vu N, Manjunath B (2008) Shape prior segmentation of multiple objects with graph cuts. In: IEEE conference on computer vision and pattern recognition, 2008 (CVPR 2008), IEEE, pp 1–8

40. Haas B, Coradi T, Scholz M, Kunz P, Huber M, Oppitz U, André L, Lengkeek V, Huyskens D, van Esch A (2008) Automatic segmentation of thoracic and pelvic CT images for radiotherapy planning using implicit anatomic knowledge and organ-specific segmentation strategies. Phys Med Biol 53(6):1751

41. Park H, Bland PH, Meyer CR (2003) Construction of an abdominal probabilistic atlas and its application in segmentation. IEEE Trans Med Imaging 22(4):483–492

42. Seifert S, Barbu A, Zhou SK, Liu D, Feulner J, Huber M, Suehling M, Cavallaro A, Comaniciu D (2009) Hierarchical parsing and semantic navigation of full body CT data. In: SPIE Medical imaging, International Society for Optics and Photonics, pp 725902–725908

43. Cootes TF, Taylor CJ, Cooper DH, Graham J (1995) Active shape models-their training and application. Comput Vis Image Underst 61(1):38–59

44. Rusinek H, Boykov Y, Kaur M, Wong S, Bokacheva L, Sajous JB, Huang AJ, Heller S, Lee VS (2007) Performance of an automated segmentation algorithm for 3D MR renography. Magn Reson Med 57(6):1159–1167

45. Boykov Y, Lee VS, Rusinek H, Bansal R (2001) Segmentation of dynamic ND data sets via graph cuts using Markov models. In: Medical image computing and computer-assisted intervention—MICCAI 2001, Springer, pp 1058–1066

46. Sun Y, Jolly M-P, Moura J (2004) Integrated registration of dynamic renal perfusion MR images. In: International conference on image processing, 2004 (ICIP'04 2004), IEEE, pp 1923–1926

47. Zöllner FG, Sance R, Rogelj P, Ledesma-Carbayo MJ, Rørvik J, Santos A, Lundervold A (2009) Assessment of 3D DCE-MRI of the kidneys using non-rigid image registration and segmentation of voxel time courses. Comput Med Imaging Graph 33(3):171–181

48. Song T, Lee VS, Rusinek H, Bokacheva L, Laine A (2008) Segmentation of 4D MR renography images using temporal dynamics in a level set framework. In: 5th IEEE international symposium on biomedical imaging: from nano to macro, 2008 (ISBI 2008), IEEE, pp 37–40

49. Freiman M, Kronman A, Esses S, Joskowicz L, Sosna J (2010) Non-parametric iterative model constraint graph min-cut for automatic kidney segmentation. In: Medical image computing and computer-assisted intervention—MICCAI 2010, Springer, pp 73–80

50. Tsagaan B, Shimizu A, Kobatake H, Miyakawa K (2002) An automated segmentation method of kidney using statistical information. In: Medical image computing and computer-assisted intervention—MICCAI 2002, Springer, pp 556–563

51. Touhami W, Boukerroui D, Cocquerez J-P (2005) Fully automatic kidneys detection in 2D ct images: a statistical approach. In: Medical image computing and computer-assisted intervention—MICCAI 2005, Springer, pp 262–269

52. Gloger O, Tonnies KD, Liebscher V, Kugelmann B, Laqua R, Volzke H (2012) Prior shape level set segmentation on multistep generated probability maps of MR datasets for fully automatic kidney parenchyma volumetry. IEEE Trans Med Imaging 31(2):312–325

53. Lin D-T, Lei C-C, Hung S-W (2006) Computer-aided kidney segmentation on abdominal CT images. IEEE Trans Inf Technol Biomed 10(1):59–65

54. Xie J, Jiang Y, Tsui H-T (2005) Segmentation of kidney from ultrasound images based on texture and shape priors. IEEE Trans Med Imaging 24(1):45–57

55. Li X, Chen X, Yao J, Zhang X, Tian J (2011) Renal cortex segmentation using optimal surface search with novel graph construction. In: Medical image computing and computer-assisted intervention—MICCAI 2011, Springer, pp 387–394
56. Spiegel M, Hahn DA, Daum V, Wasza J, Hornegger J (2009) Segmentation of kidneys using a new active shape model generation technique based on non-rigid image registration. Comput Med Imaging Graph 33(1):29–39
57. Dryden I, Mardia K (1998) Statistical analysis of shape. Wiley, Chichester
58. Mitchell SC, Bosch JG, Lelieveldt BPF, van der Geest RJ, Reiber JHC, Sonka M (2002) 3-D active appearance models: segmentation of cardiac MR and ultrasound images. IEEE Trans Med Imaging 21(9):1167–1178
59. Udupa JK, Leblanc VR, Zhuge Y, Imielinska C, Schmidt H, Currie LM, Hirsch BE, Woodburn J (2006) A framework for evaluating image segmentation algorithms. Comput Med Imaging Graph 30(2):75–87
60. Emrich T, Graf F, Kriegel H-P, Schubert M, Thoma M, Cavallaro A (2010) CT slice localization via instance-based regression. In: Proceedings of the SPIE medical imaging, p 762320
61. Chen X, Udupa JK, Bagci U, Zhuge Y, Yao J (2012) Medical image segmentation by combining graph cuts and oriented active appearance models. IEEE Trans Image Process 21(4):2035–2046
62. Maurer CR Jr, Qi R, Raghavan V (2003) A linear time algorithm for computing exact euclidean distance transforms of binary images in arbitrary dimensions. IEEE Trans Pattern Anal Mach Intell 25(2):265–270
63. Anderson R, Setubal JC (1995) A parallel implementation of the push-relabel algorithm for the maximum flow problem. J Parallel Distrib Comput 29(1):17–26
64. Liu J, Sun J (2010) Parallel graph-cuts by adaptive bottom-up merging. In: IEEE conference on computer vision and pattern recognition (CVPR), IEEE, pp 2181–2188

Biography

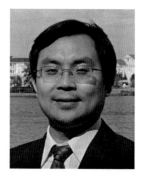

Xinjian Chen received the Ph.D. degree in 2006 from the Center for Biometrics and Security Research, Key Laboratory of Complex Systems and Intelligence Science, Institute of Automation, Chinese Academy of Sciences, Beijing, China. After graduation, he entered Microsoft Research Asia and researched on Handwriting Recognition. From January 2008 to May 2012, he has conducted the

Postdoctoral Research at several prestigious groups: Medical Image Processing Group, Department of Radiology, University of Pennsylvania (January 2008 to October 2009); Department of Radiology and Image Sciences, Clinical Center, National Institutes of Health (October 2009 to August 2011); Prof. Milan Sonka's Group, Department of Electrical and Computer Engineering, University of Iowa (September 2011 to May 2012). Currently, he is with the school of Electrical and Information Engineering, Soochow University, China, as a full professor. His research interests include medical image processing and analysis, pattern recognition, machine learning, and their applications.

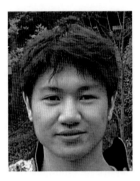

Dehui Xiang received the B.E. degree in automation from Sichuan University, China, in 2007. He received the Ph.D. degree in 2012 from the Medical Image Processing Group, State Key Laboratory of Management and Control for Complex Systems, Institute of Automation, Chinese Academy of Sciences, Beijing, China. He is with the school of Electrical and Information Engineering, Soochow University, China, as an associate professor. His current research interests include volume rendering, medical image analysis, computer vision, and pattern recognition.

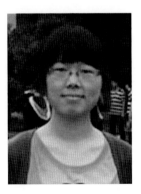

Wei Ju received the Bachelor degree in Electronic and Information Academy from Soochow University, China, in 2012. She is currently studying toward the graduate degree in the Medical Image Processing Analysis and Visualization Lab in

Electronic and Information Academy, Soochow University, Suzhou, China. Her current research interests include digital image processing, medical image analysis, computer vision, and pattern recognition.

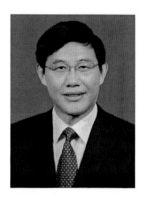

Heming Zhao is a professor and Dean of the School of Electronics and Information Engineering. He graduated from the Physics Department of Soochow University in 1982. From 1984 to 1985, he was a visiting assistant Professor in the Department of Electronic Engineering, Tsinghua University. He had conducted collaborative research in the Technical University of Munich in Germany in 1988–1990. Professor Zhao is now a member of the IEEE, the senior member of the Chinese Institute of Electronics, National Signal Processing Society of editorial board of "Signal Processing," IEEE Nanjing Section executive committee member, China Association for Artificial Intelligence Neural Networks and Computational Intelligence committee member. Chinese People's Political Consultative Conference Jiangsu Committee member.

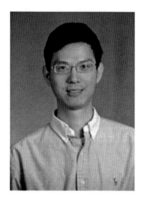

Jianhua Yao received B.S., M.S., and Ph.D. degrees in computer science from Tianjin University, Tsinghua University, and Johns Hopkins University, respectively. He joined the National Institutes of Health in 2002 as a staff scientist, where he directs a clinical image processing lab. He is also affiliated with the Imaging Biomarker and Computer-Aided Diagnosis Lab at NIH. His research interests include clinical image processing, deformable model, nonrigid registration, CAD and CT colonography. He has published over 150 papers in journals and conference proceedings and holds two patents in colon cancer CAD technique.

Diffuse Fatty Liver Disease: From Diagnosis to Quantification

Luís Curvo-Semedo, Daniel Ramos Andrade, Catarina Ruivo,
Cláudia Paulino, and Filipe Caseiro-Alves

Abstract Even though liver biopsy is considered to be the gold standard for diagnosis and quantification of liver steatosis, it is not devoid of problems, since it implicates an invasive maneuver which carries a certain amount of risk of hemorrhage. Furthermore, it suffers from sampling errors and is very dependent on the experience of the reader for quantification.

As such, noninvasive imaging methods have been increasingly used for detecting and quantifying fatty infiltration of the liver, and their growing importance is reflected on their widespread use for this purpose. Ultrasound, computed tomography, and, particularly, magnetic resonance imaging may be especially helpful in this regard. This chapter deals with their use in the assessment of liver steatosis, focusing on the main features of diffuse fatty liver infiltration on each imaging method and on their application for quantification of liver fat.

Abbreviations

ALD	Alcoholic liver disease
CT	Computed tomography
FFS	Far-field slope value
FSF	Fat signal fraction

L. Curvo-Semedo (✉) • F. Caseiro-Alves
Medical Imaging Department, Coimbra University Hospitals, Praceta Mota Pinto/Avenida Bissaya-Barreto, 3000-075 Coimbra, Portugal

Faculty of Medicine, University of Coimbra, Azinhaga de Santa Comba, 3000-075 Coimbra, Portugal
e-mail: curvosemedo@gmail.com

D.R. Andrade • C. Ruivo • C. Paulino
Medical Imaging Department, Coimbra University Hospitals, Praceta Mota Pinto/Avenida Bissaya-Barreto, 3000-075 Coimbra, Portugal

A.S. El-Baz et al. (eds.), *Abdomen and Thoracic Imaging: An Engineering & Clinical Perspective*, DOI 10.1007/978-1-4614-8498-1_4,
© Springer Science+Business Media New York 2014

HU	Hounsfield units
MDCT	Multi-detector row CT
MR	Magnetic resonance
MRI	Magnetic resonance imaging
NAFLD	Nonalcoholic fatty liver disease
NASH	Nonalcoholic steatohepatitis
ppm	Parts per million
ROI	Region of interest
SVS	Single-voxel spectroscopy
US	Ultrasonography
USS	Ultrasonographic steatosis score

Introduction

Fatty liver disease encompasses a wide spectrum of conditions which are characterized by triglyceride accumulation within the cytoplasm of hepatocytes. The two most common conditions associated with fatty liver are alcoholic liver disease (ALD) and nonalcoholic fatty liver disease (NAFLD) which is related to obesity, insulin resistance, and metabolic syndrome. NAFLD is the most prevalent chronic hepatic disease in the Western countries, affecting more than 30 % of adults and 38 % of obese children [1, 2].

Apart from "simple" steatosis with fat accumulation in the hepatocyte, more severe states exist, which are characterized by hepatic mononuclear cell infiltration, hepatocyte necrosis, and inflammation—nonalcoholic steatohepatitis (NASH)—representing an important risk factor for progression to liver failure, cirrhosis, and even hepatocellular carcinoma [2, 3].

Fatty acids in the liver promote conditions resulting in systemic subclinical inflammation, increased hepatic glucose production, and, as recently described, increased secretion of fetuin-A [4–7]. This protein is increasingly produced and secreted from the liver under hepatic steatosis [8, 9] and directly induces insulin resistance and increased cytokine expression. Both, ALD and NAFLD may lead to steatohepatitis with inflammation, cell injury, and fibrosis and may progress to irreversible cirrhosis [10–15].

Liver biopsy and histological analysis are considered the diagnostic reference standard for the assessment of fatty infiltration of the liver. Histological assessment provides information about the fat distribution within the hepatic lobules and allows a semiquantitative evaluation of steatosis. Thus the steatosis pattern can be divided into macro- and microvesicular steatosis with hepatocytes containing either one large vacuole of fat which is larger than the cell nucleus, displacing it, or many small fatty cytoplasmic inclusions without a significant nuclear displacement, respectively [16]. Macrovesicular steatosis is more common and is found not only in NAFLD but also in alcoholic fatty liver disease [17].

The extent of hepatic steatosis is visually estimated based on the percentage of hepatocytes containing visible fatty inclusions, whereas the size of the intracellular fat inclusions is not taken into account [18]. Scales representing the degree of steatosis are used, ranging from three- to six-point scales [16, 18–20]. Often, a five-point ordinal scale is used (0, 1–5, 6–33, 34–66, >67 %). However, liver biopsy is an invasive method with the risk of post-interventional hemorrhage and bleeding, even though the post-biopsy complication rate is quite low [21]. As for the mortality rate, it lies between 0.1 and 0.01 % [21]. Nevertheless, it should be emphasized that biopsy-based quantification of steatosis is derived from a small tissue sample and may, as such, be inaccurate in cases of uneven fat distribution in the liver, as it might not be a representative of the entire organ.

Therefore, noninvasive techniques are desirable in order to estimate or even quantify the degree of steatosis and eventually assess the pattern of hepatic fat distribution.

This is true, for instance, in the preoperative evaluation of liver donors for transplantation, in whom the assessment of hepatic steatosis plays an important role [22, 23]. Especially the macrovesicular subtype is critical for donor selection as it has been associated with a greater risk of primary nonfunction after liver transplantation [24, 25]. Another area of application is the monitoring of steatosis following treatment, especially after dietary and lifestyle intervention since repeated measurements are warranted [26, 27].

This chapter will focus on the usefulness of different imaging modalities (ultrasound, computed tomography, and magnetic resonance imaging (MRI)) in the diagnosis and quantitative assessment of diffuse liver steatosis in the clinical setting.

Imaging Modalities

Ultrasound

Ultrasonography (US) is widely accepted as the initial screening means for the evaluation of fatty infiltration of the liver, since it provides a noninvasive, well-tolerated, and inexpensive tool for detection and estimation of steatosis [28, 29].

In US images, diffuse hepatic steatosis manifests as a generalized increase in echogeneity compared to adjacent right kidney (Fig. 1a) or spleen, due to the intracellular accumulation of fat inclusions [28, 30]. However, US is neither highly sensitive nor specific for detection of hepatic steatosis (sensitivity ranges of 60–94 % and specificity of 66–95 % in several studies), and it cannot reliably distinguish between fibrosis and steatosis [30]. In fact, diffuse hepatic steatosis and diffuse fibrosis can have analogous appearances on US, and therefore it can sometimes be difficult to differentiate between them (Fig. 1).

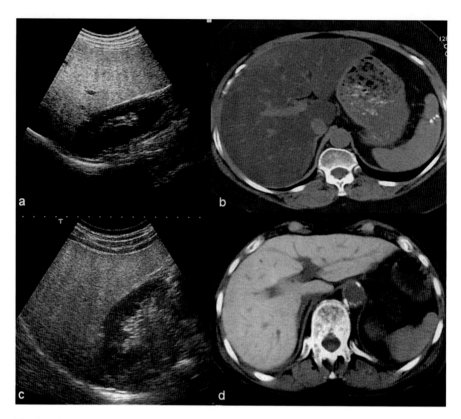

Fig. 1 US images (**a**, **c**) showing both hyperechoic livers in comparison to the parenchyma of the right kidney. Corresponding CT images of the same patients demonstrate respectively hypodense liver parenchyma due to marked fatty infiltration (**b**) and hyperattenuating liver parenchyma in a patient with liver fibrosis (**d**)

As a result, some work groups have preferred the designation "fatty fibrotic pattern" to describe this pattern of increased echogeneity, despite the fact that the echo shadows tend to be coarser in the presence of pure fibrosis [31].

As predicted, sensitivity of US raises with increasing degrees of fatty infiltration [28]. For example, in the presence of hepatic fat content of 10–19 %, it has a sensitivity of 55 %, which increases to 80 % in the presence of >30 % fatty infiltration. However, in the presence of morbid obesity (as defined by a body mass index superior to 40 kg/m^2), the sensitivity and specificity of US fall to 49 % and 75 %, respectively, possibly due to technical problems in performing US in such patients [32].

Most US studies refer to a three-point scoring system for grading hepatic steatosis (mild, moderate, and severe), based on subjective evaluation of hyperechogenic liver tissue, the increased discrepancy of echogeneity between liver and kidney, and the loss of echoes from the walls of the portal system [33]. A recent study performed in a pediatric population scored steatosis identified by US using a 0–3 scale as follows: absent steatosis (score 0)—normal liver echotexture; mild steatosis (score 1)—slight and diffuse increase in fine parenchymal echoes with normal visualization of diaphragm and portal vein borders; moderate steatosis (score 2)—moderate and diffuse increase in fine echoes with slightly impaired visualization of portal vein borders and diaphragm; and severe steatosis (score 3)—fine echoes with poor or no visualization of portal vein borders, diaphragm, and posterior portion of the right liver lobe. It was demonstrated that this ultrasonographic steatosis score (USS) had an excellent correlation with the histological grade of steatosis and a USS score of 2 had a sensitivity of almost 80 % for moderate to severe steatosis [34].

However, this visual quantification can be very subjective; in a retrospective US study of liver fat, the intra-observer agreement for severity of steatosis ranged from 55 to 68 % [35]. Therefore, it should be stressed that US visual examination is accurate for detecting moderate to severe hepatic steatosis, but the diagnosis of mild steatosis can be difficult.

In addition, recent studies demonstrated that US is very poor at discriminating small changes in hepatic fat content. For example, Fishbein and colleagues suggested from their study that an individual with hepatic steatosis undergoing a reduction of MRI hepatic fat fraction from 40 to 20 % through successful intervention would be unlikely to have a corresponding change in US appearance [19].

As mentioned above, the hyperechogenicity of the liver visually compared with that of the kidney parenchyma is well recognized as one of the most important signs of steatosis (Fig. 1a). Some studies suggested a computed hepatorenal index for quantification of liver fat, as a means of overcoming variability related to subjective evaluation [36–38]. In fact, a significant correlation was found between the hepatorenal sonographic index and magnetic resonance spectroscopy or histological steatosis in several studies, including one that showed very high concordance (sensitivity and specificity higher than 90 %) between the hepatorenal sonographic index and the degree of steatosis in biopsy [38]. Moreover, the hepatorenal sonographic index showed higher sensitivity than traditional US qualitative methods in detecting mild hepatic steatosis [38]. Furthermore, this index is reproducible and operator-independent, as shown by an interobserver agreement rate of 95.6 % for the diagnosis of hepatic steatosis [37]. There are however some drawbacks. The most important occurs in patients with inhomogeneous distribution of the liver fat, in whom sampling errors may be found (the measurements of echo intensity in only one region of interest (ROI) could not be representative of the entire liver). Another possible limitation to the use of this ratio is related to the presence of renal diseases, including structural disease or ectopic or absent right kidneys [38].

Another method available for quantitative grading of liver fat infiltration encompasses the estimation of the decrease in amplitude of the backscattered echo—the far-field slope (FFS) value. Normal liver has an FFS of 33 ± 6, and values of 38 ± 10, 44 ± 8, and 49 ± 4 are reported to be indicative of mild to severe hepatic steatosis, respectively. However, qualitative rating of steatosis at US was more accurate than quantitative estimation (sensitivity, specificity, and accuracy of 60 %–100 %, 77 %–95 %, and 96 %, in comparison with 77 %, 77 %, and 71 %, respectively) [39].

Ultimately, the US assessment of hepatic fat content is based on a subjective visual assessment rather than an objective quantification of sonographic images in the setting of the daily clinical practice. The lack of reliable quantitative methods, weak reproducibility, failure in differentiating fatty infiltration from fibrosis, and its relative inability to detect small changes in liver fat with time are impeditive of a widespread use of US in the quantification of hepatic steatosis. Further analysis on the validity of computer-aided US (hepatorenal index) should be performed in order to confirm the accuracy, reproducibility, and standardization value of this method, as it seems to be a promising effective noninvasive imaging modality that can be applied for quantifying fatty infiltration of the liver and that could be used for follow-up.

Computed Tomography

Computed tomography (CT) can be useful in the assessment of hepatic steatosis. Fatty infiltration typically results in decreased attenuation of the liver parenchyma (hypodense liver) in non-enhanced CT images (Fig. 2).

The visual assessment of liver fat usually requires an internal control in order to compare its attenuation with that of the liver (usually the spleen but also the kidney and the skeletal muscle).

In non-enhanced CT, the hepatic fat content can be assessed either subjectively by visual inspection or objectively by placing an ROI and measuring the attenuation values within it [40].

Several scales for visual assessment of the amount of steatosis on non-enhanced CT images have been suggested. A recent study used a five-point scale as follows: grade 1, hepatic vessels show lower attenuation than the hepatic parenchyma out to the peripheral third of the liver; grade 2, hepatic vessels show lower attenuation than hepatic parenchyma out to the middle third of the liver; grade 3, hepatic vessels show lower attenuation than hepatic parenchyma in the central third of the liver; grade 4, hepatic vessels show the same attenuation as that of hepatic parenchyma; and grade 5, hepatic vessels show higher attenuation than the hepatic parenchyma [41] (Fig. 2).

When placing a ROI to determine the attenuation of the liver parenchyma, three kinds of measurements have been investigated, which include (1) the absolute measurement of liver attenuation in Hounsfield units (HU), (2) the calculation of the spleen-to-liver attenuation ratio, and (3) the difference in attenuation values between liver and spleen. The comparison with the spleen permits to minimize errors in attenuation measurements caused by variations in CT parameters due to individual factors (such as body habit and metallic instruments) [30].

The placement of one or two ROIs as large as possible (at least 1 cm^2), avoiding inclusion of any large vessels or biliary structures in the right hepatic lobe, is commonly the preferred method in the measurement of hepatic attenuation (Fig. 3).

Fig 2 Non-enhanced CT scan. There is hypoattenuation of liver parenchyma relative to the hepatic vessels and the spleen, corresponding to marked fatty infiltration. Asterisk is placed over a focal area of fatty sparing in the left liver lobe

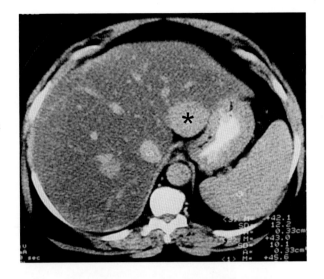

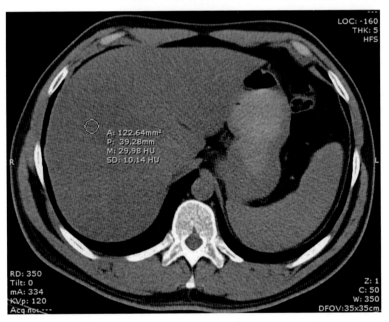

Fig. 3 ROI placing over the right liver lobe for measurement of the attenuation of the liver parenchyma. In this patient, the density value of about 30 HU reflects a marked fatty infiltration of the liver

Kodama and co-workers found that a hepatic attenuation of 40 HU represents a degree of fatty infiltration of approximately 30 % (moderate to severe steatosis). Their study showed that liver CT numbers of 64.4 HU ± 3.1, 59.1 HU ± 7.3, 41.9 HU ± 6.7, and 25.0 HU ± 15.5 at non-enhanced imaging correlated with degrees

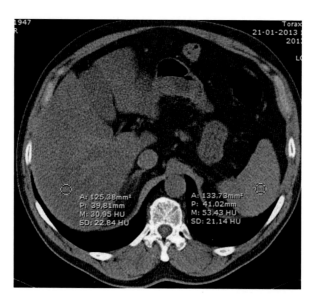

Fig. 4 Measurement of the hepatic attenuation index. Placing a ROI over the liver and other over the spleen allows determination of their attenuation values and calculation of the index. In this case, attenuation coefficients were approximately 31 and 53 HU for liver and spleen, respectively. As a result, the hepatic attenuation index was 0,58, corresponding to marked steatosis

of fatty change of 0 %, 1–25 %, 26–50 %, and more than 50 %, respectively. This retrospective study suggested that the absolute liver attenuation value on non-enhanced CT was the best predictor of pathologic fat content and that comparison methods with splenic attenuation were deemed unnecessary, as they did not contribute to accurately predict fat content and were more complex and time-consuming [42]. In clinical practice, however, the absolute value of hepatic attenuation is unreliable because most CT scanners are not appropriately calibrated for this purpose and because an overlap exists between normal and abnormal liver attenuation values. Therefore, most investigators favor a comparison between the hepatic attenuation value and an internal standard devoid of fat, such as the spleen [43].

This hepatic attenuation index can be achieved by calculating the ratio of hepatic attenuation to splenic attenuation (Fig. 4).

Several studies showed that the ratio of liver to spleen attenuation values provides a useful index of liver fat. Park and collaborators reported that a hepatic to splenic attenuation ratio of less than 0.8 had 100 % specificity for the diagnosis of moderate to severe (>30 %) macrovesicular steatosis [44]. Even in markedly obese patients (BMI of 44.4 ± 1.1), the liver to spleen index correlated strongly with histological macrosteatosis [45].

Another method of obtaining the quantification of liver fat involves the measurement of the difference between the hepatic and splenic attenuation (Fig. 5).

Attenuation value of normal healthy liver parenchyma is about 50–57 HU, which is 8–10 HU higher than that of the spleen [46]. Two studies found a specificity of 100 % for the detection of steatosis of more than 30 % when the hepatic–splenic

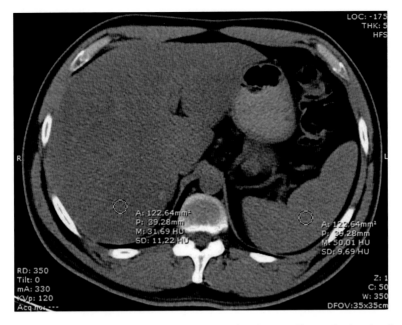

Fig. 5 Measurement of the difference in attenuation values between liver and spleen by placing ROIs over the liver and the spleen for determination of their attenuation values. In this patient, attenuation coefficients were approximately 32 and 50 HU for liver and spleen, respectively. The difference in attenuation was −18, reflecting marked fatty liver infiltration

attenuation difference was less than −9 HU [44] and less than −10 HU [24]. Limanond and co-workers showed that a hepatic–splenic attenuation difference of more than 5 HU was an accurate predictor of the absence of significant macrovesicular steatosis (0–5 %) and a difference of −10 to 5 HU was suggestive of mild to moderate steatosis (6–30 %) [24]. However, the sensitivity of these measurements for the diagnosis of macrovesicular steatosis of more than 30 % was comprehended between 73 and 82 % [24, 41, 44].

Contrast-enhanced CT plays a limited role in the diagnosis of steatosis because in this case the attenuation values of liver parenchyma depend on several factors related to the contrast and the patient, such as total volume and rate of injection, iodine concentration, body weight, cardiac output, location of intravenous access, and timing of the measurement [40, 47]. These factors lead to significant overlap between the densities of normal and fatty livers as Jacobs and colleagues found in their study [48].

However, in order to reduce the radiation burden to the patient, frequently only contrast-enhanced images are acquired. In this setting, the attenuation measurements should ideally be done 80–100 s after the beginning of contrast injection to minimize those factors [48]. Using this delay, a difference of at least 20 UH between the liver and spleen was reported to have high sensitivity and specificity (86 % and 87 %, respectively) in the diagnosis of fatty liver infiltration, when using 150 mL of iothalamate meglumine injected at a rate of 2 mL/s [48].

Panicek and co-workers suggested that when only contrast-enhanced images are available, comparing attenuation of liver to skeletal muscle is preferable as it is considered to be more specific, particularly with severe degrees of fatty infiltration. However, this hypothesis is true only if the grade of fatty infiltration is high [49].

The first studies evaluating dual-source/dual-energy CT suggest that this technique may be used to measure the extent and grade of fatty liver infiltration [50, 51], by measuring changes in hepatic attenuation between images acquired at the lower and higher energy levels (typically, 140 and 80 kVp). The attenuation of fatty liver changes more markedly with the change in tube potential than does that of normal liver [40]. Raptopoulos et al. showed that an attenuation change by more than 10 HU with a tube potential change from 140 and 80 kVp was indicative of fatty infiltration of more than 25 % [52]. The value of dual-energy CT in the quantification of steatosis, however, has to be evaluated in further studies, because attenuation difference varies significantly in the presence of iron overload.

The most important drawback of CT in the quantification of steatosis is that tissue attenuation does not depend solely on fat content. It might be influenced by an assortment of other factors, some immeasurable by CT, such as iron, copper, glycogen, fibrosis, or edema [43]. As such, underlying diffuse liver diseases may alter attenuation values of liver parenchyma so that hepatic steatosis may be misdiagnosed or concealed. For example, increased iron deposition in liver parenchyma in case of hemochromatosis may lead to a significant increase in attenuation values of the liver. Subsequently, the increase of attenuation due to iron deposition and the decrease due to fatty infiltration might add up to almost normal attenuation values, so that hepatic steatosis can be masked [52, 53].

Furthermore, it has recently been demonstrated in vitro that CT attenuation values vary significantly between different manufacturers' multi-detector row CT (MDCT) scanners, among different generations of MDCT scanners, and even with individual combinations of scanner and convolution kernel [54]. Moreover, CT is associated with radiation exposure which limits its use in longitudinal studies and in specific age groups (children).

Although non-contrast-enhanced CT is a viable option for the qualitative diagnosis of macrovesicular steatosis of 30 % or greater, it is not clinically acceptable for the diagnosis and quantification of mild to moderate hepatic steatosis, especially in living donor liver transplant candidates, in whom preoperative evaluation of fatty infiltration is critical for donor selection.

Magnetic Resonance Imaging

At present, MRI is considered to be the most sensitive and objective imaging tool for the demonstration and quantification of hepatic steatosis. Three MR techniques for the detection and quantification of steatosis are available for clinical use: chemical shift imaging, frequency-selective imaging, and MR spectroscopy [55].

These techniques help to detect fat signals on the basis of the difference in precessional frequency between water and fat.

Although fat detection may be enough to suggest the diagnosis of fatty liver, fat quantification is required to determine the severity of steatosis, actively monitor patients over time, and assess response to therapeutic intervention.

Unlike fat detection, which can be accomplished by recognizing certain qualitative imaging features, fat quantification requires quantitative analysis of the MR signal. Regardless of the MR imaging technique used, the key step is to break down the net MR signal into fat signal and water signal. Once fat and water signals have been identified and their intensities measured, the fat signal fraction (FSF) can be calculated as the ratio of the fat signal to the total MR signal:

$$\text{FSF} = S_{\text{fat}}/(S_{\text{water}} + S_{\text{fat}})$$

where S_{fat} = fat signal and S_{water} = water signal

However, all MR signals are subject to longitudinal (T1) and transverse (T2 or T2*) relaxation effects and are influenced by the imaging parameters that control T1 and T2 (or T2*) weighting. Therefore, the accuracy of quantification varies depending on the pulse sequence and imaging parameters used.

Chemical Shift

Chemical shift imaging is by far the most widely used method for the detection of steatosis in clinical practice, since in-phase and out-of-phase images are routinely acquired as part of the abdominal MR imaging protocol.

Chemical shift is related to the difference in resonance frequency between two proton MR signals, expressed in parts per million (ppm) of the resonance frequency of the static magnetic field B0. The difference of resonance frequency between protons bound to methylene groups of triglycerides (CH_2 in fatty acid chains) and water (H_2O) protons amounts to approximately 3.5 ppm. This means that when a standard nonselective radiofrequency pulse is applied to a fat–water admixture, both proton species are excited, but the water signal precesses faster than the fat signal by about 3.5 ppm (224 Hz at 1.5 T and 447 Hz at 3.0 T) [28, 30, 55].

Because of the phase interference between the fat and water signals, the gradient echoes obtained at the in-phase and out-of-phase echo times can be summarized with the equations

$$SIP = S_{\text{water}} + S_{\text{fat}}$$
$$SOP = S_{\text{water}} - S_{\text{fat}}$$

where *SIP* and *SOP* are the net signal within a given pixel in the in-phase and out-of-phase echoes, respectively, and S_{fat} and S_{water} are the contributions from fat signal and water signal, respectively.

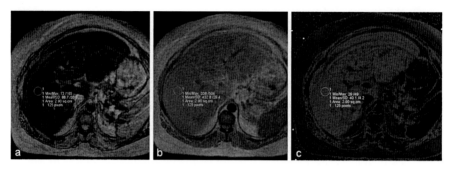

Fig. 6 Calculation of FSF. Out-of-phase (**a**) and in-phase (**b**) MR images obtained at 1.5 T show a fatty liver. Cancellation of fat and water signals causes diffuse signal intensity loss on the out-of-phase image. (**c**) FSF map. Fat–water admixture (fatty liver) appears bright, whereas subcutaneous fat (almost exclusively fat) appears similar to lean tissue (e.g., spleen) due to *fat–water dominance ambiguity*. FSF can be estimated by measuring the liver signal on the FSF map (40 % in this case). If no FSF map is available, FSF can be calculated with the equation (SIP–SOP)/2 SIP; in this case, (433–89)/(2 × 433) = 40 %

The strength of fat signal relative to water signal (FSF) can be quantified by measuring the signal on the in-phase and out-of-phase images and then applying the equation

$$FSF = S_{fat}/(S_{water} + S_{fat}) = (SIP - SOP)/2SIP$$

If out-of-phase and in-phase images are acquired with the dual-echo sequence, pixel-by-pixel computation of the FSF values over the entire image is possible by means of a simple and rapid post-processing technique to generate an "FSF map." Such an image depicts, at each pixel location, the proportion of the total signal arising from fat (Fig. 6).

While conventional spin-echo sequences possess acquisition times of several minutes for the whole liver, the development of fast gradient-echo techniques and parallel imaging [56, 57] has reduced acquisition time sufficiently enough to permit breath-hold sequences and, since the in-phase and out-of-phase images are acquired simultaneously, misregistration errors to be minimized [58]. In clinical practice, a breath-hold T1-weighted gradient-echo in-/out-of-phase sequence is used [59, 60]. The dual-echo technique is an implementation of the out-of-phase/in-phase gradient-echo sequence, in which both the out-of-phase and in-phase echoes are acquired after a single radiofrequency excitation [55].

With 1.5-T magnets, the fat and water protons are in phase or out of phase when the TE is an even or odd multiple, respectively, of 2.32 ms [16].

With an echo time at which the fat and water signals are in phase, their signals add constructively; when they are out of phase, their signals cancel [58]. Fat detection is possible by comparing the signal intensity on the in-phase and out-of-phase images. In the presence of steatosis, there is a signal loss on out-of-phase images due to phase cancellation of fat and water (Figs. 7 and 8).

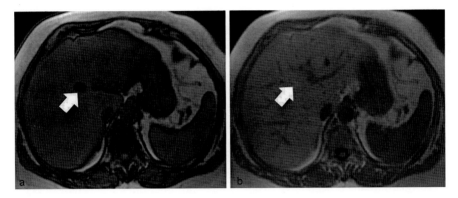

Fig. 7 Chemical shift imaging. Out-of-phase (**a**) and in-phase (**b**) MR images obtained at 1.5 T show diffuse signal intensity loss on the out-of-phase image in a fatty liver. There is a focal area of greater signal loss on out-of-phase image (*white arrow*), corresponding to a more marked focal fatty infiltration

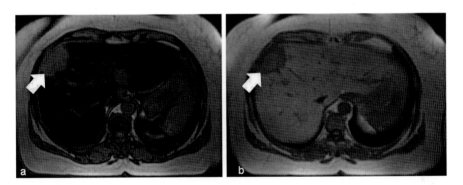

Fig. 8 Chemical shift imaging. Out-of-phase (**a**) and in-phase (**b**) MR images show marked diffuse signal intensity loss on the out-of-phase image in a fatty liver. There is a liver metastasis from a gastric cancer (*white arrow*) that does not show signal intensity changes in the out-of-phase image due to the absence of fatty components within it

This has been shown to be an accurate predictor of hepatic fat content, with very good correlation with the histological assessment of liver fat [16, 28, 61–63].

Chemical shift imaging provides a simple and rapid method for fat quantification over the entire imaging field. The method is robust because it is relatively unaffected by magnetic field inhomogeneity and works well at a variety of B0 field strengths.

Despite its conceptual simplicity and ease of implementation, however, the chemical shift method has important limitations. With standard clinical postprocessing, images are reconstructed from the signal intensity (magnitude of the magnetization vector) and not the signal phase (direction of the magnetization vector). In the out-of-phase echo, the water and fat magnetizations are opposed; consequently, the direction of the net magnetization vector is aligned with whichever signal is dominant. However, because only the signal intensity image is reconstructed, the out-of-phase intensity represents water minus fat or fat minus water, whichever value is positive. The consequence of this so-called fat–water signal dominance ambiguity is that the FSF calculated from a single pair of out-of-phase and in-phase echoes cannot distinguish water-dominant fatty tissue ("wet" fat) from fat-dominant fatty tissue ("dry" fat). For example, a tissue with 20 % fat by signal composition would appear to have the same FSF as a tissue with 80 % fat. This phenomenon is apparent on the FSF map, on which subcutaneous adipose tissue (dry fat) appears darker than the fatty liver parenchyma (wet fat) (Fig. 6). Nevertheless, this may be more of a theoretic concern rather than a practical one, since a liver fat fraction above 50 % is relatively rare.

A dual-flip-angle technique using low- and high-flip-angle gradient-echo sequences to determine the dominant component has been suggested by some authors to answer this problem [58]. Because greater T1 weighting amplifies the fat signal, a high flip angle increases the out-of-phase signal cancellation if water is the dominant component but diminishes the out-of-phase signal cancellation if fat is dominant. If the signal loss is more pronounced with a high flip angle, water is dominant; if it is more marked with a low flip angle, fat is dominant.

To overcome ambiguity, a phase-sensitive processing has also been proposed. This method (three-point Dixon method) requires the acquisition of an additional image with a phase shift of -180° or 360° and elaborated phase-correction algorithms to obtain true fat-only and true water-only images [64–71]. Unfortunately, the necessity of recording several images for the Dixon method from the liver is critical, due to the restricted duration of a breath-hold of the patient. On the other hand, several measurements in different breath-hold periods suffer from potentially variable positions of the liver in the fixed coordinate system of the scanner.

Reeder and co-workers have developed the so-called IDEAL technique [72], combining iterative decomposition of water and fat with echo asymmetry and least-squares estimation. This technique describes a multipoint fat–water separation using optimized echo shifts in order to achieve maximal signal-to-noise performance. Combined with gradient-echo imaging, it provides robust fat–water separation even in the presence of inhomogeneities of the static magnetic field [73].

Comparing chemical shift images obtained before and after gadolinium administration could also help resolve fat–water dominance ambiguity. Because gadolinium amplifies the water signal relative to the fat signal, its administration diminishes the out-of-phase signal cancellation if water is dominant but increases the out-of-phase signal cancellation if fat is dominant. Thus, if the FSF is greater after than before gadolinium administration, fat is the dominant signal component; if the reverse is true, water is the dominant signal component.

Out-of-phase/in-phase chemical shift imaging relies on the premise that the fat and water signals characteristically interfere with each other at a known frequency. However, the human fat spectrum has multiple peaks, each representing a distinct proton species. Although the dominant CH_2 peak has the greatest role in canceling the water signal in the out-of-phase echo times, other less dominant peaks may also contribute to the fat signal. Because fat quantification with a pair of in-phase and

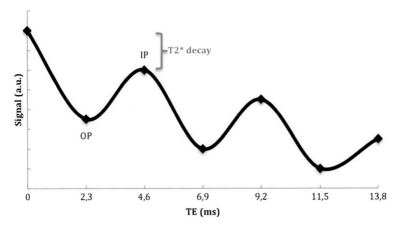

Fig. 9 Gradient-echo MR signal intensity in arbitrary units (a.u.) from fatty liver (approximately 25 % at MR spectroscopy) as a function of echo time (TE) at 1.5 T. A "best fit" biexponential curve, drawn through measured in-phase (IP) and out-of-phase (OP) signal intensities, demonstrates phase interference effect between fat and water protons and T2* decay

out-of-phase echoes is based only on the interaction between water and the CH_2 component of the total fat signal, it does not account for complex phase interference patterns from other chemical moieties and may, therefore, be somewhat inaccurate.

Another general limitation of the in-phase/out-of-phase techniques is that in the resultant fat-only and water-only images, T1 and T2* relaxation effects cannot be completely ruled out so that hepatic fat content may be misdiagnosed [47, 49, 74]. The relaxation times can be measured separately and considered in the fat calculation, but additional measurement of relaxation times leads to increased examination times [58, 75].

Heavy T1 weighting (short repetition time or high flip angle) preferentially suppresses the water signal (with longer T1), leading to relative amplification of the fat signal. Because heavily T1-weighted sequences tend to lead to overestimation of fat quantity, they are well suited for the detection of small amounts of fat and should be used if high detection sensitivity is desired. In contrast, low T1 weighting causes the T1 terms of the fat and water to be more balanced and reduces the relative amplification of the fat signal. Because minimally T1-weighted sequences are relatively unbiased by T1 effects, low T1 weighting (long repetition time or low flip angle) is recommended for fat quantification.

Yet another approach to reduce the T1 bias is to administer gadolinium [76]. At a standard clinical dose, gadolinium reduces the signal of fatty tissue relative to that of nonfatty tissues by increasing the signal of water within the fatty tissue. However, its routine use for the sole purpose of fat quantification is not recommended due to cost and potential risks.

T2* effects can also affect fat quantification. The out-of-phase/in-phase sequential design causes unavoidable underestimation of the fat signal because both fat and water signals undergo T2* signal decay during the interecho interval (Fig. 9).

The degree of underestimation depends on the amount of signal decay from out-of-phase imaging (early echo) to in-phase imaging (late echo). In tissues with very short T2* relative to the interecho interval (e.g., liver with excess iron), the T2* signal decay may overwhelm the effect of fat–water signal cancellation. A high concentration of iron within the hepatocyte can cause relevant localized magnetic field inhomogeneities, resulting in a signal loss of the liver parenchyma [16, 59, 60]. Insufficient signal yield, however, may render accurate fat quantification impossible, and the fat fraction may be grossly underestimated [60].

Therefore, Alustiza and Castiella recommend to perform a study of iron quantification in cases of markedly decreased signal intensity on in-phase images [59].

T2* effects can be minimized by selecting the earliest possible consecutive out-of-phase and in-phase echoes and the most closely spaced set of out-of-phase and in-phase echoes possible, using the out-of-phase/in-phase sequential design.

Multiple studies have found a high correlation between histological liver fat fraction and fat fraction calculated with out-of-phase/in-phase chemical shift MR imaging. However, the accuracy of this technique for liver fat quantification is influenced by the presence of hepatic iron and is poor in patients with elevated liver iron content (such as in cirrhosis and hemochromatosis). Accuracy also depends on whether an out-of-phase/in-phase (high-specificity) or in-phase/out-of-phase (low-specificity) strategy is used.

Frequency-Selective Imaging

Fat quantification may also be performed by acquiring two images, one with and one without a fat-saturation pulse, applied around the CH_2 peak to null the dominant component of the fat signal. Because other fat peaks are nearby, their signals may also be suppressed depending on the bandwidth of the saturation pulse. If complete suppression of all fat signals by the fat-saturation pulse is assumed, the FSF can be calculated as

$$NFS = S_{water} + S_{fat}$$
$$FS = S_{water}$$
$$FSF = S_{fat}/S_{water} + S_{fat} = (S_{NFS} - S_{FS})/S_{NFS}$$

where FS = fat-saturated, NFS = non-fat-saturated, and S_{NFS} and S_{FS} represent the signals obtained without and with the fat-saturation pulse, respectively.

The efficacy of the fat suppression depends on multiple factors: (a) the separation of the fat peaks from the water peak (in ppm), which increases proportionally to B0; (b) the fat-saturation pulse bandwidth, which must be sufficiently wide to cover as many fat peaks as possible without suppressing the water peak; and (c) the severity of local field inhomogeneity.

The fat-saturation technique has theoretical advantages over the two-point chemical shift approach [77, 78]. Unlike the two-point chemical shift FSF, the FSF computed with equation $(S_{NFS}-S_{FS})/S_{NFS}$ is unambiguous over the entire

0–100 % FSF range. Thus, if the saturation pulse successfully suppresses most of the fat peaks without suppressing the water peak, the measured FSF will account for the multiple components of the fat signal.

However, frequency-selective fat saturation requires precise targeting of the frequency band containing the fat peaks. In the presence of B0 magnetic field inhomogeneity, the efficacy of the suppression can be compromised. Achieving a uniform magnetic field within the abdomen can be difficult even with appropriate preparation (the so-called shimming), and the fat-saturation pulse may have unpredictable results, such as incomplete fat suppression or even inadvertent water suppression. Complete failure of fat suppression is readily apparent, but incomplete failure may be difficult to observe visually. Because it is not practical to measure field inhomogeneity in routine clinical practice, the success of fat saturation within a ROI cannot be assured, and quantification errors may occur.

The same principles discussed for chemical shift imaging apply to frequency-selective imaging. Low T1 weighting (long repetition time and, for gradient-echo sequences, low flip angle) improves accuracy for fat quantification. Therefore, single-shot fast spin-echo sequences, which have a very long effective repetition time and generate T1-independent images, are well suited for fat quantification. However, a fat fraction map obtained at a particular echo time inevitably has some T2 weighting and can be biased for the long T2 signal component. To correct for T2 effects, a two-echo single-shot fast spin-echo sequence may be performed without and with frequency-selective fat saturation. At each effective echo time, the fat-saturated image (water signal) is subtracted from the unsaturated image (water plus fat signal) to create a fat-signal image. Thus, two water-signal images and two fat-signal images are generated, one at each effective echo time. The T2 of water and fat are then estimated from the water-signal and fat-signal images, respectively, and the T2-corrected fat fraction is calculated.

Although early results with frequency-selective imaging are promising, confirmatory studies are needed before routine clinical application is recommended. The ability of this method to help detect and quantify small amounts of fat is uncertain and requires further investigation.

MR Spectroscopy

The MR imaging spectrum describes the strength of the proton signal as a function of the resonance frequency and encompasses all proton moieties in fatty acids as well as in water. Each proton moiety (H_2O, CH, CH_2, CH_3, and others) has well-known unique precession frequencies. Spectra from liver tissue recorded in vivo usually show only two dominant signal portions, namely, the water signal (positioned at 4.7 ppm) and the signal from methylene protons of fatty acids (positioned at 1.3 ppm). The signal of each chemical moiety is proportional to the area under the spectral peak at the corresponding frequency (Fig. 10).

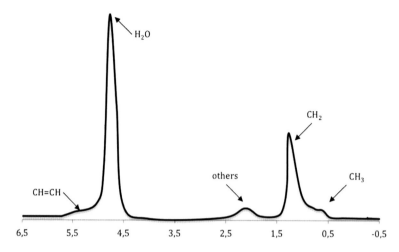

Fig. 10 MR imaging spectrum of a fatty liver. Water (H$_2$O) protons resonate at 4.7 ppm and fat (CH$_2$) protons at 1.3 ppm. Other components of triglycerides (e.g., CH$_3$, CH$_2$-COOR moieties (others), and CH=CH) possess their own characteristic resonance frequencies at 0.9, 2.1, and 5.3 ppm, respectively

The gathering of reliable spectral data and precise resolution of individual peaks require high magnetic field homogeneity. Such homogeneity is usually attainable within the 1–3-cm MR spectroscopy voxel with shimming.

Several strategies are applied for volume-selective proton MR spectroscopy in vivo: single-voxel spectroscopy (SVS) techniques, point resolved spectroscopy (PRESS) [79] or stimulated-echo acquisition mode (STEAM) sequences [80] are usually applied for recording spectra from voxel sizes in a range from 1 ccm (1 × 1 × 1 ccm) to 27 ccm (3 × 3 × 3 ccm). Suitable voxels for spectroscopy can be easily positioned in a subregion of the liver without inclusion of subcutaneous or visceral adipose tissue—and remote to lung tissue.

In most cases of NAFLD, hepatic lipids seem to be distributed relatively homogeneously in the liver [81–83], and therefore, SVS approaches are considered representative for a reliable quantification of hepatic lipids. However, it should be mentioned that Cowin and co-workers showed significant differences between different regions in right and left lobe in their study [26].

The total fat signal can be accurately modeled as the sum of the areas of the CH, CH$_2$, CH$_3$, and other peaks. The FSF can be defined as follows:

$$\text{FSF} = A_{\text{fat}}/(A_{\text{water}} + A_{\text{fat}})$$
$$A_{\text{fat}} = A_{\text{CH}} + A_{\text{CH2}} + A_{\text{CH3}} + A_{\text{others}}$$

where A is the spectral peak area for the indexed proton species, with A_{fat} equal to $A_{CH} + A_{CH2} + A_{CH3} + A_{\text{others}}$.

MR spectroscopy takes into account the multiple spectral components of fatty acids and, in theory, is the most direct method of fat quantification.

Good reproducibility of liver MR spectroscopy has been determined, revealing high intraindividual correspondence in repeated measurements [26, 82, 84].

Nevertheless, in vivo MR spectroscopy requires a skilled operator to correctly perform the examination, process the data, and interpret the results. The major disadvantage of MR spectroscopic fat quantification is the complexity of data analysis. The spectroscopy software generally requires a large amount of user input; is prone to bias; and may not permit accurate, reproducible quantification of all fat signal components. Setting up initial prior knowledge parameters in the software can be quite challenging and requires substantial expertise in proton MR spectroscopy.

Standard MR spectroscopic pulse sequences have relatively long minimum echo times, which may introduce T2 weighting between the signals of individual peaks and, unless T2 relaxation effects are taken into account, may lead to quantification errors. Also, shimming the MR spectroscopy voxel tends to be time-consuming and may lengthen overall examination time considerably.

In proton MR spectroscopy, each frequency peak represents a distinct proton species with its own longitudinal and transverse relaxation rates, and the relative signal strength of the peaks can vary depending on repetition time and echo time. Thus, a FSF calculated from a single spectrum obtained with a particular repetition time and echo time can be biased. If MR spectroscopy is performed, it should use a relatively long repetition time (≥ 3 s) to minimize T1 effects and acquire data at multiple echo times to measure and correct for T2 decay. This ensures complete or near-complete recovery of the longitudinal magnetization of most biologic tissues, including the water and fat components of a fatty liver, and generates spectra which are independent of T1 relaxation effects. However, T2 relaxation causes the intensity of individual signal components to decay at different rates, and the relative spectral peak areas vary as a function of echo time.

At multiecho MR spectroscopy with a long repetition time, bias can be removed by minimizing T1 effect and, peak by peak, correcting for T2 effect. The T2 value of each spectral peak is calculated assuming a monoexponential signal decay, and the relative proton density of each peak is estimated by extrapolating the T2 decay curve to an echo time of 0. The fat fraction calculated in this way is independent of T1 and, for every peak, is corrected for T2.

MR spectroscopy is considered the most accurate noninvasive technique for fat quantification. If both T1 and T2 relaxation effects are taken into account with use of a long repetition time and multiecho acquisition protocol, respectively, MR spectroscopy allows direct proton-density quantification of the water and fat chemical moieties, from which molecular triglyceride concentration (in micromoles per milligram) can be calculated.

It is important to note in this context that percentage values of liver steatosis from MR spectroscopy studies (and from MR imaging studies as well) are different from percentage values from histological examinations. The reason is that MR techniques determine volume fractions of lipids in the liver tissue rather than the percentage of hepatocytes showing visible fat droplets in the microscopic view [30].

Conclusion

In conclusion, several methods for noninvasive detection and quantification of liver fat are available in daily clinical practice. Although liver biopsy is still regarded as the gold standard in the assessment of fatty infiltration of the liver, since it provides a distinction between simple steatosis and steatohepatitis based on pathological assessment of the specimen, it is an invasive and a potentially risky method for the patient. At the same time, it allows a subjective estimation of the fat content in a small tissue sample, which is not necessarily representative for the whole organ.

Ultrasound is widely available, noninvasive, and cost-efficient but also operator-dependent and relatively insensitive for lower grades of fatty infiltration. Computed tomography permits a semiquantitative assessment of hepatic steatosis but is in turn influenced by iron overload and exposes patients to ionizing radiation. MRI offers imaging and spectroscopic methods for quantification of liver fat with high accuracy without many of the drawbacks related to the above mentioned imaging techniques. Despite its benefits, it is not as widely available as the other methods and is technically challenging. It seems however that MR techniques are especially helpful in many clinical settings, where mainly quantitative data of lipid content in liver are important.

References

1. Schwimmer JB, Deutsch R, Kahen T, Lavine JE, Stanley C, Behling C (2006) Prevalence of fatty liver in children and adolescents. Pediatrics 118:1388–1393
2. Angulo P (2007) Obesity and nonalcoholic fatty liver disease. Nutr Rev 65:S57–S63
3. Adams LA, Lymp JF, St Sauver J et al (2005) The natural history of nonalcoholic fatty liver disease: a population-based cohort study. Gastroenterology 129:113–121
4. Stefan N, Kantartzis K, Haring HU (2008) Causes and metabolic consequences of fatty liver. Endocr Rev 29:939–960
5. Stefan N, Kantartzis K, Machann J et al (2008) Identification and characterization of metabolically benign obesity in humans. Arch Intern Med 168:1609–1616
6. Kotronen A, Westerbacka J, Bergholm R, Pietilainen KH, Yki-Jarvinen H (2007) Liver fat in the metabolic syndrome. J Clin Endocrinol Metab 92:3490–3497
7. Roden M (2006) Mechanisms of disease: hepatic steatosis in type 2 diabetes—pathogenesis and clinical relevance. Nat Clin Pract Endocrinol Metab 2:335–348
8. Stefan N, Hennige AM, Staiger H et al (2006) Alpha2-Heremans-Schmid glycoprotein/fetuin-A is associated with insulin resistance and fat accumulation in the liver in humans. Diabetes Care 29:853–857
9. Reinehr T, Roth CL (2008) Fetuin-A and its relation to metabolic syndrome and fatty liver disease in obese children before and after weight loss. J Clin Endocrinol Metab 93:4479–4485
10. Farrell GC, Larter CZ (2006) Nonalcoholic fatty liver disease: from steatosis to cirrhosis. Hepatology 43:S99–S112
11. Kleiner DE, Brunt EM, Van Natta M et al (2005) Design and validation of a histological scoring system for nonalcoholic fatty liver disease. Hepatology 41:1313–1321
12. Lefkowitch JH (2005) Morphology of alcoholic liver disease. Clin Liver Dis 9:37–53
13. Reuben A (2007) Alcohol and the liver. Curr Opin Gastroenterol 23:283–291

14. Reuben A (2008) Alcohol and the liver. Curr Opin Gastroenterol 24:328–338
15. Wanless IR, Shiota K (2004) The pathogenesis of nonalcoholic steatohepatitis and other fatty liver diseases: a four-step model including the role of lipid release and hepatic venular obstruction in the progression to cirrhosis. Semin Liver Dis 24:99–106
16. Valls C, Iannacconne R, Alba E et al (2006) Fat in the liver: diagnosis and characterization. Eur Radiol 16:2292–2308
17. Oleszczuk A, Spannbauer M, Tannapfel A et al (2007) Regenerative capacity differs between micro and macrovesicular hepatic steatosis. Exp Toxicol Pathol 59:205–213
18. Hamer OW, Aguirre DA, Casola G, Lavine JE, Woenckhaus M, Sirlin CB (2006) Fatty liver: imaging patterns and pitfalls. Radiographics 26:1637–1653
19. Fishbein M, Castro F, Cheruku S et al (2005) Hepatic MRI for fat quantitation: its relationship to fat morphology, diagnosis, and ultrasound. J Clin Gastroenterol 39:619–625
20. Chalasani N, Wilson L, Kleiner DE, Cummings OW, Brunt EM, Unalp A (2008) Relationship of steatosis grade and zonal location to histological features of steatohepatitis in adult patients with non-alcoholic fatty liver disease. J Hepatol 48:829–834
21. Strassburg CP, Manns MP (2006) Approaches to liver biopsy techniques—revisited. Semin Liver Dis 26:318–327
22. Minervini MI, Ruppert K, Fontes P et al (2009) Liver biopsy findings from healthy potential living liver donors: reasons for disqualification, silent diseases and correlation with liver injury tests. J Hepatol 50:501–510
23. Nagai S, Fujimoto Y, Kamei H, Nakamura T, Kiuchi T (2009) Mild hepatic macrovesicular steatosis may be a risk factor for hyperbilirubinaemia in living liver donors following right hepatectomy. Br J Surg 96:437–444
24. Limanond P, Raman SS, Lassman C et al (2004) Macrovesicular hepatic steatosis in living related liver donors: correlation between CT and histologic findings. Radiology 230:276–280
25. Vetelainen R, van Vliet A, Gouma DJ, van Gulik TM (2007) Steatosis as a risk factor in liver surgery. Ann Surg 245:20–30
26. Cowin GJ, Jonsson JR, Bauer JD et al (2008) Magnetic resonance imaging and spectroscopy for monitoring liver steatosis. J Magn Reson Imaging 28:937–945
27. Wieckowska A, McCullough AJ, Feldstein AE (2007) Noninvasive diagnosis and monitoring of nonalcoholic steatohepatitis: present and future. Hepatology 46:582–589
28. Karcaaltincaba M, Akhan O (2007) Imaging of hepatic steatosis and fatty sparing. Eur J Radiol 61(1):33–43
29. Perez NE, Siddiqui FA, Mutchnick MG et al (2007) Ultrasound diagnosis of fatty liver in patients with chronic liver disease: a retrospective observational study. J Clin Gastroenterol 41:624–629
30. Schwenzer NF, Springer F, Schraml C, Stefan N, Machann J, Schick F (2009) Non-invasive assessment and quantification of liver steatosis by ultrasound, computed tomography and magnetic resonance. J Hepatol 51(3):433–445
31. Joseph AE, Saverymuttu SH, Al-Sam S, Cook MG, Maxwell JD (1991) Comparison of liver histology with ultrasonography in assessing diffuse parenchymal liver disease. Clin Radiol 43:26–31
32. Mottin CC, Moretto M, Padoin AV et al (2004) The role of ultrasound in the diagnosis of hepatic steatosis in morbidly obese patients. Obes Surg 14:635–637
33. Lall CG, Aisen AM, Bansal N, Sandrasegaran K (2008) Nonalcoholic fatty liver disease. Am J Roentgenol 190(4):993–1002
34. Shannon A, Alkhouri N, Carter-Kent C et al (2011) Ultrasonographic quantitative estimation of hepatic steatosis in children With NAFLD. J Pediatr Gastroenterol Nutr 53(2):190–195
35. Strauss S, Gavish E, Gottlieb P, Katsnelson L (2007) Interobserver and intraobserver variability in the sonographic assessment of fatty liver. Am J Roentgenol 189:W320–W323
36. Mancini M, Prinster A, Annuzzi G et al (2009) Sonographic hepatic-renal ratio as indicator of hepatic steatosis: comparison with 1H magnetic resonance spectroscopy. Metabolism 58 (12):1724–1730

37. Xia MF, Yan HM, He WY et al (2012) Standardized ultrasound hepatic/renal ratio and hepatic attenuation rate to quantify liver fat content: an improvement method. Obesity (Silver Spring) 20(2):444–452
38. Webb M, Yeshua H, Zelber-Sagi S et al (2009) Diagnostic value of a computerized hepatorenal index for sonographic quantification of liver steatosis. Am J Roentgenol 192 (4):909–914
39. Graif M, Yanuka M, Baraz M et al (2000) Quantitative estimation of attenuation in ultrasound video images: correlation with histology in diffuse liver disease. Invest Radiol 35:319–324
40. Ma X, Holalkere NS, Kambadakone RA, Mino-Kenudson M, Hahn PF, Sahani DV (2009) Imaging-based quantification of hepatic fat: methods and clinical applications. Radiographics 29(5):1253–1277
41. Lee SW, Park SH, Kim KW et al (2007) Unenhanced CT for assessment of macrovesicular hepatic steatosis in living liver donors: comparison of visual grading with liver attenuation index. Radiology 244(2):479–485
42. Kodama Y, Ng CS, Wu TT et al (2007) Comparison of CT methods for determining the fat content of the liver. Am J Roentgenol 188(5):1307–1312
43. Mazhar SM, Shiehmorteza M, Sirlin CB (2009) Noninvasive assessment of hepatic steatosis. Clin Gastroenterol Hepatol 7(2):135–140
44. Park SH, Kim PN, Kim KW et al (2006) Macrovesicular hepatic steatosis in living liver donors: use of CT for quantitative and qualitative assessment. Radiology 239:105–112
45. Shores NJ, Link K, Fernandez A et al (2011) Non-contrasted computed tomography for the accurate measurement of liver steatosis in obese patients. Dig Dis Sci 56(7):2145–2151
46. Piekarski J, Goldberg HI, Royal SA, Axel L, Moss AA (1980) Difference between liver and spleen CT numbers in the normal adult: its usefulness in predicting the presence of diffuse liver disease. Radiology 137:727–729
47. Johnston RJ, Stamm ER, Lewin JM, Hendrick RE, Archer PG (1998) Diagnosis of fatty infiltration of the liver on contrast-enhanced CT: limitations of liver-minus-spleen attenuation difference measurements. Abdom Imaging 23(4):409–415
48. Jacobs JE, Birnbaum BA, Shapiro MA et al (1998) Diagnostic criteria for fatty infiltration of the liver on contrast-enhanced helical CT. Am J Roentgenol 171:659–664
49. Panicek DM, Giess CS, Schwartz LH (1997) Qualitative assessment of liver for fatty infiltration on contrast-enhanced CT: is muscle a better standard of reference than spleen? J Comput Assist Tomogr 21:699–705
50. Flohr TG, McCollough CH, Bruder H et al (2006) First performance evaluation of a dual-source CT (DSCT) system. Eur Radiol 16:256–268
51. Wang B, Gao Z, Zou Q, Li L (2003) Quantitative diagnosis of fatty liver with dual-energy CT. An experimental study in rabbits. Acta Radiol 44:92–97
52. Raptopoulos V, Karellas A, Bernstein J, Reale FR, Constantinou C, Zawacki JK (1991) Value of dual-energy CT in differentiating focal fatty infiltration of the liver from low-density masses. Am J Roentgenol 157:721–725
53. Mendler MH, Bouillet P, Le Sidaner A et al (1998) Dual-energy CT in the diagnosis and quantification of fatty liver: limited clinical value in comparison to ultrasound scan and single-energy CT, with special reference to iron overload. J Hepatol 28:785–794
54. Birnbaum BA, Hindman N, Lee J, Babb JS (2007) Multi-detector row CT attenuation measurements: assessment of intra- and interscanner variability with an anthropomorphic body CT phantom. Radiology 242:109–119
55. Cassidy FH, Yokoo T, Aganovic L et al (2009) Fatty liver disease: MR imaging techniques for the detection and quantification of liver steatosis. Radiographics 29(1):231–260
56. Park HW, Kim YH, Cho ZH (1988) Fast gradient-echo chemical-shift imaging. Magn Reson Med 7:340–345
57. Chen Q, Stock KW, Prasad PV, Hatabu H (1999) Fast magnetic resonance imaging techniques. Eur J Radiol 29:90–100

58. Hussain HK, Chenevert TL, Londy FJ et al (2005) Hepatic fat fraction: MR imaging for quantitative measurement and display—early experience. Radiology 237:1048–1055

59. Alustiza JM, Castiella A (2008) Liver fat and iron at in-phase and opposed-phase MR imaging. Radiology 246:641

60. Westphalen AC, Qayyum A, Yeh BM et al (2007) Liver fat: effect of hepatic iron deposition on evaluation with opposed-phase MR imaging. Radiology 242:450–455

61. Fishbein MH, Gardner KG, Potter CJ, Schmalbrock P, Smith MA (1997) Introduction of fast MR imaging in the assessment of hepatic steatosis. Magn Reson Imaging 15:287–293

62. Levenson H, Greensite F, Hoefs J et al (1991) Fatty infiltration of the liver: quantification with phase-contrast MR imaging at 1.5 T vs biopsy. Am J Roentgenol 156:307–312

63. Mitchell DG, Kim I, Chang TS et al (1991) Fatty liver: chemical shift phase-difference and suppression magnetic resonance imaging techniques in animals, phantoms, and humans. Invest Radiol 26:1041–1052

64. Borrello JA, Chenevert TL, Meyer CR, Aisen AM, Glazer GM (1987) Chemical shift-based true water and fat images: regional phase correction of modified spin-echo MR images. Radiology 164:531–537

65. Glover GH, Schneider E (1991) Three-point Dixon technique for true water/fat decomposition with B0 inhomogeneity correction. Magn Reson Med 18:371–383

66. Glover GH (1991) Multipoint Dixon technique for water and fat proton and susceptibility imaging. J Magn Reson Imaging 1:521–530

67. Lodes CC, Felmlee JP, Ehman RL et al (1989) Proton MR chemical shift imaging using double and triple phase contrast acquisition methods. J Comput Assist Tomogr 13:855–861

68. Rybicki FJ, Chung T, Reid J, Jaramillo D, Mulkern RV, Ma J (2001) Fast three-point Dixon MR imaging using low-resolution images for phase correction: a comparison with chemical shift selective fat suppression for pediatric musculoskeletal imaging. Am J Roentgenol 177:1019–1023

69. Szumowski J, Coshow WR, Li F, Quinn SF (1994) Phase unwrapping in the three-point Dixon method for fat suppression MR imaging. Radiology 192:555–561

70. Szumowski J, Coshow W, Li F, Coombs B, Quinn SF (1995) Double-echo three-point-Dixon method for fat suppression MRI. Magn Reson Med 34:120–124

71. Yeung HN, Kormos DW (1986) Separation of true fat and water images by correcting magnetic field inhomogeneity in situ. Radiology 159:783–786

72. Reeder SB, Pineda AR, Wen Z et al (2005) Iterative decomposition of water and fat with echo asymmetry and least-squares estimation (IDEAL): application with fast spin-echo imaging. Magn Reson Med 54:636–644

73. Reeder SB, McKenzie CA, Pineda AR et al (2007) Water–fat separation with IDEAL gradient-echo imaging. J Magn Reson Imaging 25:644–652

74. Mehta SR, Thomas EL, Bell JD, Johnston DG, Taylor-Robinson SD (2008) Non-invasive means of measuring hepatic fat content. World J Gastroenterol 14:3476–3483

75. Guiu B, Petit JM, Loffroy R et al (2009) Quantification of liver fat content: comparison of triple-echo chemical shift gradient-echo imaging and in vivo proton MR spectroscopy. Radiology 250:95–102

76. Mitchell DG, Stolpen AH, Siegelman ES, Bolinger L, Outwater EK (1996) Fatty tissue on opposed-phase MR images: paradoxical suppression of signal intensity by paramagnetic contrast agents. Radiology 198:351–357

77. Qayyum A, Goh JS, Kakar S, Yeh BM, Merriman RB, Coakley FV (2005) Accuracy of liver fat quantification at MR imaging: comparison of out-of-phase gradient-echo and fat-saturated fast spin-echo techniques—initial experience. Radiology 237:507–511

78. Cotler SJ, Guzman G, Layden-Almer J, Mazzone T, Layden TJ, Zhou XJ (2007) Measurement of liver fat content using selective saturation at 3.0 T. J Magn Reson Imaging 25:743–748

79. Bottomley PA (1987) Spatial localization in NMR spectroscopy in vivo. Ann N Y Acad Sci 508:333–348

80. Frahm J, Bruhn H, Gyngell ML, Merboldt KD, Hanicke W, Sauter R (1989) Localized high-resolution proton NMR spectroscopy using stimulated echoes: initial applications to human brain in vivo. Magn Reson Med 9:79–93

81. Machann J, Stefan N, Schick F (2008) ^{1}H MR spectroscopy of skeletal muscle, liver and bone marrow. Eur J Radiol 67:275–284

82. Machann J, Thamer C, Schnoedt B et al (2006) Hepatic lipid accumulation in healthy subjects: a comparative study using spectral fat-selective MRI and volume-localized ^{1}H-MR spectroscopy. Magn Reson Med 55:913–917

83. Thomas EL, Hamilton G, Patel N et al (2005) Hepatic triglyceride content and its relation to body adiposity: a magnetic resonance imaging and proton magnetic resonance spectroscopy study. Gut 54:122–127

84. Szczepaniak LS, Nurenberg P, Leonard D et al (2005) Magnetic resonance spectroscopy to measure hepatic triglyceride content: prevalence of hepatic steatosis in the general population. Am J Physiol Endocrinol Metab 288:E462–E468

Multimodality Approach to Detection and Characterization of Hepatic Hemangiomas

Rajan T. Gupta and Daniele Marin

Abstract Hemangiomas are the most common benign hepatic tumor and represent a common incidental finding on routine imaging examinations of the liver. The majority of hemangiomas demonstrate classical imaging findings on grayscale ultrasound (US), multidetector-row computed tomography (MDCT), and magnetic resonance imaging (MRI). The classic appearance on contrast-enhanced cross-sectional imaging is that of centripetal nodular enhancement with progressive fill-in of the lesion over time with conventional extracellular CT and MR contrast agents. With the advent of new gadolinium-based MR contrast agents such as hepatocyte-specific contrast agents and blood pool contrast agents, some different appearances of hemangiomas are possible and familiarity with these appearances is critical in making the correct diagnosis. There are also variants of the typical hemangioma, including the flash-filling hemangioma, giant hemangioma, sclerosed or hyalinized hemangioma, as well as hemangiomas occurring on a background of hepatic steatosis and cirrhosis. Again, knowledge of these variant types of hemangiomas can prevent against misdiagnosis of these lesions in the clinical setting.

Introduction

Hemangioma represents the most common benign liver tumor, with an estimated incidence of 5–20 % in the general population [1, 2]. Although hemangiomas can occur in both sexes at all ages, middle-aged women are more frequently affected, perhaps reflecting the causative effect of female sex hormones. Hepatic hemangiomas are commonly identified in asymptomatic patients during imaging studies performed for unrelated reasons [3]. In a minority of cases, larger lesions may

R.T. Gupta, M.D. (✉) • D. Marin, M.D.
Department of Radiology, Duke University Medical Center, DUMC Box 3808, Durham, NC 27710, USA
e-mail: rajan.gupta@duke.edu; daniele.marin@duke.edu

A.S. El-Baz et al. (eds.), *Abdomen and Thoracic Imaging: An Engineering & Clinical Perspective*, DOI 10.1007/978-1-4614-8498-1_5,
© Springer Science+Business Media New York 2014

produce signs and symptoms related to mass effect, such as a palpable upper abdominal mass, abdominal discomfort, or pain. Sudden onset with acute pain owing to spontaneous or traumatic rupture has been sporadically described in larger lesions. Large hemangiomas can also present with thrombocytopenia and consumptive coagulopathy.

Pathology

Hemangiomas are usually solitary, although lesions can be multiple in approximately 15 % of cases. At macroscopic inspection, hemangiomas appear as flat, well-demarcated, lesions of red-blue color, varying in size from few millimeters to several centimeters [4]. Hepatic hemangiomas are more commonly peripheral in location, with a subcapsular location in many cases. Organized thrombi, fibrosis, and calcification may be noted at gross inspection, particularly in the central area of larger lesions. Occasionally, hemangiomas may undergo sclerosis, presenting as a firm, gray-white nodule of fibrous tissue at inspection (the so-called sclerosed hemangioma). Microscopically, hemangiomas consist of a tangle of cavernous vascular spaces lined by flattened endothelium with minimal intervening connective tissue.

Association of hemangioma with other benign liver lesions, such as focal nodular hyperplasia and hepatic adenoma, has been described.

Imaging Techniques

Ultrasonography

At grayscale ultrasonography (US), the typical appearance of hepatic hemangioma is a homogeneous, hyperechoic mass with well-defined margins and posterior acoustic enhancement [5] (Fig. 1). Occasionally, small (<3 cm) lesions may demonstrate a thick hyperechoic rim with a central hypoechoic region that, according to some authors, may correspond to areas of previous hemorrhagic necrosis, scarring, or myxomatous changes [6]. Color and power Doppler imaging has limited value in the diagnosis of hepatic hemangioma.

Contrast-enhanced US can be performed to help in the characterization of hemangiomas that present equivocal imaging findings on grayscale US [7]. Hemangiomas demonstrate a reproducible and specific enhancement pattern at contrast-enhanced US that closely reflect the imaging appearance with other contrast-enhanced cross-sectional imaging techniques. This includes demonstration of peripheral nodular enhancement of the lesion in the arterial phase that expand in a centripetal pattern during the hepatic venous phase and beyond, often progressing

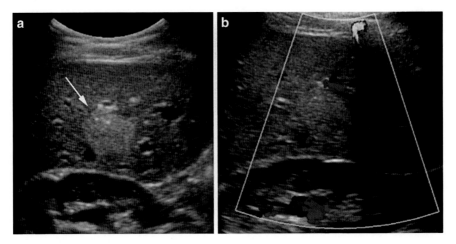

Fig. 1 Forty-five-year-old female who presents for liver ultrasound due to right upper abdominal pain. (**a**) Grayscale sonographic image demonstrates a hyperechoic lesion in the right hepatic lobe (*arrow*) with imaging characteristics of a hemangioma. (**b**) Color Doppler imaging of the lesion demonstrates no substantial central flow within the lesion and some peripheral vascularity. This appearance is common for hemangiomas and is likely related to the very slow blood flow within the central dilated vascular channels of the lesion

to complete fill-in of the lesion. Although the speed of enhancement may differ in different lesions, likely reflecting differences in the circulatory time of contrast material in various lesions, the degree of enhancement of the peripheral nodules classically exceeds that of the adjacent liver parenchyma. This sustained enhancement, in which the lesion has an echogenicity equal to or greater than that of the liver through the portal venous phase and beyond, is a requisite for a confident diagnosis. Complete enhancement does not always occur, especially in large lesions, which often undergo central thrombosis of the intralesional venous sinusoids.

Multidetector-Row Computed Tomography

With the recent advent of multidetector-row computed tomography (MDCT) scanners, substantial anatomic volumes can be acquired within a short scan time, with submillimeter section thickness and virtually no penalty in increased radiation dose. With the assistance of test bolus or bolus-tracking techniques for monitoring the contrast material bolus transit time, these technologic advances have led to image acquisition during peak vascular enhancement, with almost uniform enhancement along the entire scanned volume, reduced motion artifacts, and the capability to generate high-resolution reformations in any desired plane. As a result, the incidental detection of hemangiomas in an asymptomatic patient has become a relatively common finding during radiologic examinations performed for indications other than evaluation for liver disease. The main goal of imaging is to firmly establish a diagnosis to avoid unnecessary, aggressive management and to minimize patient distress and anxiety.

At precontrast CT, hemangiomas manifest as a hypoattenuating lesion relative to the liver. However, because hemangioma may be hyperattenuating in the setting of diffuse fatty liver disease, lesion's isoattenuation relative to aorta and intrahepatic vessels has been used as a more reliable finding for the diagnosis of hemangioma on precontrast CT. Central calcifications may occur in giant hemangiomas and are better identified before intravenous administration of iodinated contrast media. At contrast-enhanced CT, hemangiomas classically show peripheral, discontinuous, nodular enhancement, with centripetal progression of lesion's enhancement (Fig. 2). The enhancing areas of hemangiomas are isoattenuating to aorta during the hepatic arterial phase and to the blood pool during the hepatic venous and delayed phases [5, 8]. When all typical criteria are observed, lack of complete lesion enhancement on the delayed-phase imaging should not dissuade from the diagnosis of hemangioma. Giant hemangiomas usually lack complete enhancement on delayed-phase imaging owing to thrombosis or sclerosis of the central portion of the tumor or insufficient imaging time to complete lesion filling.

In rare circumstances, small hemangiomas may demonstrate very slow enhancement following administration of intravenous contrast material, showing persistent hypoattenuation relative to the liver on all imaging phases. This uncommon finding has been explained as a slow fill-in of the large vascular spaces of the lesion. Identification of even a single small focus of enhancement (also known as the "central dot sign") allows confident diagnosis in some of these atypical lesions [9].

Magnetic Resonance Imaging

With the recent introduction of fast imaging sequences that allow breath-hold imaging of the liver during short acquisition times (less than 20 s), and substantial reduction in the cost per examination, MR imaging has been advocated by some as the modality of choice in the noninvasive work-up of focal liver lesions. Compared to CT, major advantages of MR imaging include higher soft-tissue contrast resolution, greater sensitivity to intravenous gadolinium-based contrast agents, excellent depiction of fluid-containing structures (e.g., the biliary tree, gallbladder, or cystic lesions), and the absence of ionizing radiation. The latter attribute of MR imaging can be an effective strategy to limit the radiation burden from CT examinations, most importantly in children and young adults.

Most hepatic hemangiomas can be confidently characterized at MR imaging, using a combination of T2-weighted and T1-weighted sequences before and after contrast material administration. The hallmark of these lesions is the very long T1 and long T2 values derived from the blood pooling within the vascular channels,

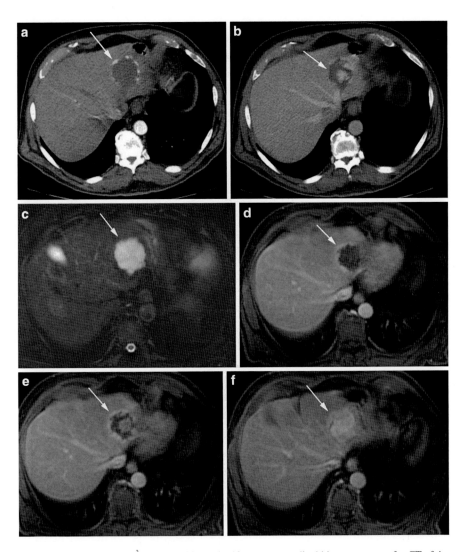

Fig. 2 Seventy-four-year-old male with no significant past medical history presents for CT of the abdomen and pelvis for follow-up of a pancreatic cystic lesion. (**a, b**) Axial contrast-enhanced CT (CECT) images of the liver, acquired in the arterial and portal venous phases, respectively, show a left hepatic lobe lesion with progressive centripetal nodular enhancement (*arrow*). (**c**) Axial T2-weighted (T2W) 3D fast spin echo (FSE) with fat saturation (FS) reveals the lesion in the left hepatic lobe to be homogeneously hyperintense (*arrow*) relative to the background liver. (**d, e**) Axial T1-weighted (T1W) 3D gradient recalled echo (GRE) images with FS acquired in the portal venous and late venous phases (approximately 70 and 120 s after administration of Gd-BOPTA, respectively) show progressive peripheral nodular enhancement within the lesion (*arrow*), similar to the CT enhancement pattern. (**f**) Axial T1W 3D GRE with FS image acquired in the equilibrium phase (approximately 5 min after administration of Gd-BOPTA) shows complete fill-in of the lesion (*arrow*), confirming that it is a hemangioma

which is responsible for lesion's low signal intensity on T1-weighted images and markedly high signal intensity on T2-weighted images. Many studies have emphasized the importance of acquiring heavily T2-weighted imaging in the diagnosis of hepatic hemangiomas at imaging [10]. While the use of fat suppression increases the conspicuity of these lesions on T2-weighted images, this improvement is not necessarily accompanied by an improved characterization of these liver tumors. Although less common, metastases from neuroendocrine tumors, mucinous colorectal cancer, and, occasionally, breast cancer may also manifest high signal intensity on T2-weighted images, thus mimicking hepatic hemangioma. Although correlation with lesion characteristics on other imaging sequences allows confident differential diagnosis, percutaneous lesion biopsy may be still necessary in a small number of indeterminate cases.

With recent advances in technology, diffusion-weighted (DW) MR imaging has been increasingly used in abdominal imaging applications, including liver lesion characterization. Black-blood diffusion images (using low b values) allow suppression of the signal from the intrahepatic vessels improving detection of focal liver lesions, as compared to a standard T2-weighted sequence. This improvement is related to improved image contrast and lack of blurring with single-shot spin-echo echo-planar imaging [11]. In addition, preliminary evidence suggests that the diffusion information provided by imaging at higher b values may also improve characterization of focal liver lesion. Previous studies showed that hepatic hemangioma (and simple hepatic cysts) manifest a typical imaging pattern on DW imaging, including high signal intensity on DW images at low b values (e.g., $b = 0$ s/mm^2), strong signal intensity on DW images at high b value (e.g., $b = 500$ s/mm^2), and substantially higher ADC values relative to the background liver. This appearance is remarkably different from that of malignant liver neoplasms, which classically demonstrate mild to moderate hyperintensity on DW images at low b values, which persist at higher b values. ADC values of malignant liver neoplasms are also typically lower compared with those of the surrounding liver parenchyma.

The enhancement pattern of hepatic hemangioma on contrast-enhanced MR imaging using conventional extracellular gadolinium contrast agents is comparable to that seen at multiphasic contrast-enhanced CT (Fig. 3). The greater sensitivity of MR to intravenous gadolinium-based contrast agents, particularly with the use of optimized fat-suppressed T1-weighted sequences, may improve visualization of smaller peripheral foci of enhancement in small hemangiomas with slow flow and conceivably result in better characterization of these lesions.

More recently, the introduction into daily clinical practice of hepatocyte-specific gadolinium-based MR contrast media has offered the possibility to simultaneously provide information of a standard MR imaging examination with the additional functional data during the liver-specific phase of imaging. The combination of functional and morphologic information improves the detection and characterization of liver tumors. Gadolinium benzyloxypropionictetraacetate, or Gd-BOPTA (MultiHance, Bracco Diagnostics Inc., Princeton, NJ), and gadolinium ethoxybenzyl diethylenetriaminepentaacetic acid, or Gd-EOB-DTPA (Eovist/Primovist,

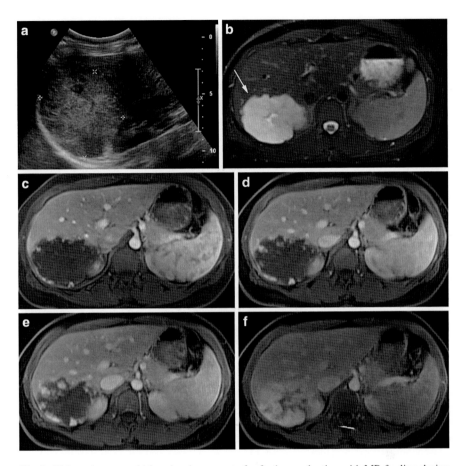

Fig. 3 Thirty-nine-year-old female who presents for further evaluation with MR for liver lesion seen on ultrasound. (**a**) Grayscale sonographic image demonstrates a hyperechoic lesion in the right hepatic lobe without any evidence of a hypoechoic halo. (**b**) Axial T2W FSE with FS image prior to the administration of Gd-BOPTA reveals a large hyperintense lesion in the posterior segment of the right hepatic lobe (*arrow*) with area of increased signal centrally. (**c**) Axial T1W 3D GRE with FS image acquired in the arterial phase (approximately 25 s after administration of Gd-BOPTA) shows peripheral nodular enhancement with this lesion. (**d**) Axial T1W 3D GRE with FS image acquired in the portal venous phase (approximately 70 s after administration of Gd-BOPTA) shows some increased nodular enhancement of the lesion. (**e**) Axial T1W 3D GRE with FS image acquired in the late venous phase (approximately 3 min after administration of Gd-BOPTA) shows the lesion to progressively fill in with contrast. (**f**) Axial T1W 3D GRE with FS image acquired in the delayed phase (approximately 10 min after administration of Gd-BOPTA) shows the lesion to nearly completely fill with contrast. This is the characteristic appearance of hemangiomas using extracellular contrast agents. Note that the blood pool remains bright on these images, compatible with the fact that hemangiomas will follow the signal of the blood pool

Bayer Pharmaceuticals, Wayne, NJ), are two commonly used examples of this category of contrast agent. Gd-EOB-DTPA, which was approved by US Food and Drug Administration (FDA) for focal liver lesion detection and characterization in 2008, has a substantially greater uptake by the hepatocyte and excretion through the hepatobiliary pathway compared to Gd-BOPTA (approximately 50 % compared to 5 % in patients without impaired hepatic function) [12]. This contrast dynamic characteristics result in stronger and more rapid enhancement of the liver and biliary system during the hepatobiliary phase, with a peak enhancement approximately 20 min after contrast material injection [13–15] compared to 40–120 min for gadobenate dimeglumine [16–20]. While early imaging during the hepatobiliary phase is beneficial, theoretically leading to improved workflow considerations [21] and possible decreased examination costs due to the potential ability to characterize lesions in a single MR time slot, the rapid hepatic uptake of Gd-EOB-DTPA may potentially create a pitfall in the assessment of the enhancement pattern of hepatic hemangiomas [22]. Recent evidence has shown that these lesions are commonly hypointense relative to the high signal intensity background liver on images acquired during the delayed and, in some cases, the portal venous phases. This appearance can be confusing and be potentially misinterpreted as evidence of washout within a lesion, a finding commonly associated with other liver lesions such as adenoma, hepatocellular carcinoma, and liver metastases (Figs. 4, 5, and 6). Consideration of imaging characteristics during the other imaging phases of enhancement as well as on the precontrast T2-weighted and DW images is critical for the confident differential diagnosis of these hepatic lesions.

Of note, our preliminary clinical experience suggests that the enhancement pattern of hemangiomas in not substantially altered from conventional extracellular agents when using some of the newer blood pool contrast agents, such as gadofosveset trisodium (Ablavar, Lantheus Medical Imaging, North Billerica, Massachusetts, USA) (Fig. 7). Hemangiomas are again noted to follow the blood pool, a finding consistent with the pathologic composition of hemangioma, constituted almost entirely by multiple vascular channels with minimal interposed connective fibrous tissue.

Nuclear Medicine

Technetium-99m pertechnetate-labeled red blood cell scintigraphy was previously regarded as a reference standard for the diagnosis of hemangiomas. Because hemangiomas have increased blood volume relative to the liver, they manifest as a hot spot on blood pool scanning (30–50 min after injection of the radiotracer).

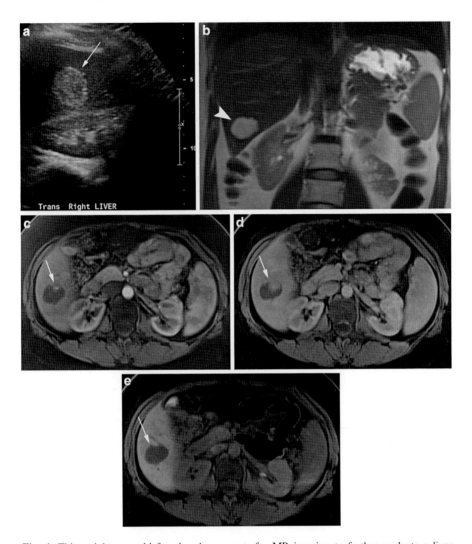

Fig. 4 Thirty-eight-year-old female who presents for MR imaging to further evaluate a liver lesion seen on ultrasound. (**a**) Grayscale sonographic image demonstrates a homogeneously hyperechoic lesion in the right hepatic lobe (*arrow*) adjacent to the right kidney. (**b**) Coronal half-Fourier acquisition single-shot turbo spin-echo (HASTE) images reveal a corresponding well-circumscribed T2 hyperintense lesion in the right hepatic lobe (*arrowhead*). (**c**) Axial T1W 3D GRE with FS image acquired in the arterial phase (approximately 25 s after administration of Gd-EOB-DTPA) shows a small amount of peripheral nodular enhancement within this lesion (*arrow*). (**d**) Axial T1W 3D GRE with FS image acquired in the portal venous phase (approximately 70 s after administration of Gd-EOB-DTPA) shows additional high signal within the lesion, corresponding to progressive enhancement (*arrow*). (**e**) Axial T1W 3D GRE with FS image acquired in the hepatocyte phase (approximately 10 min after administration of Gd-EOB-DTPA) shows the lesion to be hypointense to the liver parenchyma (*arrow*), related to the decreased dose of Gd-EOB-DTPA versus conventional extracellular agents, shorter plasma half-life as well as increased hepatobiliary uptake [22]

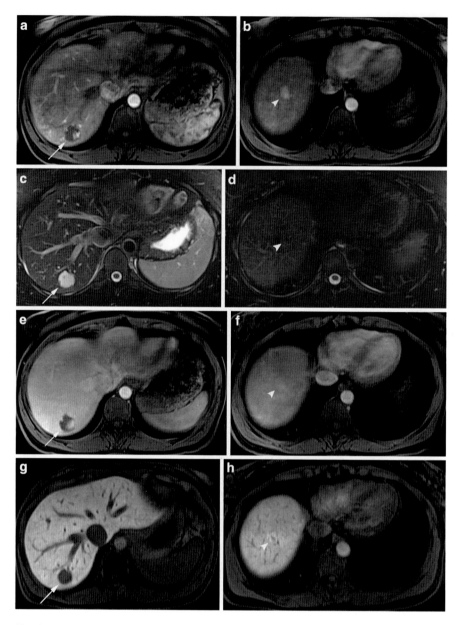

Fig. 5 Thirty-eight-year-old female who presents abdominal MR examination due to elevated total serum bilirubin. (**a, b**) Axial T1W 3D GRE with FS images at two different levels of the liver acquired in the arterial phase (approximately 25 s after administration of Gd-EOB-DTPA) shows a lesion with peripheral nodular enhancement in the posterior segment of the right hepatic lobe (*arrow*) as well as a hyperenhancing lesion in the hepatic dome (*arrowhead*). (**c, d**) Axial T2W FSE with FS images at the same levels in the liver reveals a hyperintense lesion in the right hepatic lobe (*arrow*) corresponding to the first lesion on the arterial phase images. Note that the

Atypical Appearances of Hepatic Hemangioma

Flash-Filling Hemangioma

Small hemangiomas frequently have atypical features that make their diagnosis challenging at imaging. In approximately 40 % of cases, small hemangiomas can demonstrate vivid and uniform enhancement during the late hepatic arterial phase (the so-called flash-filling hemangioma pattern) [23]. This appearance is frequently associated with lack of lesion's isoattenuation relative to the blood pool during contrast-enhanced imaging. These imaging findings may overlap with those of other hypervascular liver tumors (most notably, hepatocellular carcinoma and hypervascular liver metastases [24]), thus precluding a confident diagnosis of these lesions at imaging (Fig. 8). Demonstration of vivid and homogeneous enhancement similar to the aorta during the late hepatic arterial phase and high signal intensity on T2-weighted MR images provide useful diagnostic clues in the diagnosis of these challenging lesions. Areas of transient perilesional enhancement during the hepatic arterial phase caused by arteriovenous shunt have been described in association with flash-filling hemangiomas and other hypervascular liver tumors [25].

Grayscale US has a limited role in the diagnosis of flash-filling hemangiomas. A large number of lesions demonstrate atypical imaging findings (i.e., hypoechoic appearance relative to the liver). On the other hand, the high temporal resolution of real-time contrast-enhanced US may allow better visualization of small peripheral areas of early enhancement with rapid centripetal progression in some flash-filling hemangiomas, thus allowing confident characterization of the lesion.

Fig. 5 (continued) hyperenhancing focus more superiorly in the liver is not definitely seen on the T2W image (*arrowhead* denoting the region of interest). (**e, f**) Axial T1W 3D GRE with FS images acquired in the portal venous phase (approximately 70 s after administration of Gd-EOB-DTPA) shows more nodular enhancement of the first lesion in the posterior segment of the right hepatic lobe and near isointensity of the second lesion in the hepatic dome to the surrounding parenchyma. (**g, h**) Axial T1W 3D GRE with FS image acquired in the hepatocyte phase (approximately 15 min after administration of Gd-EOB-DTPA) shows the posterior right hepatic lesion to be relatively hypointense compared to the hyperintense liver parenchyma. The lesion in the hepatic dome is mildly hyperintense to the surrounding liver parenchyma. Based on these signal characteristics, the lesion in the posterior right hepatic lobe represents a hemangioma and the lesion in the hepatic dome represents focal nodular hyperplasia (FNH). The FNH is hyperintense to the liver parenchyma in the delayed hepatocyte phase with Gd-EOB-DTPA due to the fact that it contains hepatocytes and malformed biliary ductules [21]

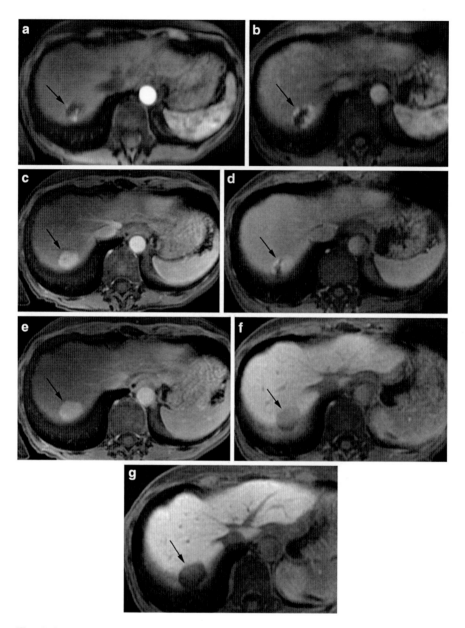

Fig. 6 Seventy-five-year-old female with history of gastrointestinal stromal tumor and liver lesion. MR examinations were performed with Gd-BOPTA and Gd-EOB-DTPA approximately 7 months apart. (**a**) Axial T1W 3D GRE with FS image acquired in the arterial phase (approximately 25 s) after administration of Gd-BOPTA shows a hypointense lesion in the right hepatic lobe with centripetal nodular enhancement (*arrow*). (**b**) Axial T1W 3D GRE with FS image acquired in the arterial phase (approximately 25 s after administration of Gd-EOB-DTPA) shows similar findings as the study using Gd-BOPTA. (**c, d**) Axial T1W 3D GRE with FS images

Giant Hemangioma

Hemangiomas measuring 4 cm or greater in diameter have been also referred to as giant hemangiomas [5, 26]. Giant hemangiomas are often heterogeneous on all imaging modalities, due to internal areas of hemorrhage, thrombosis, extensive hyalinization, liquefaction, and fibrosis. After intravenous administration of contrast material, the typical early, peripheral, globular enhancement of hemangiomas is generally observed in these large lesions, allowing confident diagnosis at imaging. Incomplete contrast enhancement of the lesion on delayed imaging is not uncommon due to central cleft-like area of cystic degeneration and stellate fibrous septa (Fig. 7).

Sclerosed or Hyalinized Hemangioma

Sclerosed or hyalinized hemangiomas are rare [27, 28]. Some authors have suggested that hyalinized hemangiomas represent an end stage of hemangioma involution [29]. Sclerosed hemangiomas demonstrate atypical features, including minimal increase in T2 signal intensity and lack of early enhancement on dynamic contrast-enhanced image (Figs. 9 and 10). Diagnosis cannot always be made at imaging, and liver biopsy may occasionally be necessary for definitive confirmation.

Fig. 6 (continued) acquired in the portal venous phase approximately 90 s after administration of Gd-BOPTA (**c**) and Gd-EOB-DTPA (**d**) shows the lesion to demonstrate progressive fill-in with contrast (*arrow*). Some relatively increased signal noted in the liver parenchyma is also noted on (**d**). (**e, f**) Axial T1W 3D GRE with FS image acquired approximately 8 min after administration of Gd-BOPTA (**e**) shows the lesion to be substantially brighter than the adjacent liver parenchyma. This is in contrast to the findings on (**f**) which is an axial T1W 3D GRE with FS image acquired approximately 8 min after administration of Gd-EOB-DTPA. In this image, the lesion is noted to be hypointense to the adjacent liver parenchyma. Note also the markedly different signal of the hepatic parenchyma between the comparison studies acquired at similar time points with the two contrast agents. This likely indicates that the liver is in the hepatocyte phase with Gd-EOB-DTPA (**f**) but not yet in the hepatocyte phase with Gd-BOPTA (**e**). This is an expected finding based on the pharmacokinetics of these contrast agents. (**g**) Axial T1W 3D GRE with FS image acquired 21 min after administration of Gd-EOB-DTPA shows the effects of the negative contrast to noise ratio of the hemangioma to the liver in the delayed phase (figures and legend reprinted from European Journal of Radiology, Volume 81(10), Gupta RT, Marin D, Boll DT, et al., "Hepatic hemangiomas: Difference in enhancement pattern on 3T MR imaging with gadobenate dimeglumine versus gadoxetate disodium," pp. 2457–2462, Copyright 2012 with permission of Elsevier)

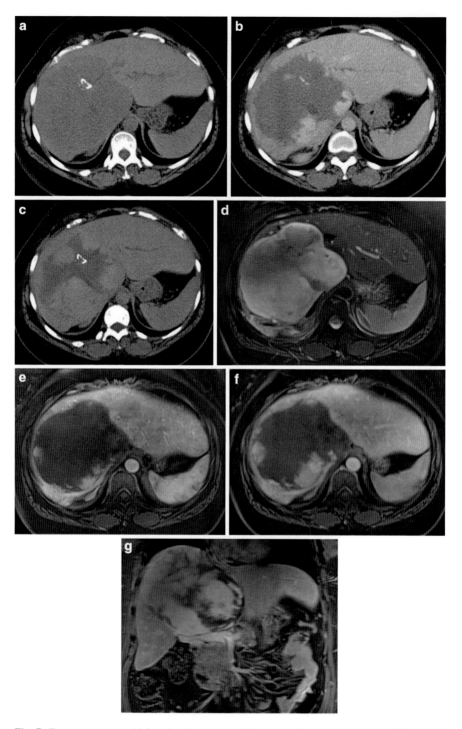

Fig. 7 Forty-seven-year-old female who presents follow-up of liver lesion seen on CT. Patient underwent MR examination approximately 6 months after initial scan using gadofosveset trisodium (Ablavar, Lantheus Medical Imaging, North Billerica, Massachusetts, USA). (a) Noncontrast-enhanced axial CT (NECT) of the liver reveals a large low-attenuation lesion in the

Hemangioma in Fatty Liver

Severe fatty liver may confound the assessment of the enhancement pattern of focal hepatic lesions. In severe fatty liver, the attenuation of hemangioma may reverse to even hyperattenuation relative to the liver on precontrast CT. Hemangiomas may also be accompanied by a focal spared zone as seen in malignant tumors in fatty liver. On grayscale US, this finding could mimic the hypoechoic halo seen in metastatic liver lesions. MR imaging with the combination of T2-weighted imaging and fat-suppressed T1-weighted imaging before and following administration of gadolinium contrast agents almost invariably allows confident diagnosis of hemangioma in the setting of diffuse fatty liver disease.

Hemangioma in Cirrhotic Liver

Hemangiomas are less commonly detected or are generally smaller when occurring within a cirrhotic liver [27]. This observation is likely related to a progressive shrinkage of the lesion in the fibrotic liver. Capsular retraction may occur over peripheral hemangiomas that regressed [27, 28]. Larger lesions typically demonstrate classic imaging characteristics, thus allowing confident diagnosis at cross-section imaging. Smaller hemangiomas, on the other hand, frequently demonstrate an atypical enhancement pattern, including early homogenous enhancement during the arterial phase, which could not always reflect the blood pool on more delayed imaging phases. In the setting of cirrhosis, this appearance is concerning for hepatocellular carcinoma. The multiparametric characteristics of MR imaging could help in the differential diagnosis of these challenging cases.

Fig. 7 (continued) right hepatic lobe with some central dystrophic calcifications. (**b**) Axial CECT of the liver, acquired in the portal venous phase, shows the right hepatic lobe lesion with centripetal nodular enhancement. (**c**) Axial CECT of the liver, acquired approximately 5 min after administration of intravenous contrast media, shows the right hepatic lobe lesion to be progressively filling in with contrast, confirming the diagnosis of hemangioma. (**d**) Axial T2W 3D FSE with FS image prior to the administration of intravenous gadolinium reveals a large homogenously hyperintense lesion in the right hepatic lobe. (**e**) Axial T1W 3D GRE with FS image acquired in the arterial phase (approximately 25 s after administration of gadofosveset) shows the lesion in the right hepatic lobe beginning to show subtle peripheral nodular enhancement. (**f**) Axial T1W 3D GRE with FS image acquired in the portal venous phase (approximately 70 s after administration of gadofosveset) shows the lesion in the right hepatic lobe demonstrating increased peripheral nodular enhancement. (**g**) Coronal T1W 3D GRE with FS acquired approximately 11 min after administration of gadofosveset shows puddling of contrast and near-complete fill-in of the right hepatic lobe lesion. Note how the lesion follows the blood pool as is characteristic of hemangiomas

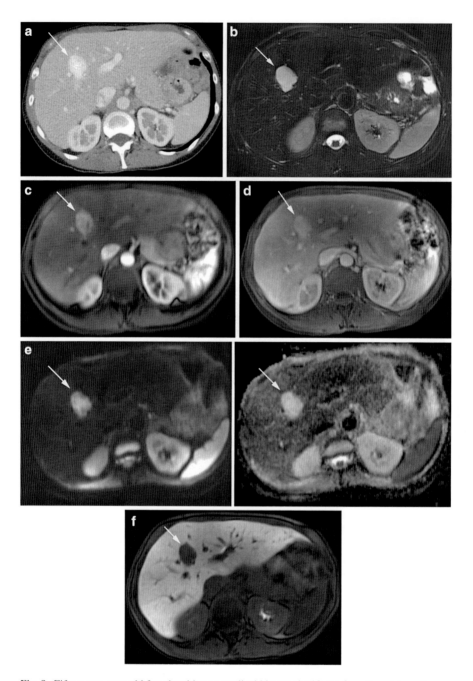

Fig. 8 Fifty-seven-year-old female with past medical history significant for colorectal carcinoma presents with an incidental hepatic lesion seen on CT. (**a**) Axial CECT images of the liver, acquired in the portal venous phase, shows a hyperdense lesion in the right hepatic lobe (*arrow*). (**b**) Axial T2W FSE with FS image reveals the lesion in the right hepatic lobe to be

Recommendations for Follow-up or Surgery

Hepatic hemangiomas virtually never cause complications and should be treated conservatively. In rare circumstances, larger lesions may become clinically symptomatic, requiring surgical enucleation or resection. If the appearance is classic for hepatic hemangioma at US, no further evaluation should be required in patients without a history of underlying malignancy. MR imaging should represent the modality of choice for the characterization of atypical lesions or lesions that occur in the setting of chronic liver disease or if there is any clinical concerns for metastatic disease.

Despite the high diagnostic accuracy of imaging in the diagnosis of hepatic hemangioma, a minority of lesions may still remain indeterminate due to atypical findings at imaging. In the absence of prior evidence of stability, 6–12 months imaging follow-up is frequently recommended in patients with a low index of suspicion for liver malignancy. While the large majority of hemangiomas demonstrate a stable appearance at follow-up, a slight interval increase in size of a lesion has been occasionally described and should not be necessarily regarded as evidence of malignancy. Percutaneous liver biopsy may be indicated for the definitive diagnosis of atypical hemangiomas in patients at high risk for malignancy. This procedure is not associated with an increased complication rate when compared to percutaneous biopsy of other liver lesions.

Conclusions

Hemangiomas are the most common benign hepatic tumor and represent a common incidental finding on routine imaging examinations of the liver. The majority of lesions demonstrate typical imaging finding on grayscale US and no further investigation is needed in patients with low risk of malignancy. In some cases, further

---

Fig. 8 (continued) well circumscribed, mildly lobulated, and homogeneously hyperintense (*arrow*). (**c**) Axial T1W 3D GRE with FS image acquired in the arterial phase (approximately 25 s after administration of Gd-EOB-DTPA) shows the lesion to be hyperenhancing (*arrow*). (**d**) Axial T1W 3D GRE with FS image acquired in the portal venous phase (approximately 70 s after administration of Gd-EOB-DTPA) shows the lesion to be persistently hyperintense to the surrounding liver parenchyma (*arrow*). (**e**) Axial diffusion-weighted imaging (DWI) and corresponding automated diffusion coefficient (ADC) maps show the lesion to not demonstrate restricted diffusion, but rather "T2 shine through" as it is bright on both DWI and ADC. This supports the diagnosis of a flash-filling hemangioma as opposed to a metastatic focus, which would likely demonstrate restricted diffusion (i.e., bright on DWI, dark on ADC maps). (**f**) Axial T1W 3D GRE with FS image acquired in the hepatocyte phase (approximately 15 min after administration of Gd-EOB-DTPA) shows the lesion to be hypointense to the liver parenchyma (*arrow*), compatible with the expected appearance of a hemangioma using this MR contrast agent

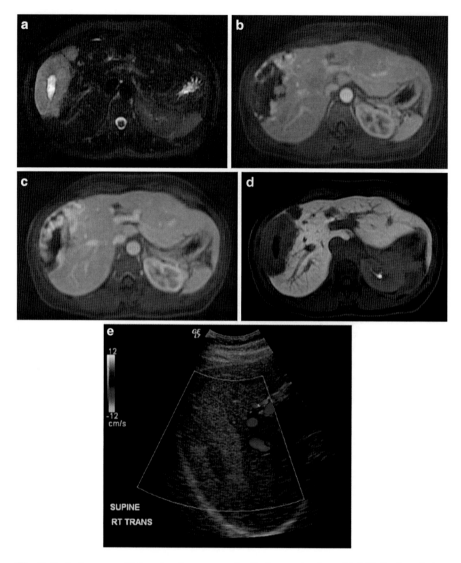

Fig. 9 Forty-five-year-old female who presents for further evaluation with MR for liver lesion seen on CT. (**a**) Axial T2W 3D FSE with FS image prior to the administration of Gd-EOB-DTPA reveals a large hyperintense lesion in the right hepatic lobe with area of increased signal centrally. This T2 hyperintensity with focal-increased signal centrally can be seen with sclerosing hemangiomas. (**b**) Axial T1W 3D GRE with FS image acquired in the arterial phase (approximately 25 s after administration of Gd-EOB-DTPA) shows peripheral nodular enhancement that is characteristic of hemangiomas. (**c**) Axial T1W 3D GRE with FS image acquired in the portal venous phase (approximately 70 s after administration of Gd-EOB-DTPA) shows progressive fill-in of the lesion. (**d**) Axial T1W 3D GRE with FS image acquired in the hepatocyte phase (approximately 25 min after administration of Gd-EOB-DTPA) shows the lesion to be relatively hypointense compared to the hyperintense liver parenchyma. The central portion of the lesion is more hypointense compared to the surrounding lesion, likely related to sclerosis. (**e**) Grayscale sonographic image with color Doppler signal of the lesion demonstrates similar morphology as noted on the MR

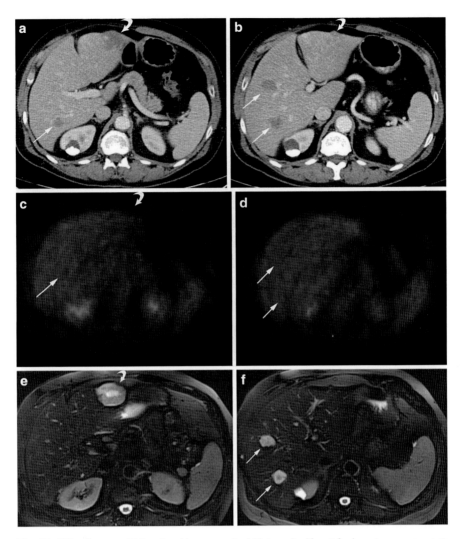

Fig. 10 Fifty-six-year-old female with past medical history significant for breast cancer presents for further evaluation of hepatic lesions seen on PET-CT. Patient underwent MR examination immediately after initial PET-CT scan using Gd-EOB-DTPA for lesion characterization. (**a, b**) Axial CECT images through the liver in the portal venous phase demonstrate at least four low-attenuation lesions in the liver, including a lesion in the lateral segment of the left hepatic lobe (*curved arrow*) and two lesions in the posterior segment of the right hepatic lobe (*straight arrows*). (**c, d**) Positron-emission tomographic (PET) images at the same level as the CT images in (**a, b**) reveal no substantial FDG uptake in the expected location of the left hepatic lobe lesion (*curved arrow*) and right hepatic lobe lesions (*straight arrows*). (**e, f**) Axial T2W 3D FSE with FS image reveals the lesions to be hyperintense. (**g**) Axial T1W 3D GRE with FS image acquired in the portal venous phase (approximately 70 s after administration of Gd-EOB-DTPA) shows the lesions with peripheral nodular enhancement. (**h**) Axial T1W 3D GRE with FS image acquired in the late venous phase (approximately 3 min after administration of Gd-EOB-DTPA) shows the lesions with progressive fill-in of contrast. (**i, j**) Axial T1W 3D GRE with FS images acquired in the hepatocyte phase (approximately 15 min after administration of Gd-EOB-DTPA) shows the lesions to be hypointense to the hyperintense liver parenchyma. Note that the left hepatic lobe lesion (*curved arrow*) is more hypointense centrally which could suggest that this is a sclerosing hemangioma. This is in contrast to the lesions in the right hepatic lobe (*straight arrows*) which look more homogeneously hypointense; this likely indicates that these lesions are not sclerosed and are following the blood pool signal

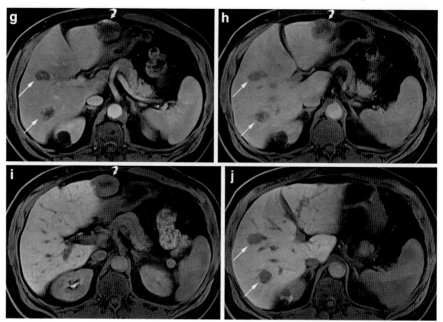

Fig. 10 (continued)

imaging investigation is necessary to establish an accurate diagnosis of hemangioma. In the absence of a relative or absolute contraindication, MR imaging is generally preferred over contrast-enhanced multiphase CT, due to the higher diagnostic performance and lack of ionizing radiation exposure to the patient. Radiologists should be familiar with the potentially confusing enhancement pattern of hepatic hemangiomas at contrast-enhanced MR using new liver-specific contrast agents. Imaging follow-up or percutaneous liver biopsy is occasionally necessary for the diagnosis of the small number of lesions that remain indeterminate at imaging.

References

1. Karhunen P (1986) Benign hepatic tumours and tumour like conditions in men. J Clin Pathol 39(2):183–188
2. Jang H, Kim T, Lim H et al (2003) Hepatic hemangioma: atypical appearances on CT, MR imaging, and sonography. AJR Am J Roentgenol 180(1):135–141
3. Mergo PJ, Ros PR (1998) Benign lesions of the liver. Radiol Clin North Am 36(2):319–331
4. Ishak KJ et al (2001) Benign mesenchymal tumors and pseudotumors. In: Ishak KJ, Goodman ZD, Stocsker JT (eds) Tumours of the liver and intrahepatic bile ducts. Armed Forces Institute of Pathology, Washington, DC, pp 113–114
5. Nelson RC, Chezmar JL (1990) Diagnostic approach to hepatic hemangiomas. Radiology 176(1):11–13
6. Moody A, Wilson S (1993) Atypical hepatic hemangioma: a suggestive sonographic morphology. Radiology 188(2):413–417

7. Lee JY, Choi BI, Han JK et al (2002) Improved sonographic imaging of hepatic hemangioma with contrast-enhanced coded harmonic angiography: comparison with MR imaging. Ultrasound Med Biol 28(3):287–295
8. Quinn SF, Benjamin G (1992) Hepatic cavernous hemangiomas: simple diagnostic sign with dynamic bolus CT. Radiology 182(2):545–548
9. Jang HJ, Choi B, Kim T et al (1998) Atypical small hemangiomas of the liver: "bright dot" sign at two-phase spiral CT. Radiology 208(2):543–548
10. Itai Y, Ohtomo K, Furui S et al (1985) Noninvasive diagnosis of small cavernous hemangioma of the liver: advantage of MRI. AJR Am J Roentgenol 145(6):1195–1199
11. Taouli B, Koh DM (2010) Diffusion-weighted MR imaging of the liver. Radiology 254 (1):47–66
12. Dahlstrom N, Persson A, Albiin N et al (2007) Contrast-enhanced magnetic resonance cholangiography with Gd-BOPTA and Gd-EOB-DTPA in healthy subjects. Acta Radiol 48 (4):362–368
13. Carlos RC, Hussain HK, Song JH et al (2002) Gadolinium-ethoxybenzyl-diethylenetriamine pentaacetic acid as an intrabiliary contrast agent: preliminary assessment. AJR Am J Roentgenol 179(1):87–92
14. Hamm B, Staks T, Muhler A et al (1995) Phase I clinical evaluation of Gd-EOB-DTPA as a hepatobiliary MR contrast agent: safety, pharmacokinetics, and MR imaging. Radiology 195 (3):785–792
15. Carlos RC, Branam JD, Dong Q et al (2002) Biliary imaging with Gd-EOB-DTPA: is a 20-minute delay sufficient? Acad Radiol 9(11):1322–1325
16. Tschirch FT, Struwe A, Petrowsky H et al (2008) Contrast-enhanced MR cholangiography with Gd-EOB-DTPA in patients with liver cirrhosis: visualization of the biliary ducts in comparison with patients with normal liver parenchyma. Eur Radiol 18(8):1577–1586
17. Lim JS, Kim MJ, Jung YY et al (2005) Gadobenate dimeglumine as an intrabiliary contrast agent: comparison with mangafodipir trisodium with respect to non-dilated biliary tree depiction. Korean J Radiol 6(4):229
18. Petersein J, Spinazzi A, Giovagnoni A et al (2000) Focal liver lesions: evaluation of the efficacy of gadobenate dimeglumine in MR imaging-a multicenter phase III clinical study. Radiology 215(3):727–736
19. Seale M, Catalano O, Saini S et al (2009) Hepatobiliary-specific MR contrast agents: role in imaging the liver and biliary tree. Radiographics 29(6):1725–1748
20. Schneider G, Maas R, Schultze KL et al (2003) Low-dose gadobenate dimeglumine versus standard dose gadopentetate dimeglumine for contrast-enhanced magnetic resonance imaging of the liver: an intra-individual crossover comparison. Invest Radiol 38(2):85
21. Gupta RT, Iseman CM, Leyendecker JR et al (2012) Diagnosis of focal nodular hyperplasia with MRI: multicenter retrospective study comparing gadobenate dimeglumine to gadoxetate disodium. AJR Am J Roentgenol 199(1):35–43
22. Gupta RT, Marin D, Boll DT et al (2012) Hepatic hemangiomas: difference in enhancement pattern on 3T MR imaging with gadobenate dimeglumine versus gadoxetate disodium. Eur J Radiol 81(10):2457–2462
23. Hanafusa K, Ohashi I, Himeno Y et al (1995) Hepatic hemangioma: findings with two-phase CT. Radiology 196(2):465–469
24. Larson RE, Semelka RC, Bagley AS et al (1994) Hypervascular malignant liver lesions: comparison of various MR imaging pulse sequences and dynamic CT. Radiology 192 (2):393–399
25. Byun JH, Kim TK, Lee CW et al (2004) Arterioportal shunt: prevalence in small hemangiomas versus that in hepatocellular carcinomas 3 cm or smaller at two-phase helical CT. Radiology 232(2):354–360
26. Valls C, Rene M, Gil M et al (1996) Giant cavernous hemangioma of the liver: atypical CT and MR findings. Eur Radiol 6(4):448–450

27. Brancatelli G, Federle MP, Blachar A et al (2001) Hemangioma in the cirrhotic liver: diagnosis and natural history. Radiology 219(1):69–74
28. Vilgrain V, Boulos L, Vullierme MP et al (2000) Imaging of atypical hemangiomas of the liver with pathologic correlation. Radiographics 20(2):379–397
29. Soyer P, Bluemke DA, Vissuzaine C et al (1994) CT of hepatic tumors: prevalence and specificity of retraction of the adjacent liver capsule. AJR Am J Roentgenol 162(5):1119–1122

Biography

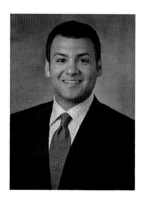

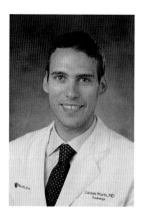

Rajan T. Gupta, M.D., and **Daniele Marin, M.D.**, are both Assistant Professors of Radiology in the Division of Abdominal Imaging at Duke University Medical Center in Durham, North Carolina. Dr. Gupta also serves as the Director of the Abdominal Imaging Fellowship Program at Duke. Liver MRI is an area of clinical and research interest for both Drs. Gupta and Marin, particularly the use of the newer hepatobiliary-specific MR contrast agents and their application in clinical practice for diagnosis and characterization of focal liver lesions.

Ultrasound Liver Surface and Textural Characterization for the Detection of Liver Cirrhosis

Ricardo Ribeiro, Rui T. Marinho, Jasjit Suri, and J. Miguel Sanches

Abstract This chapter addresses the problem of liver cirrhosis classification via ultrasound imaging. For this classification problem, a liver semiautomatic contour segmentation algorithm to characterize the morphology and a textural feature extraction scheme for the characterization of liver parenchyma are proposed. Phase congruency is used to enhance liver contour and help medical doctor in the inspection of liver surface. The regularity of the enhanced liver contour is characterized from geometrical features that are used together with US textural features in the classification process. The classification of the proposed method is tested by using *support vector machine*, *Bayesian*, Parzen and *k-nearest neighbor* classifiers and their performance are compared. The *Bayes* classifier outperformed the compared classifiers, attaining an overall accuracy of 87.22 %, with a detection rate of 88.52 % and 86.11 % for the non-cirrhotic and cirrhotic class, respectively.

R. Ribeiro (✉)
Institute for Systems and Robotics/Instituto Superior Técnico, Escola Superior de Tecnologia da Saúde de Lisboa, Lisboa, Portugal
e-mail: ricardo.ribeiro@estesl.ipl.pt

R.T. Marinho
Liver Unit, Department of Gastroenterology and Hepatology, Hospital de Santa Maria, Medical School of Lisbon, Lisbon, Portugal
e-mail: rui.marinho@mail.telepac.pt

J. Suri
Point of Care Division-Healthcare Solutions Global Biomedical Technologies, Inc., Roseville, CA, USA
e-mail: jsuri@comcast.net

J.M. Sanches
Instituto de Sistemas e Robótica, Instituto Superior Técnico, Torre Norte, 6 Piso, Av. Rovisco Pais, 1049-001 Lisboa, Portugal
e-mail: jmrs@ist.utl.pt

A.S. El-Baz et al. (eds.), *Abdomen and Thoracic Imaging: An Engineering & Clinical Perspective*, DOI 10.1007/978-1-4614-8498-1_6,
© Springer Science+Business Media New York 2014

Introduction

Chronic liver disease (CLD) is an oncogenic disease where most likely developments, if not treated, are *hepatocellular carcinoma* (HCC) or death. Major progress in the knowledge and management of liver disease has been observed in the past 30 years; however, still 29 million people in the European Union suffer from a chronic liver condition [1].

Cirrhosis is the end-stage of every CLD [2], defined as the histological development of regenerative nodules surrounded by fibrous bands in response to chronic liver injury [3] and has a variety of clinical manifestations and complications [4]. The most probable outcome of cirrhosis is HCC, which is the fifth most common cause of cancer in Europe [1]. There are 14–26 new cirrhosis cases per 100,000 inhabitants per year or an estimated 170,000 deaths per year [1].

Four leading causes of cirrhosis have been identified, namely chronic alcohol consumption, chronic viral hepatitis B, chronic viral hepatitis C, and *non-alcoholic fatty liver disease* (NAFLD). If detected in time, each of these causes is responsive to treatment. The problem is, in part, related to the fact that CLD is characterized by a silent and asymptomatic phase. Thus, the solution relies on early detection and staging.

Liver fibrosis results from a repeated healing response, leading to an abnormal fibrogenesis (connective tissue production and deposition). The progression rate of fibrosis depends on the disease cause, environmental and host factors. Cirrhosis is an advanced stage of liver fibrosis that is accompanied by distortion of the hepatic vasculature. It leads to hemodynamic changes, compromising exchange between hepatic sinusoids and hepatocytes [3]. The major clinical consequences of cirrhosis are impaired hepatocyte (liver) function, an increased intrahepatic resistance (portal hypertension) and the development of HCC [3].

As the disease progresses, portal pressure increases and liver function decreases, resulting in the development of ascites, portal hypertensive gastrointestinal (GI) bleeding, encephalopathy, and jaundice. The development of any of these complications marks the transition from a *compensated* to a *decompensated* phase [2].

Decompensated cirrhosis is defined by the presence of ascites, variceal bleeding, encephalopathy, and/or jaundice. Ascites is considered the landmark sign of decompensated cirrhosis. Transition from a compensated to a decompensated stage occurs at a rate of 57 % per year [2].

The survival of patients with compensated cirrhosis (> 12 years) is significantly longer than that of decompensated patients (~ 2 years). Death in compensated patients occurs mostly after transition to a decompensated stage [2].

In CLD, clinical and biochemical evaluation are often irrelevant. Thus, *liver biopsy* (LB) is considered a key role for the diagnosis and follow-up of CLD, particularly in HCV chronic infected patients. The role of LB is to confirm the diagnosis of chronic hepatitis, to assess the necro-inflamatory activity (grading) and the severity of fibrosis (staging), to exclude another hepatopathy or an associated disease, and to certify the diagnosis of cirrhosis (when present) [5]. However, LB is

Table 1 Liver surface contour characteristics used to detect cirrhosis from US images

Class	US findings
Normal	Hyperechoic straight [10, 12] and regular [12] line, with a thickness less than 1 mm [10].
Cirrhosis	Liver surface with diffuse irregularity [10].
	Nodular aspect of the liver surface [13].
	Multiple nodular irregularities on the ventral liver freely mobile, during respiratory excursion [9].
	Dotted or irregular line and/or heterogenous liver parenchyma [12].
	Curved line superior to 2.04 cm in a straight 2 cm segment line [11].

an imperfect technique, highly invasive, prone to errors and clinical complications, with a sensibility ranging 80 % [6]. Also, practical issues are also raised, since the size of a biopsy specimen, which should be > 2.5 cm in length and between 1.2 to 1.8 mm in diameter, representing only a 1/50000 of the total liver mass.

Clinical trends are leading to alternative, simple, and noninvasive methods. A direct consequence of this trend is a decrease in the performed LB of more than 90 %. The main advantages of these methods are the good cost/effective relation and wide accessibility. Among the noninvasive methods, ultrasound (US) is considered very promising and it is typically a frontline exam.

Cirrhosis is detected on US images by liver surface coarseness, portal mean flow velocity from Doppler, and changes of the liver parenchyma observed on the speckle textural characteristics [7]. As in clinical examination, US liver surface coarseness is a reliable indicator [8], directly correlated with the gross appearance of the cirrhotic liver, as seen at laparoscopy [9]. This morphological feature is best observed when ascites is present or when a high-frequency linear transducer (5–12 MHz) is used [9–13].

Most of the proposed US CAD systems for cirrhosis detection are based on linear transducers instead of the convex ones. Linear US transducers are able to achieve higher frequencies and thus increase image spatial resolution, enhancing the perception of image edges and details (e.g., liver surface) [14, 15], while reducing speckle noise. Nevertheless, Gaiani et al. [8] has reported the ability to detect this surface irregularity with low-frequency convex transducer (3.5–5 MHz). This possibility will be further studied in this work, since low-frequency convex transducers are normally used in abdominal US exams, performed in clinical practice.

Visual inspection of liver surface is the preferred approach in the majority of the studies. Table 1 summarizes the visual features used to characterize liver surface contour via US images. As referred in [16], these approaches are subjective, non-reproducible, and qualitative. Berzigotti et al. [11] is an example of the extraction of quantitative features, directly from the US image, with a dedicated software, for cirrhosis contour.

The goal of this chapter is to provide objective US morphological assessment of liver surface and textural information of the liver parenchyma for the detection of liver cirrhosis. The method is based on common US images (e.g., acquired with a low-frequency convex transducer), to be as reproducible as possible. To enhance liver surface details on US images, while avoiding noise amplification, a novel enhancement algorithm based on a phase congruency (PC) map computed from a *de-speckled* field is presented. This topic will be further discussed in section "Methods".

To increase the robustness of the method, US textural features extracted from the liver parenchyma are combined with the morphological ones. Textural analysis of US liver parenchyma is a powerful tool for CLD diagnosis and staging. Image texture may be viewed as a global pattern arising from a deterministic or random repetition of local subpatterns or primitives. The structure resulting from this repetition is very useful for discriminating between the contents of the image of a complex scene [17].

Common features used for liver parenchyma analysis are: (1) textural based, e.g. first order statistic [18–20], co-occurrence matrix [20–22], wavelet transform [21, 23] and (2) depth attenuation and intensity related, e.g. attenuation along the depth [20, 24, 25] and backscattering [20, 24, 25] parameters and coefficients. In this chapter, we introduce the monogenic decomposition as a feature extractor from US images of the liver parenchyma, as well as the co-occurrence matrix.

A binomial classification is then considered, cirrhosis or non-cirrhosis, and several classifiers are used to assess the discriminative power of the selected features: (1) the *support vector machine* (SVM), (2) the *Bayes classifier*, and (3) the *k-nearest neighbor* (kNN). Several figures of merit were computed to assess and compare the performance of each classifier.

The remainder of this chapter is organized as follows. "Methods" formulates the problem discussed and it is organized in the following topics: "US Image Pre-processing" introduces the pre-processing algorithm used, the "Liver Surface Enhancement" describes the methods applied to enhance liver surface, with particular relevance to the use of phase congruency edge detection on the *de-speckle* field; "Liver Surface Detection and Feature Extraction" describes the algorithm used to detect liver surface and posterior extraction of morphological and textural features; and "Feature Selection and Classification Procedure" outlines the feature selection and classification techniques. The experimental results are given in the "Results" section and discussed in the section "Discussion and conclusions" which also summarizes the chapter.

Methods

In this section, a detailed description of the algorithms and methods used to formulate the problem is presented. In short, by using PC algorithm, a liver surface map is developed from the *de-speckle* field. Based on this, contour points are collected and morphological features extracted for cirrhosis detection. The performances of the detection algorithm are tested with four different classifiers.

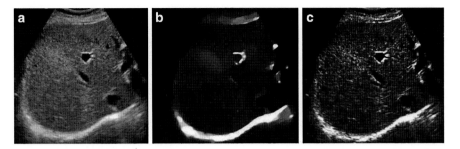

Fig. 1 Decomposition procedure of US liver parenchyma. (**a**) Observed *B-mode* US image. Estimated (**b**) *de-speckle* and (**c**) *speckle* fields

US Image Pre-processing

To eliminate the influence of the US scanner and operator, US images are normalized and decomposed. The procedure described in [26] to separate the textural and intensity information within US images is here adopted. In this, an estimation of the *radio frequency* (RF) raw data is firstly done based on physical considerations about the data generation process, namely, by taking into account the US scanner parameters tuned by the clinician during the US exam.

The estimated RF image is decomposed in *de-speckled* and *speckle* fields according to the following model [26]

$$y(i,j) = x(i,j)\eta(i,j), \tag{1}$$

where $\eta(i,j)$ are considered independent and identically distributed (i.i.d.) random variables with *Rayleigh* distribution. This image describes the noise and textural information and is called *speckle* field. In this model, the noise is multiplicative in the sense that its variance, observed in the original image, depends on the underlying signal, $x(i,j)$. Figure 1 illustrates an example of the decomposition methodology in a US liver image of a patient with decompensated cirrhosis.

Liver Surface Enhancement

Speckle noise present in US images decreases the discriminative perception of meaningful details, namely, edges. Besides this difficulty, in clinical practice the perceived liver capsule and the adjacent overlying membranous structures (peritoneum, transverse fascia, pre-peritoneal fat) are not always clear and irregularities due to subfascial or sub-peritoneal pathology may be falsely described as abnormalities of the liver surface [9].

To reduce these drawbacks, the use of the *de-speckle* field is proposed to outline liver surface. This field is obtained in a Bayesian framework using a total variation edge preserving prior, with the ability to maintain the tissue interfaces and, therefore, the geometric shape of liver boundaries [26].

PC-based algorithm for edge detection is used to study liver surface detection accuracy. The results obtained with *de-speckle* images outperform the ones obtained with the common methods based on the B-mode US images, directly provided by the US scanner. Next a short description of the phase congruency algorithm [27] is given.

Contour regularity/smothness can be characterized from the PC map. PC is related to the local energy and it is invariant to image brightness and contrast [28]. Local Energy Model postulates that features are perceived at point in an image where the Fourier components are maximally in phase [29]. The local Fourier components at a location, x, in a signal will each have an amplitude $A_m(x)$ and a phase angle $\phi_m(x)$.

The magnitude of the vector from the origin to the end point is the *local energy*, $|E(x)|$. The measure of PC developed by Morrone [30] is:

$$PC = \frac{|E(x)|}{\sum_m A_m(x)} \tag{2}$$

If all Fourier components are in phase, all the complex vectors would be aligned and the ratio of $|E(x)| = \sum_m A_m(x)$ would be 1. If there is no PC, the ratio falls to a minimum of 0 [29].

The wavelet transform is used to obtain frequency information to a point in a signal. To preserve phase information, linear-phase filters must be used like non-orthogonal wavelets that are in symmetric/anti-symmetric quadrature pairs. Let $\eta(x)$, M_s^e and M_s^o denote the one-dimensional signal, even-symmetric (cosine) and odd-symmetric (sine) wavelets at scale s, respectively. The response vector, formed by the responses of each quadrature pair of filters, is as follows,

$$[e_s(x), o_s(x)] = [\eta(x) * M_s^e, \eta(x) * M_s^o]. \tag{3}$$

The amplitude of the transform at a given wavelet scale is given by

$$A_s(x) = \sqrt{e_s(x)^2 + o_s(x)^2}, \tag{4}$$

and the phase is given by

$$\phi_s(x) = atan2(e_s(x), o_s(x)). \tag{5}$$

At each point x in the η signal, there is an array of these response vectors, one vector for each scale of filter. These response vectors form the basis of the localized representation of the signal, and they can be used in exactly the same way as Fourier components can be used to calculate PC.

A difficulty with phase congruency is its response to noise [27]. If the distribution of the noise response is determined, the noise T is taken to be:

$$T = \mu_r + k\sigma_r, \tag{6}$$

where μ_r and σ_r describe the mean and standard deviation of the distribution describing the noise energy response, respectively, and k is typically in the range 2 to 3.

Taking the noise in consideration, the expression for PC is

$$PC = \frac{W(x)\lfloor E(x) - T \rfloor}{\sum_s A_s(x) + \varepsilon} \tag{7}$$

where $\lfloor \rfloor$ denotes that the enclosed quantity is equal to itself when its value is positive and zero otherwise, $W(x)$ is a weighting function and ε is a small positive constant to avoid PC to became ill conditioned when all Fourier amplitudes are very small.

PC extension to a two-dimensional signal requires the formation of a 90 degree phase shift of the signal, which is accomplished using odd-symmetric filters. As one cannot construct rotationally symmetric odd-symmetric filters, one is forced to analyze a two-dimensional signal by applying the one-dimensional analysis over several orientations and combining the results.

To detect edges at all orientations, a bak of filters must be designed to tile the frequency plane uniformly. In the frequency plane, the filters appear as 2-D Gaussians symmetrically or anti-symmetrically placed around the origin, depending on the spatial symmetry of the filters. The length-to-width ratio of the 2-D wavelets controls their directional selectivity. This ratio can be varied in conjunction with the number of filter orientations used in order to achieve an even coverage of the 2-D spectrum. A more sensitive phase deviation function on which to base the calculation of PC is

$$\Delta\Phi_{s\theta}(x, y) = \cos(\phi_{s\theta}(x, y) - \bar{\phi}_\theta(x, y)) - |\sin(\phi_{s\theta}(x, y) - \bar{\phi}_\theta(x, y)), \tag{8}$$

where $\bar{\phi}_\theta(x, y)$ denotes the mean phase angle at orientation θ.

The approach of [27] produces the following equation for 2D phase congruency:

$$PC(x, y) = \frac{\sum_\theta \sum_s W(x)\lfloor A_{s\theta}(x, y)\Delta\Phi_{s\theta}(x, y) - T \rfloor}{\sum_\theta \sum_s A_{s\theta}(x, y) + \varepsilon}, \tag{9}$$

PC algorithm [27] was implemented with the following parameters. Six orientations and five scales were used. The wavelength of the smallest scale filters was 3 pixels, the scaling factor between successive filters was 2. A noise compensation k value of 2 was used. The cutoff c was set at 0.5 and γ at 10.

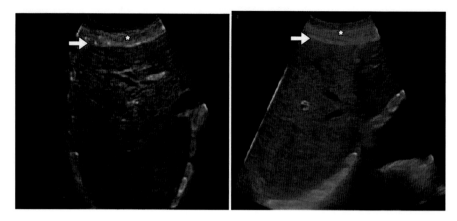

Fig. 2 Examples of the US liver surface enhanced image. The *white arrow* indicates the highlight given to the anterior liver surface, which aids in the inspection of the liver contour. The *white star* points to the fat/muscle layers that typically increase the difficulty in a correct identification of the contour

The performance of the PC detector for the original US image and *de-speckle* field was analyzed by estimated noise T value and by visual inspection, particularly inspecting the continuity of the detected contour line. Based on PC noise estimation it is expected that, due to the presence of speckle corruption, the original US image leads to more blurred definition of liver surface when compared with the *de-splecke* field.

Liver Surface Detection and Feature Extraction

PC contour from the *de-speckle* field is then overlaid on the original US image to generate a liver surface enhancement. The aim of this overlay image is to aid the physician in the evaluation and selection of liver contour points. Figure 2 shows examples of the resultant US liver surface enhanced image obtained from the conducted experiments.

The liver surface contour is then extracted, for characterization purposes, using the snake technique proposed by [31], which computes one iteration of the energy-minimization of active contour models. To initialize the snake, the operator selects at least four points in the liver surface, as exemplified in Fig. 3.

Liver contour is characterized with respect to spatial coordinates and inclination angles. Based on the detected liver contour, the following features were extracted:

1. *root mean square* (rms) of the different angles produced by the points that characterize the contour, rms_α, where the first point was assumed the reference point (as shown in Fig. 3),

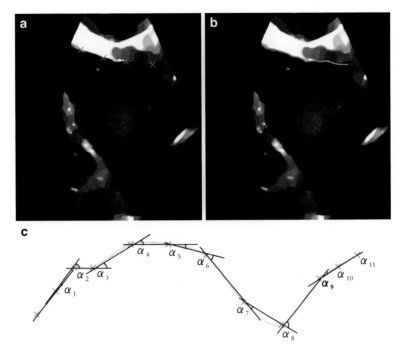

Fig. 3 Example of the snake method in the *de-speckle* field: the initialization step (**a**), the resulting contour detection (**b**), and a scheme of the extracted angles and contour points (**c**)

2. root mean square of the variation of the points of the contour in the y-axis (image depth), rms_y,
3. the mean (μ) and variance (σ^2) of the referred angles, μ_α and σ_α^2,
4. the variance of the y-axis coordinates at each point, σ_y^2, and
5. the correlation coefficient of the y-axis coordinates, R_y.

Thus, the morphological feature set, used in this thesis, is composed by a total of 6 features,

$$Morphological\ set \in \{rms_\alpha, rms_y, \mu_\alpha, \sigma_\alpha^2, \sigma_y^2, R_y\}.$$

To increase the discriminative power of the method, textural features extracted from the US liver parenchyma are also considered for feature selection. From each *speckle* field, an ROI, of 128×128 pixels, is manually selected by an expert operator along medial axis, as exemplified in Fig. 4 with the criteria: (1) representative of liver parenchyma; (2) avoid major vessels and ligaments; and (3) as superficial as possible, to avoid US beam distortions. The following textural features are then extracted.

Fig. 4 Example of correct
positioning of the ROI
within an US image

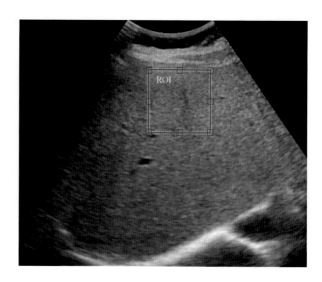

Co-occurrence Matrix

A common approach for texture characterization is using the co-occurrence matrix, which is based on the definition of the joint probability distributions of pairs of pixels. The second-order histogram is defined as the co-occurrence matrix [32].

The elements of the *Co-occurrence* tensor, $Co = \{c_{i,j}(\Delta_l, \Delta_c)\}$, describe the gray level spatial correlation in the image [32]. More precisely, element $c_{i,j}(\Delta_l, \Delta_c)$ represents the joint probability of the pixel intensities i and j in relative spatial position of (Δ_l, Δ_c) [32] and can be computed as follows

$$c_{i,j}(\Delta_l, \Delta_c) = \sum_{l=1}^{N} \sum_{c=1}^{M} \begin{cases} 1 & \text{if} (\eta_{l,c} = i) \wedge (\eta_{l+\Delta l, c+\Delta c} = j) \\ 0 & \text{otherwise} \end{cases} \tag{10}$$

For instance, let us assume a pixel distance of 6 and four directions $[0°, 45°, 90°, 135°]$. In this case, the displacement vector, used for co-occurrence computation, is $(\Delta_l, \Delta_c) \in \{(0, 6), (-6, 6), (-6, 0), (-6, -6)\}$. Here, we calculate the most commonly statistical features, based on [33], namely:

- *Contrast*: measure the local variations in the co-occurrence matrix,

$$contrast(\Delta_l, \Delta_c) = \sum_{i,j} |i - j|^2 c_{i,j}(\Delta_l, \Delta_c) \tag{11}$$

- *Correlation*: measure the joint probability occurrence of the specified pixel pairs,

$$correlation(\Delta_l, \Delta_c) = \sum_{i,j} \frac{(i - \mu_i)(j - \mu_j) c_{i,j}(\Delta_l, \Delta_c)}{\sigma_i \sigma_j} \tag{12}$$

- *Energy*: also known as the angular second moment [20],

$$energy(\Delta_l, \Delta_c) = \sum_{i,j} c_{i,j}(\Delta_l, \Delta_c)^2 \qquad (13)$$

- *Homogeneity*: measures the closeness of the distribution of elements in the matrix to the matrix diagonal,

$$homogeneity(\Delta_l, \Delta_c) = \sum_{i,j} \frac{c_{i,j}(\Delta_l, \Delta_c)}{(1 + |i - j|)} \qquad (14)$$

A set of 4 features, for each (Δ_l, Δ_c) pair, is extracted from the co-occurrence matrix, in a total of 16 features:

$$co\text{-}occurrence\ matrix\ set \in \{contrast, correlation, energy, homogeneity\}.$$

2-D Monogenic Signal Decomposition

In the polar representation of a complex signal, the modulus of the complex signal is identified as a local quantitative measure of the *local amplitude*, and the argument of the complex signal is identified as a local measure of its variation, called the *local phase* [34]. From the image processing and recognition points of view, the magnitude of the monogenic image is strongly related to the intensity of the images. The phase fields reveal local and global spatial variations of these intensities and therefore are very discriminative and powerful for textural characterization purposes.

Given a two-dimensional signal $f(\mathbf{x})$, $\mathbf{x} \in \mathbb{R}^2$, Felsberg and Sommer [34] define the three-component monogenic signal as [35]

$$f_m(\mathbf{x}) = (f(\mathbf{x}), Re(\mathbb{R}f(\mathbf{x})), Im(\mathbb{R}f(\mathbf{x}))) = (f, f_1, f_2). \qquad (15)$$

The local amplitude of the signal is given by $A(\mathbf{x}) = \|f_m(\mathbf{x})\| = \sqrt{f^2 + f_1^2 + f_2^2}$, while its local orientation θ and local phase ψ are specified by the following relations

$$f = A \cos\psi, \quad f_1 = A \sin\psi \cos\theta, \quad f_2 = A \sin\psi \sin\theta. \qquad (16)$$

In the *monogenic decomposition* (MD), the local amplitude includes energetic information, and the phase includes structural information. If the monogenic phase is decomposed into local orientation and local phase, the split of identity is also preserved with respect to geometric and structural information. The local phase is invariant to changes of the local orientation, and the local orientation is invariant to changes of the local structure [34]. This decomposition is particularly useful for feature extraction and classification in image processing.

Here, a third order decomposition is used, as proposed by [27]. From each response $(A, \psi, \theta)_\tau$, where $\tau \in \{1,2,3\}$, the AR coefficients of a first order 2D model $\{a_{1,1}, a_{1,0}, a_{0,1}\}$, energy and μ are extracted. A total of 45 features are extracted in the MD set,

$$MD \; set \in \{(A, \psi, \theta)_\tau (a_{0,1}, a_{1,0}, a_{1,1}, energy, \mu)\},$$

where $\tau \in \{1, 2, 3\}$.

The textural set, *co-occurrence matrix set* and *MD set*, is composed by a total of 61 US features, extracted from the liver parenchyma. To avoid overfitting, feature selection is performed, as explained in the next section.

Feature Selection and Classification Procedure

The proposed features are incorporated in a forward feature selection method, using as criterion the performance of a kNN classifier, where $k = 1$, in a leave-one-out cross-validation basis, to select the most significant features to characterize liver contour and textural changes in this classification problem.

Four different classifiers were implemented and tested: the SVM, *Bayes*, Parzen, and kNN classifier. A short description of each is now provided.

The aim of SVM is to find a decision plane that has a maximum distance (margin) from the nearest training pattern This is performed by mapping the feature vector in a higher-dimensional space. In this new space the SVM finds a hyperplane to separate the two classes with a decision boundary set by support vectors [21, 36]. The computationally intensive mapping process can be reduced with an appropriate kernel function. In this work, the *radial-basis* kernel (SVM_R) is used.

The implementation of the *Bayes* classifier assumes that the vector of features are multivariate normal distributed [36, 37] with different means, $\{\mu_1, \mu_2\}$ and covariance matrices, $\{\Sigma_1, \Sigma_2\}$. The corresponding quadratic discriminant functions

$$g_\tau(\mathbf{x}) = -\frac{1}{2}(\mathbf{x} - \mu_\tau)^T \Sigma_\tau (\mathbf{x} - \mu_\tau) - \frac{1}{2}\ln|\Sigma_\tau| + \ln P(\omega_\tau), \qquad (17)$$

with $\tau \in \{1, 2\}$ and where $P(\omega_\tau)$ is the prior probability of the ζ-*th* class. The probability of each class from the data as follows,

$$P(\omega_\tau) = \frac{N_\tau}{N_S}, \qquad (18)$$

where N_τ is the number of samples within class ω_τ and N_s the number of samples of the population. The classification of a given feature vector $\mathbf{x}$ is performed according to

$$
\begin{cases}
2 & \text{if } g_2(\mathbf{x}) > g_1(\mathbf{x}) \\
1 & \text{otherwise}
\end{cases}
\tag{19}
$$

The *Parzen* classifier estimates the distribution density of the samples that constitute each class by summing the distance-weighed contributions of each sample in a class and classify a test sample by the label corresponding to the maximum posterior [37].

The nonparametric kNN classifier is also tested in this work. It classifies a test sample to a class according to the majority of the training neighbors in the feature space by using the minimum Euclidean distance criterion [20].

All classifiers were implemented using the algorithm proposed by [38]. The comparison of the proposed classifiers is based on their performance. The classifier performance is measured based on the *overall accuracy* (OA),

$$
OA = \frac{TP + TN}{TP + FN + FP + TN},
\tag{20}
$$

the *sensitivity* (sens),

$$
sens = \frac{TP}{TP + FN},
\tag{21}
$$

and *specificity* (spec),

$$
spec = \frac{TN}{FP + TN},
\tag{22}
$$

where TP, FP, FN, and TN are *true-positives, false-positives, false-negatives,* and *true-negatives,* respectively. The table displayed in Fig. 5, containing these classification performance metrics, is the confusion matrix.

Moreover, for the classifier that yields the best performance, the *positive likelihood ratio* (+LR) and *negative likelihood ratio* (−LR) are calculated, as follows

$$
+LR = \frac{TP/(TP + FN)}{FP/(FP + TN)} = \frac{sens}{1 - spec}
\tag{23}
$$

and

$$
-FR = \frac{FN/(TP + FN)}{TN/(FP + TN)} = \frac{1 - sens}{spec}.
\tag{24}
$$

True diagnosis

		Positive	Negative	
Classification	Positive	TP	FP	*TP + FP*
	Negative	FN	TN	*FN + TN*
		TP + FN	*FP + TN*	

Fig. 5 Example of a confusion matrix. A confusion matrix is a 2×2 table showing actual values (*columns*) versus classified values (*rows*), where TP, FP, FN, and TN are *true-positives*, *false-positives*, *false-negatives*, and *true-negatives*, respectively

Data Set

We enrolled 72 patients with cirrhosis, confirmed by liver biopsy. A non-cirrhotic group with 61 patients (31 patients belonging to the normal class and 30 from the chronic hepatitis one) was submitted to the same examination. The database ($n = 133$) was divided into two classes; *non-cirrhosis*, ω_{NC}, and *cirrhosis*, ω_C.

All patients were outpatients coming for a routine visit and registered at the Liver Unit, Gastroenterology Department, of Santa Maria Hospital in Lisbon, Portugal. The study protocol was approved by the Ethics Committee of the referred hospital, according to the principles of the Declaration of Helsinki. All participants gave their informed and written consent before entering the study.

Data collection was performed between October 2010 and April 2011. The same data acquisition protocol was used for each patient, which includes US examination, biochemical tests, and clinical history. Whenever possible, data from each patient was collected in the same day, to avoid intra-patient variability.

Results

The first experiment conducted here aims to study the advantage of using the *de-speckle* field for the detection of liver contour, over the traditional B-mode US image. PC was computed in both images and the estimated noise was calculated. Figure 6 shows a plot of the noise values, T, for the original US image and the correspondent *de-speckle* field. The mean (σ) values obtained for the original US image and *de-speckle* field are 10.94 (4.60) and 0.26 (0.49), respectively. Statistical differences ($p < 0.01$) were observed. As expected, US images are highly associated with noise, which corrupt the detected shape of the liver contour.

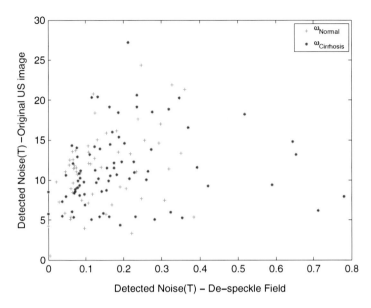

Fig. 6 Scatter plot of the detected noise, T, in the original US image and in the *de-speckle* field

The presence of noise also affected the performance of the PC edge detector. The improvement achieved with the use of the *de-speckle* field is observed in Fig. 7. Under the *de-speckle* field, PC map marked prominently the liver contour, whereas in the map computed from the original US image confusion between the definition of the contour and noise is observed. To standardize the proceedings, and as reported in the literature, the study is focused on the anterior surface of the liver.

From the proposed morphological feature set, 2 features were selected, namely: rms_α and R_y. rms_α measures the angle variation in the contour points, achieving a mean (σ) value for ω_{NC} and ω_C of 1.19 (0.59) and 1.80 (0.90), respectively. In R_y, the mean (σ) values for ω_{NC} and ω_C are $-$ 0.01 (0.02) and 0.01 (0.01), respectively. The probability density functions of the selected features are displayed in Fig. 8, where it is possible to observe a significantly inter-class overlap.

To evaluate the discriminant power of the selected morphological features, four different classifiers were tested, namely a kNN, a *Bayes* classifier, and an SVM classifier with radial-basis (SVM_R) kernels. The results are summarized in Table 3.

The *Bayes* classifier outperformed the other considered classifiers, achieving an overall accuracy of 73.30 %, a sensitivity of 83.67 %, and a specificity of 54.09 %. Figure 9 demonstrates the difficulty of defining an acceptable classification boundary, due to inter-class feature overlap.

Despite the low accuracy of the classification, the detection rate achieved for ω_C outperforms the studies of [12, 16, 39–43], which reported a sensitivity ranging from 12.5 % [16] to 73.0 % [43]. The opposite behavior is observed in the specificity, where all the stated studies outperform the present study. This may be related to the fact that ω_{NC} incorporates normal liver volunteers and chronic hepatitis ones, which can increase the variability in the detected liver contour.

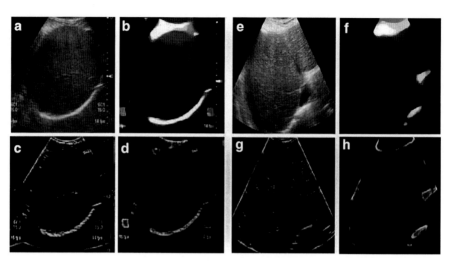

Fig. 7 Examples of the detected liver surface via phase congruency. (**a**), (**b**), (**c**), and (**d**) represent an example from a normal samples of the original US image, *de-speckle* field, PC map obtained from the original US image and PC map from the *de-speckle* field, respectively. A cirrhotic example is also given from (**e**) to (**h**), where (**e**) is the original US image, (**f**) the correspondent *de-speckle* field, (**g**) the PC map computed from the original US image, and (**h**) the PC map computed from the *de-speckle* field

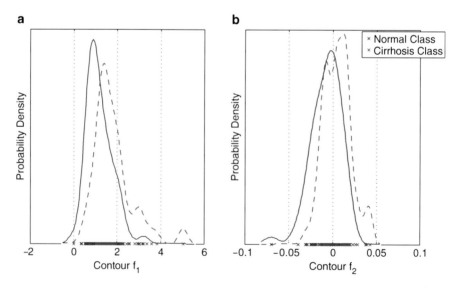

Fig. 8 Plot of the estimated probability density function of the selected contour features ((**a**) rms_α and (**b**) R_y). Individual inspection reveals that exists a significant overlap between the considered classes

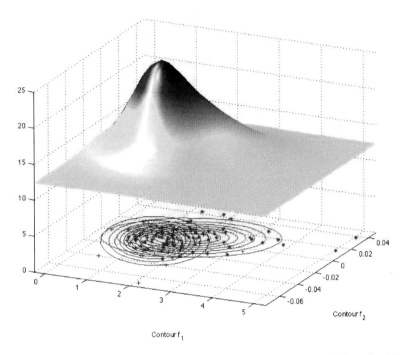

Fig. 9 Approximation of a two-dimensional probability density function via the trained *Bayes* classifier

		ω_{NC}		ω_C	
Table 2 Mean (μ) and standard deviation (σ) of the selected US textural features	Features	μ	σ	μ	σ
	$a_{1,0} A_1$	0.11	0.08	0.05	0.10
	energy (0,6)	0.61	0.32	0.78	0.24
	energy A_1	3.39	0.04	3.38	0.03
	energy ψ_2	3.39	0.05	3.39	0.06
	$a_{0,1} A_2$	0.86	0.03	0.89	0.02

To improve the robustness of the method and its discrimination power, liver parenchyma US textural features were included. Physiologically, the irregularities observed in liver surface should corroborate with changes in liver parenchyma.

After feature selection, a subset of 5 textural features was obtained: $a_{1,0} A_1$, *energy* (0,6), energy A_1, energy ψ_2 and $a_{0,1} A_2$. The great majority of the selected features are extracted from the monogenic decomposition. Table 2 summarizes the statistical characteristics (μ and σ) of the selected features for ω_{NC} and ω_C.

As in the morphological feature subset, the same classification procedure was applied to the textural feature subset. Table 3 outlines the classification results. Textural feature subset yields better classification performances than the

Table 3 Overall and individual class accuracies (%) for each classifiers, with the morphological subset, textural subset, and the combination of both

Classifier	Morphological subset			Textural subset			Morphological + Textural		
	ω_{NC}	ω_C	OA	ω_{NC}	ω_C	OA	ω_{NC}	ω_C	OA
Bayes	54.09	83.67	73.30	67.21	76.39	72.18	88.52	86.11	87.22
Parzen	40.98	40.81	53.46	42.62	93.06	69.92	60.66	83.33	72.93
3-NN	44.26	68.37	59.12	65.57	88.89	78.20	86.90	81.90	84.20
SVM_R	6.56	92.85	59.75	75.41	77.78	76.69	87.50	70.49	79.70

morphological subset. The best overall performance was achieved with the kNN classifier, $k = 3$, which attained an OA of 78.20 %. However, the best individual performance, that jointly maximize the sensitivity and specificity, was observed with the SVM classifier, radial-basis kernel ($r = 0.4$), with a sensitivity and specificity of 77.78 % and 75.41 %, respectively.

Combining the subsets of features further improves the classifiers performance, as summarized in Table 3. With feature combination, the best overall performance was obtained with the *Bayes* classifier. This result outperforms the results obtained individually for each subset, morphological and textural, which reinforce the idea that both changes are present in liver cirrhosis and are detectable by US.

In the individual class performance, *Bayes* classifier correctly identified 54 of the 61 patients of ω_{NC}, corresponding to a specificity of 88.52 %. For ω_C, the results show a probability that the test is positive on cirrhotic patients of 86.11 %, corresponding to a feasibility of 62 correct diagnosis in 72 patients. A $+LR$ (95 % confidence interval) of 6.2 (5.4–7.2) and a $-LR$ of 0.21 (0.18–0.24) were achieved.

Discussion and Conclusions

Patients with CLD have a higher risk of death or oncogenesis. Most HCC cases are associated with cirrhosis related to chronic HBV or HCV infection. Southern European countries tend to have mid-incidence levels of HCC (10–20 per 100,000 individuals). The 5-year cumulative risk of developing HCC for patients with cirrhosis ranges between 5 % and 30 % [44]. Thus, noninvasive methods for CLD detection and staging are a key feature for this clinical problem.

In this scope, the present work sought to know whether US imaging information, morphological and textural one, can better discriminate cirrhosis.

A semiautomatic detection of liver surface, based on US images, is proposed to discriminate liver cirrhosis. The post-processing algorithm was able to enhance the contour information in common low-frequency abdominal US examinations (2.8–5.0 MHz) with a convex probe. The implementation of the phase congruency algorithm computed in the *de-speckled* field allowed an enhancement of liver surface. PC map was then overlaid to the original B-mode US image, to work as

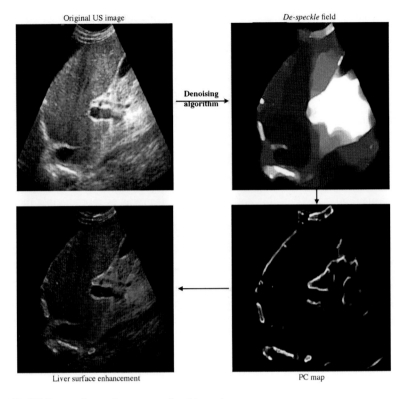

Fig. 10 US liver surface enhancement algorithm scheme

a guide to outline liver contour. The proposed enhancement algorithm is schematically represented in Fig. 10.

The results stress that US image decomposition in its *speckle* and *de-speckle* fields enhanced the discrimination power of the extracted features, improving the reliability of the proposed algorithm.

Morphological information extracted via phase congruency algorithm from the *de-speckle* field positively characterizes liver surface changes in liver cirrhosis. Changes produced by liver cirrhosis in the liver surface appear to be related to the relation of the contour points in depth and its inclination variation. Similar results were obtained in [9–13]; however, this work presents two major innovations: (i) the use of low-frequency US transducer and (ii) the extraction of objective and reproducible US morphological features.

The inclusion of textural information obtained from the liver parenchyma improved the classification performance. Textural features extracted from the *speckle* field peak the architectural changes observed in liver parenchyma.

Monogenic decomposition feature set is dominant in the feature selection process. A novelty in this work is the introduction of this set as a US feature extractor.

Relevant information was found to be in the second and third US decomposition levels of this technique.

The outlines of this approach are resumed as follows:

- The *de-speckle* field allows edges preservation of the anatomical structures, while smoothing homogenous regions contaminated by speckle, in accordance with the results of [45]. By this, it is possible to use low-frequency US transducers (3.5 MHz) and thus maintaining the normal US protocol used in clinical facilities.
- Edge perception via phase congruency computed from the *de-speckle* image highlights liver surface. By overlaying the resultant PC edge image over the original US image we proposed the *US liver surface enhanced image*.
- One main advantage of this approach is that it produces reproducible morphological features for the detection of liver cirrhosis and does not depend on ROI positioning.
- The combination of morphological (extracted from the *de-speckle* field) and textural (extracted from the *speckle* field) information can accurately detect cirrhosis.

Future studies in the area of liver surface detection should include other features to increase diagnostic accuracy, perform a more exhaustive analysis in terms of classifiers, such as using a combination of classifiers and use state-of-the-art automatic snakes, in order to create a fully automatic detection method. Also, more robust classification techniques should be attempted, particularly classifiers combinations.

In conclusion, liver cirrhosis can accurately be detected by US images based on morphological and textural features. When cirrhosis is present, liver surface is characterized by its uncorrelated variation in depth and its inclination angles. Characteristic textural changes are also present in cirrhotic liver parenchyma, particularly related to a multi-resolution spatial analysis. These findings describe the commonly referred *liver with coarse and heterogenous appearance*, present in US clinical reports in cirrhotic patients.

References

1. Martin B, Henri L, Markus P-R, Dominique-Charles V, Françoise R-T (2013) The burden of liver disease in europe - a review of available epidemiological data. Technical report, European Association for the Study of the Liver
2. D'Amico G, Garcia-Tsao G, Pagliaro L (2006) Natural history and prognostic indicators of survival in cirrhosis: Systematic review of 118 studies. J Hepatol 44(1):217–231
3. Schuppan D, Afdhal N (2008) Liver cirrhosis. Lancet 371:838–851
4. Fauci AS, Braunwald E, Kasper DL, Hauser SL, Longo DL, Jameson JL, Loscalzo J (2008) Harrison's principles of internal medicine, 17th edn. McGraw-Hill's, New York
5. Sporea I, Popescu A, Sirli R (2008) Why, who and how should perform liver biopsy in chronic liver diseases. World J Gastroenterol 14(21):3396–3402

6. Denzer UW, Luth S (2009) Non–invasive diagnosis and monitoring of liver fibrosis and cirrhosis. Best Pract Res Clin Gastroenterol 23:453–460
7. Allan R, Thoirs K, Phillipsm (2010) Accuracy of ultrasound to identify chronic liver disease. World J Gastroenterol 28(16):3510–3520
8. Gaiani S, Gramantieri L, Venturoli N, Piscaglia F, Siringo S, D'Errico A, Zironi G, Grigioni W, Bolondi L (1997) What is the criterion for differentiating chronic hepatitis from compensated cirrhosis? a prospective study comparing ultrasonography and percutaneous liver biopsy. J Hepatol 27(6):979–985
9. Simonovsky V (1999) The diagnosis of cirrhosis by high resolution ultrasound of the liver surface. Br J Radiol 72(853):29–34
10. Ferral H, Male R, Cardiel M, Munoz L, Ferrari FQ (1992) Cirrhosis: Diagnosis by liver surface analysis with high-frequency ultrasound. Gastrointest Radiol 17:74–78
11. Berzigotti A, Abraldes JG, Tandon P, Erice E, Gilabert R, Garca-Pagan JC, Bosch J (2010) Ultrasonographic evaluation of liver surface and transient elastography in clinically doubtful cirrhosis. J Hepatol 52(6):846–853
12. Colli A, Fraquelli M, Andreoletti M, Marino B, Zuccoli E, Conte D (2003) Severe liver fibrosis or cirrhosis: accuracy of us for detection - analysis of 300 cases. Radiology 227:89–94
13. Aube C, Oberti F, Korali N, Namour M-A, Loisel D, Tanguy J-Y, Valsesia E, Pilette C, Rousselet MC, Bedossa P, Rifflet H, Maiga MY, Penneau-Fontbonne D, Caron C, Cales P (1999) Ultrasonographic diagnosis of hepatic fibrosis or cirrhosis. J Hepatol 30(3):472–478
14. Pitas I, Venetsunopoulos AN (1990) Nonlinear digital filters: principles and application. Kluwer, Dordecht
15. Levine MD (1985) Vision in man and machine. McGraw-Hill, New York
16. Ladenheim JA, Luba DG, Yao F, Gregory PB, Jeffrey RB, Garcia G (1992) Limitations of liver surface US in the diagnosis of cirrhosis. Radiology 185(1):21–23
17. sam shanmugan K, Narayanan V, Frost VS, Stiles JA, Holtzman JC (1981) Textural features for radar image alaysis. IEEE Trans Geosci Remote Sens GE-19(3):153–156
18. Maeda K, Utsu M, Kihaile PE (1998) Quantification of sonographic echogenicity with grey-level histogram width: A clinical tissue characterization. Ultrasound Med Biol 24(2):225–234
19. Lee C, Choi J, Kim K, Seo T, Lee J, Park C (2006) Usefulness of standard deviation on the histogram of ultrasound as a quantitative value for hepatic parenchymal echo texture; preliminary study. Ultrasound Med Biol 32(12):1817–1826
20. Kadah Y, Farag A, Zurada JM, Badawi AM, Youssef AM (1996) Classification algorithms for quantitative tissue characterization of diffuse liver disease from ultrasound images. IEEE Trans Med Imag 15:466–478
21. Yeh W, Jeng Y, Li C, Lee P, Li P (2003) Liver fibrosis grade classification with B-mode ultrasound. Ultrasound Med Biol 29:1229–1235
22. Yeh W, Jeng Y, Li C, Lee P, Li P (2005) Liver steatosis classification using high-frequency ultrasound. Ultrasound Med Biol 31(5):599–605
23. Mojsilovic A, Markovic S, Popovic M (1997) Characterization of visually similar diffuse diseases from b-scan liver images with the nonseparable wavelet transform. Image Process Int Conf 3:547
24. Gaitini D, Baruch Y, Ghersin E, Veitsman E, Kerner H, Shalem B, Yaniv G, Sarfaty C, Azhari H (2004) Feasibility study of ultrasonic fatty liver biopsy: Texture vs. attenuation and backscatter. Ultrasound Med Biol 30(10):1321–1327
25. Meziri M, Pereira W, Abdelwahab A, Degott C, Laugier P (2005) In vitro chronic hepatic disease characterization with a multiparametric ultrasonic approach. Ultrasonics 43 (5):305–313
26. Seabra JC, Sanches JM (2010) On estimating de-speckled and speckle components from B-mode ultrasound images. In Proceedings of the 2010 I.E. international conference on Biomedical imaging: from nano to Macro, ISBI'10, pp 284–287. IEEE, New York
27. Kovesi P (2000) Phase congruency: A low-level image invariant. Psychol Res 136–148

28. Kovesi P (1999) Image features from phase congruency. Videre: J Comput Vision Res 1 (3):1–26
29. Burlacu A, Lazar C (2008) Image features detection using phase congruency and its application in visual servoing. In: 4th international conference on intelligent computer communication and processing, ICCP 2008, pp 47–52. IEEE Computer Society, Washington, DC
30. Morrone MC, Owens RA (1987) Feature detection from local energy. Pattern Recognit Lett (6):303–313
31. Bregler C, Slaney M (1995) Snakes-A MatLab MEX file to demonstrate snake contour-following
32. Haralick RM, Shanmugam K, Dinstein I (1973) Textural features for image classification. IEEE Trans Syst Man Cybern SMC-3(6):610–621
33. Valckx FMJ, Thijssen JM (1997) Characterization of echographic image texture by cooccurrence matrix parameters. Ultrasound Med Biol 23(4):559–571
34. Felsberg M, Sommer G (2001) The monogenic signal. IEEE Trans Signal Process 49 (12):3136–3144
35. Unser M, Sage D, Van De Ville D (2009) Multiresolution monogenic signal analysis using the riesz-laplace wavelet tranform. IEEE Trans Image Process 18(11):2402–2418
36. Duda RO, Hart PE, Stork DG (2000) Pattern classification, 2nd edn. Wiley-Interscience, New York
37. Theodoridis S, Koutroumbas K (2008) Pattern recognition, 4th edn. Academic, New York
38. van der Heijden F, Duin R, de Ridder D, Tax DMJ (2004) Classification, parameter estimation and state estimation: an engineering approach using MATLAB, 1st edn. Wiley, New York
39. Colli A, Colucci A, Paggi S, Fraquelli M, Massironi S, Andreoletti M, Michela V, Conte D (2005) Accuracy of a predictive model for severe hepatic fibrosis or cirrhosis in chronic hepatitis C. World J Gastroenterol 11:7318–7322
40. DOnofrio M, Martone E, Brunelli S, Faccioli N, Zamboni G, Zagni I, Fattovichm G, Mucelli RP (2005) Accuracy of ultrasound in the detection of liver fibrosis in chronic viral hepatitis. Radiol Med 110:341–348
41. Vigano M, Visentin S, Aghemo A, Rumi MG, Ronchi G (2005) Ultrasound features of liver surface nodularity as a predictor of severe fibrosis in chronic hepatitis C. Radiology 234:641
42. Gaia S, Cocuzza C, Rolle E, Bugianesi E, Carucci P, Vanni E, Evangelista A, Rizzetto M, Brunello F (2009) A comparative study between ultrasound evaluation, liver stiffness and biopsy for staging of hepatic fibrosis in patients with chronic liver disease. J Hepatol 50 (Suppl1):S361
43. Paggi S, Colli A, Fraquelli M, Vigano M, Del Poggio P, Facciotto C, Colombo M, Ronchi G, Conte D (2009) A non-invasive algorithm accurately predicts advanced fibrosis in hepatitis C: a comparison using histology with internal-external validation. J Hepatol 49:564–571
44. El-Serag HB (2012) Epidemiology of viral hepatitis and hepatocellular carcinoma. Gastroenterology (142):1264–1273
45. Seabra J (2011) Medical Ultrasound B-Mode Modeling, De-speckling and Tissue Characterization - Assessing the Atherosclerotic Disease. PhD thesis, Instituto Superio Técnico

Biography

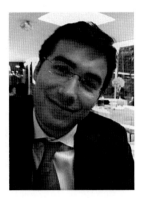

Ricardo T. Ribeiro received his B.Sc. degree in radiology from the Lisbon School of Health Technology, Polytechnic Institute of Lisbon, M.Sc. degree from the University of Evora and Ph.D. degree in biomedical engineering at the Institute for Systems and Robotics, Instituto Superior Técnico from the Technical University of Lisbon in collaboration with the University of Lisbon Medical School. He is currently an Adjunct Professor at Lisbon School of Health Technology. His current research interests include the use of machine learning, computer vision, and tissue characterization for the classification of ultrasound imaging. He is also engaged in clinical research in ultrasound imaging.

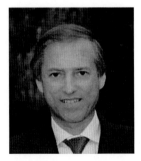

Rui Tato Marinho M.D., Ph.D., is a Gastroenterologist and Hepatologist at the Medical School of Lisbon, Hospital Santa Maria. He is also the editor-in-chief of *Acta Médica Portuguesa*, the Scientific Journal of Portuguese Medical Association (Ordem dos Médicos), adviser of the Viral Hepatitis Prevention Board, and president of Portuguese College of Hepatology of the Portuguese Medical Association.

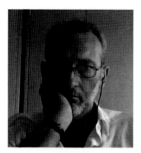

J. Miguel Sanches received the E.E., M.Sc., and Ph.D. degrees from the Instituto Superior Técnico (IST), Technical University of Lisbon, Portugal, in 1991, 1996, and 2003, respectively. He is a Professor of the Bioengineering Department at the Instituto Superior Técnico and researcher at the Institute for Systems and Robotics. He is also a senior member of the IEEE Engineering in Medicine and Biology Society and Member of the Bio Imaging and Signal Processing Technical Committee (BISP-TC) of the IEEE Signal Processing Society and president of the Portuguese Association of Pattern Recognition (APRP), affiliated to the International Association of Pattern Recognition (IAPR). His work has been focused in Biomedical Engineering, namely, in Biomedical Signal and Image Processing and Physiological Modeling of Biological Systems.

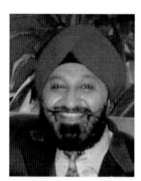

Jasjit Suri, Ph.D., MBA is an innovator, visionary, scientist, and an internationally known world leader. Dr. Suri was crowned with Director General's Gold medal in 1980 and the *Fellow of American Institute of Medical and Biological Engineering* (AIMBE), awarded by National Academy of Sciences, Washington DC in 2004. Dr. Suri has been the chairman of IEEE Denver section and has won over 50 awards during his career and has held executive positions.

MR Imaging of Hepatocellular Carcinoma

Dong Ho Lee and Jeong Min Lee

Abstract Liver cirrhosis is a major public health problem worldwide and is the end result of chronic liver disease. Cirrhotic liver is characterized by advanced hepatic fibrosis and formation of a spectrum of hepatocellular nodules ranging from benign regenerative nodules to overt HCC. Screening and early detection of HCC in cirrhotic liver are highly important because the treatment result for HCC is optimal when the tumor is small. With the technical development of MR scanners and recent advances in MR contrast agent for liver imaging as well as dedicated MR exam protocol including functional assessment, MR imaging has emerged as an important modality for assessing liver cirrhosis and detecting HCC. Therefore, the radiologist should be familiar with the MR imaging features of HCC.

Introduction

Hepatocellular carcinoma (HCC) is the fifth most common tumor in the world and is the third most common cause of cancer-related death, after lung cancer and stomach cancer [1]. The incidence rates of HCC are varied: 20–150/100,000/year in high-risk area in Asia and Africa, 5–20/100,000/year in the areas with intermediate risk in Japan and the Mediterranean countries, and <5/100,000/year in areas with low risk in Northern Europe and the USA [2]. However, the incidence of HCC in

D.H. Lee, M.D.
Department of Radiology, Seoul National University Hospital, 101 Daehangno,
Jongno-gu, Seoul 110-744, South Korea

J.M. Lee, M.D. (✉)
Department of Radiology, Seoul National University Hospital, 101 Daehangno,
Jongno-gu, Seoul 110-744, South Korea

Institute of Radiation Medicine, Seoul National University Hospital, 101 Daehangno,
Jongno-gu, Seoul 110-744, South Korea
e-mail: jmsh@snu.ac.kr

A.S. El-Baz et al. (eds.), *Abdomen and Thoracic Imaging: An Engineering
& Clinical Perspective*, DOI 10.1007/978-1-4614-8498-1_7,
© Springer Science+Business Media New York 2014

USA has been raised over the last 10 years [3] and is expected to increase on the next 2 decades [4], mainly due to the increase of hepatitis C or B virus (HCV/HBV) infections [5]. The strongest predisposing factor for developing HCC is liver cirrhosis and approximately 80 % of cases of HCC have been developed in a cirrhotic liver [6]. The annual incidence of HCC is 2.0–6.6 % in patients with liver cirrhosis, while 0.4 % in patients without liver cirrhosis [6]. All kinds of chronic liver disease can cause liver cirrhosis, and the etiologic agents of liver cirrhosis are different among the different areas. The most common etiologic agents are HBV infection in Asia, except Japan and Africa [7, 8], and HCV infection in the West and Japan. Other lesser common causes of liver cirrhosis including hereditary hemochromatosis, alcohol abuse, and biliary cirrhosis have variable but usually lower rates of HCC [9]. In viral-related cirrhosis, co-infection with other viruses and alcohol abuse significantly increase the risk of developing HCC [10]. Liver cirrhosis is characterized by irreversible remodeling of the hepatic architecture with bridging fibrosis and formation of a spectrum of hepatocellular nodules, including regenerative nodules (RN), dysplastic nodules (DN), and HCCs [11]. These cirrhosis-associated hepatocellular nodules result from the localized proliferation of hepatocytes and their supporting stroma in response to liver injury [12]. The development of HCC in a cirrhotic liver is described as a multistep progression, from low-grade DN to high-grade DN, then to DN with microscopic foci of HCC, then to small well-differentiated HCC, and finally to overt carcinoma [13, 14]. However, also a de novo development of HCC can occur, and it has been usually seen on normal liver parenchyma without evidence of cirrhosis or nodules in European and American people who have low incidence of chronic liver disease [15, 16].

HCC meets the criteria established by the World Health Organization for performing surveillance [17]. Currently, various therapeutic options for HCCs are available, including liver transplantation, surgical resection, local ablation therapy, and transcatheter arterial chemoembolization (TACE), all of which contribute to improvements in patients survival rates [18, 19]. The 5-year survival rates of patients undergoing curative therapy such as liver transplantation, hepatic resection, and percutaneous ablation therapy range between 40 and 75 % [20]. Therefore, screening the cirrhosis patients and differentiation of cirrhosis-associated hepatocellular nodules, early detection of HCC is important, because the most effective treatment of HCC is curative therapy when the tumor is small [21–23]. However, detection of small and early stage HCCs remains the most challenging area in liver imaging [9]. Currently, various imaging modalities such as ultrasound (US), computed tomography (CT), magnetic resonance imaging (MRI), and positron-emission tomography (PET) have been used for the detection and diagnosis of HCC [9, 24, 25]. Among these, dynamic contrast-enhanced CT is considered as a first-line modality for the diagnosis and therapeutic planning in HCC [24, 25]. However, MRI is an upcoming alternative as a modality for liver imaging and seems to be more useful than other modalities for detecting and assessing the cirrhosis-associated hepatocellular nodules because it provides better soft-tissue contrast and a more nuanced depiction of different tissue properties, without ionizing radiation [23, 26]. In addition, MRI can demonstrate some unique pathologic features of HCC, which cannot be easily accessed by other imaging modalities. For example, chemical shift gradient-echo imaging can depict intratumoral steatosis (by the accumulation of triglycerides within cytoplasm of hepatocytes) and these imaging features are helpful to predict malignant transformation of a DN to HCC [19, 27]. Dynamic contrast-enhanced MRI also provides reliable information regarding tumor vascularity which is related to sinusoid capillarization and neoangiogenesis of the HCC during the hepatocarcinogenesis [28]. Furthermore, recent advances in MR imaging techniques such as parallel acquisition imaging, a powerful gradient system with increased speed, rapid high-quality MR technique, and functional MRI tools such as diffusion-weighted imaging (DWI) and elastography have facilitated the detection and characterization of small HCCs and optimal management of cirrhotic patients [23]. Newly developed dedicated MR contrast agents that target the reticuloendothelial system (RES) or hepatocyte have also been introduced in liver MR imaging, providing better chance to detect and assess the cirrhosis-associated hepatocellular nodules. With these developments in MR technology, MRI has dramatic changes with regard to artifact robustness, spatial resolution, and scan speed in the liver imaging area [25]. As imaging has the crucial role in detection, characterization, therapeutic planning, and posttreatment follow-up for HCC, the radiologists should know the MR imaging features of HCC.

Liver MR Imaging Technique

Imaging of the cirrhotic liver can be performed at 1.5-T or 3.0-T field strength [9, 29]. A phased-array coil should routinely be used [9]. In a standard protocol for liver MR, study should always include T1-weighted gradient recalled echo (GRE) in-phase and opposed-phase sequences, a moderately T2-weighted turbo spin-echo (TSE) or fast spin-echo (FSE) sequence, and multiphase T1-weighted three-dimensional (3D) spoiled GRE sequence with fat suppression before and after contrast medium administration [23]. The rationale for the acquisition of pre-contrast T1- and T2-weighted images is to emphasize the presence of different tissue components both in the normal liver parenchyma as well as in a focal lesion, such as the presence of water, the entity of vascularization, fibrotic changes, fat, and metabolites [30]. A heavily T2-weighted sequence (echo time > 120 ms) helps distinguish between solid and cystic lesions, and a fast sequence such as single-shot FSE or half-Fourier acquisition TSE is used for this purpose [9, 23].

The sequences used can vary according to vendor and personal preferences [31], but several guidelines should be kept: First, to improve image quality, sequences should be performed during suspended respiration or should be respiratory averaged (some T2-weighted sequences) [9]. Suspending respiration at end expiration produces more consistent breath holding compared with end inspiration but is more difficult for patients. Second, three-dimensional (3D) gadolinium-enhanced GRE sequences are preferred to two-dimensional (2D) GRE sequences because of the thinner sections obtained, which improve lesion detection and permit multiplanar image reconstructions [9, 32–35]. Section thickness being lesser than 4 mm for 3D sequences should be used. Third, contrast agent bolus timing is strongly recommended. Appropriate evaluation of the liver parenchyma and focal lesion requires imaging during the hepatic arterial phase of contrast enhancement, especially late hepatic arterial phase, when the portal vein is only slightly enhanced [36, 37]. However, late hepatic arterial phase continues only for approximately 15–20 s [38–41]. Therefore, well-timed acquisition of late arterial phase images is crucial, and there has been three methods which may be used to determined the acquisition delay necessary to obtain images during the late hepatic arterial phase: hazarding a "best" guess with fixed delay, MR fluoroscopic triggering, and timing with a test bolus [42–44]. Based on previous reports [9, 37, 45], a best guess with fixed delay is not a reliable method for consistently resulting in optimal timing in patients with liver cirrhosis and is not recommended. Hypervascular HCC is most obvious in the late arterial phase and can be missed if the hepatic arterial-dominant phase images are obtained early [36]. Therefore, as a general rule, it is better to perform the image acquisition too late than too early; if in doubt about optimal timing for late hepatic arterial phase, one should error on the side of a longer acquisition delay [37]. The use of fluoroscopic triggering is appropriate only for MR sequences with which the high-contrast central portion of k-space is filled first, at the beginning of the acquisition [44]. A test bolus, or timing run, can provide the most accurate determination of the acquisition delay [37, 42, 43, 46]. However, if rapid multiphase arterial images are acquired, a timing bolus may not be essential [9]. Fourth, for the improvement of lesion characterization—for example, to detect the washout of HCC on delayed phase or to visualize delayed contrast retention of hemangioma or cholangiocarcinoma—multiphase dynamic gadolinium contrast-enhanced imaging should include three contrast-enhanced phases or more [9]. Nowadays, late hepatic arterial phase, portal venous phase, and delayed or equilibrium phase images are routinely obtained in many institutes including ours. In addition, in case of application of hepatocyte-targeting contrast agent, it is necessary that a further 3D-GRE breath-hold T1-weighted sequence be obtained at different delayed times, depending on applied contrast agent. Fifth, unless signal intensity is not compromised, the highest spatial resolution should be used. For this purpose, parallel imaging techniques can be applied with the possibility of reducing the acquisition time. However, parallel imaging techniques should be used with care, because they can result in image artifacts and reduced lesion conspicuity [47]. Patients' breath-holding capacity is also taken into account for the high spatial resolution image acquisition and reducing the breathing-related motion artifact.

Post-processed images, such as subtracted image which derived from arterial phase gadolinium-enhanced image and unenhanced image, are sometimes useful to assess the real presence of hypervascularization of nodule showing as hyperintense also on baseline T1-weighted image [48, 49]. Subtraction can be performed if the unenhanced and gadolinium-enhanced imaging sequences are identical, if the MR scanner is not retuned between acquisitions, and if there are no image rescaling issues [9].

Patients should be instructed to hold their breath in a similar fashion during all sequences to minimize misregistration artifacts, which appear as a bright line at the edge of organ due to incomplete overlap [9].

Recently, functional MRI tools such as DWI and elastography have been introduced and facilitated the detection and characterization of small cirrhosis-associated hepatocellular nodules. The DWI is an imaging technique which provides tissue contrast by measuring the diffusion properties of water molecules within tissue [50]. Diffusion is a physical process that results from the thermally driven, random motion of water molecules [51–53]. DWI is based on intravoxel incoherent motion (IVIM) and provides noninvasive quantification of water diffusion and microcapillary-blood perfusion [23, 54]. DWI uses a T2-weighted spin-echo sequence and two strong motion sensitizing gradients on either side of the 180° refocusing pulse, known as the Stejskal-Tanner sequence [50]. In the tissue with restricted water diffusion, the effect of the dephasing gradient is cancelled out by the rephasing gradient, which reflected as a maintained T2 signal intensity in the tissue. On the contrary, in the tissue with free water diffusion, the mobile water molecules are not fully rephased and a reduction in overall T2 signal intensity follows [23, 52]. The sensitivity of a DWI sequence is characterized by its b value, which summarizes the influence of the motion-sensitizing gradients. The higher the b value, the more sensitive the sequence is to diffusion effects [23]. For the quantification of diffusion property reflected in an apparent diffusion coefficient (ADC), DWI acquisition with at least two different b values are required. Low ADC values mean restricted water diffusion, thus in tissue which are higher cellular. On the contrary, high ADC values are seen in areas with relatively free diffusion, thus in tissue with low cellularity [23, 55]. Therefore, DWI images can provide information regarding tissue cellularity. As DWI does not require gadolinium contrast material, DWI is attractive in patients with renal dysfunction at high risk for nephrogenic systemic fibrosis [23, 54]. However, DWI has played only a minor role in abdominal imaging for a long time, as DWI in the body suffers from low signal-to-noise ratio (SNR), low spatial resolution, and significant artifact caused by patient-related motion. With advanced technologic development, including new scanner generations with homogenous magnetic fields and with introduction of high-grade amplitudes and parallel imaging, DWI with echo-planar images is suitable for a high-quality and robustness [52, 55]. The DWI of the liver is usually performed before contrast material administration, although performing DWI after administration of gadolinium chelates did not appear to significantly affect ADC calculations [54]. DWI can help to increase the detection rate of focal liver lesions and show added value increasing the detection rate for HCC with gadolinium-enhanced dynamic MR in patients with liver cirrhosis [25, 54, 56].

MR elastography (MRE) is an emerging technique which can assess the tissue mechanical properties quantitatively [57, 58]. Using modified phase-contrast MR sequences to image propagating shear waves in tissue, MRE is the proposed noninvasive method for measuring the stiffness value of the liver parenchyma and focal liver lesions [59–61]. The technique is used to obtain spatial maps and measurements of shear wave displacement patterns [23]. The wave images are processed to generate maps known as elastograms, which show local quantitative values of the shear modulus of the tissues [58]. There have been several reports concerning the feasibility of MRE of the liver, and these studies offered promising results indicating that MRE of the liver can be used as a successful quantitative method for the noninvasive diagnosis of liver fibrosis [61–64]. Inspired by these successful application of MRE to noninvasive evaluation of hepatic fibrosis, recent study tried to evaluate the usability of MRE to characterize solid liver tumors [58].

MR Contrast Agent for Liver Imaging

The major classes of contrast agents currently used for assessing cirrhosis-associated hepatocellular nodules include the three classes: gadolinium chelates with low molecular weight extracellular agent, reticuloendothelial system (RES)-targeting agent including superparamagnetic iron oxide (SPIO) particles, and hepatobiliary contrast agents. Low molecular weight gadolinium chelates are extracellular paramagnetic contrast agents distributed within the extracellular interstitial space [26]. Gadolinium has seven unpaired electrons and thus is highly paramagnetic. Gadolinium causes T1 shortening of adjacent water protons, and these T1 shortening effects tend to cause signal enhancement at T1-weighted imaging [65, 66]. Gadolinium chelates and iodinated contrast media have the similar pharmacokinetics in the liver as well as throughout the body and enter the liver via the hepatic artery and portal vein and are freely redistributed from the vascular to the interstitial space [37]. Therefore, gadolinium chelate-enhanced T1-weighted image can be understood as the manner used for the interpretation of iodinated contrast-enhanced CT imaging. The important difference between gadolinium chelates and iodinated contrast is that the iodine molecule itself is imaged at computed tomography, whereas in MR it is the effect of gadolinium that is assessed rather than molecule itself [37]. For exact assessment of liver tissue or hepatic tumor vascularity using gadolinium chelates with T1-weighted image, well-timed arterial phase imaging is crucial. Therefore, dynamic contrast-enhanced T1-image acquisition and variable methods for determining the acquisition timing are widely used for liver MRI.

Reticuloendothelial agents target the RES, particularly liver and spleen. The uptake of such agents, like that of technetium 99 m sulfur colloid in nuclear medicine, reflects the number of functioning macrophages [67, 68]. RES-targeting agents in clinical use include superparamagnetic iron oxide (SPIO) particles [37]. These dextran-coated iron-based particles are 30–150 nm in diameter [69]. SPIO particles are phagocytosed by macrophages throughout the whole body but are preferentially entrapped by Kupffer cells taking up more than 80 % of circulating particles, which line the hepatic sinusoids [37]. SPIO particles act as a negative contrast agent. Their superparamagnetic properties cause local magnetic field inhomogeneity and result in considerable T2 and T2* shortening [37, 67].

Tissues that accumulate SPIO particle thus reduced signal intensity, particularly on T2- and T2*-weighted images [66, 70]. Therefore, T2- or T2*-weighted sequences must be needed for evaluation of focal liver lesion after administration of SPIO particles. Most focal hepatic lesions including liver tumors are deficient in Kupffer cells and do not accumulate SPIO particles [71, 72]. Therefore, after administration of SPIO particles, focal hepatic lesions appear relatively hyperintense as the background liver which accumulates the SPIO particle darkens preferentially [37]. In some institutions, SPIO particles are used in combination with gadolinium chelates to create a dual-contrast effect. With this technique so called as dual-contrast liver MRI, the SPIO particles are administrated first and are followed later by an infusion of gadolinium chelates [37]. The two agents synergistically improve lesion-to-liver contrast on dynamic T1-weighted images because background liver is darkened by the SPIO particles uptake by Kupffer cells whereas the focal liver lesion of interest including HCC is highlighted by gadolinium chelates [73–75]. For exact evaluation of focal liver lesion with dual-contrast liver MRI protocol, both T2- and T2*-weighted images after SPIO particle administration and before infusion of gadolinium chelates and dynamic T1-weighted images after gadolinium chelates administration are required. However, the appearance on subsequent dynamic gadolinium chelate-enhanced images may be altered due to the previously injected SPIO particles, and the assessment of venous washout may be impaired [26, 75]. In case of severe liver dysfunction with or without cirrhosis, the ability of SPIO particle accumulation by Kupffer cell is decreased, which would limit the utility of this agent [76]. In such cases, the spleen is the site of preferential SPIO uptake. SPIO particles cause signal intensity loss; thus, SPIO-enhanced images tend to be signal poor [37]. To compensate this drawback of SPIO particles, the voxel size or the acquisition time may have to be increased depending on the indication of liver MRI. Signal intensity loss in the liver also may lead to obscuration of the intrahepatic bile ducts by blooming artifacts [37]. Accordingly, MR cholangiographic sequences should be obtained before SPIO particle administration. Hepatic signal intensity loss may also result in the partial obscuration of focal liver lesions, and this is another drawback of SPIO particles.

Hepatobiliary contrast agents are paramagnetic compounds that are taken up by functioning hepatocytes and excreted in bile. Agents of this class increase the signal intensity of the liver, bile duct, and some hepatocyte-containing lesions at T1-weighted imaging [74, 77, 78]. Manganese is chelated to dipyridoxyl diphosphate to produce the prototype hepatobiliary agent known as mangafodipir trisodium [37]. Nowadays, new gadolinium-based contrast agents having both extracellular and hepatobiliary properties are developed and introduced in liver MR imaging: gadobenate dimeglumine (Gd-BOPTA) and gadolinium ethoxybenzyl diethylenetriaminepentaacetic acid (Gd-EOB-DTPA). These contrast media are commonly applied for the study of liver vascular supply during the dynamic studies on the first part of image acquisition [49, 79]. Moreover, thanks to their lipophilic characteristics, these media, after the intravascular and interstitial distribution, are taken up by functioning hepatocytes, metabolized, and excreted into the bile through the so-called canalicular multispecific organic anion transporter, shared with bilirubin [80]. The main difference between Gd-BOPTA and Gd-EOB-DTPA consists in the fact that approximately 50 % of Gd-EOB-DTPA is excreted by the biliary tract, while regarding Gd-BOPTA, this percentage is much lower, being approximately 5 % of the administered dose [78]. The peak of intracellular concentration of these contrast agents ranges from 20 to 60 min after injection, depending on the biliary excretion rate of contrast medium and on the hepatic function of the patient [81, 82]. Therefore, although two imaging sessions are typically required with Gd-BOPTA if dynamic imaging and hepatobiliary phase imaging are desired, one imaging session is necessary with Gd-EOB-DTPA for assessment of lesion vascularity using dynamic images and hepatocellular function using hepatobiliary phase [23]. Thanks to their dual function, these newly developed gadolinium-based hepatobiliary contrast agents are nowadays applied for a number of clinical purposes such as characterization of focal liver lesions, the correct assessment of hepatic metastasis, as well as the characterization of cirrhosis-associated hepatocellular nodules [83–88].

Hepatocarcinogenesis and MR Imaging Features of Hepatocellular Nodules

Liver cirrhosis is the end result of chronic liver disease and is characterized by destruction of the normal hepatic architecture, which is replaced by fibrotic septa and formation of a spectrum of hepatocellular nodules ranging from benign regenerative nodules to overt HCC [89, 90]. The development of HCC in a cirrhotic liver is described as a multistep progression, from low-grade DN to high-grade DN, then to DN with microscopic foci of HCC, then to small well-differentiated HCC, and finally to overt carcinoma [13, 14]. High-grade DN is considered as premalignant lesion, and patients with high-grade DN are at the greatest risk of developing HCC [14]. The differentiation of these cirrhosis-associated hepatocellular nodules and early detection of HCC are important, because the most effective treatment for HCC is surgical resection or transplantation and local ablation therapy when the HCC is small [21, 22]. However, their accurate characterization may be difficult even at histopathologic analysis, because of the multistep process that features of these cirrhosis-associated hepatocellular nodules overlap, particularly with regard to differentiation of DN and small HCC [9, 26]. Several important changes within the hepatocellular nodules can occur during the progression of hepatocarcinogenesis toward to HCC, and these changes can provide the clue for the differential diagnosis for cirrhosis-associated hepatocellular nodules. Therefore, the radiologist should know these important changes and be familiar with these imaging features.

Regenerative Nodule

A regenerative nodule is defined as a hepatocellular nodule containing one (monoacinar regenerative nodule) or more portal tracts (multiacinar regenerative nodule) in a liver that is otherwise abnormal due to either cirrhosis or other severe liver disease [12]. Regenerative nodules form in response to necrosis, altered circulation, or other stimuli [12]. These nodules are the most common cirrhosis-associated hepatocellular nodules [91, 92] and are presented eventually in all cirrhotic livers and are surrounded by fibrous septa [12, 93]. Cirrhosis is classified, on the basis of the size of these nodules in the pathologic specimen, into micronodular ($\leq$3 mm), macronodular (>3 mm), and mixed types [12]. Although most regenerative nodules have a diameter of less than 2 cm, regenerative nodules with a diameter of more than 2 cm have been observed in patients with long-standing Budd-Chiari syndrome [12] and in patients with cirrhosis due to autoimmune hepatitis [94]. Giant regenerative nodules with a diameter of 5 cm have also been described, but they are rare [12]. The largest nodules are usually located near major vessels [26]. Regenerative nodules are constituted by proliferating normal hepatocytes that maintain all metabolic activity of normal hepatocytes [49]. At histologic analysis, regenerative nodules have an intact reticulin framework, a normal vascular profile, and preserved hepatocellular and phagocytic functions [95]. Portal tracts are present, but due to the periportal fibrosis and scarring, ductular proliferation and portal vein obliteration may occur [26]. Because regenerative nodules consist of proliferating normal hepatocytes with surrounding fibrous septa, most of these nodules are indistinct and invisible on T1-weighted and T2-weighted images [89]. Less commonly, they can be hyperintense to surrounding liver parenchyma on T1-weighted images. The exact cause for this T1 hyperintensity is unknown; it may be due to the intranodular presence of lipid, protein, or possibly copper [96, 97]. Lipid-containing regenerative nodules also display a signal loss on opposed-phase GRE images in comparison with in-phase images. Steatotic regenerative nodules tend to occur in multiples [26]. A single fatty nodule may be suggestive of a dysplastic or malignant process [26]. Some regenerative nodules can contain iron (the so-called siderotic nodules), and these iron-containing regenerative nodules may have decreased signal intensity on both T1- and T2-weighted images due to susceptibility effects of iron [89, 92, 98, 99]. Generally, the blood supply of a regenerative nodule continues to be largely from the portal vein with minimal contribution from the hepatic artery and overlays that of liver parenchyma [100]. Therefore, such a blood supply pattern can explain why there is no enhancement during the hepatic arterial phase on MR images (Fig. 1). Hepatic arterial phase enhancement in regenerative nodules has been reported in few cases and can be mistaken for HCC [93, 101]; however, the lack of washout during the portal venous and late equilibrium phases enables the differentiation between the capillarization of sinusoids and a true neoangiogenesis, which characterizes the HCC blood supply [95]. As most regenerative nodules have a preserved phagocytic action by functioning Kupffer cell, they can accumulate

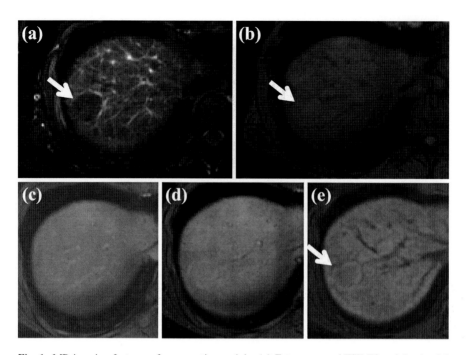

Fig. 1 MR imaging features of regenerative nodule. (**a**) Fat-suppressed FSE T2-weighted axial MR image shows approximately 2 cm-sized subtle low-signal-intensity nodule in segment VIII of the liver (*white arrow*). (**b**) On T1-weighted image, this nodule shows iso-signal intensity to surrounding liver parenchyma (*white arrow*). (**c**) On arterial phase Gd-EOB-DTPA-enhanced image, this nodule shows no arterial enhancement. (**d**) On portal venous phase, this nodule shows iso-signal intensity. (**e**) On hepatobiliary phase image obtained 20 min after administration of Gd-EOB-DTPA, this nodule shows iso-signal intensity. Subtle hyperintensity is also seen at the periphery of this nodule. On pathologic exam, this nodule is diagnosed with regenerative nodule

SPIO particle like a normal liver parenchyma and appear hypointense on SPIO-enhanced T2- and T2*-weighted images and isointense to surrounding liver parenchyma. Uptake and excretion of hepatobiliary contrast agents by these regenerative nodules is usually preserved, and on hepatobiliary phase, virtually all regenerative nodules have a similar signal intensity to surrounding liver parenchyma, which gives the liver a homogeneous appearance [26]. Occasionally, some regenerative nodules show hyperintense signal on hepatobiliary phase, and this can be explained as follow: regenerative nodules may have sufficient hepatocellular function to take up the hepatobiliary contrast agent but not to excrete it (i.e., excretion function of hepatocyte is impaired firstly) [26]. Regenerative nodules with a diameter of more than 15 mm at imaging have an increased likelihood of being dysplastic or malignant and can be mistaken for HCC [26]. However, an absence of hepatic arterial phase gadolinium contrast enhancement, preserved uptake function of hepatobiliary contrast agents, and accumulation of SPIO particles are findings suggestive of benignity [26].

Dysplastic Nodule

A dysplastic nodule is defined as a nodule of hepatocytes of at least 1 mm in diameter, and is composed of hepatocytes that display histologic characteristics of abnormal growth but do not meet the histologic criteria for malignancy [12]. Dysplastic nodules usually occur in the setting of cirrhosis and may be classified as low or high grade, according to the degree of dysplasia [12, 26]. Dysplastic nodules are found in 15–25 % of cirrhotic livers [102]. Dysplastic nodules are characterized histologically by progressive architectural derangement, nuclear crowding, atypia, and a variable number of unpaired arterioles or capillaries [26]. Low-grade dysplastic nodules closely resemble the regenerative nodules histologically. These nodules are composed of hepatocytes with minimal atypia, including slightly increased nuclear/cytoplasmic ratio, minimal nuclear atypia, and absent mitosis as well as have the normal vascular profile, hepatocellular function, and Kupffer cell density [12]. Low-grade dysplastic nodules are considered to have low malignant potential with slow, infrequent progression to HCC and are not thought to be premalignant [103]. To the contrary, high-grade dysplastic nodules show at least moderate dysplasia, some architectural distortion, and occasional mitosis, with sinusoidal capillarization and an increased density of unpaired arteries [104]. They may even express alpha-fetoprotein (AFP) but are not frankly malignant [105]. The Kupffer cell density is variable; it may be increased, normal, or diminished [106–108]. High-grade dysplastic nodules are thought to progress to HCC more frequently than low-grade dysplastic nodules [103]. They are considered as premalignant, and development of HCC within a dysplastic nodule has been reported within as little as 4 months [109, 110]. However, the rate of malignant transformation of dysplastic nodules is relatively slow, and it has been suggested that both high- and low-grade dysplastic nodules may disappear on follow-up studies and that only a small percentage of high-grade dysplastic nodules progress to HCC [26, 111]. As expected on the basis of their heterogeneous histologic characteristics, dysplastic nodules have variable appearance on MR images, and their signal intensity characteristics overlap with those of regenerative nodules and well-differentiated HCC [26] (Figs. 2 and 3). However, many of dysplastic nodules usually have similar signal intensity on T1- and T2-weighted images to regenerative nodules; thus, they are isointense to surrounding liver parenchyma [9]. Some dysplastic nodules can retain copper, which causes them to have hyperintensity on T1-weighted images [89]. If siderotic, these nodules are hypointense to surrounding liver parenchyma on T1- and T2-weighted images due to susceptibility effects of iron. Occasionally, both regenerative and dysplastic nodules can infract, leading to high signal intensity on T2-weighted images, and therefore are often mistaken for HCC [112]. Regarding blood supply to dysplastic nodules, low-grade dysplastic nodules are normally supplied by the portal vein, and therefore are isointense to liver parenchyma during the hepatic arterial phase [9]. Whereas some high-grade dysplastic nodules can receive increasing arterial blood supply [113–116], this feature of high-grade dysplastic nodules may overlap with those of HCC nodules

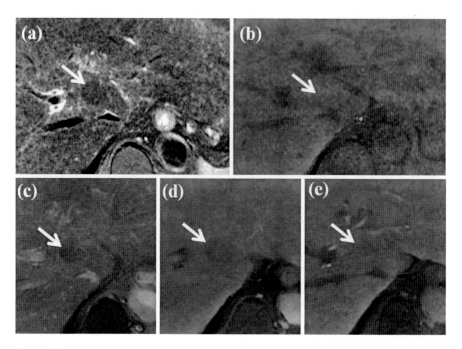

Fig. 2 MR imaging features of dysplastic nodule. (**a**) T2-weighted FSE axial MR image shows approximately 2 cm-sized low-signal-intensity nodule in segment I of the liver (*white arrow*). (**b**) On T1-weighted image, this nodule shows iso- or slightly high signal intensity (*white arrow*). (**c**, **d**, **e**) On dynamic contrast enhancement, this nodule (*white arrow*) reveals low signal intensity on arterial (**c**), portal (**d**), and equilibrium image (**e**)

during the process of hepatocarcinogenesis. These nodules can reveal the contrast enhancement on hepatic arterial phase, and therefore can be mistaken for HCC [9]. In case of high-grade dysplastic nodules showing an arterial enhancement, the differential diagnosis with an HCC is mainly demanded by the lack of washout on portal venous and late equilibrium phase images [49]. Regarding RES-targeting agents, dysplastic nodules usually accumulate the SPIO particles, therefore appear as hypointense on SPIO-enhanced T2- or T2*-weighted images and as isointense to surrounding liver parenchyma. However, the density of Kupffer cells in high-grade dysplastic nodules may vary, thus explaining the different signal intensities, ranging from slightly hypointense to iso- or even slightly hyperintense [49]. Regarding hepatobiliary contrast agents, it is not yet clear whether this class of contrast agent permits the characterization of dysplastic nodules [26]. A dysplastic nodule with a focal focus of HCC was first described on T2-weighted images as "a nodule within a nodule" appearance [117]. The classic MR appearance is a focus of high signal intensity within a low-signal-intensity nodule on T2-weighted images, and this focus of HCC may also show arterial enhancement [118] (Figs. 4 and 5).

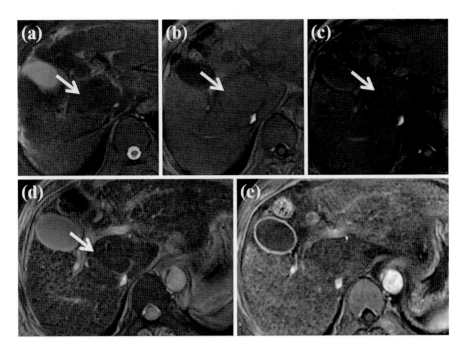

Fig. 3 Large fat-containing dysplastic nodule. (**a**) T2-weighted FSE axial MR image shows approximately 3 cm-sized low-signal-intensity nodule in segment I of the liver (*white arrow*). (**b**) On in-phase T1-weighted image, this nodule shows iso-signal intensity (*white arrow*). (**c**) On opposed-phase T1-weighted image, signal drop is seen for this nodule when compared with in-phase image (*white arrow*), suggesting fat-containing nodule. (**d**) On SPIO-enhanced T2*-weighted image, this nodule shows accumulation of SPIO particle, resulting in signal drop (*white arrow*). (**e**) On arterial phase-contrast-enhanced image, no arterial enhancement is seen on this nodule

Hepatocellular Carcinoma

HCC is defined as a malignant neoplasm composed of cells with hepatocellular differentiation [12]. HCC generally are describes as small (<2 cm in diameter) or large (≥2 cm in diameter). The classic system of macroscopic classification of HCC, in use since 1901, includes three major types: nodular when there are small lesions with distinct margins, massive when there is a single large mass with or without small satellite nodules, and diffuse when there are multiple infiltrative tumors [119]. Large HCCs tend to show evidence of necrosis and often have a mosaic appearance characterized by a seemingly random distribution of confluent small nodules with intervening fibrous septa and areas of necrosis [12, 26]. Tumor capsules, irregular margins, satellite nodules, and vascular invasion are frequently found with such large HCCs [12, 120, 121]. All these features of large HCCs can provide the clue for the MR imaging diagnosis of HCCs. However, regarding small

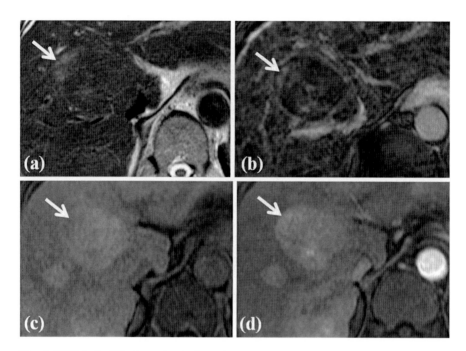

Fig. 4 HCC foci within large dysplastic nodule. (**a**) T2-weighted FSE axial MR image shows approximately 4 cm-sized heterogeneous signal intensity mass in segment IV of the liver. Right upper portion of this nodule shows high signal intensity (*white arrow*) within the surrounding low-signal-intensity nodule. This feature of nodule is called as nodule-in-nodule appearance. (**b**) On SPIO-enhanced T2*-weighted image, right upper portion of nodule does not accumulate SPIO particle, resulting in high signal intensity (*white arrow*). (**c**) On T1-weighted image, this nodule shows high signal intensity except right upper portion (*white arrow*). (**d**) On arterial phase-contrast-enhanced image, arterial enhancement is seen for right upper portion of this nodule (*white arrow*). On pathologic exam, this right upper portion of nodule is diagnosed with HCC foci

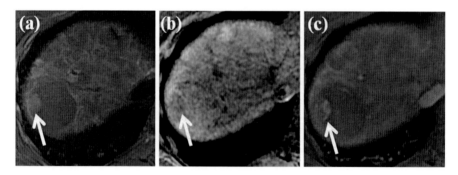

Fig. 5 HCC foci within large dysplastic nodule. (**a**) T2-weighted FSE axial MR image shows approximately 4 cm-sized low-signal-intensity nodule in segment VII of the liver. However, right lateral portion of this nodule shows high signal intensity (*white arrow*). (**b**) On T1-weighted image, this right lateral portion of nodule shows slightly low signal intensity (*white arrow*). (**c**) On arterial phase-contrast-enhanced image, arterial enhancement is seen for right lateral portion of this nodule (*white arrow*). On pathologic exam, this right lateral portion of nodule is diagnosed with HCC foci

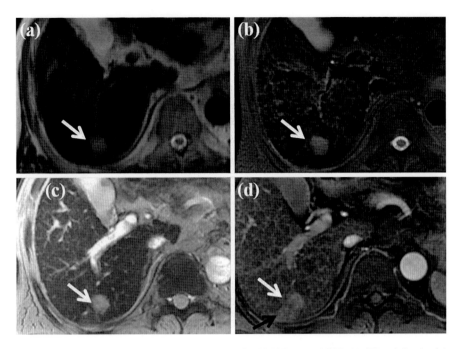

Fig. 6 Typical MR features of small HCC. (**a, b**) On SSFSE (**a**) and FSE (**b**), T2-weighted axial MR images show approximately 2 cm-sized nodule in segment VII of the liver (*white arrow*). (**c**) On SPIO-enhanced T2*-weighted image, this nodule shows high signal intensity (*white arrow*), suggesting no accumulation of SPIO particle. (**d**) On arterial phase-contrast-enhanced image, this nodule shows arterial enhancement (*white arrow*). Arterioportal shunt is also seen adjacent to this nodule (*black arrow*). All these image features are typical for HCC

(<2 cm in diameter) and early stage of HCC, these features are almost absent (Figs. 6, 7, 8, and 9). Histologic features of HCC include advanced architectural distortion (widening and irregularity of hepatocyte plates, presence of pseudoglandular structures, absence of portal tracts, and increased density of unpaired arteries), nuclear atypia, necrosis, and microscopic invasion of stroma and portal tracts [26]. Kupffer cells are also eventually absent in HCC; however, well-differentiated HCCs can contain some Kupffer cells. Normal hepatocyte uptake and excretion function are also disappeared in HCCs. However, some well-differentiated HCCs preserve some uptake function of hepatocytes. A tumor capsule composed of an inner fibrous tissue layer and an outer layer of compressed vessels and bile ducts is evident at histologic examination in 65–82 % of larger HCCs [26]. However, regenerative nodules and dysplastic nodules may also have a tumor capsule. Small HCCs tend to be well differentiated, and large HCCs are most often moderately or poorly differentiated [12]. The presence of extracapsular extension or macrovascular invasion, the absence of tumor capsule, and poor histologic differentiation are associated with a higher risk of tumor recurrence after treatment [26].

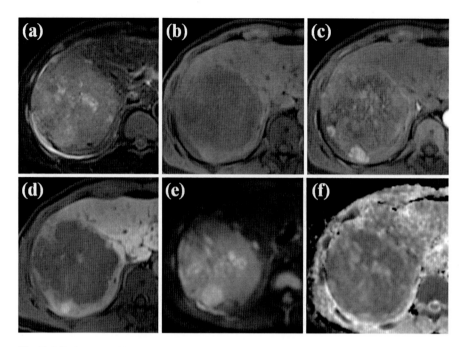

Fig. 7 MR features of large HCC with diffusion and hepatobiliary phase. (**a**) FSE T2-weighted axial MR image shows large heterogeneous high-signal-intensity mass lesion at right lobe of the liver. (**b**) On T1-weighted images, this mass shows low signal intensity. (**c**) On arterial phase Gd-EOB-DTPA-enhanced image, heterogeneous arterial enhancement is seen within this nodule. (**d**) On hepatobiliary phase image obtained 20 min after administration of Gd-EOB-DTPA, this mass shows low signal intensity. (**e**) On diffusion-weighted image, this mass shows high signal intensity. (**f**) On ADC map, this mass reveals low signal intensity. Considering diffusion-weighted image and ADC map, this mass has diffusion restriction, suggesting high cellularity, one of the typical features of HCC

The signal intensity characteristics of HCCs depend on their size, histologic grade, and biologic features, and therefore are variable on T1- and T2-weighted images [122, 123]. Some HCCs show hypersignal intensity to surrounding liver parenchyma on T1-weighted images, and these T1 hyperintensities are attributed to intratumoral fat, to copper, or to glycogen [122, 124]. Intratumoral fat content leads to loss of signal intensity on opposed-phase GRE images in comparison with in-phase GRE images, thus easily identified with dual echo imaging [125]. Moderate hyperintensity on T2-weighted images is one of key imaging features of HCC, as dysplastic nodules do not show T2 hyperintensity unless they are infracted [89, 112, 122]. However, small HCC can be difficult to detect on T2-weighted images because of heterogeneity of cirrhotic liver, which obscures mildly hyperintense tumors. Breathing-related artifacts, particularly in patients with ascites, can also keep HCC from being detected [126, 127]. Also, some well-differentiated HCCs may appear isointense or even hypointense on T2-weighted images to

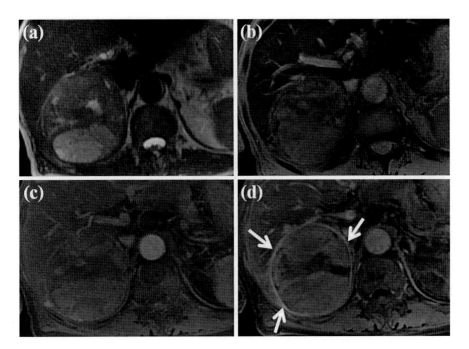

Fig. 8 Large HCC with mosaic pattern and capsular enhancement. (**a**) T2-weighted FSE axial MR image shows approximately 5 cm-sized heterogeneous high-signal-intensity mass lesion in right posterior segment of the liver. (**b**) On SPIO-enhanced T2*-weighted image, this mass shows heterogeneous high signal intensity. (**c**) On arterial phase-contrast-enhanced image, this mass shows heterogeneous arterial enhancement. (**d**) On portal phase image, peripheral capsular enhancement is seen (*white arrows*)

surrounding liver parenchyma [26]. Large HCCs can exhibit a greater variability of signal intensity, mainly caused by necrosis and hemorrhage. Hemorrhagic HCCs may show marked high signal intensity on T1-weighted images and low signal intensity on T2- and T2*-weighted images. Intratumoral necrosis typically manifests as one or more areas of low signal intensity on T1-weighted images and high signal intensity onT2-weighted images [26].

In nature of blood supply to the cirrhosis-associated hepatocellular nodules, as the progression of multistep carcinogenesis from regenerative nodules to overt HCC, gradual reduction of the normal hepatic arterial and portal venous blood supply to the nodule, and followed by an increase in the abnormal arterial supply via newly formed abnormal arteries (neoangiogenesis) are the key features of change occurring within the nodules, and these features were reported by some investigators with CT during hepatic arteriography (CTHA) and CT during arterial portography (CTAP) [116, 128]. Histologically, this feature corresponds to a diminution in the portal tracts (portal vein and hepatic artery), which are virtually absent in HCC [128]. Moreover, unpaired arteries and sinusoidal capillarization are most common in HCC, less common in dysplastic nodules, and rare in regenerative

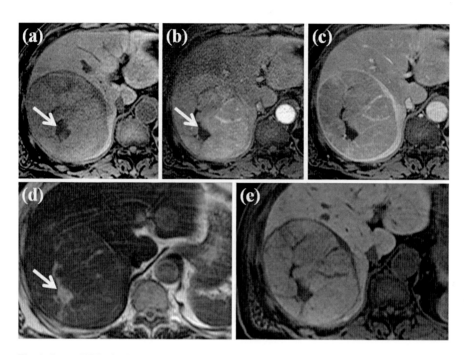

Fig. 9 Large HCC with inner necrosis. (**a**) On T1-weighted axial MR image shows approximately 7 cm-sized mass lesion in right posterior segment of the liver. More prominent hypointensity is seen at central portion of mass (*white arrow*). (**b**) On arterial phase-contrast-enhanced image, contrast enhancement of mass is seen except for the central portion (*white arrow*). (**c**) Portal phase image shows peripheral capsular enhancement of this mass. (**d**) On FSE T2-weighted image, this mass shows moderate-degree high signal intensity. More prominent hyperintensity is also seen at central portion of mass (*white arrow*). On pathologic exam, this portion is diagnosed as internal necrosis of HCC. (**e**) On mangafodipir trisodium-enhanced T1-weighted MR image, this mass shows low signal intensity

nodules [9, 104]. Therefore, overt HCCs provide their blood supply wholly from newly formed abnormal arteries. This process of neoangiogenesis of arterial recruitment during the hepatocarcinogenesis reflects the one of key imaging features of HCC, which is arterial enhancement [129, 130]. With moderate hyperintensity on T2-weighted images, arterial enhancement (hypervascularity) is considered as essential characteristic of HCC. Enhancement tends to be heterogeneous in large HCCs and is homogeneous in small HCCs [123, 131]. However, all HCCs are not hypervascular, and approximately 80–90 % of HCCs are hypervascular and show intense enhancement on hepatic arterial phase after an injection of gadolinium contrast agents [26]. About 10–20 % of HCCs are hypovascular and show contrast enhancement slightly less than that in surrounding liver parenchyma on hepatic arterial phase. Typically, hypovascular HCCs are small, well-differentiated tumors [26]. This feature probably reflects the stage of hepatocarcinogenesis within nodule where there has been partial or complete loss of the normal portal tract, with no associated increased neo-arterializations to cause hyperintensity in the hepatic arterial phase [128, 132]. However, poorly differentiated and diffusely infiltrative hypovascular HCC also may occur [133, 134]. In such cases, despite large size and aggressive behavior, HCCs may be difficult to detect on gadolinium-enhanced MR images. In such cases, T2-weighted images or SPIO-enhanced images can help the visualization of these tumors [26]. Since portal venous blood supply to HCC is reduced, HCCs usually become hypointense in the portal venous phase, the so-called washout. These washouts and hypointensity to liver parenchyma of HCCs are more evident on delayed phase images and highly specific for HCCs with a reported overall sensitivity of 89 % and specificity of 96 % for delayed hypointensity [129]. Rarely, some HCCs may remain hyperintense to surrounding liver parenchyma on portal venous and delayed phase images [9]. On portal venous and delayed phase images, HCC can show a delayed enhancing outer rim "capsule," and these features are also highly specific for HCCs [9, 89, 101]. Ueda et al. reported that all 32 HCCs (mean diameter, 2.5 cm) in their study using single-level dynamic CT hepatic arteriography (CTHA) showed surrounding halo of enhancement or "corona enhancement" in the venous phase [135]. This finding can be explained by portal venous drainage of the HCCs, and the portal venous drainage of HCCs may explain the high incidence of portal vein thrombosis associated with HCC [9]. A tumor capsule can appear as a thin circumferential rim at the periphery of an HCC nodule on MR images and typically thickens with increasing tumor size [136]. On unenhanced T1- and T2-weighted images, the tumor capsule often shows low signal intensity. As tumor capsules are composed of fibrous inner tissue and compressed outer vessels, they enhance progressively after gadolinium contrast administration and retain contrast agent longer, therefore showing hyperintensity to the surrounding liver parenchyma on delayed phase images [136–138]. Therefore, delayed capsular rim enhancement of HCCs can be explained by either portal venous drainage of the HCC or tumor capsule delayed enhancement.

Regarding SPIO particles, moderately and poorly differentiated HCCs characteristically accumulate less or eventually no SPIO particles when comparing with the surrounding liver parenchyma, and therefore show no signal drop in SPIO-enhanced T2- and T2*-weighted images, revealing the relatively high signal intensity to surrounding liver parenchyma. The neoplastic sinusoid capillarization and formation of unpaired arteries lead to progressive loss of Kupffer cells within nodules [139]. However, well-differentiated HCCs can contain Kupffer cells and may accumulate SPIO particles, and therefore tend to be iso- or hypointense on SPIO-enhanced T2- and T2*-weighted images compared with the surrounding liver parenchyma [106–108]. Large HCCs may have nonuniform Kupffer cells density and show heterogeneous uptake of SPIO particles [26]. HCCs are lacking of functioning hepatocytes within the nodules, so they do not accumulate or excrete hepatobiliary contrast agents. Therefore, on hepatobiliary phase images obtained after administration of hepatobiliary contrast agents, HCCs appear as low signal intensity in comparison with the surrounding liver parenchyma [133, 140]. According to recent study, hepatobiliary phase images obtained using Gd-EOB-DTPA can increase the sensitivity for detecting HCCs [85]. Rarely, some small HCCs can show iso- or even hyperintensity on hepatobiliary phase, especially in case of well-differentiated HCCs. These findings can be explained as follows: well-differentiated small HCCs may preserve hepatocellular function to take up the hepatobiliary contrast agent but have impaired excreting function, and therefore the hepatobiliary contrast agents can be retained within these nodules.

Functional MRI tools such as DWI and elastography can also help the detection and diagnosis of HCC in cirrhotic liver. As other malignant tumor, HCCs have increased cellularity. Increased cellularities within the HCCs prevent water from freely diffusing, and this restricted water molecule diffusion of HCCs can be detected on DWI as hyperintensity lesions. There are compelling data that show better performance of DWI compared with T2-weighted imaging for lesion characterization [23, 54]. DWI can help to increase the detection rate of focal liver lesions and show added value increasing the detection rate for HCC with gadolinium-enhanced MR in cirrhotic liver [25, 54, 56]. In addition, the quantification of restricted diffusion with the ADC maps helps to differentiate malignant lesion from benign lesion [141–143]. Different ADC cutoffs ($1.4–1.6 \times 10^{-3}$ mm^2/s) have been suggested in the literature, with a reported sensitivity of 74–100 % and specificity of 77–100 % [23, 53]. However, up to now there is no evidence in the literature in how far DWI might be a feasible approach to differentiate among regenerative nodules, dysplastic nodules, and HCCs [23, 25]. Malignant tumors including HCCs are also harder in comparison with surrounding normal tissues and have increased stiffness values. MR elastography (MRE) can detect focal liver lesions with increased stiffness values and measure the tissue stiffness value quantitatively. According to a previous study [57], HCCs have greater stiffness value than benign tumor or surrounding liver parenchyma, and a cutoff value of 5 kPa for differentiation of benign tumors form malignant hepatic tumors is suggested. Use of MRE may lead to new quantitative tissue characterization parameters for differentiating benign and malignant hepatocellular nodules in a cirrhotic liver [23, 57]. Further studies are needed to validate the possible application of MRE in the diagnosis and monitoring of HCCs [23, 57, 144].

Large HCCs show a more variable pattern. A mosaic pattern is created by confluent nodules separated by fibrous septa and area of necrosis [9]. These tumors usually show high signal intensity on T2-weighted images and enhance heterogeneously [145, 146]. Large HCCs do not pose a diagnostic problem.

Diffuse-type HCC constitutes up to 13 % of cases of HCC [147] and appears as an extensive, heterogeneous, permeative hepatic tumor, often associated with an elevated serum AFP level [9]. These tumors have a patchy or nodular early enhancement pattern and can be difficult to detect on unenhanced T1- or T2-weighted images but become hypointense in the late phase of enhancement [147]. Contour deformity of liver surface can also be a clue for the diagnosis of these tumors.

Portal vein invasion is another important characteristic of HCC and is thought to be associated with the portal venous drainage of HCC [135, 148]. However, patients

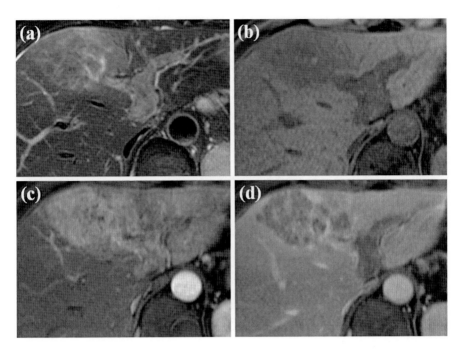

Fig. 10 HCC with left portal vein invasion. (**a**) T2-weighted FSE axial MR image shows diffuse high signal intensity at left medial segment of the liver. Expansion of left portal vein with inner high signal intensity is also seen. (**b**) T1-weighted image shows diffuse low signal intensity at left medial segment with expansion of left portal vein with inner low signal intensity. (**c**) On arterial phase-contrast-enhanced image, diffuse arterial enhancement of left medial segment is seen. Expanded left portal vein also shows arterial enhancement. (**d**) Portal phase image shows diffuse low signal intensity in left medial segment. The expanded left portal vein also shows low signal intensity, suggesting washout. All these imaging features are typical for HCC with left portal vein invasion

with cirrhosis can also develop benign portal vein thrombosis secondary to portal hypertension and venous stasis [149]. Malignant portal vein thrombosis in HCC occurs by means of direct invasion of vein [149]. The incidence of malignant portal vein thrombosis in association with HCC is reported from 5 to 44 % [150–153], and at autopsy, the reported rate has been increased [154]. A malignant portal vein thrombus is always contiguous with or directly in contact with a parenchymal HCC [9]. Increased signal intensity on T2-weighted images is highly suggestive of malignant thrombosis. Malignant portal vein thrombosis is characterized by dramatic expansion of the vein, compared with near-normal-diameter veins in benign bland thrombosis [155] (Fig. 10). The enhancement of intravascular tumor tissue during the arterial phase and filling defect on later phase images is also highly specific for malignant thrombosis and is due to the presence of neovascularization of tumor [155]. Therefore, assessment of the dynamic gadolinium-enhanced gradient-echo images can help distinguish between bland portal vein thrombosis and malignant ones. A bland thrombus has very low signal intensity due to

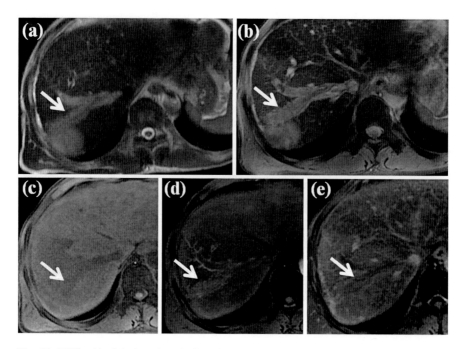

Fig. 11 HCC with right hepatic vein invasion. (**a**) T2-weighted FSE axial MR image shows approximately 3 cm-sized high-signal-intensity mass lesion in segment VII of the liver. Expansion of adjacent right hepatic vein with inner high signal intensity (*white arrow*) is also seen. (**b**) On SPIO-enhanced T2*-weighted image, expansion of right hepatic vein with high signal intensity is also noted (*white arrow*). (**c**) On T1-weighted image, expanded right hepatic vein shows low signal intensity (*white arrow*). (**d**) On arterial phase-contrast-enhanced image, arterial enhancement of expanded right hepatic vein is seen (*white arrow*). (**e**) Portal phase image shows low signal intensity of expanded right hepatic vein, suggesting washout (*white arrow*). All these imaging features are typical for HCC with right hepatic vein invasion

hemosiderin content, whereas malignant thrombus has the same signal intensity and contrast enhancement pattern as the HCC [9, 156]. However, some rare cases with enhancement of bland benign thrombi have also been reported [155]. Differentiation of these two types of thrombi is critical in clinical practice. The presence of a tumor thrombus also carries a higher risk of hematogenous dissemination of HCC and precludes liver transplantation for treatment options. However, a bland thrombus is a frequent finding in the setting of liver cirrhosis, may occur in the absence of HCC, and depending on its location and extent, may be of minimal importance for decision making with regard to disease management [26].

Invasion of HCC into the hepatic veins occurs less frequently than and is often associated with invasion of the portal vein [9] (Fig. 11). In rare cases, HCC may grow into the major bile ducts, resulting in obstructive jaundice, and is frequently associated with concomitant portal vein tumor invasion [154] (Fig. 12).

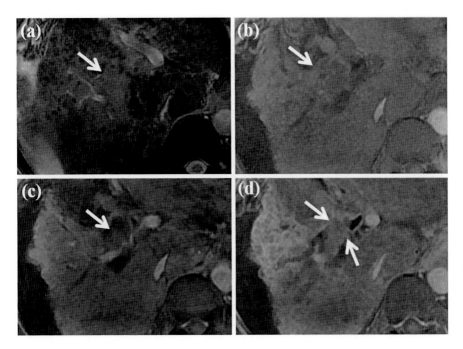

Fig. 12 HCC with bile duct invasion. (**a**) On SPIO-enhanced T2*-weighted image, diffuse high signal intensity at right anterior segment of the liver is seen (*white arrow*). (**b**) T1-weighted image also shows diffuse subtle low signal intensity at right anterior segment (*white arrow*). (**c, d**) On arterial phase (**a**) and portal phase (**b**), contrast-enhanced images show expansion of right anterior bile duct with intraluminal enhancing mass (*white arrows*). This intraluminal enhancing mass is HCC which invades right anterior bile duct

Lesions Mimicking HCC

Among the MR imaging characteristics of HCC, arterial enhancement is considered the most consistent feature of HCC. However, other arterial enhancing nonmalignant lesions can also be seen in the cirrhotic liver, especially those measuring smaller than 2 cm in diameter, which may be regarded as HCC and explains the high incidence of false-positive results for HCC [157–159] (Figs. 13, 14, 15, and 16). Transient arterial enhancement due to non-tumorous arterioportal shunts [160, 161] or focal obstruction of a distal parenchymal portal vein [38] is often seen in the cirrhotic liver. Usually these shunts are isointense to surrounding liver parenchyma on T1- and T2-weighted images and are commonly located in the liver periphery, wedge shaped. However, shunts can be seen as nodular or irregularly outlined shape and may also show minimally hyperintensity on T2-weighted images [38, 160, 162]. In such cases, the differentiation between small HCC and arterioportal shunts is difficult, and shunt can be misinterpreted as small HCC. On dynamic contrast-enhanced MR images, shunts are isointense to the surrounding liver parenchyma on portal venous and delayed phase. Aberrant venous drainage and

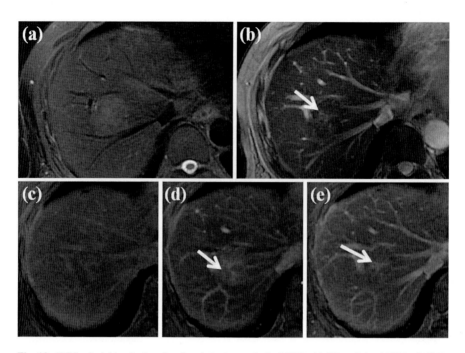

Fig. 13 HCC mimicking lesion: focal nodular hyperplasia (FNH). (**a**) T2-weighted FSE axial MR image shows approximately 3 cm-sized high-signal-intensity lesion. (**b**) On SPIO-enhanced T2*-weighted image, this nodule shows low signal intensity suggesting accumulation of SPIO particle. However, central portion of this nodule corresponding to central scar does not accumulate SPIO particle, resulting in high signal intensity (*arrow*). (**c**) On precontrast T1-weighted image, this nodule shows subtle low signal intensity. (**d**) On arterial phase-contrast-enhanced image, arterial enhancement of this nodule is seen. However, central portion of this nodule does not show enhancement on this phase (*white arrow*). (**e**) On equilibrium phase, delayed enhancement of central scar is clearly seen (*white arrow*). These imaging findings are consistent with FNH, which can mimic HCC considering T2 high signal intensity and arterial enhancement

early drainage by a subcapsular vein have all been described as hypervascular areas which are seen hyperintense on hepatic arterial phase images and mimicking small HCCs [9, 160, 163]. As shunts and vascular changes are not true mass or tumor, functional MR imaging including DWI can also help the differential diagnosis. However, the ability of DWI differentiating HCCs from non-tumorous lesions has not been fully investigated. Further study has to be needed for this issue.

Fibrosis is frequently found in cirrhotic liver and usually in a lattice-like network throughout the liver. Focal confluent hepatic fibrosis, observed in end-stage liver disease, can have mass-like appearance, and therefore may be mistaken for HCC [164]. Areas of confluent fibrosis can be diffuse but more often focal, wedge shaped with the wide base toward the liver capsule, and usually located in the anterior and medial segment of the liver, either involving the entire segment or a portion of it [164]. Confluent fibrosis is usually associated with atrophy of the affected segment, and capsular retraction over the area is common [93]. Confluent fibrosis is usually of

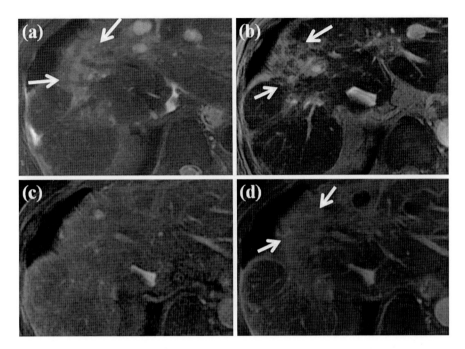

Fig. 14 HCC mimicking lesion: confluent hepatic fibrosis. (**a**) T2-weighted FSE axial MR image shows diffuse high signal intensity at right anterior segment of the liver (*white arrows*). Volume loss of affected segment and capsular retraction are also seen. (**b**) On SPIO-enhanced T2*-weighted image, diffuse wedge-shaped high signal intensity at right anterior segment is seen (*white arrows*), suggesting no accumulation of SPIO particle in this area. (**c**) On arterial phase-contrast-enhanced image, arterial enhancement of this area is not evident. (**d**) On equilibrium phase, diffuse delayed enhancement at right anterior segment is clearly seen (*white arrow*). These features are consistent with confluent hepatic fibrosis, which can mimic HCC considering T2 high signal intensity and no accumulation of SPIO particles

low signal intensity to the surrounding liver parenchyma in T1-weighted images and hyperintense on T2-weighted images. Confluent fibrosis do not contain Kupffer cells, therefore hyperintense on SPIO-enhanced T2- and T2*-weighted images. These hyperintensity on T2-weighted images and SPIO-enhanced images may lead to misclassification of focal confluent hepatic fibrosis as HCCs. On dynamic MR images after gadolinium contrast administration, delayed enhancement of fibrosis is characteristic [9]. However, occasionally confluent fibrosis shows contrast enhancement during the hepatic arterial phase, mimicking small HCCs and requiring biopsy for exact diagnosis [164, 165]. The characteristic shape, location, volume loss, and enhancement pattern can help differentiate focal confluent fibrosis from an HCC [166].

Other arterial enhancing hepatic tumor such as hemangioma, focal nodular hyperplasia (FNH), hepatic adenoma, and hypervascular metastasis can also mimic an HCC [167–169]. Hemangiomas, commonly found in normal livers, are rare in end-stage cirrhosis, probably because the process of cirrhosis can obliterate existing hemangiomas [9]. Therefore, hemangiomas are often atypical in

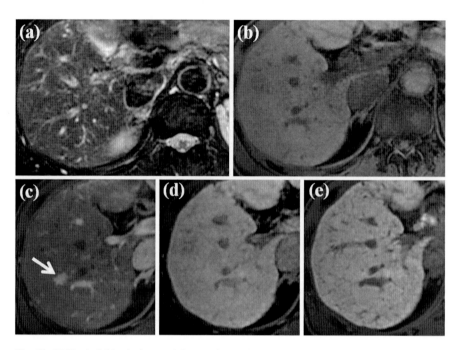

Fig. 15 HCC mimicking lesion: nodular arterioportal (AP) shunt. (**a, b**) There is no focal lesion in the liver on FSE T2-weighted (**a**) and T1-weighted (**b**) axial MR images. (**c**) However, on EOB-DTPA-enhanced arterial phase image, nodular-enhancing lesion is clearly seen (*arrow*). (**d**) On equilibrium phase, however, this nodule is not visualized. (**e**) On hepatobiliary phase image, there is no focal lesion in the liver. This is the case of nodular AP shunt which can mimic HCC considering nodular arterial enhancement

appearance in cirrhotic livers and contain large regions of fibrosis [164]. Especially, with the concomitant use of gadolinium chelates and SPIO particles using dual-contrast protocol, enhancement pattern of hemangioma after gadolinium administration can be impaired due to the previously injected SPIO particle and may lead to misclassification of hemangioma as HCCs [75]. Some FNH and hepatic adenoma have Kupffer cell, therefore can accumulate SPIO particle, and show low signal intensity on SPIO-enhanced T2- and T2*-weighted images. These characteristic can help differentiate these nodules from HCCs [170].

It is important to distinguish HCC from benign large regenerative nodules, which occurs secondary to liver damage without cirrhosis, for example, in case of Budd-Chiari syndrome or severe disease of the portal veins or hepatic sinusoid. These nodules often appear as multiple well-defined arterially enhancing nodules with high signal intensity on T2-weighted images and sometimes delayed hypointensity [171, 172]. They sometimes contain a central scar [173]. Information about patient's history can be helpful [9].

Mass-forming intrahepatic cholangiocarcinoma is also occasionally misinterpreted as an HCC. Mass-forming intrahepatic cholangiocarcinoma usually shows thin or thick rim enhancement in the arterial and venous phases, with progressive

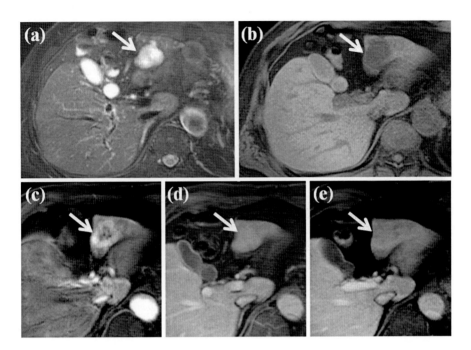

Fig. 16 HCC mimicking lesion: hemangioma. (**a**) FSE T2-weighted axial MR image shows approximately 3 cm-sized high-signal-intensity lesion at segment III of the liver (*white arrow*). (**b**) On T1-weighted image, this lesion shows low signal intensity (*white arrow*). (**c**) On arterial phase-contrast-enhanced image, arterial enhancement is seen on the peripheral portion of this lesion. (**d**) On portal venous phase, complete fill-in-type enhancement of this lesion is also seen (*white arrow*). (**e**) On equilibrium phase, this lesion shows subtle persistent enhancement (*white arrow*). This is the typical MR features of hemangioma which can mimic HCC considering T2 high-signal-intensity arterial contrast enhancement

and concentric filling of contrast agent in the later phases [174]. This pattern of contrast enhancement is atypical for HCC. However, in case of small mass-forming intrahepatic cholangiocarcinoma, arterial enhancement can be seen. Intrahepatic biliary duct dilation distal to the tumor and associated capsular retraction are features more commonly associated with mass-forming intrahepatic cholangiocarcinoma and are rarely seen in association with HCC [174, 175].

Difficulty in Diagnosis of Small ($\leq$2 cm) Arterial Enhancing Lesion

Key MR features for the diagnosis of HCC are as follows: (1) contrast enhancement during the hepatic arterial phase and washout during the later portal venous and equilibrium phase, (2) capsular rim enhancement on portal venous and delayed phase images, (3) moderately hyperintensity on T2-weighted images, (4) hyperintensity on SPIO-enhanced T2- and T2*-weighted images, (5) hypointensity on hepatobiliary phase after administration of hepatobiliary contrast agent, (6) and restricted diffusion on DWI. Large HCCs (>2 cm) usually show all of these features and do not pose a diagnostic problem. However, small HCCs (≤2 cm) tend not to have these entire features but have some of them. Therefore, small nodules are often difficult to characterize as benign or malignant. In addition, small arterially enhancing nodules are not uncommon in the cirrhotic liver, and the majority of these nodules are benign [101, 132, 157, 158, 176–178]. However, detection and characterization of small HCCs is important because curative treatment options such as transplantation or percutaneous ablation are optimally beneficial when the tumor is small [179, 180]. In patients with cirrhosis and small HCC, the 5-year survival rate after transplantation is 80 % compared with less than 5 % in those with untreated symptomatic HCC [6, 178, 181]. If small HCCs are left alone, these HCCs can grow aggressively. Invasion of tumor can also occur before tumors reach the 2 cm cutoff size for small HCC [129]. Therefore, every attempt should be made to characterize these small nodules [9]. If exact characterization of these nodules is not possible with MR images, follow-up imaging or biopsy should be considered to verify their nature. The management of small enhancing nodules (≤2 cm) is mainly dependent on their imaging features [9]. If the imaging features are highly suggestive of malignancy (i.e., hypointensity on delayed image, capsular rim enhancement on portal venous and delayed phase images, moderate hyperintensity on T2-weighted images, restricted diffusion, absence of uptake of SPIO particles and hepatobiliary contrast agent), the diagnosis of HCC should be made at either imaging or biopsy, because resection or ablation therapy is more effective and beneficial than surveillance. However, more often than not, the imaging features of these nodules are nonspecific, and biopsy or follow-up imaging becomes necessary to confirm their nature [9]. The optimal follow-up interval is yet to be established and is influenced by the tumor volume doubling time. Reported doubling time for HCC ranges from 18 to 605 days, and smaller HCCs tend to grow rapidly and to have a shorter doubling time [182–188]. Therefore, a follow-up interval of 3–6 months has been suggested and used in many institute nowadays.

References

1. Parkin DM, Bray F, Ferlay J, Pisani P (2001) Estimating the world cancer burden: Globocan 2000. Int J Cancer 94(2):153–156
2. MacSween RNM, Anthony PP, Scheuer PJ (1979) Pathology of the liver. Churchill Livingstone; distributed in U.S. by Longman, Edinburgh; New York, New York
3. El-Serag HB, Mason AC (1999) Rising incidence of hepatocellular carcinoma in the United States. N Eng J Med 340(10):745–750. doi:10.1056/NEJM199903113401001
4. El-Serag HB (2004) Hepatocellular carcinoma: recent trends in the United States. Gastroenterology 127(5 Suppl 1):S27–S34

5. Bosch FX, Ribes J, Cleries R, Diaz M (2005) Epidemiology of hepatocellular carcinoma. Clin Liver Dis 9(2):191–211, v. doi:10.1016/j.cld.2004.12.009
6. Llovet JM, Burroughs A, Bruix J (2003) Hepatocellular carcinoma. Lancet 362 (9399):1907–1917. doi:10.1016/S0140-6736(03)14964-1
7. Beasley RP, Hwang LY, Lin CC, Chien CS (1981) Hepatocellular carcinoma and hepatitis B virus. A prospective study of 22 707 men in Taiwan. Lancet 2(8256):1129–1133
8. Fattovich G, Giustina G, Schalm SW, Hadziyannis S, Sanchez-Tapias J, Almasio P, Christensen E, Krogsgaard K, Degos F, Carneiro de Moura M et al (1995) Occurrence of hepatocellular carcinoma and decompensation in western European patients with cirrhosis type B. The EUROHEP Study Group on Hepatitis B Virus and Cirrhosis. Hepatology 21 (1):77–82
9. Willatt JM, Hussain HK, Adusumilli S, Marrero JA (2008) MR Imaging of hepatocellular carcinoma in the cirrhotic liver: challenges and controversies. Radiology 247(2):311–330. doi:10.1148/radiol.2472061331
10. Fattovich G, Stroffolini T, Zagni I, Donato F (2004) Hepatocellular carcinoma in cirrhosis: incidence and risk factors. Gastroenterology 127(5 Suppl 1):S35–S50
11. Popper H (1977) Pathologic aspects of cirrhosis. A review. Am J Pathol 87(1):228–264
12. Terminology of nodular hepatocellular lesions. International Working Party (1995). Hepatology 22(3):983–993
13. Coleman WB (2003) Mechanisms of human hepatocarcinogenesis. Curr Mol Med 3 (6):573–588
14. Shah TU, Semelka RC, Pamuklar E, Firat Z, Gerber RD, Shrestha R, Russo MW (2006) The risk of hepatocellular carcinoma in cirrhotic patients with small liver nodules on MRI. Am J Gastroenterol 101(3):533–540. doi:10.1111/j.1572-0241.2006.00450.x
15. Freeny PC, Baron RL, Teefey SA (1992) Hepatocellular carcinoma: reduced frequency of typical findings with dynamic contrast-enhanced CT in a non-Asian population. Radiology 182(1):143–148
16. Fernandez MP, Redvanly RD (1998) Primary hepatic malignant neoplasms. Radiologic Clin 36(2):333–348
17. Meissner HI, Smith RA, Rimer BK, Wilson KM, Rakowski W, Vernon SW, Briss PA (2004) Promoting cancer screening: learning from experience. Cancer 101(5 Suppl):1107–1117. doi:10.1002/cncr.20507
18. Pleguezuelo M, Germani G, Marelli L, Xiruochakis E, Misseri M, Pinelopi M, Arvaniti V, Burroughs AK (2008) Evidence-based diagnosis and locoregional therapy for hepatocellular carcinoma. Expert Rev Gastroenterol Hepatol 2(6):761–784. doi:10.1586/17474124.2.6.761
19. Shimofusa R, Ueda T, Kishimoto T, Nakajima M, Yoshikawa M, Kondo F, Ito H (2010) Magnetic resonance imaging of hepatocellular carcinoma: a pictorial review of novel insights into pathophysiological features revealed by magnetic resonance imaging. J Hepatobiliary Pancreat Sci 17(5):583–589. doi:10.1007/s00534-009-0198-z
20. Llovet JM, Schwartz M, Mazzaferro V (2005) Resection and liver transplantation for hepatocellular carcinoma. Semin Liver Dis 25(2):181–200. doi:10.1055/s-2005-871198
21. Choi BI (2004) The current status of imaging diagnosis of hepatocellular carcinoma. Liver Transpl 10(2 Suppl 1):S20–S25. doi:10.1002/lt.20038
22. Bruix J, Sherman M (2005) Management of hepatocellular carcinoma. Hepatology 42 (5):1208–1236. doi:10.1002/hep.20933
23. Lee JM, Choi BI (2011) Hepatocellular nodules in liver cirrhosis: MR evaluation. Abdom Imaging 36(3):282–289. doi:10.1007/s00261-011-9692-2
24. Ariff B, Lloyd CR, Khan S, Shariff M, Thillainayagam AV, Bansi DS, Khan SA, Taylor-Robinson SD, Lim AK (2009) Imaging of liver cancer. World J Gastroenterol 15 (11):1289–1300
25. Zech CJ, Reiser MF, Herrmann KA (2009) Imaging of hepatocellular carcinoma by computed tomography and magnetic resonance imaging: state of the art. Dig Dis 27 (2):114–124. doi:10.1159/000218343

26. Hanna RF, Aguirre DA, Kased N, Emery SC, Peterson MR, Sirlin CB (2008) Cirrhosis-associated hepatocellular nodules: correlation of histopathologic and MR imaging features. Radiographics 28(3):747–769. doi:10.1148/rg.283055108

27. Karcaaltincaba M, Akhan O (2007) Imaging of hepatic steatosis and fatty sparing. Eur J Radiol 61(1):33–43. doi:10.1016/j.ejrad.2006.11.005

28. Bhartia B, Ward J, Guthrie JA, Robinson PJ (2003) Hepatocellular carcinoma in cirrhotic livers: double-contrast thin-section MR imaging with pathologic correlation of explanted tissue. AJR Am J Roentgenol 180(3):577–584

29. Hussain SM, Wielopolski PA, Martin DR (2005) Abdominal magnetic resonance imaging at 3.0 T: problem or a promise for the future? Top Magn Reson Imaging 16(4):325–335. doi:10.1097/01.rmr.0000224689.06501.16

30. Bartolozzi C, Battaglia V, Bozzi E (2009) HCC diagnosis with liver-specific MRI–close to histopathology. Dig Dis 27(2):125–130. doi:10.1159/000218344

31. Martin DR, Danrad R, Hussain SM (2005) MR imaging of the liver. Radiol Clin North Am 43 (5):861–886, viii. doi:10.1016/j.rcl.2005.05.001

32. Rofsky NM, Lee VS, Laub G, Pollack MA, Krinsky GA, Thomasson D, Ambrosino MM, Weinreb JC (1999) Abdominal MR imaging with a volumetric interpolated breath-hold examination. Radiology 212(3):876–884

33. Blasbalg R, Mitchell DG, Outwater EK, Ito K, Gabata T, Chiowanich P (2000) Free MRA of the abdomen: postprocessing dynamic gadolinium-enhanced 3D axial MR images. Abdom Imaging 25(1):62–66

34. Lee VS, Lavelle MT, Rofsky NM, Laub G, Thomasson DM, Krinsky GA, Weinreb JC (2000) Hepatic MR imaging with a dynamic contrast-enhanced isotropic volumetric interpolated breath-hold examination: feasibility, reproducibility, and technical quality. Radiology 215 (2):365–372

35. Lavelle MT, Lee VS, Rofsky NM, Krinsky GA, Weinreb JC (2001) Dynamic contrast-enhanced three-dimensional MR imaging of liver parenchyma: source images and angiographic reconstructions to define hepatic arterial anatomy. Radiology 218(2):389–394

36. Mori K, Yoshioka H, Takahashi N, Yamaguchi M, Ueno T, Yamaki T, Saida Y (2005) Triple arterial phase dynamic MRI with sensitivity encoding for hypervascular hepatocellular carcinoma: comparison of the diagnostic accuracy among the early, middle, late, and whole triple arterial phase imaging. AJR Am J Roentgenol 184(1):63–69

37. Gandhi SN, Brown MA, Wong JG, Aguirre DA, Sirlin CB (2006) MR contrast agents for liver imaging: what, when, how. Radiographics 26(6):1621–1636. doi:10.1148/rg.266065014

38. Baron RL (1994) Understanding and optimizing use of contrast material for CT of the liver. AJR Am J Roentgenol 163(2):323–331

39. Hollett MD, Jeffrey RB Jr, Nino-Murcia M, Jorgensen MJ, Harris DP (1995) Dual-phase helical CT of the liver: value of arterial phase scans in the detection of small (< or = 1.5 cm) malignant hepatic neoplasms. AJR Am J Roentgenol 164(4):879–884

40. Baron RL, Oliver JH III, Dodd GD III, Nalesnik M, Holbert BL, Carr B (1996) Hepatocellular carcinoma: evaluation with biphasic, contrast-enhanced, helical CT. Radiology 199 (2):505–511

41. Oi H, Murakami T, Kim T, Matsushita M, Kishimoto H, Nakamura H (1996) Dynamic MR imaging and early-phase helical CT for detecting small intrahepatic metastases of hepatocellular carcinoma. AJR Am J Roentgenol 166(2):369–374

42. Earls JP, Rofsky NM, DeCorato DR, Krinsky GA, Weinreb JC (1997) Hepatic arterial-phase dynamic gadolinium-enhanced MR imaging: optimization with a test examination and a power injector. Radiology 202(1):268–273

43. Van Beers BE, Materne R, Lacrosse M, Jamart J, Smith AM, Horsmans Y, Gigot JF, Gilon R, Pringot J (1999) MR imaging of hypervascular liver tumors: timing optimization during the arterial phase. J Magn Reson Imaging 9(4):562–567

44. Hussain HK, Londy FJ, Francis IR, Nghiem HV, Weadock WJ, Gebremariam A, Chenevert TL (2003) Hepatic arterial phase MR imaging with automated bolus-detection three-

dimensional fast gradient-recalled-echo sequence: comparison with test-bolus method. Radiology 226(2):558–566

45. Martin DR, Semelka RC (2005) Magnetic resonance imaging of the liver: review of techniques and approach to common diseases. Semin Ultrasound CT MR 26(3):116–131

46. del Frate C, Bazzocchi M, Mortele KJ, Zuiani C, Londero V, Como G, Zanardi R, Ros PR (2002) Detection of liver metastases: comparison of gadobenate dimeglumine-enhanced and ferumoxides-enhanced MR imaging examinations. Radiology 225(3):766–772

47. Vogt FM, Antoch G, Hunold P, Maderwald S, Ladd ME, Debatin JF, Ruehm SG (2005) Parallel acquisition techniques for accelerated volumetric interpolated breath-hold examination magnetic resonance imaging of the upper abdomen: assessment of image quality and lesion conspicuity. J Magn Reson Imag 21(4):376–382. doi:10.1002/jmri.20288

48. Yu JS, Kim YH, Rofsky NM (2005) Dynamic subtraction magnetic resonance imaging of cirrhotic liver: assessment of high signal intensity lesions on nonenhanced T1-weighted images. J Comput Assist Tomogr 29(1):51–58

49. Bartolozzi C, Battaglia V, Bozzi E (2011) Hepatocellular nodules in liver cirrhosis: contrast-enhanced MR. Abdom Imaging 36(3):290–299. doi:10.1007/s00261-011-9687-z

50. Kele PG, van der Jagt EJ (2010) Diffusion weighted imaging in the liver. World J Gastroenterol 16(13):1567–1576

51. Le Bihan D (1991) Molecular diffusion nuclear magnetic resonance imaging. Magn Reson Q 7(1):1–30

52. Bammer R (2003) Basic principles of diffusion-weighted imaging. Eur J Radiol 45 (3):169–184

53. Taouli B, Koh DM (2010) Diffusion-weighted MR imaging of the liver. Radiology 254 (1):47–66. doi:10.1148/radiol.09090021

54. Taouli B, Ehman RL, Reeder SB (2009) Advanced MRI methods for assessment of chronic liver disease. AJR Am J Roentgenol 193(1):14–27. doi:10.2214/AJR.09.2601

55. Charles-Edwards EM, deSouza NM (2006) Diffusion-weighted magnetic resonance imaging and its application to cancer. Cancer Imaging 6:135–143. doi:10.1102/1470-7330.2006.0021

56. Vandecaveye V, De Keyzer F, Verslype C, Op de Beeck K, Komuta M, Topal B, Roebben I, Bielen D, Roskams T, Nevens F, Dymarkowski S (2009) Diffusion-weighted MRI provides additional value to conventional dynamic contrast-enhanced MRI for detection of hepatocellular carcinoma. Eur Radiol 19(10):2456–2466. doi:10.1007/s00330-009-1431-5

57. Venkatesh SK, Yin M, Glockner JF, Takahashi N, Araoz PA, Talwalkar JA, Ehman RL (2008) MR elastography of liver tumors: preliminary results. AJR Am J Roentgenol 190 (6):1534–1540. doi:10.2214/AJR.07.3123

58. Mariappan YK, Glaser KJ, Ehman RL (2010) Magnetic resonance elastography: a review. Clin Anat 23(5):497–511. doi:10.1002/ca.21006

59. Muthupillai R, Lomas DJ, Rossman PJ, Greenleaf JF, Manduca A, Ehman RL (1995) Magnetic resonance elastography by direct visualization of propagating acoustic strain waves. Science 269(5232):1854–1857

60. Muthupillai R, Rossman PJ, Lomas DJ, Greenleaf JF, Riederer SJ, Ehman RL (1996) Magnetic resonance imaging of transverse acoustic strain waves. Magn Reson Med 36 (2):266–274

61. Rouviere O, Yin M, Dresner MA, Rossman PJ, Burgart LJ, Fidler JL, Ehman RL (2006) MR elastography of the liver: preliminary results. Radiology 240(2):440–448. doi:10.1148/radiol. 2402050606

62. Huwart L, Sempoux C, Salameh N, Jamart J, Annet L, Sinkus R, Peeters F, ter Beek LC, Horsmans Y, Van Beers BE (2007) Liver fibrosis: noninvasive assessment with MR elastography versus aspartate aminotransferase-to-platelet ratio index. Radiology 245 (2):458–466. doi:10.1148/radiol.2452061673

63. Huwart L, Sempoux C, Vicaut E, Salameh N, Annet L, Danse E, Peeters F, ter Beek LC, Rahier J, Sinkus R, Horsmans Y, Van Beers BE (2008) Magnetic resonance elastography for

the noninvasive staging of liver fibrosis. Gastroenterology 135(1):32–40. doi:10.1053/j. gastro.2008.03.076

64. Asbach P, Klatt D, Schlosser B, Biermer M, Muche M, Rieger A, Loddenkemper C, Somasundaram R, Berg T, Hamm B, Braun J, Sack I (2010) Viscoelasticity-based staging of hepatic fibrosis with multifrequency MR elastography. Radiology 257(1):80–86. doi:10. 1148/radiol.10092489

65. Wood ML, Hardy PA (1993) Proton relaxation enhancement. J Magn Reson Imaging 3 (1):149–156

66. Semelka RC, Helmberger TK (2001) Contrast agents for MR imaging of the liver. Radiology 218(1):27–38

67. Ferrucci JT, Stark DD (1990) Iron oxide-enhanced MR imaging of the liver and spleen: review of the first 5 years. AJR Am J Roentgenol 155(5):943–950

68. Chambon C, Clement O, Le Blanche A, Schouman-Claeys E, Frija G (1993) Superparamagnetic iron oxides as positive MR contrast agents: in vitro and in vivo evidence. Magn Reson Imaging 11(4):509–519

69. Sjogren CE, Johansson C, Naevestad A, Sontum PC, Briley-Saebo K, Fahlvik AK (1997) Crystal size and properties of superparamagnetic iron oxide (SPIO) particles. Magn Reson Imaging 15(1):55–67

70. Weissleder R, Stark DD, Engelstad BL, Bacon BR, Compton CC, White DL, Jacobs P, Lewis J (1989) Superparamagnetic iron oxide: pharmacokinetics and toxicity. AJR Am J Roentgenol 152(1):167–173

71. Araki T (2000) SPIO-MRI in the detection of hepatocellular carcinoma. J Gastroenterol 35 (11):874–876

72. Kim YK, Kwak HS, Kim CS, Chung GH, Han YM, Lee JM (2006) Hepatocellular carcinoma in patients with chronic liver disease: comparison of SPIO-enhanced MR imaging and 16-detector row CT. Radiology 238(2):531–541. doi:10.1148/radiol.2381042193

73. Ward J, Guthrie JA, Scott DJ, Atchley J, Wilson D, Davies MH, Wyatt JI, Robinson PJ (2000) Hepatocellular carcinoma in the cirrhotic liver: double-contrast MR imaging for diagnosis. Radiology 216(1):154–162

74. Reimer P, Schneider G, Schima W (2004) Hepatobiliary contrast agents for contrast-enhanced MRI of the liver: properties, clinical development and applications. Eur Radiol 14(4):559–578. doi:10.1007/s00330-004-2236-1

75. Lee DH, Kim SH, Lee JM, Park HS, Lee JY, Yi NJ, Suh KS, Jang JJ, Han JK, Choi BI (2009) Diagnostic performance of multidetector row computed tomography, superparamagnetic iron oxide-enhanced magnetic resonance imaging, and dual-contrast magnetic resonance imaging in predicting the appropriateness of a transplant recipient based on milan criteria: correlation with histopathological findings. Invest Radiol 44(6):311–321

76. Yamashita Y, Yamamoto H, Hirai A, Yoshimatsu S, Baba Y, Takahashi M (1996) MR imaging enhancement with superparamagnetic iron oxide in chronic liver disease: influence of liver dysfunction and parenchymal pathology. Abdom Imaging 21(4):318–323

77. Lim KO, Stark DD, Leese PT, Pfefferbaum A, Rocklage SM, Quay SC (1991) Hepatobiliary MR imaging: first human experience with MnDPDP. Radiology 178(1):79–82

78. Giovagnoni A, Paci E (1996) Liver. III: Gadolinium-based hepatobiliary contrast agents (Gd-EOB-DTPA and Gd-BOPTA/Dimeg). Magn Reson Imaging Clin N Am 4(1):61–72

79. Kim SH, Lee J, Kim MJ, Jeon YH, Park Y, Choi D, Lee WJ, Lim HK (2009) Gadoxetic acid-enhanced MRI versus triple-phase MDCT for the preoperative detection of hepatocellular carcinoma. AJR Am J Roentgenol 192(6):1675–1681. doi:10.2214/AJR.08.1262

80. Kirchin MA, Pirovano GP, Spinazzi A (1998) Gadobenate dimeglumine (Gd-BOPTA). An overview. Invest Radiol 33(11):798–809

81. Hamm B, Staks T, Muhler A, Bollow M, Taupitz M, Frenzel T, Wolf KJ, Weinmann HJ, Lange L (1995) Phase I clinical evaluation of Gd-EOB-DTPA as a hepatobiliary MR contrast agent: safety, pharmacokinetics, and MR imaging. Radiology 195(3):785–792

82. Spinazzi A, Lorusso V, Pirovano G, Taroni P, Kirchin M, Davies A (1998) Multihance clinical pharmacology: biodistribution and MR enhancement of the liver. Academic radiology 5 Suppl 1:S86–S89; discussion S93–84

83. Jung G, Breuer J, Poll LW, Koch JA, Balzer T, Chang S, Modder U (2006) Imaging characteristics of hepatocellular carcinoma using the hepatobiliary contrast agent Gd-EOB-DTPA. Acta Radiol 47(1):15–23

84. Hammerstingl R, Huppertz A, Breuer J, Balzer T, Blakeborough A, Carter R, Fuste LC, Heinz-Peer G, Judmaier W, Laniado M, Manfredi RM, Mathieu DG, Muller D, Mortele K, Reimer P, Reiser MF, Robinson PJ, Shamsi K, Strotzer M, Taupitz M, Tombach B, Valeri G, van Beers BE, Vogl TJ (2008) Diagnostic efficacy of gadoxetic acid (Primovist)-enhanced MRI and spiral CT for a therapeutic strategy: comparison with intraoperative and histopathologic findings in focal liver lesions. Eur Radiol 18(3):457–467. doi:10.1007/s00330-007-0716-9

85. Ahn SS, Kim MJ, Lim JS, Hong HS, Chung YE, Choi JY (2010) Added value of gadoxetic acid-enhanced hepatobiliary phase MR imaging in the diagnosis of hepatocellular carcinoma. Radiology 255(2):459–466. doi:10.1148/radiol.10091388

86. Ichikawa T, Saito K, Yoshioka N, Tanimoto A, Gokan T, Takehara Y, Kamura T, Gabata T, Murakami T, Ito K, Hirohashi S, Nishie A, Saito Y, Onaya H, Kuwatsuru R, Morimoto A, Ueda K, Kurauchi M, Breuer J (2010) Detection and characterization of focal liver lesions: a Japanese phase III, multicenter comparison between gadoxetic acid disodium-enhanced magnetic resonance imaging and contrast-enhanced computed tomography predominantly in patients with hepatocellular carcinoma and chronic liver disease. Invest Radiol 45(3):133–141. doi:10.1097/RLI.0b013e3181caea5b

87. Raman SS, Leary C, Bluemke DA, Amendola M, Sahani D, McTavish JD, Brody J, Outwater E, Mitchell D, Sheafor DH, Fidler J, Francis IR, Semelka RC, Shamsi K, Gschwend S, Feldman DR, Breuer J (2010) Improved characterization of focal liver lesions with liver-specific gadoxetic acid disodium-enhanced magnetic resonance imaging: a multicenter phase 3 clinical trial. J Comput Assist Tomogr 34(2):163–172. doi:10.1097/RCT.0b013e3181c89d87

88. Sun HY, Lee JM, Shin CI, Lee DH, Moon SK, Kim KW, Han JK, Choi BI (2010) Gadoxetic acid-enhanced magnetic resonance imaging for differentiating small hepatocellular carcinomas (< or =2 cm in diameter) from arterial enhancing pseudolesions: special emphasis on hepatobiliary phase imaging. Invest Radiol 45(2):96–103. doi:10.1097/RLI.0b013e3181c5faf7

89. Krinsky GA, Lee VS (2000) MR imaging of cirrhotic nodules. Abdom Imaging 25(5):471–482

90. Ito K, Mitchell DG (2004) Imaging diagnosis of cirrhosis and chronic hepatitis. Intervirology 47(3–5):134–143. doi:10.1159/000078465

91. Kanematsu M, Hoshi H, Yamada T, Murakami T, Kim T, Kato M, Yokoyama R, Nakamura H (1999) Small hepatic nodules in cirrhosis: ultrasonographic, CT, and MR imaging findings. Abdom Imaging 24(1):47–55

92. Zhang J, Krinsky GA (2004) Iron-containing nodules of cirrhosis. NMR Biomed 17(7):459–464. doi:10.1002/nbm.926

93. Baron RL, Peterson MS (2001) From the RSNA refresher courses: screening the cirrhotic liver for hepatocellular carcinoma with CT and MR imaging: opportunities and pitfalls. Radiographics: a review publication of the Radiological Society of North America, Inc 21 Spec No:S117–132

94. Qayyum A, Graser A, Westphalen A, Merriman RB, Ferrell LD, Yeh BM, Coakley FV (2004) CT of benign hypervascular liver nodules in autoimmune hepatitis. AJR Am J Roentgenol 183(6):1573–1576

95. Roncalli M, Roz E, Coggi G, Di Rocco MG, Bossi P, Minola E, Gambacorta M, Borzio M (1999) The vascular profile of regenerative and dysplastic nodules of the cirrhotic liver: implications for diagnosis and classification. Hepatology 30(5):1174–1178. doi:10.1002/hep.510300507

96. Mathieu D, Paret M, Mahfouz AE, Caseiro-Alves F, Tran Van Nhieu J, Anglade MC, Rahmouni A, Vasile N (1997) Hyperintense benign liver lesions on spin-echo T1-weighted MR images: pathologic correlations. Abdom Imaging 22(4):410–417

97. Krinsky GA, Israel G (2003) Nondysplastic nodules that are hyperintense on T1-weighted gradient-echo MR imaging: frequency in cirrhotic patients undergoing transplantation. AJR Am J Roentgenol 180(4):1023–1027

98. Ito K, Mitchell DG, Gabata T, Hann HW, Kim PN, Fujita T, Awaya H, Honjo K, Matsunaga N (1999) Hepatocellular carcinoma: association with increased iron deposition in the cirrhotic liver at MR imaging. Radiology 212(1):235–240

99. Krinsky GA, Lee VS, Nguyen MT, Rofsky NM, Theise ND, Morgan GR, Teperman LW, Weinreb JC (2001) Siderotic nodules in the cirrhotic liver at MR imaging with explant correlation: no increased frequency of dysplastic nodules and hepatocellular carcinoma. Radiology 218(1):47–53

100. Lim JH, Kim EY, Lee WJ, Lim HK, Do YS, Choo IW, Park CK (1999) Regenerative nodules in liver cirrhosis: findings at CT during arterial portography and CT hepatic arteriography with histopathologic correlation. Radiology 210(2):451–458

101. Freeny PC, Grossholz M, Kaakaji K, Schmiedl UP (2003) Significance of hyperattenuating and contrast-enhancing hepatic nodules detected in the cirrhotic liver during arterial phase helical CT in pre-liver transplant patients: radiologic-histopathologic correlation of explanted livers. Abdom Imaging 28(3):333–346. doi:10.1007/s00261-002-0053-z

102. Theise ND, Schwartz M, Miller C, Thung SN (1992) Macroregenerative nodules and hepatocellular carcinoma in forty-four sequential adult liver explants with cirrhosis. Hepatology 16(4):949–955

103. Borzio M, Fargion S, Borzio F, Fracanzani AL, Croce AM, Stroffolini T, Oldani S, Cotichini R, Roncalli M (2003) Impact of large regenerative, low grade and high grade dysplastic nodules in hepatocellular carcinoma development. J Hepatol 39(2):208–214

104. Park YN, Yang CP, Fernandez GJ, Cubukcu O, Thung SN, Theise ND (1998) Neoangiogenesis and sinusoidal "capillarization" in dysplastic nodules of the liver. Am J Surg Pathol 22(6):656–662

105. Theise ND, Fiel IM, Hytiroglou P, Ferrell L, Schwartz M, Miller C, Thung SN (1995) Macroregenerative nodules in cirrhosis are not associated with elevated serum or stainable tissue alpha-fetoprotein. Liver 15(1):30–34

106. Imai Y, Murakami T, Yoshida S, Nishikawa M, Ohsawa M, Tokunaga K, Murata M, Shibata K, Zushi S, Kurokawa M, Yonezawa T, Kawata S, Takamura M, Nagano H, Sakon M, Monden M, Wakasa K, Nakamura H (2000) Superparamagnetic iron oxide-enhanced magnetic resonance images of hepatocellular carcinoma: correlation with histological grading. Hepatology 32(2):205–212. doi:10.1053/jhep.2000.9113

107. Lim JH, Choi D, Cho SK, Kim SH, Lee WJ, Lim HK, Park CK, Paik SW, Kim YI (2001) Conspicuity of hepatocellular nodular lesions in cirrhotic livers at ferumoxides-enhanced MR imaging: importance of Kupffer cell number. Radiology 220(3):669–676

108. Asahina Y, Izumi N, Uchihara M, Noguchi O, Ueda K, Inoue K, Nishimura Y, Tsuchiya K, Hamano K, Itakura J, Himeno Y, Koike M, Miyake S (2003) Assessment of Kupffer cells by ferumoxides-enhanced MR imaging is beneficial for diagnosis of hepatocellular carcinoma: comparison of pathological diagnosis and perfusion patterns assessed by CT hepatic arteriography and CT arterioportography. Hepatol Res 27(3):196–204

109. Takayama T, Makuuchi M, Hirohashi S, Sakamoto M, Okazaki N, Takayasu K, Kosuge T, Motoo Y, Yamazaki S, Hasegawa H (1990) Malignant transformation of adenomatous hyperplasia to hepatocellular carcinoma. Lancet 336(8724):1150–1153

110. Sakamoto M, Hirohashi S, Shimosato Y (1991) Early stages of multistep hepatocarcinogenesis: adenomatous hyperplasia and early hepatocellular carcinoma. Hum Pathol 22(2):172–178

111. Seki S, Sakaguchi H, Kitada T, Tamori A, Takeda T, Kawada N, Habu D, Nakatani K, Nishiguchi S, Shiomi S (2000) Outcomes of dysplastic nodules in human cirrhotic liver: a clinicopathological study. Clin Cancer Res 6(9):3469–3473

112. Kim T, Baron RL, Nalesnik MA (2000) Infarcted regenerative nodules in cirrhosis: CT and MR imaging findings with pathologic correlation. AJR Am J Roentgenol 175(4):1121–1125

113. Matsui O, Kadoya M, Kameyama T, Yoshikawa J, Takashima T, Nakanuma Y, Unoura M, Kobayashi K, Izumi R, Ida M et al (1991) Benign and malignant nodules in cirrhotic livers: distinction based on blood supply. Radiology 178(2):493–497

114. Krinsky GA, Theise ND, Rofsky NM, Mizrachi H, Tepperman LW, Weinreb JC (1998) Dysplastic nodules in cirrhotic liver: arterial phase enhancement at CT and MR imaging–a case report. Radiology 209(2):461–464

115. Choi BI, Han JK, Hong SH, Kim TK, Song CS, Kim KW, Kim MJ, Han MC (1999) Dysplastic nodules of the liver: imaging findings. Abdom Imaging 24(3):250–257

116. Hayashi M, Matsui O, Ueda K, Kawamori Y, Kadoya M, Yoshikawa J, Gabata T, Takashima T, Nonomura A, Nakanuma Y (1999) Correlation between the blood supply and grade of malignancy of hepatocellular nodules associated with liver cirrhosis: evaluation by CT during intraarterial injection of contrast medium. AJR Am J Roentgenol 172 (4):969–976

117. Mitchell DG, Rubin R, Siegelman ES, Burk DL Jr, Rifkin MD (1991) Hepatocellular carcinoma within siderotic regenerative nodules: appearance as a nodule within a nodule on MR images. Radiology 178(1):101–103

118. Goshima S, Kanematsu M, Matsuo M, Kondo H, Kato H, Yokoyama R, Hoshi H, Moriyama N (2004) Nodule-in-nodule appearance of hepatocellular carcinomas: comparison of gadolinium-enhanced and ferumoxides-enhanced magnetic resonance imaging. J Magn Reson Imaging 20(2):250–255. doi:10.1002/jmri.20100

119. Edmondson HA, Steiner PE (1954) Primary carcinoma of the liver: a study of 100 cases among 48,900 necropsies. Cancer 7(3):462–503

120. Hussain SM, Semelka RC, Mitchell DG (2002) MR imaging of hepatocellular carcinoma. Magn Reson Imaging Clin N Am 10(1):31–52, v

121. Hussain SM, Zondervan PE, IJzermans JN, Schalm SW, de Man RA, Krestin GP (2002) Benign versus malignant hepatic nodules: MR imaging findings with pathologic correlation. Radiographics 22(5):1023–1036, discussion 1037–1029

122. Earls JP, Theise ND, Weinreb JC, DeCorato DR, Krinsky GA, Rofsky NM, Mizrachi H, Teperman LW (1996) Dysplastic nodules and hepatocellular carcinoma: thin-section MR imaging of explanted cirrhotic livers with pathologic correlation. Radiology 201(1):207–214

123. Kelekis NL, Semelka RC, Worawattanakul S, de Lange EE, Ascher SM, Ahn IO, Reinhold C, Remer EM, Brown JJ, Bis KG, Woosley JT, Mitchell DG (1998) Hepatocellular carcinoma in North America: a multiinstitutional study of appearance on T1-weighted, T2-weighted, and serial gadolinium-enhanced gradient-echo images. AJR Am J Roentgenol 170(4):1005–1013

124. Kelekis NL, Semelka RC, Woosley JT (1996) Malignant lesions of the liver with high signal intensity on T1-weighted MR images. J Magn Reson Imaging 6(2):291–294

125. Mitchell DG, Palazzo J, Hann HW, Rifkin MD, Burk DL Jr, Rubin R (1991) Hepatocellular tumors with high signal on T1-weighted MR images: chemical shift MR imaging and histologic correlation. J Comput Assist Tomogr 15(5):762–769

126. Hussain HK, Syed I, Nghiem HV, Johnson TD, Carlos RC, Weadock WJ, Francis IR (2004) T2-weighted MR imaging in the assessment of cirrhotic liver. Radiology 230(3):637–644. doi:10.1148/radiol.2303020921

127. Hecht EM, Holland AE, Israel GM, Hahn WY, Kim DC, West AB, Babb JS, Taouli B, Lee VS, Krinsky GA (2006) Hepatocellular carcinoma in the cirrhotic liver: gadolinium-enhanced 3D T1-weighted MR imaging as a stand-alone sequence for diagnosis. Radiology 239(2):438–447. doi:10.1148/radiol.2392050551

128. Matsui O (2004) Imaging of multistep human hepatocarcinogenesis by CT during intra-arterial contrast injection. Intervirology 47(3–5):271–276. doi:10.1159/000078478

129. Marrero JA, Hussain HK, Nghiem HV, Umar R, Fontana RJ, Lok AS (2005) Improving the prediction of hepatocellular carcinoma in cirrhotic patients with an arterially-enhancing liver mass. Liver Transpl 11(3):281–289. doi:10.1002/lt.20357

130. Shinmura R, Matsui O, Kobayashi S, Terayama N, Sanada J, Ueda K, Gabata T, Kadoya M, Miyayama S (2005) Cirrhotic nodules: association between MR imaging signal intensity and intranodular blood supply. Radiology 237(2):512–519. doi:10.1148/radiol.2372041389

131. Yamashita Y, Mitsuzaki K, Yi T, Ogata I, Nishiharu T, Urata J, Takahashi M (1996) Small hepatocellular carcinoma in patients with chronic liver damage: prospective comparison of detection with dynamic MR imaging and helical CT of the whole liver. Radiology 200 (1):79–84

132. Holland AE, Hecht EM, Hahn WY, Kim DC, Babb JS, Lee VS, West AB, Krinsky GA (2005) Importance of small (< or = 20-mm) enhancing lesions seen only during the hepatic arterial phase at MR imaging of the cirrhotic liver: evaluation and comparison with whole explanted liver. Radiology 237(3):938–944. doi:10.1148/radiol.2373041364

133. Vogl TJ, Stupavsky A, Pegios W, Hammerstingl R, Mack M, Diebold T, Lodemann KP, Neuhaus P, Felix R (1997) Hepatocellular carcinoma: evaluation with dynamic and static gadobenate dimeglumine-enhanced MR imaging and histopathologic correlation. Radiology 205(3):721–728

134. Lutz AM, Willmann JK, Goepfert K, Marincek B, Weishaupt D (2005) Hepatocellular carcinoma in cirrhosis: enhancement patterns at dynamic gadolinium- and superparamagnetic iron oxide-enhanced T1-weighted MR imaging. Radiology 237(2):520–528. doi:10.1148/radiol.2372041183

135. Ueda K, Matsui O, Kawamori Y, Nakanuma Y, Kadoya M, Yoshikawa J, Gabata T, Nonomura A, Takashima T (1998) Hypervascular hepatocellular carcinoma: evaluation of hemodynamics with dynamic CT during hepatic arteriography. Radiology 206(1):161–166

136. Kadoya M, Matsui O, Takashima T, Nonomura A (1992) Hepatocellular carcinoma: correlation of MR imaging and histopathologic findings. Radiology 183(3):819–825

137. Itai Y (1999) Capsule of hepatocellular carcinoma: where and how does the capsule show enhancement? Radiology 210(2):577–579

138. Ishizaki M, Ashida K, Higashi T, Nakatsukasa H, Kaneyoshi T, Fujiwara K, Nouso K, Kobayashi Y, Uemura M, Nakamura S, Tsuji T (2001) The formation of capsule and septum in human hepatocellular carcinoma. Virchows Arch 438(6):574–580

139. Chen RC, Lii JM, Chou CT, Chang TA, Chen WT, Li CS, Tu HY (2008) T2-weighted and T1-weighted dynamic superparamagnetic iron oxide (ferucarbotran) enhanced MRI of hepatocellular carcinoma and hyperplastic nodules. J Formos Med Assoc 107(10):798–805. doi:10.1016/S0929-6646(08)60193-X

140. Tanimoto A, Kuwatsuru R, Kadoya M, Ohtomo K, Hirohashi S, Murakami T, Hiramatsu K, Yoshikawa K, Katayama H (1999) Evaluation of gadobenate dimeglumine in hepatocellular carcinoma: results from phase II and phase III clinical trials in Japan. J Magn Reson Imaging 10(3):450–460

141. Bruegel M, Holzapfel K, Gaa J, Woertler K, Waldt S, Kiefer B, Stemmer A, Ganter C, Rummeny EJ (2008) Characterization of focal liver lesions by ADC measurements using a respiratory triggered diffusion-weighted single-shot echo-planar MR imaging technique. Eur Radiol 18(3):477–485. doi:10.1007/s00330-007-0785-9

142. Taouli B, Sandberg A, Stemmer A, Parikh T, Wong S, Xu J, Lee VS (2009) Diffusion-weighted imaging of the liver: comparison of navigator triggered and breathhold acquisitions. J Magn Reson Imaging 30(3):561–568. doi:10.1002/jmri.21876

143. Miller FH, Hammond N, Siddiqi AJ, Shroff S, Khatri G, Wang Y, Merrick LB, Nikolaidis P (2010) Utility of diffusion-weighted MRI in distinguishing benign and malignant hepatic lesions. J Magn Reson Imaging 32(1):138–147. doi:10.1002/jmri.22235

144. Yin M, Chen J, Glaser KJ, Talwalkar JA, Ehman RL (2009) Abdominal magnetic resonance elastography. Top Magn Reson Imaging 20(2):79–87. doi:10.1097/RMR.0b013e3181c4737e

145. Stevens WR, Gulino SP, Batts KP, Stephens DH, Johnson CD (1996) Mosaic pattern of hepatocellular carcinoma: histologic basis for a characteristic CT appearance. J Comput Assist Tomogr 20(3):337–342

146. Ito K (2006) Hepatocellular carcinoma: conventional MRI findings including gadolinium-enhanced dynamic imaging. Eur J Radiol 58(2):186–199. doi:10.1016/j.ejrad.2005.11.039

147. Kanematsu M, Semelka RC, Leonardou P, Mastropasqua M, Lee JK (2003) Hepatocellular carcinoma of diffuse type: MR imaging findings and clinical manifestations. J Magn Reson Imaging 18(2):189–195. doi:10.1002/jmri.10336

148. Pawlik TM, Poon RT, Abdalla EK, Ikai I, Nagorney DM, Belghiti J, Kianmanesh R, Ng IO, Curley SA, Yamaoka Y, Lauwers GY, Vauthey JN (2005) Hepatectomy for hepatocellular carcinoma with major portal or hepatic vein invasion: results of a multicenter study. Surgery 137(4):403–410. doi:10.1016/j.surg.2004.12.012

149. Dodd GD III, Memel DS, Baron RL, Eichner L, Santiguida LA (1995) Portal vein thrombosis in patients with cirrhosis: does sonographic detection of intrathrombus flow allow differentiation of benign and malignant thrombus? AJR Am J Roentgenol 165(3):573–577

150. Pirisi M, Avellini C, Fabris C, Scott C, Bardus P, Soardo G, Beltrami CA, Bartoli E (1998) Portal vein thrombosis in hepatocellular carcinoma: age and sex distribution in an autopsy study. J Cancer Res Clin Oncol 124(7):397–400

151. Llovet JM, Bustamante J, Castells A, Vilana R, Ayuso Mdel C, Sala M, Bru C, Rodes J, Bruix J (1999) Natural history of untreated nonsurgical hepatocellular carcinoma: rationale for the design and evaluation of therapeutic trials. Hepatology 29(1):62–67. doi:10.1002/hep.510290145

152. Koike Y, Nakagawa K, Shiratori Y, Shiina S, Imamura M, Sato S, Obi S, Teratani T, Hamamura K, Yoshida H, Omata M (2003) Factors affecting the prognosis of patients with hepatocellular carcinoma invading the portal vein–a retrospective analysis using 952 consecutive HCC patients. Hepato-gastroenterology 50(54):2035–2039

153. Takayasu K, Arii S, Ikai I, Omata M, Okita K, Ichida T, Matsuyama Y, Nakanuma Y, Kojiro M, Makuuchi M, Yamaoka Y (2006) Prospective cohort study of transarterial chemoembolization for unresectable hepatocellular carcinoma in 8510 patients. Gastroenterology 131(2):461–469. doi:10.1053/j.gastro.2006.05.021

154. Nakashima T, Okuda K, Kojiro M, Jimi A, Yamaguchi R, Sakamoto K, Ikari T (1983) Pathology of hepatocellular carcinoma in Japan. 232 Consecutive cases autopsied in ten years. Cancer 51(5):863–877

155. Tublin ME, Dodd GD III, Baron RL (1997) Benign and malignant portal vein thrombosis: differentiation by CT characteristics. AJR Am J Roentgenol 168(3):719–723

156. Aslam Sohaib SA, Teh J, Nargund VH, Lumley JS, Hendry WF, Reznek RH (2002) Assessment of tumor invasion of the vena caval wall in renal cell carcinoma cases by magnetic resonance imaging. J Urol 167(3):1271–1275

157. Krinsky GA, Lee VS, Theise ND, Weinreb JC, Rofsky NM, Diflo T, Teperman LW (2001) Hepatocellular carcinoma and dysplastic nodules in patients with cirrhosis: prospective diagnosis with MR imaging and explantation correlation. Radiology 219(2):445–454

158. Brancatelli G, Baron RL, Peterson MS, Marsh W (2003) Helical CT screening for hepatocellular carcinoma in patients with cirrhosis: frequency and causes of false-positive interpretation. AJR Am J Roentgenol 180(4):1007–1014

159. Wiesner RH, Freeman RB, Mulligan DC (2004) Liver transplantation for hepatocellular cancer: the impact of the MELD allocation policy. Gastroenterology 127(5 Suppl 1): S261–S267

160. Yu JS, Kim KW, Jeong MG, Lee JT, Yoo HS (2000) Nontumorous hepatic arterial-portal venous shunts: MR imaging findings. Radiology 217(3):750–756

161. Choi BI, Lee KH, Han JK, Lee JM (2002) Hepatic arterioportal shunts: dynamic CT and MR features. Korean J Radiol 3(1):1–15

162. Yu JS, Kim KW, Sung KB, Lee JT, Yoo HS (1997) Small arterial-portal venous shunts: a cause of pseudolesions at hepatic imaging. Radiology 203(3):737–742

163. Ito K, Honjo K, Fujita T, Awaya H, Matsumoto T, Matsunaga N (1996) Hepatic parenchymal hyperperfusion abnormalities detected with multisection dynamic MR imaging: appearance and interpretation. J Magn Reson Imaging 6(6):861–867
164. Dodd GD III, Baron RL, Oliver JH III, Federle MP (1999) Spectrum of imaging findings of the liver in end-stage cirrhosis: part I, gross morphology and diffuse abnormalities. AJR Am J Roentgenol 173(4):1031–1036
165. Ahn IO, de Lange EE (1998) Early hyperenhancement of confluent hepatic fibrosis on dynamic MR imaging. AJR Am J Roentgenol 171(3):901–902
166. Brancatelli G, Federle MP, Baron RL, Lagalla R, Midiri M, Vilgrain V (2007) Arterially enhancing liver lesions: significance of sustained enhancement on hepatic venous and delayed phase with magnetic resonance imaging. J Comput Assist Tomogr 31(1):116–124. doi:10.1097/01.rct.0000232474.30033.06
167. Ruiz Guinaldo A, Martin Herrera L, Roldan Cuadra R (1997) Hepatic tumors in patients with cirrhosis: an autopsy study. Revista espanola de enfermedades digestivas 89(10):771–780
168. Seymour K, Charnley RM (1999) Evidence that metastasis is less common in cirrhotic than normal liver: a systematic review of post-mortem case–control studies. Br J Surg 86 (10):1237–1242. doi:10.1046/j.1365-2168.1999.01228.x
169. Quaglia A, Tibballs J, Grasso A, Prasad N, Nozza P, Davies SE, Burroughs AK, Watkinson A, Dhillon AP (2003) Focal nodular hyperplasia-like areas in cirrhosis. Histopathology 42(1):14–21
170. Zheng WW, Zhou KR, Chen ZW, Shen JZ, Chen CZ, Zhang SJ (2002) Characterization of focal hepatic lesions with SPIO-enhanced MRI. World J Gastroenterol 8(1):82–86
171. Vilgrain V, Lewin M, Vons C, Denys A, Valla D, Flejou JF, Belghiti J, Menu Y (1999) Hepatic nodules in Budd-Chiari syndrome: imaging features. Radiology 210(2):443–450
172. Reshamwala PA, Kleiner DE, Heller T (2006) Nodular regenerative hyperplasia: not all nodules are created equal. Hepatology 44(1):7–14. doi:10.1002/hep.21258
173. Maetani Y, Itoh K, Egawa H, Haga H, Sakurai T, Nishida N, Ametani F, Shibata T, Kubo T, Tanaka K, Konishi J (2002) Benign hepatic nodules in Budd-Chiari syndrome: radiologic-pathologic correlation with emphasis on the central scar. AJR Am J Roentgenol 178 (4):869–875
174. Choi BI, Lee JM, Han JK (2004) Imaging of intrahepatic and hilar cholangiocarcinoma. Abdom Imaging 29(5):548–557. doi:10.1007/s00261-004-0188-1
175. Blachar A, Federle MP, Brancatelli G (2002) Hepatic capsular retraction: spectrum of benign and malignant etiologies. Abdom Imaging 27(6):690–699. doi:10.1007/s00261-001-0094-8
176. Jeong YY, Mitchell DG, Kamishima T (2002) Small (<20 mm) enhancing hepatic nodules seen on arterial phase MR imaging of the cirrhotic liver: clinical implications. AJR Am J Roentgenol 178(6):1327–1334
177. Shimizu A, Ito K, Koike S, Fujita T, Shimizu K, Matsunaga N (2003) Cirrhosis or chronic hepatitis: evaluation of small (<or=2-cm) early-enhancing hepatic lesions with serial contrast-enhanced dynamic MR imaging. Radiology 226(2):550–555
178. Taouli B, Goh JS, Lu Y, Qayyum A, Yeh BM, Merriman RB, Coakley FV (2005) Growth rate of hepatocellular carcinoma: evaluation with serial computed tomography or magnetic resonance imaging. J Comput Assist Tomogr 29(4):425–429
179. Arii S, Yamaoka Y, Futagawa S, Inoue K, Kobayashi K, Kojiro M, Makuuchi M, Nakamura Y, Okita K, Yamada R (2000) Results of surgical and nonsurgical treatment for small-sized hepatocellular carcinomas: a retrospective and nationwide survey in Japan. The Liver Cancer Study Group of Japan. Hepatology 32(6):1224–1229. doi:10.1053/jhep.2000. 20456
180. Ikai I, Arii S, Kojiro M, Ichida T, Makuuchi M, Matsuyama Y, Nakanuma Y, Okita K, Omata M, Takayasu K, Yamaoka Y (2004) Reevaluation of prognostic factors for survival after liver resection in patients with hepatocellular carcinoma in a Japanese nationwide survey. Cancer 101(4):796–802. doi:10.1002/cncr.20426

181. Mazzaferro V, Regalia E, Doci R, Andreola S, Pulvirenti A, Bozzetti F, Montalto F, Ammatuna M, Morabito A, Gennari L (1996) Liver transplantation for the treatment of small hepatocellular carcinomas in patients with cirrhosis. N Eng J Med 334(11):693–699. doi:10.1056/NEJM199603143341104

182. Sheu JC, Sung JL, Chen DS, Yang PM, Lai MY, Lee CS, Hsu HC, Chuang CN, Yang PC, Wang TH et al (1985) Growth rate of asymptomatic hepatocellular carcinoma and its clinical implications. Gastroenterology 89(2):259–266

183. Ebara M, Ohto M, Shinagawa T, Sugiura N, Kimura K, Matsutani S, Morita M, Saisho H, Tsuchiya Y, Okuda K (1986) Natural history of minute hepatocellular carcinoma smaller than three centimeters complicating cirrhosis. A study in 22 patients. Gastroenterology 90 (2):289–298

184. Okazaki N, Yoshino M, Yoshida T, Suzuki M, Moriyama N, Takayasu K, Makuuchi M, Yamazaki S, Hasegawa H, Noguchi M et al (1989) Evaluation of the prognosis for small hepatocellular carcinoma based on tumor volume doubling time. A preliminary report. Cancer 63(11):2207–2210

185. Barbara L, Benzi G, Gaiani S, Fusconi F, Zironi G, Siringo S, Rigamonti A, Barbara C, Grigioni W, Mazziotti A et al (1992) Natural history of small untreated hepatocellular carcinoma in cirrhosis: a multivariate analysis of prognostic factors of tumor growth rate and patient survival. Hepatology 16(1):132–137

186. Bruix J, Sherman M, Llovet JM, Beaugrand M, Lencioni R, Burroughs AK, Christensen E, Pagliaro L, Colombo M, Rodes J (2001) Clinical management of hepatocellular carcinoma. Conclusions of the Barcelona-2000 EASL conference. European Association for the Study of the Liver. J Hepatol 35(3):421–430

187. Chang S, Kim SH, Lim HK, Lee WJ, Choi D, Lim JH (2005) Needle tract implantation after sonographically guided percutaneous biopsy of hepatocellular carcinoma: evaluation of doubling time, frequency, and features on CT. AJR Am J Roentgenol 185(2):400–405

188. O'Malley ME, Takayama Y, Sherman M (2005) Outcome of small (10–20 mm) arterial phase-enhancing nodules seen on triphasic liver CT in patients with cirrhosis or chronic liver disease. Am J Gastroenterol 100(7):1523–1528. doi:10.1111/j.1572-0241.2005.41814.x

Dong Ho Lee Board-certificated radiologist in South Korea.
Fellowship in Department of Radiology Seoul National University Hospital.

Magnetic Resonance Imaging of Adenocarcinoma of the Pancreas

Richard C. Semelka, Luz Adriana Escobar, Najwa Al Ansari, and Charles Thomas Alexander Semelka

Abstract Technical advances of magnetic resonance imaging (MRI), including ultrahigh-field magnetic resonance at 3.0 T, parallel imaging techniques, and multichannel receive coils of the abdomen, are valuable tools in the assessment of the pancreatic disease. A standard MR protocol including non-contrast T1-weighted fat-suppressed and dynamic gadolinium-enhanced gradient-echo imaging is sensitive for the evaluation of pancreatic cancer. Optimal use of MRI in the investigation of pancreatic cancer occurs in the following circumstances: (1) detection of small non-contour deforming tumors, (2) evaluation of local extension and vascular encasement, (3) determination of the presence of lymph node and peritoneal metastases, and (4) determination and characterization of associated liver lesions and liver metastases.

Introduction

Epidemiology and Risk Factors

Pancreatic ductal adenocarcinoma, referring to carcinoma arising in the exocrine portion of the gland, accounts for 95 % of malignant tumors of the pancreas and is the fourth most common cause of cancer death in the United States [1].

The lesion is more common in men and blacks, most frequently in the eighth decade of the life [2, 3].

Several predisposing factors have been related with an increased incidence of pancreatic cancer. Heavy alcohol drinking may result in chronic pancreatitis, which

R.C. Semelka, M.D. (✉) • L.A. Escobar, M.D. • N. Al Ansari, M.D. • C.T.A. Semelka, B.Sc.
UNC Department of Radiology, 101 Manning Drive, CB# 7510 2001 Old Clinic Bldg,
Chapel Hill, NC 27599-7510, USA
e-mail: richsem@med.unc.edu; luchis80@yahoo.com; najwaalansari@yahoo.it;
ctasemelka@yahoo.com

A.S. El-Baz et al. (eds.), *Abdomen and Thoracic Imaging: An Engineering & Clinical Perspective*, DOI 10.1007/978-1-4614-8498-1_8,
© Springer Science+Business Media New York 2014

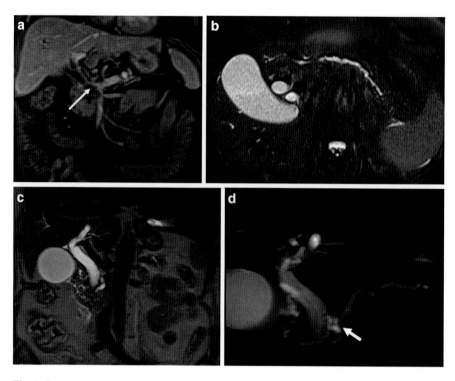

Fig. 1 Pancreatic cancer, arising in the head of the pancreas with biliary tree dilatation and main pancreatic duct dilatation, "double duct sign." Immediate postgadolinium T1-weighted fat-suppressed SGE images (**a**) fat-suppressed T2-weighted SS-ETSE, (**b**) coronal T2-weighted SS-ETSE (**c**) thick section MRCP (**d**). A 2-cm tumor is shown in the pancreatic head with minimal peripheral enhancement on the early post-contrast images (*arrow* (**a**)), causing proximal dilatation and abrupt distal narrowing of the common bile duct (CBD), with simultaneous dilatation of the main pancreatic duct (MPD), which represents the "double duct sign" (**d**)

is a risk factor for pancreatic cancer. A strong family history of pancreatic cancer is also likely a risk factor, although the association is not as great as for breast or colon cancer.

Pancreatic adenocarcinoma has a poor prognosis, with a 5-year survival rate of only 5 % [2, 3].

Approximately 60–70 % of pancreatic adenocarcinomas involve the pancreatic head (Fig. 1), 10–20 % area located in the body (Fig. 2) and 5–10 % in the tail. Diffuse glandular involvement occurs in 5 % of cases [4].

Pancreatic cancer arising in the head of the pancreas may cause obstruction of the CBD and pancreatic duct, with the MR cholangiopancreatography (MRCP) appearance of a "double duct sign" (Fig. 1), which was first described on ERCP studies. This sign can be also appreciated, although less commonly, in patients with focal pancreatitis. Painless jaundice is the classical presenting feature of carcinomas within the pancreatic head. It should be noted that cancer arising in the uncinate process may not obstruct the CBD until very late in the course of disease.

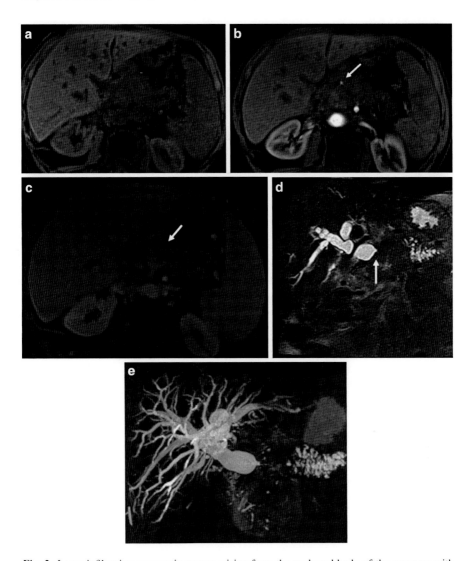

Fig. 2 Large infiltrative pancreatic cancer arising from the neck and body of the pancreas with biliary tree and pancreatic duct dilatation and vascular encasement. Fat-suppressed T1-weighted SGE (**a**), immediate postgadolinium T1-weighted fat-suppressed SGE (**b**), 90-s postgadolinium fat-suppressed SGE (**c**), non-breath hold 3D MRCP; and (**d**) MRCP with MIP reconstruction (**e**) images. A 5-cm poorly differentiated infiltrative adenocarcinoma of the neck and body of the pancreas (*arrow* (**c**)), causing a marked dilatation of the intrahepatic ducts and obstruction of the common bile duct (CBD) visualizing and abrupt narrowing of the distal CBD (*arrow* (**d**)). Dilatation CBD, the main pancreatic duct and side branches of the body and tail of the pancreas are best depicted on MRCP images (**d, e**). The tumor has low signal intensity on immediate post-contrast (**b**) showing encasement of the hepatic artery (*arrow* (**b**)). The portal vein and proximal SMV are encased by the mass and there is a filling defect in the SMV, compatible with thrombus (**c**)

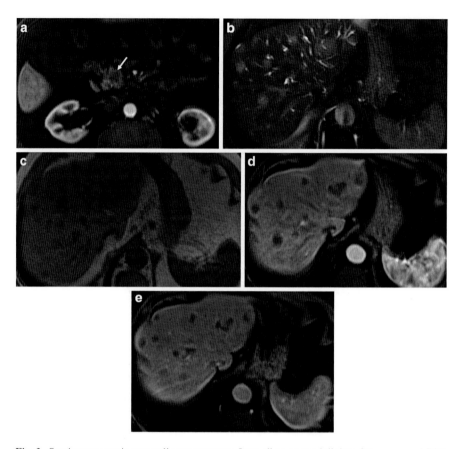

Fig. 3 Staging pancreatic cancer liver metastases. Immediate postgadolinium fat-suppressed SGE (**a**), T2-weighted fat-suppressed spin-echo (**b**), T1-weighted in-phase SGE (**c**), immediate, and (**d**) and 90-s postgadolinium T1-weighted fat-suppressed SGE images (**e**). Small tumor in the head of the pancreas (*arrow* (**a**)) with the presence of multiple liver metastases that are mildly hyperintense on T2 (**b**) hypointense on T1-weighted images (**c**), and have a discrete ring enhancement on the immediate postgadolinium images (**d**)

Carcinoma involving the body and tail of the pancreas grows insidiously and often has already metastasized widely at the time of diagnosis [5]. The most common sites of metastases are the liver, regional lymph nodes, peritoneum, and lungs.

The rich lymphatic supply and lack of pancreatic capsule account for the early spread of cancer into regional nodes. The nodal groups most frequently involved include paraortic, parapancreatic, paracaval, celiac, and paraportal.

Clinical manifestations may be nonspecific, including abdominal pain, weight loss, and painless jaundice caused by obstruction of the common bile duct.

Nonresectable disease is seen at presentation in 75 % of patients, with liver (Fig. 3) and peritoneal metastases as the most frequent secondary organ involvement [4].

Surgery remains the sole curative treatment for patients with pancreatic carcinoma, with postoperative 5-year survival rate of 20 % [6].

Accurate detection and staging of pancreatic cancer are essential to ensure appropriate selection of patients who will benefit from surgery.

One study regarding prognostic factors after a Whipple procedure found that the 5-year survival rate was greater for patients with node-negative and small tumors (<3 cm) than for those with node-positive and large tumors [7]. Another study demonstrated a 5-year survival of 100 % for patients with a tumor smaller than 1 cm and limited to the intraductal epithelium [8].

Advances in magnetic resonance imaging (MRI) including fast acquisition methods and sequences, parallel imaging techniques, multichannel phased-array torso coil, and high-field MR systems (1.5 and 3.0 T) have provided high-quality images of the pancreas, which are sufficient to detect and characterize focal pancreatic lesions smaller than 1 cm. Tumors that measure <1 cm in size that are resected are associated with a 95 % 5-year survival. Hence, detection of these small tumors is critical to improve patient survival.

Magnetic Resonance Imaging Technique

New MRI techniques in the abdomen that limit artifacts have improved the role of MRI in the diagnosis and characterization of pancreatic disease.

MRI of the pancreas should always be performed with a high-field (1.5 or 3.0 T) magnetic resonance unit with a phased-array torso coil to maximize signal to noise ratio, improving breath hold and increased fat-water frequency shift, which facilitates chemically selective excitation-spoiling fat suppression or water excitation.

The use of high spatial resolution MR imaging at 3.0 T will provide the highest image quality and spatial resolution of the pancreas, allowing for the detection of small focal pancreatic lesions [9].

Breath-hold T1-weighted gradient-echo sequences obtained either as a 2D or 3D gradient echo, fat suppression techniques, and dynamic administration of gadolinium chelate provide a high-quality study of the pancreas sufficient to evaluate and characterize focal pancreatic mass lesions smaller than 1 cm in diameter and to evaluate diffuse pancreatic disease [10–12].

MRCP depicts well the biliary and pancreatic ducts to evaluate ductal dilatation (Fig. 1) and abnormal duct pathways [13–15]. Combining the tissue imaging sequences and MRCP gives comprehensive information of the full range of pancreatic disease.

The standard MR protocol for the evaluation of the pancreatic cancer used in our institution includes coronal and transverse T2-weighted single-shot echo train spin-echo (SS-ETSE), transverse T2-weighted fat-suppressed SS-ETSE, transverse T1-weighted spoiled gradient echo (SGE) in-phase and out-of-phase, and transverse T1-weighted fat-suppressed 3-dimensional gradient echo (3D GE) acquired before and after contrast administration during the hepatic arterial dominant (15–20 s), early hepatic venous (45 s), and the interstitial phase (120 s), with the interstitial phase images acquired in transverse and coronal plane.

Magnetic resonance cholangiopancreatography (MRCP) acquired in a coronal oblique projection can delineate the pancreatic and bile ducts [10] (Fig. 2).

MRCP images can be used to position in plane the pancreatic duct, in an oblique coronal projection, to delineate longer segments of the pancreatic duct in continuity.

T2-weighted echo train spin-echo sequences such as T2-weighted half-Fourier acquisition snapshot turbo spin-echo (HASTE) provide anatomic display of the common bile duct (CBD) and pancreatic duct on coronal and transverse plane images. This sequence also provides information about the complexity of pancreatic fluid collections in the presence of complications.

T2-weighted fat-suppressed images are useful in demonstrating liver metastases, islet cell, and cystic pancreatic tumors.

Performing postgadolinium gradient-echo imaging as a 3D gradient-echo technique has advantages such as: (a) thinner sections (3 vs. 5 mm for 2D-SGE) and (b) absence of mirror artifacts from the aorta, which is problematic at 2D-SGE. The thinner sections obtainable at 3 T permit high spatial resolution reconstructions in alternative planes, which can be helpful to evaluate the portal vein.

Evaluation of Pancreatic Cancer Using MRI

Tumor Detection

The normal pancreas is high in signal intensity on non-contrast T1-weighted fat-suppressed images because of the presence of aqueous protein in the acini of the pancreatic parenchyma (Fig. 4) [10]. In elderly patients the signal intensity of the pancreas can diminish and be lower than that of the liver, reflecting changes of fibrosis secondary to the aging process [12].

On the gadolinium contrast-enhanced images, the pancreas demonstrates a uniform capillary blush on immediate post-contrast images, becoming isointense in signal to the liver on interstitial phase images (Fig. 4) [7].

Pancreatic cancer usually appears as a low-signal-intensity mass on non-contrast T1-weighted fat-suppressed images [10, 17, 18], with decreased enhancement on immediate post-contrast images and mild progression of enhancement on interstitial phase images (Fig. 5). In the majority of cases, the tumors show margination with decreased enhancement on immediate post-contrast with a higher signal intensity of the adjacent pancreas [19]. This appearance is commonly observed in pancreatic cancer treated with chemotherapy and radiation therapy, but may also be seen at initial presentation in 27 % of the patients, which is a feature of both anaplastic and very well-differentiated tumors [19].

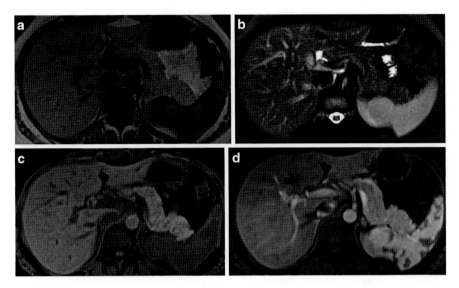

Fig. 4 A normal pancreas at 3T MRI, In-phase T1-weighted SGE (**a**), fat-suppressed T2-weighted SS-ETSE (**b**), T1-weighted fat-suppressed SGE (**c**), immediate postgadolinium T1-weighted fat-suppressed 3D GE images (**d**). Images of the pancreatic body and tail illustrates the normal appearance of the pancreas with a high intensity on T1-weighted fat-suppressed images due to the presence of aqueous protein in the acini of the pancreas (**c**). A uniform capillary blush is seen on the immediate postgadolinium images, which renders a higher in signal intensity comparing to the enhancement of the adjacent liver, bowel, and abdominal fat (**d**)

Conventional spin-echo images are generally limited in the detection of pancreatic cancer. On T2-weighted images, tumors are usually minimally hypointense relative to pancreas and therefore difficult to visualize.

Detection of carcinoma is best performed on immediate postgadolinium T1-weighted gradient-echo images, on which the lesion will enhance to a lesser extent than the surrounding normal tissue due to the abundant fibrous stroma and sparse tumor vascularity of the lesion [17]. The appearance of adenocarcinoma on the interstitial phase (>1 min postgadolinium) of mild progressive enhancement reflects the increased volume of the extracellular space and the venous drainage of cancers compared to normal pancreatic tissue (Fig. 5) [17].

In general, large pancreatic tumors tend to remain mildly low in signal intensity on interstitial phase images, whereas the signal intensity of smaller tumors may range from hypointense to mildly hyperintense on this phase.

Pancreatic cancers appear as mildly low-signal-intensity masses on non-contrast T1-weighted fat-suppressed images and distinct from normal pancreatic tissue, which is high in signal intensity (Fig. 5) [7, 17, 18].

Obstruction of the main pancreatic duct caused by the neoplasm, results in tumor-associated pancreatitis, which is most often observed in large tumors as the time delay during growth of the tumor allows progressive duct obstruction, atrophy,

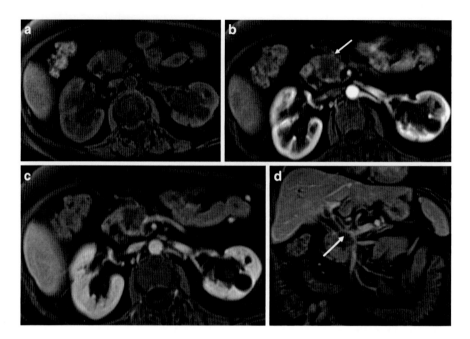

Fig. 5 Pancreatic cancer located in the pancreatic head. T1-weighted fat-suppressed SGE (**a**), immediate postgadolinium T1-weighted SGE (**b**), and transverse (**c**) and coronal (**d**) interstitial postgadolinium fat-suppressed SGE images. There is a 2-cm hypoenhancing mass in the pancreatic head clearly shown in the immediate postgadolinium image (*arrow* (**b**)) with discrete progressive enhancement on the interstitial phase gadolinium-enhanced fat-suppressed images (**c**). The tumor infiltrates distally the CBD, causing biliary obstruction and vascular infiltration of the main portal vein and SMV best visualized in the coronal image (*arrow* (**d**))

and resultant chronic pancreatitis. Pancreatic tissue distal to pancreatic cancer is often atrophic in volume and lower in signal intensity compared to normal pancreatic parenchyma due to chronic inflammation associated with progressive fibrosis and diminished proteinaceous fluid of the gland (Fig. 6) [17, 18].

In these cases, depiction of cancer is poor on non-contrast T1-weighted fat-suppressed images. However, immediate post-contrast images can define the size and extent of adenocarcinomas that obstruct the pancreatic duct, as tumors almost always enhance less than adjacent chronically inflamed pancreas [17, 18].

Chronic pancreatitis can be seen as a focal mass-like lesion in the head of the pancreas, which appears as a low-signal-intensity mass on non-contrast and immediate post-contrast T1-weighted images. This MRI feature causes difficulty distinguishing between pancreatic cancer from chronic pancreatitis on the basis of extent of enhancement of the lesion [20, 21].

One study evaluated the accuracy of MRI, emphasizing on the T1-weighted 3D GE sequence, in the differential diagnosis between pancreatic carcinoma and chronic pancreatitis, in patients with focal pancreatic mass [22]. The study results showed a sensitivity of 93 % and specificity 75 %. The most discriminative finding for pancreatic adenocarcinoma was a relative demarcation of the mass compared to

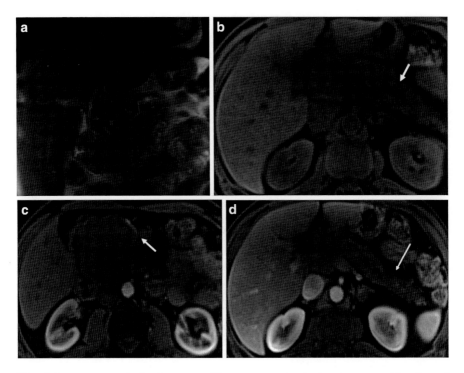

Fig. 6 Large pancreatic head cancer with tumor-associated chronic pancreatitis. Coronal T2-weighted single-shot echo train spin-echo (**a**), T1-weighted fat-suppressed SGE (**b**), immediate (**c**), and 90-s postgadolinium T1-weighted fat-suppressed SGE images (**d**). A 9-cm hypoenhancing mass located in the head and uncinate process of the pancreas encasing the superior mesenteric artery (*arrow* (**c**)) and obstruction of the distal CBD. Note the atrophy of pancreatic body and tail of the pancreas with mild dilatation of main pancreatic duct (*arrow* (**b**)). There is a diffusely low signal intensity on the precontrast T1-weighted fat-suppressed images (**b**), and diffuse diminished enhancement of the body and tail of the pancreas on the 90-s postgadolinium T1-weighted fat-suppressed SGE images (*long arrow* (**d**)). These findings are related to a long-term evolution pancreatic tumor-associated chronic pancreatitis

background pancreas in contrast to chronic pancreatitis. In contrast, the discriminative feature of chronic pancreatitis was an ill-defined demarcation with relatively increased signal intensity and enhancement compared with the background pancreas on early hepatic venous phase images reflecting a more progressive enhancement of inflammatory tissue compared to cancer from early to late postcontrast images. An additional helpful imaging feature is effacement of the fine, lobular architectural pattern of the pancreas in pancreatic adenocarcinoma [22], which is often preserved in pancreatitis.

The presence of encasement of the celiac axis, superior mesenteric artery (SMA), lymphadenopathy, and liver metastases are all helpful to establish the diagnosis of pancreatic cancer [23, 24].

MRI is a more reliable diagnostic technique than computed tomography (CT) in the detection of pancreatic cancer due to the superior soft tissue contrast and the multiple types of data acquired. This is especially important for small non-contour deforming pancreatic cancer, which may be difficult to identify even with multi-detector row CT [25, 26]. According to a previous study [18], the immediate post-contrast gradient-echo sequence was found to be the most sensitive approach to detect pancreatic cancer, particularly in the head region, compared to spiral CT.

Staging

Preoperative staging of pancreatic cancer is important in order to correctly select surgical candidates.

Advanced stage of disease precludes radical tumor resection in most patients with pancreatic cancer. There are several MRI findings that radiologists should address to determine resectability in the MRI report, such as: (1) distant metastases: liver, lung, and distant paraortic lymph nodes; (2) regional lymph nodes; (3) peritoneal disease; (4) direct invasion of adjacent organs: stomach, colon, spleen; (5) invasion into the peripancreatic arteries: celiac trunk, hepatic artery, SMA; and (6) invasion into peripancreatic veins: portal and superior mesenteric vein [24].

Local extension of cancer and lymphovascular involvement can be evaluated on non-suppressed T1-weighted images [26]. Low-signal-intensity tumors that extend beyond the pancreas and invade adjacent organs are detected in the background of high-signal-intensity fat tissue on nonfat-suppressed T1-weighted images [17]. Gadolinium-enhanced fat-suppressed GE images acquired in the interstitial phase demonstrate an intermediate-signal-intensity tumor with enhancement extending into low-signal-intensity suppressed fat. Thus, a combination of both sequences is of value to detect the local tumor extension beyond the pancreas.

Vascular Encasement

Pancreatic cancer has a tendency to encase adjacent vessels including the main portal vein, the superior mesenteric vein, celiac trunk, and its branches as well as arterial vessels such as the SMA.

On MRI, vascular encasement is observed as a loss of fat plane around vessels and as an encasing soft tissue lesion, which in advanced disease will result in luminal narrowing of the involved vessel (Figs. 2 and 5) [27].

Vascular encasement by the tumor is best evaluated on thin-section 3D GE images, which can be analyzed both as source images in the transverse plane and reformatted images in the coronal plane [28].

When the tumor-vessel contact is less than 90° of the vessel circumference or even absent, the likelihood of vessel invasion is low. A tumor-vessel contact of 90–180°, of the vessel circumference, means intermediate probability of vessel invasion.

Coronal plane reformatted images are useful to determine the relationships between tumor and the portal vein as it enters the porta hepatis and between a tumor and the superior mesenteric vein along the medial margin of the pancreatic head (Fig. 5).

Lymph Node Metastases

The presence of a rich lymphatic network and the lack of capsule of the pancreatic tissue accounts for the early spread of cancer to the regional lymph nodes in the setting of pancreatic carcinoma [29].

Lymph node metastases are observed in up to two thirds of patients with adenocarcinoma. Peripancreatic, celiac, paraportal, paracaval, and paraortic lymph node groups are the most common involved.

Lymph nodes are well demonstrated on T2-weighted fat-suppressed images and interstitial phase post-contrast fat-suppressed T1-weighted images as moderately high-signal-intensity foci in background of low-signal-intensity suppressed fat on both sequences.

T2-weighted fat-suppressed imaging is particularly useful for the demonstration of lymph nodes near the liver or in the portal hepatic region because of the signal intensity difference between moderately high-signal-intensity nodes and moderately low-signal-intensity liver and low-signal-intensity fat [30]. Nonfat-suppressed T1-weighted images, in which lymph nodes are seen as low-signal-intensity foci in a background of high-signal-intensity fat, are useful to detect mesenteric or retroperitoneal nodes in the setting of abundant fat in these locations [30]. Coronal plane images can provide a good visualization of the nodal groups involved as well.

Liver Metastases

Detection of liver metastases in the clinical context of pancreatic adenocarcinoma is crucial, because their presence makes the patient ineligible for curative resection.

Liver metastases from pancreatic cancers are generally refounded in shape, mildly low in signal intensity on T1-weighted images, and minimally hyperintense on T2-weighted images (Fig. 3). The low-signal-intensity center of the metastatic lesions reflects the desmoplasic nature of the primary cancer [10]. On immediate post-contrast gradient-echo images, they usually demonstrate ring enhancement. Wedge-shape perilesional enhancement can be seen associated with the liver metastases on the immediate postgadolinium images [28].

For small metastatic lesions, homogeneous early enhancement with rapid fading is commonly seen in the subcapsular location. These small subcapsular hypervascular metastases are observed in more than 80 % of patients with pancreatic cancer liver metastases [31].

Peritoneal Metastases

The peritoneum is often involved in metastatic pancreatic carcinoma. Detection of peritoneal metastases is critical because it excludes patients from curative surgery [16].

Peritoneal metastases appear as moderately high-signal peritoneal lesions in a dark background of suppressed fat on an interstitial phase gadolinium-enhanced fat-suppressed sequence [17]. They can be recognized both by the presence or absence of ascites and are very conspicuous even if the lesions have thin volumes or have a linear shape, because of the relatively high signal of these lesions.

Interstitial phase gadolinium-enhanced fat-suppressed sequences have been shown to be an effective technique to delineate peritoneal metastases compared with CT images [32].

Chemotherapy and Radiation Therapy Treated Pancreatic Ductal Adenocarcinoma

After treatment with chemotherapy and radiation therapy, morphologic and physiologic changes occur in the tumor, the pancreas, and peripancreatic fatty tissue.

There is a decrease in tumor size in approximately 50 % of cases, and the development of fibrogenic tissue as a sign of clinical response.

Assessment of treatment response is a challenging task because in most of the cases, the interface between the tumor margin and the surrounding background pancreatic tissue is indistinct. In these instances evaluation of tumor dimensions is extremely difficult.

Postreatment images can show signs of acute chronic pancreatitis. The presence of pancreatic tumor and pancreatitis can show an increase in abnormal pancreatic tissue even though the tumor itself has decreased in size. Follow-up imaging after pancreatitis has resolved is important.

Lesions That Simulate Pancreatic Cancer

Nonneoplastic Solid Lesions

Focal Fat Replacement

Pancreatic lipomatosis or fatty infiltration replacement is a common finding in the adult pancreas, especially in elderly and obese patients. Involvement is normally diffuse but in rare cases focal fat can simulate a neoplastic lesion.

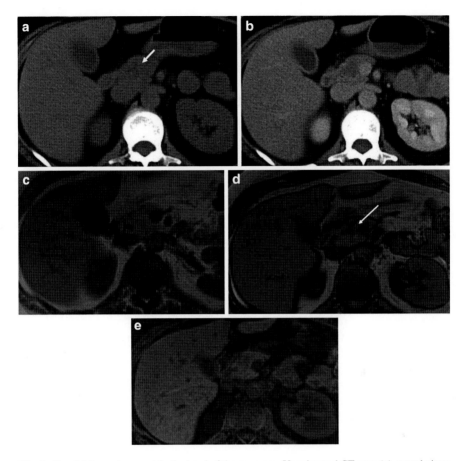

Fig. 7 Focal fatty replacement in the head of the pancreas. Unenhanced CT scan (**a**), portal phase contrast-enhanced CT scan, (**b**), transverse in-phase (**c**), and opposed-phase T1-weighted SGE (**d**) and T1-weighted fat-suppressed 3D GE images (**e**). A nondeforming 1-cm oval lesion in the anterior aspect of the head of the pancreas, showing a low attenuation (attenuation value:-17 UH) on the unenhanced CT scan (*arrow* (**a**)), mild heterogeneous enhancement on the enhanced CT scan (**b**), and marked signal loss with the opposed-phase T1-weighted sequence relative to the in-phase (*long arrow* (**d**)). There is also a signal intensity loss on the T1-weighted fat-suppressed 3D GE images (**e**). There is absent of ductal obstruction or vascular infiltration in this pancreatic lesion

The anterior aspect of the head of the pancreas is the most common location for focal fat infiltration.

Non-enhanced CT can suggest the diagnosis if the lesion contains sufficient macroscopic fat to exhibit characteristics of fat attenuation (negative Hounsfield units) (Fig. 7) [33]. Enhanced CT is not always helpful because normal parenchyma is demarcated as higher density adjacent to foci of fatty infiltration, which may simulate cancer.

The absence of mass effect, ductal, or vascular displacement, is an important clue for the diagnosis.

MR imaging is the modality of choice for the assessment of this entity due to its high specificity in the detection of fat [34]. There will be a moderate to marked signal loss with the opposed-phase T1-weighted sequence relative to the in-phase weighted sequence (Fig. 7) [35].

Macroscopic fatty replacement of the pancreas will have a high signal intensity with T1- and T2-weighted sequences and signal loss with fat-suppressed sequences.

Acute Focal Pancreatitis

Acute pancreatitis is an acute inflammatory condition typically presenting with abdominal pain and elevation in pancreatic enzymes, secondary most often to alcoholism or cholelithiasis. Autoimmune pancreatitis is a condition that is achieving greater recognition in recent years.

MRI is a very sensitive technique for detection of subtle changes of acute pancreatitis even in the setting of a morphologically normal pancreas. CT imaging examinations appear normal in 15–30 % of patients with clinical features of acute pancreatitis [36].

The sensitivity of MRI exceeds that of CT imaging, supporting the role of MRI in the evaluation of patients with a nonconclusive CT or a suspected focal lesion to differentiate inflammatory from neoplastic lesion of the pancreas.

The acutely inflamed pancreas shows either focal or diffuse enlargement of the parenchyma, with signal intensity similar to that of normal pancreatic tissue in non-complicated pancreatitis. Peripancreatic fluid is an important sign visualized in acute pancreatitis, best depicted in the T2-weighted fat-suppressed images, seen as high signal in a background of intermediate- to low-signal-pancreas and fat (Fig. 8).

Focal Chronic Pancreatitis

Chronic pancreatitis is defined pathologically by continuous or relapsing inflammation of the organ leading to irreversible morphologic injury, and typically leads to impairment of function. This clinical condition can be acquired either as a disease process distinct from acute pancreatitis or as a complication of repeated attacks of acute pancreatitis.

Distinction between focal pancreatitis and adenocarcinoma is difficult because both entities may cause focal enlargement of the pancreatic head, obstruction of the common bile duct and pancreatic duct, atrophy of the tail of the pancreas, and obliteration of the fat plane around the SMA.

It is difficult to differentiate focal enlargement of the pancreatic head due to chronic pancreatitis from pancreatic cancer based only on CT images due to the similar appearance as hypoattenuated lesions.

MRI imaging provides more accurate detail in chronic pancreatitis, not only in the morphologic findings but also distinguishing fibrosis. Fibrosis in chronic pancreatitis is shown by diminished signal intensity on T1-weighted fat-suppressed

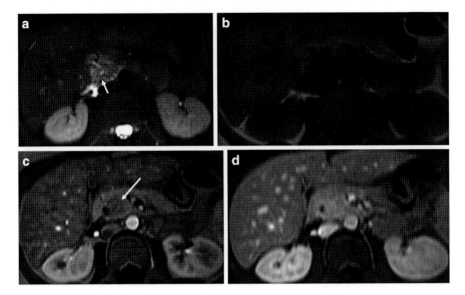

Fig. 8 Mild focal acute pancreatitis. Fat-suppressed T2-weighted single-shot echo train spin-echo (SS-ETSE) (**a**), T1-weighted SGE (**b**), immediate and interstitial postgadolinium T1-weighted fat-suppressed 3D GE images (**c**, **d**). Focal pancreatitis shows a mild focal enlargement of the posterior aspect of the head of the pancreas with high signal intensity on T2-weighted fat-suppressed images, due to minimal free fluid (*arrow* (**a**)). The intensity of the pancreatic head enhancement is less than normal for pancreas on the capillary phase (*long arrow* (**c**)) and shows progressive enhancement on the interstitial-phase images (**d**). There is a preservation of the lobular architecture of the pancreatic head

images, as well as diminished heterogeneous enhancement on immediate postgadolinium gradient-echo images, with enhancement that progresses to greater than background pancreas.

Both adenocarcinoma and chronic pancreatitis show similar signal intensity changes of the enlarged region of pancreas on non-contrast T1-weighted fat-suppressed and T2-weighted images: generally mildly hypointense on T1-weighted images and heterogeneous and mildly hyperintense on T2-weighted images.

On immediate postgadolinium images, focal chronic pancreatitis shows heterogeneous enhancement with presence of signal voids, from cysts and calcifications, without evidence of a definable mass lesion. Usually in this entity, the focally enlarged portion of the pancreas shows preservation of the glandular, feathery texture similar to that of the remaining pancreas [22]. In contrast, in pancreatic cancer, the focally enlarged portion of the pancreas loses its usual architectural detail.

Diffuse low signal intensity of the entire pancreas, including the area of focal enlargement, on T1-weighted fat-suppressed and immediate postgadolinium SGE images are characteristic for chronic pancreatitis. In the setting of pancreatic cancer, the enhancement of the tumor is less than the adjacent pancreatic parenchyma [38].

Features that favor a diagnosis of focal pancreatitis include non-dilated or smoothly tapering of pancreatic and bile ducts coursing through the mass ("duct penetrating sign") [37, 38], pancreatic calcifications, and pancreatic duct irregularities.

Abrupt interruption of a smoothly dilated pancreatic duct, upstream pancreatic gland atrophy, and a high ratio of duct caliber to the pancreatic gland width are features recognized in adenocarcinoma [39].

Acute pancreatitis superimposed on the chronic disease is well shown on MR images. Pancreatic pseudocysts are observed in patients with chronic pancreatitis as a sequel of episodes of acute inflammation. Pseudocysts are generally seen as high signal intensity on T2-weighted images, but they can have variable signal intensity depending on the presence of blood, protein, infection, or debris. Lack of enhancement on early and late postgadolinium images is therefore critical to demonstrate that a complex T2-signal lesion is a pseudocyst.

Neoplastic Lesions

Pancreatic Endocrine Tumors

Pancreatic endocrine tumors (ET) were previously called islet cell tumor, because they were thought to have originated from the islets of Langerhans; however, recent evidence suggests that these tumors originate from pluripotential stem cells in the ductal epithelium [40]. They account for 1–2 % of all pancreatic neoplasms. Most cases are sporadic, but association with syndromes such as multiples endocrine neoplasia type 1, von Hippel-Lindau syndrome, neurofibromatosis type 1, and tuberous sclerosis has been observed. ETs are classified into functioning and nonfunctioning tumors. The functioning tumors may present with an endocrine abnormality resulting from the secretion of hormones [41].

The most common pancreatic endocrine tumors are insulinomas and gastrinomas, followed in frequency by nonfunctional or untyped tumors.

Nonfunctional tumors account for at least 15–20 % of pancreatic endocrine tumors and tend to present with symptoms owing to large tumor mass or metastatic disease. In general, functioning tumors manifest early in the course of disease when they are small due to the clinical manifestations of excessive hormone production.

Malignancy cannot be diagnosed on the basis of histological appearance of pancreatic endocrine tumors instead it is determined by the presence of metastases or local invasion beyond the pancreas. The liver is the most common organ for metastatic spread.

Insulinomas are most commonly benign tumors, gastrinomas are malignant in approximately 60 % of cases, and almost all other nonfunctioning tumors are malignant in most cases.

Tumor morphologic features are variable. Small tumors are generally solid and homogeneous, whereas larger tumors are heterogeneous with presence of cystic degeneration and calcifications.

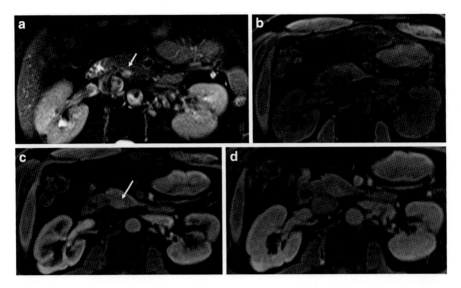

Fig. 9 Small neuroendocrine pancreatic tumor in the uncinate process. Fat-suppressed T2-weighted single-shot echo train spin-echo (SS-ETSE) (**a**), T1-weighted fat-suppressed 3D GE (**b**) immediate (**c**) and interstitial postgadolinium T1-weighted fat-suppressed 3D GE images (**d**). There is a 1-cm well-defined lesion with a high signal intensity on the T2-weighted fat-suppressed image (*arrow* (**a**)), low signal intensity on T1-weighted fat-suppressed 3D GE (**b**) showing homogeneous enhancement on the hepatic arterial dominate phase (*long arrow* (**c**)) and fading in the hepatic venous phase

In MR imaging, endocrine tumors are moderately low in signal intensity on T1-weighted fat-suppressed and intermediate to high signal intensity on T2-weighted fat-suppressed images [42]. The more distinctive feature of ET is their behavior in contrast-enhanced imaging, where they enhance avidly during the arterial phase, enhancing more rapidly and intensely than the normal pancreas (Fig. 9).

Insulinomas most often appear as small tumors (<2 cm), with intense and homogeneous enhancement on immediate postgadolinium images (Fig. 10), whereas gastrinomas most commonly are large lesions (2.5–4 cm approximately), with peripheral ring like enhancement on immediate postgadolinium images. Homogeneous enhancement is typical for small tumors less than 2 cm, whereas larger lesions tend to show heterogeneous enhancement.

Metastases to lymph nodes and solid organs such as the liver may have an enhancement pattern similar to that of the primary tumor.

It is important to differentiate endocrine tumors from other neoplasms of the pancreas, particularly adenocarcinoma, since the prognoses and treatment options are different for both entities.

Features that distinguish most pancreatic endocrine tumors from pancreatic adenocarcinoma include high signal intensity on T2-weighted sequences (Figs. 9 and 10), increased enhancement on immediate postgadolinium images,

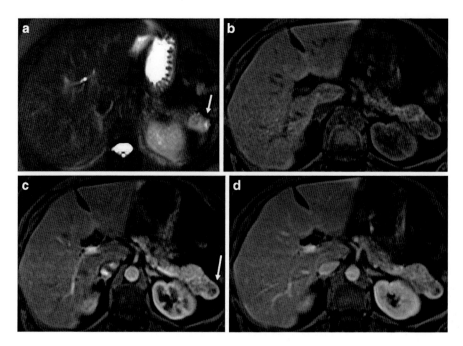

Fig. 10 Insulinoma on the tail of the pancreas. Fat-suppressed T2-weighted SS-ETSE (**a**), T1-weighted fat-suppressed 3D GE (**b**), T1-weighted postgadolinium hepatic arterial dominant and hepatic venous phase fat-suppressed 3D GE images (**c, d**) demonstrates a 2-cm lobulated mass located in the tail of the pancreas, showing high signal intensity on T2-weighted fat-suppressed images (*arrow* (**a**)), intense heterogeneous enhancement on immediate postgadolinium images (*long arrow* (**c**))

hypervascular liver metastases, lack of pancreatic duct obstruction, or vascular encasement [43].

Venous thrombosis, peritoneal regional node enlargement, are characteristic features of pancreatic ductal adenocarcinoma, are generally not present in endocrine tumors.

Periampullary and Ampullary Carcinoma

Tumors arising from the ampulla of Vater, periampullary duodenum, or distal common bile duct are termed periampullary carcinomas.

Their presentation is similar to that of pancreatic head ductal adenocarcinoma, including obstruction of both the CBD and pancreatic duct. MRCP is very effective for the visualization of biliary and pancreatic ductal dilatation as well for the level of obstruction [48].

Periampullary carcinomas can cause ampullary obstruction and become clinically symptomatic even when they are only a few millimeters in size.

The prognosis of periampullary carcinoma is significantly better than that of pancreatic carcinoma, with a 5-year survival rate up to 85 % [48].

Magnetic resonance images for periampullary carcinoma demonstrate a similar appearance to that of pancreatic adenocarcinoma. Periampullary and ampullary carcinomas have low signal intensity on T1- and T2-weighted images and diminished enhancement on early postgadolinium images because of their hypovascular character. On 2-min postgadolinium fat-suppressed images, delayed enhancement is a typical finding [48]. A thin ring of enhancement is commonly observed along the periphery of theses tumors and may also be a relatively specific finding.

Pancreatic Lymphoma

Non-Hodgkin lymphoma may involve peripancreatic lymph nodes or may directly invade the pancreas. Intermediate-signal-intensity peripancreatic lymph nodes are distinguished from high-signal-intensity normal pancreas on non-contrast T1-weighted fat-suppressed images [44].

Primary pancreatic lymphoma is a rare entity, representing less than 2 % of extranodal lymphomas and 0.5 % of pancreatic tumors [45].

Pancreatic lymphoma carries a better prognosis than pancreatic adenocarcinoma because first-line treatment with chemotherapy is generally effective, producing long-term disease regression or remission. Surgery is not required in most cases.

Two morphologic patterns of pancreatic lymphoma are recognized [46]: focal and diffuse form. The focal form occurs in the pancreatic head in 80 % of the cases and has a mean size of 8 cm (range: 2–15 cm). At MRI imaging lymphoma has a low signal intensity on T1-weighted images and intermediate signal intensity on T2-weighted images.

The diffuse form is infiltrative, leading to glandular enlargement and poor definition. These features can simulate the appearance of acute pancreatitis, showing a low signal intensity on T1- and T2-weighted MR images with homogeneous contrast enhancement, although small foci of reduced or absent enhancement are sometimes seen.

Several features that may help distinguish pancreatic lymphoma from adenocarcinoma are the presence of a bulky localized tumor in the pancreatic head without significant main pancreatic duct dilatation, enlarged lymph nodes below the level of the renal vein, and invasive tumor growth with infiltration of retroperitoneal and upper abdominal organs.

Vascular invasion is less common in lymphoma than in pancreatic adenocarcinoma.

Metastases of the Pancreas

Involvement of the pancreas by metastatic tumor may be the result of spread by direct extension or hematogenous metastases. Direct invasion from stomach and transverse colon carcinoma are not rare.

Metastases are most frequently from renal cell carcinoma and lung cancer followed by breast, colon, prostate, and malignant melanoma.

Three morphological patterns of metastatic involvement of the pancreas have been described: solitary lesion (50–70 % of cases), multifocal (5–10 %), and diffuse (15–44 %) [47].

Metastases generally have low signal intensity on T1-weighted, mildly high signal intensity on T2-weighted images. The enhancement of most metastases follows a ring pattern, with a variable degree of enhancement depending on the angiogenic properties of the primary neoplasm. Small metastases (<1 cm in diameter) enhance uniformly on immediate postgadolinium gradient-echo images.

Renal cancer metastases resemble the appearance of islet cell tumors. Melanoma metastases may be high in signal intensity on T1-weighted images because of paramagnetic properties of melanin pigment.

Ductal obstruction is uncommon even with larger tumors, which is an important feature distinguishing metastases from pancreatic ductal adenocarcinoma. Chronic pancreatitis that arises secondary to ductal obstruction is not present, and therefore background pancreas is moderately high signal intensity, creating a sharp contrast and good delineation with hypointense tumors on non-contrast T1-weighted fat-suppressed images.

Conclusions

– MRI may be the optimal method to evaluate pancreatic cancer.
– Detection of small tumors is best made with MRI.
– Staging is also performed well, with good detection and characterization of metastases.
– The full range of other pancreatic disease is well shown.

References

1. Jemal A, Siegel R, Ward E (2008) Cancer statistics. Ca Cancer J Clin 58:71–96
2. Warshaw AL, Fernandez-del Castillo C (1992) Pancreatic carcinoma. N Engl J Med 326:455–465
3. Moossa AR (1982) Pancreatic cancer: approach to diagnosis, selection for surgery and choice of operation. Cancer 50:2689–2698
4. Low G, Anukul P, Noam M (2011) Multimodality imaging of neoplastic and nonneoplastic solid lesions of the pancreas. Radiographics 31:993–1015
5. Baron R, Stanley R, Lee J (1983) Computed tomographic features of biliary obstruction. AJR Am J Roentgenol 140:1173–1178
6. Ros P, Mortelé K (2001) Imaging features of pancreatic neoplasms. JBR-BTR 84:239–249
7. Semelka RC, Kroeker M, Shoenut JP (1991) Pancreatic disease: prospective comparison of CT, ERCP, and 1.5-T MR imaging with dynamic gadolinium enhancement and fat suppression. Radiology 181(3):785–791

8. Benassai G, Mastrorilli M, Quarto G (2000) Factors influencing survival after resection for ductal adenocarcinoma of the head of the pancreas. J Surg Oncol 73:212–218

9. Zapparoli M, Semelka R, Altun E (2008) 3T MRI evaluation of patients with chronic liver diseases: initial observations. Magn Reson Imaging 26:650–660

10. Semelka RC, Ascher S (1993) MR imaging of the pancreas-state of the art. Radiology 188 (3):593–602

11. Winston CB, Mitchell D, Outwater E (1995) Pancreatic signal intensity on T1-weighted fat saturation MR images: clinical correlation. J Magn Reson Imaging 5(3):267–271

12. Mitchell D, Vinitski S, Saponaro S (1991) Liver and pancreas: improved spin-echo T1 contrast by shorter echo time and fat suppression at 1.5T. Radiology 178(1):67–71

13. Takehara Y, Ichido K, Tooyama N (1994) Breath-hold MR cholangiopancreatography with long echo train fast spin-echo sequence and a surface coil in chronic pancreatitis. Radiology 1192:73–78

14. Bret P, Reinhold C, Taourel P (1996) Pancreas divisum: evaluation with MR cholangiopancreatography. Radiology 199(1):99–103

15. Soto JA, Barish M, Yucel E (1995) Pancreatic duct: MR cholangiopancreatography with a three–dimensional fast spin-echo technique. Radiology 196:459–464

16. Vachiranubhap B, Kim YH, Balci NC, Semelka RC (2009) Magnetic resonance imaging of adenocarcinoma of the páncreas. Top Magn Reson Imaging 20:3–9

17. Gabata T, Matsui O, Kadoya M (1994) Small pancreatic adenocarcinoma: efficacy of MR imaging with fat suppression and gadolinium enhanced. Radiology 193:683–688

18. Semelka RC, Kelekis NL, Molina PL (1996) Pancreatic masses with inconclusive findings on spiral CT: is there a role for MRI? Magn Reson Imaging 6:585–588

19. Elias J, Semelka RC, Altun E (2007) Pancreatic cancer: correlation of MR findings, clinical features and tumor grade. J Magn Reson Imaging 26:1556–1563

20. Kim T, Murakami T, Takamura M (2001) Pancreatic mass due to chronic pancreatitis: correlation of CT and MR imaging features with pathologic findings. AJR Am J Roentgenol 177:367–371

21. Johnson PT, Outwater E (1999) Pancreatic carcinoma versus chronic pancreatitis: dynamic MR imaging. Radiology 212:21–218

22. Kim JK, Altun E, Elias J (2007) Focal pancreatic mass: distinction of pancreatic cancer from chronic pancreatitis using gadolinium-enhanced 3D-gradient echo MRI. J Magn Reson Imaging 26:313–322

23. Wittenberg J, Simeone J, Ferruci JT (1982) Non-focal enlargement in pancreatic carcinoma. Radiology 144:131–135

24. Clark L, Jaffe M, Choyke P (1985) Pancreatic imaging. Radiol Clin North Am 23:489–501

25. Saisho H, Yamagushi T (2004) Diagnostic imaging for pancreatic cancer: computed tomography, magnetic resonance imaging and positron emission tomography. Pancreas 28:273–278

26. Vellet AD, Romano W, Bach D (1992) Adenocarcinoma of the pancreatic ducts: comparative evaluation with CT and MRI imaging at 1.5 T. Radiology 183:87–95

27. Megibow A, Bosniak MA, Ambos MA (1981) Thickening of the celiac axis and/or superior mesenteric artery: a sign of pancreatic carcinoma on computed tomography. Radiology 141:449–453

28. Birchard KR, Semelka R, Hyslop WB (2005) Suspected pancreatic cancer: evaluation by dynamic gadolinium–enhanced 3D gradient-echo MRI. AJR Am J Roentgenol 185:700–703

29. Rosai J (1996) Pancreas and ampullary region. In: Rosai J (ed) Ackerman's surgical pathology. Mosby, St. Louis

30. Semelka RC, Pamuklar E, Firat Z (2006) Pancreas. In: Semelka RC (ed) Abdominal pelvic MRI. Wiley-Liss, New York

31. Danet IM, Semelka R, Nagase L (2003) Liver metastases from pancreatic adenocarcinoma: MR imaging characteristics. J Magn Reson Imaging 18:181–188

32. Low R, Semelka R, Worawattanakul S (2000) Extrahepatic abdominal imaging in patients with malignancy: comparison of MR imaging and helical CT in 164 patients. J Magn Reson Imaging 12:269–277
33. Kawamoto S, Siegelman S, Bluemke D, Fishman E (2009) Focal fatty infiltration in the head of the pancreas: evaluation with multidetector computed tomography with multiplanar reformation imaging. J Comput Assist Tomogr 33:90–95
34. Kim HJ, Lee JM, Ham J (2007) Focal fatty replacement of the pancreas: usefulness of chemical shift MRI. AJR Am J Roentgenol 188:429–432
35. Isserow JA, Siegelman ES, Mammone J (1999) Focal fatty infiltration of the pancreas: MR characterization with chemical shift imaging. AJR Am J Roentgenol 183:1263–1265
36. Balthazar E (1989) CT diagnosis and staging of acute pancreatitis. Radiol Clin North Am 27:19–37
37. Ichikawa T, Sou H, Araki T (2001) Duct-penetrating sign at MRCP: usefulness for differentiating inflammatory pancreatic mass from pancreatic carcinomas. Radiology 221:107–116
38. Semelka RC, Shoenut JP, Kroeker MA (1993) Chronic pancreatitis: MR imaging features before and after administration of gadopentate dimeglumine. J Magn Reson Imaging 1:79–82
39. Sissiqi AJ, Miller F (2007) Chronic pancreatitis: ultrasound, computed tomography and magnetic resonance imaging features. Semin Ultrasound CT MR 5:384–394
40. Oberg K, Ericksson B (2005) Endocrine tumors of the pancreas. Best Pract Res Clin Gastroenterol 19:753–781
41. Mozell E, Stenzel P, Woltering E (1990) Functional endocrine tumors of the pancreas: clinical presentation, diagnosis, and treatment. Curr Probl Surg 27:301–386
42. Semelka RC, Custodio CM, Cem Balci N (2000) Neuroendocrine tumors of the pancreas: spectrum of appearances on MRI. J Magn Reson Imaging 11:141–148
43. Semelka RC, Cumming M, Shoenut J (1993) Islet cell tumors: comparison of dynamic contrast-enhanced CT and MRI imaging with dynamic gadolinium enhancement and fat suppression. Radiology 186:799–802
44. Zeman R, Schiebler M, Clark L (1985) The clinical and imaging spectrum of pancreatico-duodenal lymph node enlargement. AJR Am J Roentgenol 144:1223–1227
45. Zucca E, Roggero E, Bertoni F (1997) Primary extranodal non-Hodgkin's lymphomas. Gastrointestinal, cutaneous and genitourinary lymphomas. Ann Oncol 8:727–737
46. Merkle E, Bender G, Brambs H (2000) Imaging findings in pancreatic lymphoma: differential aspects. AJR Am J Roentgnol 174:671–675
47. Tsitouridis I, Diamantopoulou A, Michaelides M (2010) Pancreatic metastases: CT and MRI findings. Diagn Interv Radiol 16:45–51
48. Irie H, Honda H, Shinozaki K (2002) MR imaging of ampullary carcinomas. J Comput Assist Tomogr 26:711–717

Richard Semelka is the Vice Chair of Quality and Safety, Director of MR services, and Professor of Radiology at the University of North Carolina at Chapel Hill. His areas of expertise are abdominal diseases, MRI, patient safety, and medicolegal matters. He has written 9 textbooks and over 300 peer-reviewed papers on these subjects.

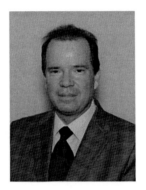

Quantitative Evaluation of Liver Function Within MR Imaging

Akira Yamada

Abstract Hepatocellular uptake index (HUI) is a quantitative indicator of excretory liver function, which is obtained from signal intensity of the liver and spleen and liver volume on gadoxetate disodium-enhanced MR images. HUI correlates well with existing quantitative liver function test results, such as indocyanine green clearance, and allows segmental liver function to be evaluated even if there are regional differences in liver function.

Introduction

Quantification of liver function is important not only for monitoring liver function but also for preoperative diagnosis of reserved liver function with the goal of preventing postoperative liver failure. Currently, the indocyanine green (ICG) clearance test is considered to be the most reliable method for such quantification [1]. This test is based on properties of the colorant compound ICG: after ICG is administered into blood, it is specifically incorporated into hepatocytes, and almost 100 % of it is excreted in bile. Thus, for example, the plasma disappearance rate of ICG (ICG-PDR) and the retention rate 15 min after intravenous administration (ICG-R15) are used as quantitative indicators of liver function [2]. However, the ICG clearance test has a disadvantage, because although it reflects total liver function, it is unable to evaluate segmental liver function. Therefore, it would be highly desirable to establish a quantitative method for evaluation of liver function using imaging modalities such as computed tomography (CT) and magnetic resonance (MR) imaging.

A. Yamada, M.D., Ph.D. (✉)
Department of Radiology, Shinshu University School of Medicine, 3-1-1 Asahi,
Matsumoto, Nagano 390-8621, Japan
e-mail: a_yamada@shinshu-u.ac.jp

A.S. El-Baz et al. (eds.), *Abdomen and Thoracic Imaging: An Engineering
& Clinical Perspective*, DOI 10.1007/978-1-4614-8498-1_9,
© Springer Science+Business Media New York 2014

An example of such a method is MR perfusion study using a gadolinium (Gd)-based extracellular fluid contrast agent. This technique has been applied to quantitative evaluation of blood flow dynamics of the liver and also to diagnosis of liver function and liver fibrosis [3]. However, the information obtained from contrast-enhanced MR imaging with a Gd-based extracellular fluid contrast agent is still an indirect indicator of liver function; using the data obtained by this method, it is still difficult to evaluate the function of the hepatocytes themselves.

On the other hand, gadoxetate disodium (Gd-EOB-DTPA) is a tissue-specific Gd contrast agent that was introduced only recently for clinical application. In this compound, a lipophilic branched-chain ethoxybenzyl (EOB) moiety is linked to an extracellular fluid contrast agent, Gd-DTPA. Because of the presence of the lipophilic branched chain, Gd-EOB-DTPA has properties of both an extracellular fluid contrast agent and a hepatocyte-specific contrast agent. Because the compound is incorporated into hepatocytes, gadoxetate disodium-enhanced MR imaging is capable of reflecting hepatocyte function. A study aimed at applying this method to quantitative evaluation of liver function has been performed [4].

Here, we describe Gd-based extracellular fluid contrast agents, which are essential for an understanding of quantitative evaluation of liver function in gadoxetate disodium-enhanced MR imaging, and discuss the pharmacokinetics of gadoxetate sodium. We also review the quantitative methods that have been proposed for diagnosis of liver function using gadoxetate disodium-enhanced MR imaging, along with the future prospects for clinical applications of these methods.

Quantitative Evaluation of Blood Flow Dynamics of the Liver, Using a Gd-Based Extracellular Fluid Contrast Agent

1. Linear two-compartment model

Among the paramagnetic ions, Gd has the most unpaired electrons (seven) and exhibits the strongest T1-shortening. However, because Gd alone is highly toxic, it must be administered as a compound with a chelating agent [5]. After administration into systemically circulating blood and arrival at the blood vessel of the target tissue, a Gd-based extracellular fluid contrast agent diffuses rapidly along the concentration gradient and reaches equilibrium between the interior and exterior of the blood vessel. Most of the contrast agent that is not incorporated into the cells and re-diffuses into the blood vessel is excreted from the kidney into the urine when kidney function is normal [5]. The disappearance of the Gd-based extracellular fluid contrast agent from the blood occurs in two phases: a distribution phase, in which it mainly diffuses from blood to tissue, and a disappearance phase, in which it is mainly excreted from blood into urine. These pharmacokinetics can be explained by a two-compartment model. In addition, because the diffusion along the concentration gradient is proportional to the concentration, the pharmacokinetics of a Gd-based extracellular fluid contrast

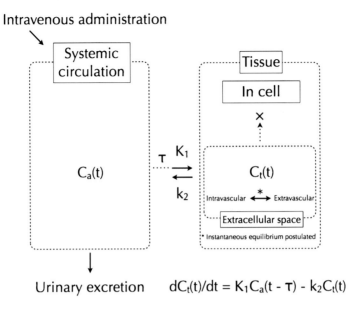

Intravenous administration

Systemic circulation

Tissue

In cell

$\times$

$C_a(t)$

τ K_1

k_2

$C_t(t)$

Intravascular $\longleftrightarrow$ Extravascular

Extracellular space

* Instantaneous equilibrium postulated

Urinary excretion

$$dC_t(t)/dt = K_1 C_a(t - \tau) - k_2 C_t(t)$$

Fig. 1 Linear two-compartment model of gadolinium-based extracellular fluid contrast agent. $C_a(t)$, concentration of the contrast agent in systemically circulating blood at time t; $C_t(t)$, concentration of the contrast agent in tissue extracellular space at time t; τ, time required for the contrast agent to arrive at tissue via the systemic circulation; K1, rate coefficient for diffusion of contrast agent from systemic circulation to tissue; and k2, rate coefficient for diffusion of contrast agent from tissue to systemic circulation. The contrast agent, administered intravenously into systemically circulating blood, reaches a tissue after a period τ, diffuses into the tissue at a velocity proportional to the concentration in systemically circulating blood $C_a(t)$ and the diffusion rate coefficient K1, and diffuses out of the tissue at a velocity proportional to the concentration in the tissue extracellular space $C_t(t)$ and the diffusion rate coefficient k2. The contrast agent is not incorporated into the cell and is excreted from the kidney into urine

agent can be explained by a linear two-compartment model consisting of a central compartment (systemic circulation) and a peripheral compartment (tissue) (Fig. 1). Strictly speaking, there are two compartments in the extracellular space of the tissue, namely, the interior and exterior of the blood vessels; in the liver, these correspond to the sinusoids and the Disse space, respectively. However, if one postulates the establishment of an instantaneous equilibrium, based on the assumption that diffusion of substances between the two extracellular spaces is extremely fast, then the two extracellular spaces may be modeled as the same compartment. (If an instantaneous equilibrium between the two extracellular spaces is not established, then a more complicated model must be considered. Details have been described in the literature [6].) If $C_a(t)$ is the concentration of the contrast agent in the systemically circulating blood (e.g., aorta) at time t, $C_t(t)$ is the concentration of the contrast agent in the tissue extracellular space (e.g., in the liver, sinusoids, and Disse space), τ is the time needed for the contrast agent to reach the tissue from systemic circulation, K1 is the rate coefficient for diffusion of the contrast agent from the systemic circulation to the tissue, and k2 is the rate coefficient for diffusion from the tissue to the systemic circulation, then the change over time in the concentration of the contrast agent in the tissue can be described by the following differential equation [6, 7]:

$$dC_t(t)/dt = K1 \times C_a(t - \tau) - k2 \times C_t(t)$$

Then, the T1 relaxation rate of the tissue after imaging (1/T1) can be expressed by the sum of the T1 relaxation rate inherent to the tissue ($1/T1_0$) and the T1-shortening caused by the contrast agent present in the extracellular fluid ($1/T1_{ECF}$) [5].

$$1/T1 = 1/T1_0 + 1/T1_{ECF}$$
$$1/T1_{ECF} = R1 \times C_t(t)$$

where R1 is an indicator termed "T1 relaxivity," which reflects the degree of T1-shortening of the contrast agent; the enhancement effect on the T1-weighted image is stronger when R1 is larger. For example, in the case of the spin echo method, the following equation describes the relationship between the T1 relaxation rate (1/T1) and the MR signal strength (S) [8]:

$$S = \kappa \times \rho \times \left(1 - 2e^{-(TR-TE/2)T1} + e^{-TR/T1}\right) \times e^{-TE/T2}$$

κ is a proportionality factor, ρ is proton density, TR is repetition time, and TE is echo time. Therefore, there is no linear proportional relationship between MRI contrast agent concentration and the MR signal intensity similar to that between the iodine contrast agent concentration and CT value. However, because there is an exponential correlation between the MRI contrast agent concentration and the signal intensity up to a certain concentration (about 5 mmol/L in a 1.5 T MR apparatus) [9], the enhancement effect on MR images is considered to mostly reflect the concentration of the contrast agent. As $C_a(t)$ and $C_t(t)$ can be determined on MR images in this way, it is possible to determine the parameters τ, K1, and k2 by curve fitting, using the time-intensity curves (TIC) of the systemic circulation and tissue obtained by multiphase imaging [10].

In the following subsections, we discuss the significance of each parameter determined in the linear two-compartment model of the Gd-based extracellular fluid contrast agent, in terms of diagnostic imaging.

2. τ

τ is the time required for the contrast agent to arrive at tissue via the systemic circulation. The contrast agent arrives more slowly at a tissue with large τ than at a tissue with small τ. A difference in τ is observed as a difference in the upward flexion point of the TIC (Fig. 2) [7].

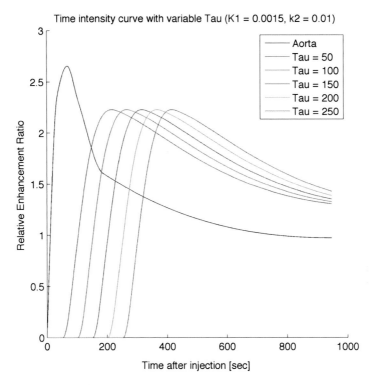

Fig. 2 Influence of τ on time-intensity curve. Shown are time-intensity curves obtained as K1 and k2 were kept constant and τ was altered. The upward flexion point of the time-intensity curve is delayed when τ is large, compared to when τ is small

3. K1

K1 is the rate coefficient for diffusion of the contrast agent from the systemic circulation into the tissue. Therefore, it can be said that within a particular period, more contrast agent flows into a tissue with larger K1 than into a tissue with smaller K1. The diffusion of the contrast agent into the tissue is influenced both by blood flow rate and by blood vessel permeability [6]. Differences in K1 are observed as differences in the peak height of the TIC during early-phase imaging (Fig. 3) [11]. The usefulness of K1 as a factor for estimating the outcome of patients with hepatocellular carcinoma, and also as an indicator for evaluation of therapeutic effects, has been reported [12].

4. k2

k2 is the rate coefficient for diffusion of the contrast agent from the tissue into the systemic circulation. It is also expressed as the inverse of mean transit time, and it can be said that the contrast agent diffuses more rapidly out of a tissue with larger k2 than out of a tissue with smaller k2 [6]. Differences in k2 are observed

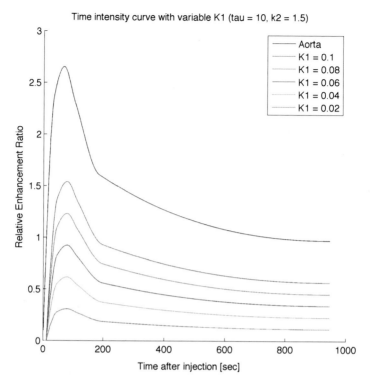

Fig. 3 Influence of K1 on time-intensity curve. Shown are time-intensity curves obtained as τ and k2 were kept constant and K1 was altered. The peak of the time-intensity curve is higher when K1 is large, compared to when K1 is small

as differences in the slope of the TIC between early- and late-phase imaging (Fig. 4) [11]. Similarly to K1, k2 has also been reported to be useful as a factor for estimating the outcome of patients with hepatocellular carcinoma and as an indicator for evaluating therapeutic effects [12].

5. K1/k2

K1/k2 is also expressed as distribution volume (V_d), which is defined as the volume of all tissues and organs in the body where the drug is distributed, assuming that it is distributed at the concentration identical to that in the systemically circulating blood [3]. It can be said that a tissue with large K1/k2 contains more contrast agent in the extracellular space than a tissue with small K1/k2. However, note should be taken of the fact that K1/k2 does not indicate the actual volume of the tissue where the contrast agent is distributed. Differences in K1/k2 are observed as differences in the height of the TIC during late-phase imaging and reflect the contrast-enhancement effect in the equilibrium-phase imaging (Fig. 5) [11].

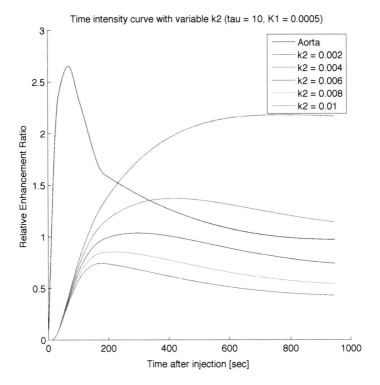

Fig. 4 Influence of k2 on time-intensity curve. Shown are time-intensity curves obtained as τ and K1 were kept constant and k2 was altered. The time-intensity curve declines more rapidly when k2 is large, compared to when k2 is small

6. Two-in-one-outlinear compartment model

Because hepatic blood flow is supplied by both the hepatic artery and the portal vein, a 2-in-1-outlinear compartment model should be considered, in order to evaluate hepatic blood flow dynamics in detail [7]. Such a model takes into the account the influence of portal blood flow in a linear two-compartment model:

$$dC_t(t)/dt = K1_a \times C_a(t - \tau_a) + K1_p \times C_p(t - \tau_p) - k2 \times C_t(t)$$

where $C_a(t)$, $C_p(t)$, τ_a, τ_p, $K1_a$, and $K1_p$ are arterial and portal concentrations of the contrast agent, time to arrival, and transfer rate coefficient. It is possible to determine the arterial blood flow rate $[K1_a/(K1_a + K1_p)]$, V_d $[(K1_a + K1_p)/k2]$, and other parameters by analyzing these values, which have been used for evaluation of liver fibrosis [3].

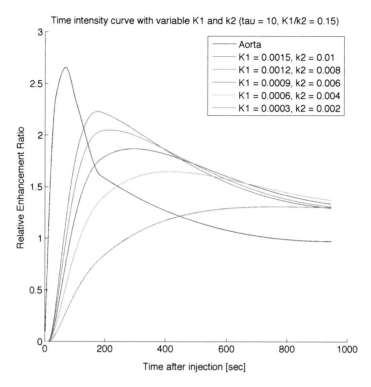

Fig. 5 Influence of magnitudes of K1 and k2 on time-intensity curve. Shown are time-intensity curves obtained as τ and K1/k2 were kept constant and K1 and k2 were altered. Various peak heights and decay patterns are observable, depending on the values of K1 and k2, but the contrast enhancement is constant in late-phase imaging

Quantitative Evaluation of Liver Function Using Gadoxetate Disodium

Gadoxetate disodium is a tissue-specific Gd contrast agent consisting of a Gd-based extracellular fluid contrast agent, Gd-DTPA, linked to a lipophilic branched-chain EOB moiety. When administered intravenously, this compound is transferred from the systemic circulation into the tissue, distributed into the extracellular fluid, and incorporated specifically into hepatocytes by the organic anion transporter peptide (OATP) expressed on the hepatocyte membrane. About 40 % of the administered agent is excreted into bile, while about 60 % of it is excreted into urine. Thus, the pharmacokinetics of gadoxetate disodium and the resulting imaging findings are easily explained by a nonlinear compartment model, in which the model of the extracellular fluid Gd-based contrast agent is modified to take into account incorporation into cells (Fig. 6) [13]:

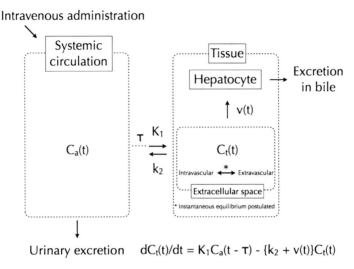

Fig. 6 Nonlinear two-compartment model of hepatocyte-specific gadolinium contrast agent. $C_a(t)$: concentration of the contrast agent in systemically circulating blood at time t; $C_t(t)$: concentration of the contrast agent in tissue extracellular space at time t; τ: time required for the contrast agent to arrive at tissue via the systemic circulation; K1: rate coefficient for diffusion of contrast agent from systemic circulation to tissue; k2: rate coefficient for diffusion of contrast agent from tissue to systemic circulation; $v(t)$: rate coefficient for uptake of contrast agent from hepatic extracellular space into cell; V_{max}: maximum reaction rate; and K_m: Michaelis-Menten constant. The contrast agent, administered intravenously into systemically circulating blood, reaches a tissue after a period τ, diffuses into the tissue at a velocity proportional to the concentration in systemically circulating blood $C_a(t)$ and the diffusion rate coefficient K1, and diffuses out of the tissue at a velocity proportional to the concentration in the tissue extracellular space $C_t(t)$ and the diffusion rate coefficient k2. The contrast agent is excreted from the kidney into urine and is also incorporated from the extracellular space into hepatocytes, via a nonlinear process $v(t)$ characterized by V_{max} and K_m, and excreted into bile

$$dC_t(t)/dt = K1 \times C_a(t - \tau) - \{k2 + v(t)\} \times C_t(t)$$

where $v(t)$ is the nonlinear rate coefficient at time t, representing the incorporation from the tissue extracellular space into cells. $v(t)$ can be expressed by the following Michaelis-Menten equation:

$$v(t) = V_{max}/\{K_m + C_t(t)\}$$

where V_{max} is the maximum rate of incorporation, and K_m is the Michaelis-Menten constant, which is defined as the substrate concentration giving an incorporation rate of half V_{max}. Normally, gadoxetate disodium-enhanced MRI is carried out within 20 min after administration of the contrast agent; if it is postulated that excretion of the contrast agent into bile is negligibly small, then the intracellular concentration of the contrast agent at time t can be expressed by $\int \{v(t) \times C_t(t)\} \cdot dt$.

In other words, gadoxetate disodium uptake into hepatocytes is governed by the amount of the contrast agent delivered to the tissue extracellular space and the uptake rate into hepatocytes, thus reflecting both blood flow and transporter function. Furthermore, in view of the fact that R1 of EOB differs between extracellular fluid ($R1_{\text{extracellular fluid}} = 8.7$ L mmol^{-1} s^{-1}) and hepatocytes ($R1_{\text{HC}} = 16.6$ L mmol^{-1} s^{-1}) [21], the T1 relaxation rate in tissue ($1/T1$) at time t can be expressed by the sum of the T1 relaxation rate specific to the tissue ($1/T1_0$), the T1-shortening by the contrast agent present in the extracellular fluid ($1/T1_{\text{extracellular fluid}}$) and the T1-shortening of the contrast agent present in the hepatocytes ($1/T1_{\text{HC}}$):

$$1/T1 = 1/T1_0 + 1/T1_{\text{extracellular fluid}} + 1/T1_{\text{HC}}$$
$$1/T1_{\text{extracellular fluid}} = R1_{\text{extracellular fluid}} \times C_t(t)$$
$$1/T1_{\text{HC}} = R1_{\text{HC}} \times \int \{v(t) \times C_t(t)\} \cdot dt$$

Thus, the hepatic enhancement effect in gadoxetate disodium-enhanced MR imaging can be assumed to reflect the sum of the concentration of gadoxetate disodium present in the extracellular fluid and the integral concentration of gadoxetate disodium incorporated into hepatocytes.

Several attempts have been made to perform quantitative evaluation of liver function by applying the pharmacokinetics of gadoxetate disodium, thereby correcting the liver signal intensity on gadoxetate disodium-enhanced MR images.

1. Correction of liver signal intensity before contrast-enhanced MR imaging

Kim et al. [14] determined liver signal intensities (SIs) on T1-weighted images using the spin echo method, before and after gadoxetate disodium-enhanced MR imaging, in a rat model of artificially induced hepatitis, to examine their correlation with the half-life of ICG in blood (ICG-$T_{1/2}$). Relative enhancement (RE), used as an indicator for evaluating the signal intensity, can be calculated according to the following equation:

$$\text{RE } (\%) = \left(\text{SI}_{\text{postcontrast}} - \text{SI}_{\text{precontrast}} \right) / \text{SI}_{\text{precontrast}} \times 100$$

The correlation coefficients of ICG-$T_{1/2}$ with RE-max (the maximum RE until 60 min after contrast-enhanced imaging) and with RE-$T_{1/2}$ (the half-life after RE-max) were -0.98 and 0.97, respectively, indicating that compromised liver function leads to a decrease in liver signal intensity in gadoxetate disodium-enhanced MR imaging and delay of excretion of gadoxetate disodium into bile [14].

Shimizu et al. [15] determined liver signal intensities on spin echo T1-weighted images before and after gadoxetate disodium-enhanced imaging, to examine the correlation between the ischemic period and RE-$T_{1/2}$ in a rat model of artificially induced local hepatic ischemia reperfusion. The results showed that RE-$T_{1/2}$ varied statistically significantly, depending on the difference of ischemic period. Furthermore, RE-$T_{1/2}$ was longer, i.e., excretion of gadoxetate disodium into bile was

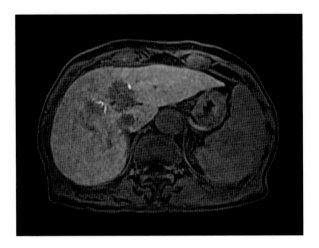

Fig. 7 Fat-suppressed T1-weighted 3-dimensional gradient echo image 20 min after Gd-EOB-DTPA administration (TR/TE/ FA = 3.5/1.42/15), in a case of chronic hepatitis (ICG-PDR* = 0.08 s^{-1}, liver volume = 1,024 mL). The contrast of the liver and spleen is reduced, and the signal intensity of the liver is uneven. *ICG-PDR = indocyanine green plasma disappearance rate

delayed, when the ischemic period was longer. The RE-T$_{1/2}$ values in the ischemic and non-ischemic regions were statistically significantly different from each other, indicating that it might be possible to diagnose segmental liver function using gadoxetate disodium-enhanced MR imaging [15].

Because gadoxetate disodium exhibits a stronger enhancement effect in hepatocytes than in extracellular fluid, the effect of the gadoxetate disodium present in the extracellular fluid on the liver signal intensity becomes insignificant sufficiently late after administration, when excretion from the kidney has progressed. Therefore, it should be possible to evaluate uptake of gadoxetate disodium into hepatocytes by subtracting the signal intensity before contrast-enhanced imaging. However, even when MR images were acquired 20 min after gadoxetate disodium administration (the time point when the maximum enhancement effect may be obtained in humans), the correlation of RE with ICG-PDR was small ($r = 0.48$) [16]. Therefore, it would be necessary to correct for the extracellular fluid-based enhancement effect in the clinical setting.

2. Correction for the extracellular fluid-based enhancement effect

Motosugi et al. [17] measured signal intensities of the liver and spleen on fat-suppressed T1-weighted 3D gradient echo images 20 min after the administration of gadoxetate disodium to patients, in order to examine the correlation of these values with various indicators of liver function (ICG-R15, serum albumin-bilirubin concentration, prothrombin time, and Child classification). Quantitative liver-to-spleen contrast ratio (Q-LSC = SI$_{liver}$/SI$_{spleen}$), which is determined from the ratio of liver and spleen signal intensities, showed the best correlation with ICG-R15. Furthermore, Q-LSC values varied statistically significantly, depending on the severity of hepatopathy by Child classification, indicating that the Q-LSC value declines, i.e., the contrast of liver and spleen becomes weaker, with progression of hepatic disease (Figs. 7 and 8). [17].

Fig. 8 Fat-suppressed
T1-weighted 3-dimensional
gradient echo image 20 min
after Gd-EOB-DTPA
administration (TR/TE/
FA = 3.5/1.42/15), in a
case of normal liver
(ICG-PDR* = 0.23 s^{-1},
liver volume = 1,091 mL).
The contrast of the liver
and spleen is strong,
and the signal intensity
of the liver is uniform.
*ICG-PDR = indocyanine
green plasma
disappearance rate

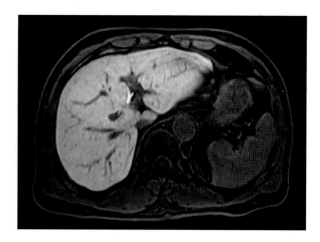

Because gadoxetate disodium is present not only in hepatocytes but also in extracellular fluid, it is necessary to correct for the extracellular fluid-based enhancement effect when hepatocyte function is evaluated from the liver signal intensity in the hepatocyte phase. On the other hand, the distribution volume (V_d = K1/k2) of extracellular fluid is significantly similar in normal liver and spleen tissues [18], with the difference between normal liver and liver cirrhosis being approximately 10 % [3]. Thus, in hepatocyte-phase imaging, when the concentration of the contrast agent in the extracellular fluid is in equilibrium, the contrast-enhancement effect ($1/T1_{extracellular\ fluid}$) of the gadoxetate disodium present in the extracellular space of the liver can be approximated by the contrast-enhancement effect of the spleen. Liver signal intensity corrected by spleen signal intensity might be used as an effective indicator of liver function (Fig. 9). However, the coefficient of determination obtained in the regression analysis of Q-LSC and liver function indicators (ICG-R15 and Child classification) was small, at 0.34 [17], suggesting that further improvement is needed in order to achieve quantitative determination of liver function with gadoxetate disodium-enhanced MR imaging. It is also possible to use the hepatic extraction fraction (HEF), which is determined by deconvolution analysis of the signal intensities of the liver and aorta over time, as an indicator for correction of the extracellular fluid-based contrast-enhancement effect and evaluation of gadoxetate disodium uptake into the liver. HEF is reported to be significantly lower in patients with primary biliary cirrhosis than in healthy subjects, and there is a correlation between HEF and the severity of PBC. However, no comparison of quantitative methods for determination of liver function (e.g., ICG clearance test) has been made in human beings [19, 20].

3. Correction for liver volume

All liver function diagnostic methods that employ conventional gadoxetate disodium contrast-enhanced MR imaging, such as RE, Q-LSC, and HEF, focus

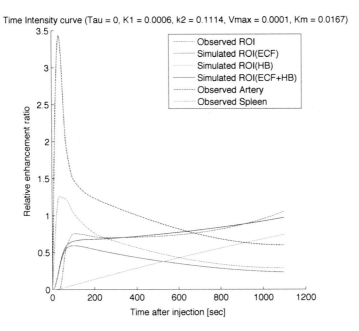

Fig. 9 Time-intensity curves of liver and kidney in gadoxetate disodium contrast-enhanced MRI. Shown are the time concentration curves observed in an actual dynamic study and simulation results obtained in the nonlinear two-compartment model analysis. Hepatocyte enhancement effect (*green*) is observed even in the early-phase imaging, contributing to a gradual increase of the time-intensity curve of the entire liver (*red*). The hepatic extracellular fluid-based enhancement effect (*blue*) shows a decay similar to those of spleen (*purple*) and aorta (*black*); the extracellular fluid-based enhancement effects of liver and spleen are quite similar to each other in the late-phase imaging

only on the local signal intensity and make no correction for liver volume. Thus, these methods may be useful in evaluating the severity of local fibrosis [21] and in qualitative diagnosis of liver function [22]. For quantitative diagnosis of liver function, however, the regional signal intensity as well as liver volume should also be taken into consideration (Figs. 10 and 11) [23]. In addition, conventional methods use the regional signal intensity as representative of the signal intensity of the entire liver, on the assumption that there are no regional differences in liver function. Thus, in cases where there are regional differences in liver function, for example, under the influence of obstructive jaundice or obstructed blood flow in the portal vein, it is necessary to use an indicator that correctly reflects these regional differences (Fig. 12). The hepatocellular uptake index (HUI) has been proposed as a quantitative indicator of liver function that takes such regional differences into account. HUI is calculated according to the following equation, which corrects for the extracellular fluid-based contrast enhancement and liver volume [24]:

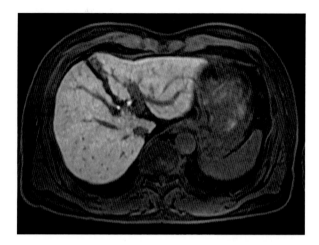

Fig. 10 Fat-suppressed T1-weighted 3-dimensional gradient echo image obtained 20 min after Gd-EOB-DTPA administration (TR/TE/FA = 3.5/1.42/15), in a case of mild hepatopathy (ICG-PDR* = 0.19 s^{-1}, liver volume = 1,045 mL). The contrast of the liver and spleen is strong but the signal intensity of the liver is uneven. Note that although the liver volume is larger and the ICG-PDR higher compared to the case of Fig. 11, the ratio of liver and spleen signal intensity is low. *ICG-PDR = indocyanine green plasma disappearance rate

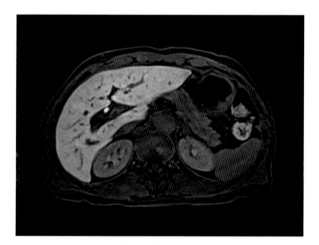

Fig. 11 Fat-suppressed T1-weighted 3-dimensional gradient echo image obtained 20 min after Gd-EOB-DTPA administration (TR/TE/FA = 3.5/1.42/15), in a case of normal liver (ICG-PDR* = 0.15 s^{-1}, liver volume = 749 mL). The contrast of the liver and spleen is strong, and the signal intensity of the liver is uniform. Note that although liver volume is smaller and ICG-PDR is lower compared to the case of Fig. 10, the ratio of liver and spleen signal intensity is high. *ICG-PDR = indocyanine green plasma disappearance rate

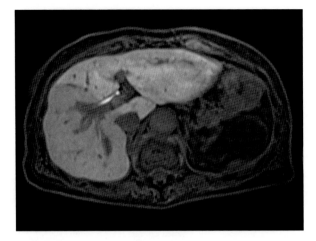

Fig. 12 Fat-suppressed T1-weighted 3-dimensional gradient echo image obtained 20 min after Gd-EOB-DTPA administration (TR/TE/FA = 3.5/1.42/15), in a case undergoing right portal vein branch embolization (ICG-PDR* = 0.21 s^{-1}, liver volume = 957 mL). Decreases are observed in the signal intensity and volume of the right hepatic lobe, which was subjected to portal vein embolization. Compensatory hypertrophy is observed in the left hepatic lobe. *ICG-PDR = indocyanine green plasma disappearance rate

$$HUI = V \times (L_{20} - S_{20})/S_{20}$$

The HUI equation above can be interpreted as follows: if the difference in signal intensity before imaging is considered negligible, then the difference between the average signal intensity of the entire liver on the fat-suppressed T1-weighted image ($L20$), and the mean signal intensity of the spleen ($S20$) 20 min after administration of gadoxetate disodium represents the enhancement effect of gadoxetate disodium uptake into hepatocytes. The amount of gadoxetate disodium uptake into hepatocytes per unit volume is determined approximately, normalizing it against the signal intensity of the spleen ($S20$), and the amount of gadoxetate disodium uptake into hepatocytes in the entire liver is estimated by integrating the concentration over the liver volume (V). HUI correlates well with the ICG plasma disappearance rate, an indicator of substrate incorporation into the same hepatocytes via OATP [24]. As HUI is determined directly from the signal intensity and the liver volume in the region of interest, it would be applicable to cases in which there are regional differences in liver function and would therefore allow more accurate estimation of segmental liver reserve function [24]. HUI has been shown to be useful in predicting reserve liver function after transarterial chemoembolization therapy [25]. Manual identification of the liver region of interest demands time and labor. However, if advances in computer-assisted diagnostic imaging allow blood supply regions and anatomical regions of interest to be

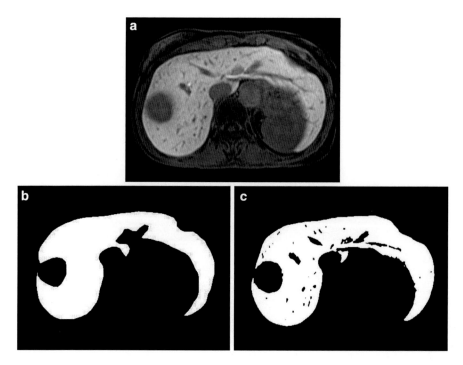

Fig. 13 Automatic extraction of liver using Gd-EOB-DTPA contrast-enhanced MRI. (**a**) F Fat-suppressed T1-weighted 3-dimensional gradient echo image obtained 20 min after Gd-EOB-DTPA administration (TR/TE/FA = 3.5/1.42/15). Original image before contour extraction. (**b**) Contour of liver manually extracted from (**a**). (**c**) Contour of liver automatically extracted from (**a**). The automatically extracted contour is more accurate than the manually extracted contour (**b**), because the latter omits fine branches of the liver

defined automatically, it will be possible to achieve more efficient and sophisticated diagnosis of reserve liver function (Fig. 13) [26].

Summary

We have presented here quantitative methods for diagnosis of liver function using MR imaging, with special reference to a gadolinium-based extracellular fluid contrast agent, the pharmacokinetics of gadoxetate disodium, and previously proposed various quantitative methods for liver function diagnosis. However, clinical application of such quantitative MR imaging for the diagnosis of reserved liver function is still challenging, and further research is required to establish a standard imaging method, correct for the effect of iron–fat deposition, and overcome any other problems.

References

1. Seyama Y, Kokudo N (2009) Assessment of liver function for safe hepatic resection. Hepatol Res 39:107–116
2. Sakka SG (2007) Assessing liver function. Curr Opin Crit Care 13:207–214
3. Hagiwara M, Rusinek H, Lee VS et al (2008) Advanced liver fibrosis: diagnosis with 3D whole-liver perfusion MR imaging—initial experience. Radiology 246:926–934
4. Reimer P, Schneider G, Schima W (2004) Hepatobiliary contrast agents for contrast-enhanced MRI of the liver: properties, clinical development and applications. Eur Radiol 14:559–578
5. Weinmann HJ, Brasch RC, Press WR et al (1984) Characteristics of gadolinium-DTPA complex: a potential NMR contrast agent. AJR 142:619–624
6. Tofts PS, Brix G, Buckley DL et al (1999) Estimating kinetic parameters from dynamic contrast-enhanced T(1)-weighted MRI of diffusable tracer: standardized quantities and symbols. J Magn Reson Imaging 10:223–232
7. Miyazaki S, Murase K, Yoshikawa T et al (2008) A quantitative method for estimating hepatic blood flow using a dual-input single-compartment model. Br J Radiol 81:790–800
8. Wehrli FW, MacFall JR, Glover GH et al (1984) The dependence of nuclear magnetic resonance (NMR) image contrast on intrinsic and pulse sequence timing parameters. Magn Reson Imaging 2:3–16
9. Mørkenborg J, Pedersen M, Jensen FT et al (2003) Quantitative assessment of Gd-DTPA contrast agent from signal enhancement: an in-vitro study. Magn Reson Imaging 21:637–643
10. Sourbron S, Sommer WH, Reiser MF et al (2012) Combined quantification of liver perfusion and function with dynamic gadoxetic acid-enhanced MR imaging. Radiology 263:874–883
11. Tofts PS (2010) T1-weighted DCE imaging concepts: modelling, acquisition and analysis. MAGNETOM Flash 45:30–39
12. Jarnagin WR, Schwartz LH, Gultekin DH et al (2009) Regional chemotherapy for unresectable primary liver cancer: results of a phase II clinical trial and assessment of DCE-MRI as a biomarker of survival. Ann Oncol 20:1589–1595
13. Schuhmann-Giampieri G (1993) Nonlinear pharmacokinetic modeling of a gadolinium chelate used as a liver-specific contrast agent for magnetic resonance imaging. Arzneimittelforschung 43:1020–1024
14. Kim T, Murakami T, Hasuike Y et al (1997) Experimental hepatic dysfunction: evaluation by MRI with Gd-EOB-DTPA. J Magn Reson Imaging 7:683–688
15. Shimizu J, Dono K, Gotoh M et al (1999) Evaluation of regional liver function by gadolinium-EOB-DTPA-enhanced MR imaging. Dig Dis Sci 44:1330–1337
16. Yamada A, Hara T, Li F et al (2010) Evaluation of liver function using gadoxetate disodium (Gd-EOB-DTPA) enhanced MR imaging. In: Molthen RC, Weaver JB (eds) Proc. SPIE 7626, Medical Imaging 2010: Biomedical Applications in Molecular, Structural, and Functional Imaging, San Diego, California, pp 762604–762610 (March 4, 2010) doi: 10.1117/12.843722
17. Motosugi U, Ichikawa T, Sou H et al (2009) Liver parenchymal enhancement of hepatocyte-phase images in Gd-EOB-DTPA-enhanced MR imaging: which biological markers of the liver function affect the enhancement? J Magn Reson Imaging 30:1042–1046
18. Kötz B, West C, Saleem A et al (2009) Blood flow and Vd(water): both biomarkers required for interpreting the effects of vascular targeting agents on tumor and normal tissue. Mol Cancer Ther 8:303–309
19. Ryeom HK, Kim SH, Kim JY et al (2004) Quantitative evaluation of liver function with MRI Using Gd-EOB-DTPA. Korean J Radiol 5:231–239
20. Nilsson H, Blomqvist L, Douglas L et al (2010) Assessment of liver fraction in primary biliary cirrhosis using Gd-EOB-DTPA-enhanced liver MRI. HPB 12:567–576
21. Tsuda N, Okada M, Murakami T (2010) New proposal for the staging of nonalcoholic steatohepatitis: evaluation of liver fibrosis on Gd-EOB-DTPA-enhanced MRI. Eur J Radiol 73:137–142

22. Motosugi U, Ichikawa T, Tominaga L et al (2009) Delay before the hepatocyte phase of Gd-EOB-DTPA-enhanced MR imaging: is it possible to shorten the examination time? Eur Radiol 19:2623–2629
23. Hashimoto M, Watanabe G (2000) Hepatic parenchymal cell volume and the indocyanine green tolerance test. J Surg Res 92:222–227
24. Yamada A, Hara T, Li F et al (2011) Quantitative evaluation of liver function with use of gadoxetate disodium–enhanced MR imaging. Radiology 260:727–733
25. Yamada A, Kadoya M, Ueda K et al (2011) Computerized estimation of quantitative segmental liver reserve after transcatheter arterial chemoembolization by use of gadoxetate. In: RSNA. McCormick Place Convention Center, Chicago. Radiological Society of North America

26. Yamada A, Hara T, Li F et al (2010) Computerized analysis of liver function using gadoxetate disodium–enhanced MR Imaging. In: RSNA. McCormick Place Convention Center, Chicago. Radiological Society of North America

Biography

Akira Yamada, MD, PhD is Assistant Professor of Department of Radiology, Shinshu University School of Medicine in Japan. He received Grant-in-Aid for Young Scientists from Japan Society for the Promotion of Science to develop his research project in functional imaging from 2011 to 2013. He is currently specializing and focusing his research in computer application for abdominal imaging and interventional radiology.

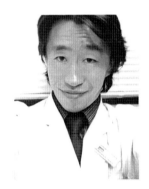

Diffusion-Weighted Imaging of the Liver

Ali Muhi, Tomoaki Ichikawa, and Utaroh Motosugi

Abstract Diffusion-weighted imaging (DWI) has been more frequently used in abdominal imaging after recent advances in technology including parallel imaging and EPI, particularly for assessment of liver. These advances in technology have reduced examination time and artifacts. DWI is quick and can be performed in a single breath-hold. It can be easily incorporated to the conventional MRI sequences. It is useful for the evaluation of focal and diffuse liver disease and has the potential for evaluation of tumor response to treatment.

DWI Acquisition Techniques

Diffusion-weighted imaging (DWI) is usually performed using a single-shot spin-echo EPI sequence. DWI can be performed using other sequences including gradient-echo EPI, single-shot fast spin echo, and some view-sharing techniques such as PROPELLER. However, spin-echo EPI is still the most efficient and appropriate sequence for abdominal DWI.

When performing DWI, combination with parallel imaging is essential because it minimizes echo time and acquisition time, which increases SNR and reduces motion-related artifacts. Keeping a long TR, for example longer than 7,000 ms can help avoid signal decay caused by insufficient T1-relaxation.

Abdominal DWI methods can be divided into three categories according to respiratory control. These are the breath-holding method, the free-breathing method, and the respiratory-triggered method (Table 1).

A. Muhi, M.B.Ch.B., Ph.D. (✉)
Department of Radiology, Muthanna University, Muthanna, Iraq
e-mail: ali_muhi@yahoo.com

T. Ichikawa, M.D., Ph.D. • U. Motosugi, M.D., Ph.D.
Department of Radiology, University of Yamanashi, Yamanshi, Japan
e-mail: ichikawaykn@yahoo.co.jp; utaroh-motosugi@nifty.com

A.S. El-Baz et al. (eds.), *Abdomen and Thoracic Imaging: An Engineering & Clinical Perspective*, DOI 10.1007/978-1-4614-8498-1_10,
© Springer Science+Business Media New York 2014

Table 1 Suggested sequence parameters for performing liver DWI (PHILIPS Achiva 1.5 T)

	Breath-hold acquisition	Free-breathing/respiratory-triggered acquisition
Sequence	SE	SE
Field of view (cm)	37.5 × 30	37.5 × 30
Matrix	152 × 120	124 × 120
Repetition time (TR)	≥980	≥1,230
Echo time (TE)	Minimum (~34)	Minimum (~59)
EPI factor	63	53
Number of averages	2	4
Slice thickness (mm)	7	5
Number of slices	25	25
Slice orientation	Axial	Axial
Direction of motion probing gradient	Phase, frequency, and slice	Phase, frequency, and slice
Fat suppression	Yes	Yes
b-Values (s/mm^2)	One or more	3 or more
Acquisition time	15	2–3 min (free-breathing), 4–5 min (respiratory-triggering)

Breath-holding DWI is the simplest method. One or two breath holds are required for about 20 s. This is done with a single acquisition to obtain maximum anatomical coverage. The advantage of breath-holding DWI is the minimal acquisition time. The disadvantages include low SNR, low spatial resolution, and high sensitivity to distortion.

Free-breathing multiple averaging DWI was first described by Dr. Takahara and is also known as DWIBS. In this technique, signal averaging is performed more than 4 times to obtain a sufficiently high SNR. ADC measurement is possible in this technique because the respiratory motion is bulky and slow that it can be considered as a coherent motion.

The advantages of free-breathing DWI are the high SNR, ability to obtain multiple b-values that enables ADC measurements, high spatial resolution, and thin slice sections. It can be performed even for uncooperative patients including pediatric cases. The disadvantages include long acquisition times, usually requires more than 3 min, and image blurring. Another disadvantage is that it is suboptimal for assessing small lesions.

Respiratory-triggered DWI is the most sophisticated method. Multiple averaging of 3 or 4 times is essential to obtain a sufficiently high SNR. Respiratory-triggered DWI shares all of the advantages of the free-breathing method. Additionally, minimal motion artifacts in this technique enable assessments of small lesions. Minimal slice misalignment is useful for preparing a fusion image. Accurate ADC measurements can be performed by eliminating the signal drop due to respiratory motion. The main disadvantage is the long acquisition time. It may take more than 5 min if the breathing of the patient is irregular. The time-consuming nature of this method limits the number of slices and anatomical coverage.

Signal intensity of both liver lobes is affected by cardiac motion in DWI. The signal loss ratio is more on the left lobe than right lobe (25.5 % vs. 17.3 %) [1].

Fat Suppression

Fat suppression is essential to reduce chemical shift-induced ghosting in EPI-based DWI. Short tau inversion recovery (STIR) has several advantages including complete fat suppression. STIR also suppresses signals from materials with short T1-relaxation times, for example, feces in the colon or rectum. Low SNR is a disadvantage. Chemical fat-selective saturation (CHESS) is more commonly used for abdominal DWI to obtain high SNR.

Choice of b-Values and Sequence Optimization

The choice of b-value is a matter of great importance and depends on the purpose of the DWI.

When DWI is performed for lesion detection, an image with $b = 0$ is not required. A single or two b-values, including low and high b-values, are enough for this purpose. However, two or more b-values including $b = 0$ may be the most common choice, yielding both detection and ADC measurements. If 3 or more b-value images are obtained, the ADC measurement is more accurate.

When 8 or more b-values are used, a more complicated and sophisticated analysis can be performed, which is known as intra-voxel incoherent motion (IVIM) imaging.

Low b-value ($b = 20$–150 s/mm^2) suppresses the intrahepatic blood vessels signal yielding a black blood images, which improve focal liver lesion detection.

High b-values (≥ 600 s/mm^2) are considered appropriate to reduce T2 shine-through ghosting, minimize the perfusion, and suppress unfavorable background signals. Of course, SNR is a key parameter to be considered when increasing the b-value. Disadvantage of high b-values is low SNR. In routine clinical practice obtaining two b-values, including one low and one high, is necessary to improve lesion detection and characterization.

Qualitative and Quantitative Assessment

Trace DWI for each b-value and ADC map is displayed. Visual assessment of DWI trace images is useful for focal liver lesion detection and characterization. Low b-value images are evaluated for lesion detection, whereas high b-value images are assessed for lesion restricted diffusion and characterization. The signal observed on

DWI is related to tissue diffusion, perfusion, and tissue T2 relaxation time. There-fore DWI has some T2 weighting and lesions such as cysts or hemangiomas, which have long T2 relaxation time, usually show high signal (T2 shine-through). To reduce T2 shine-through, high b-value images and ADC maps should be assessed. On high b-value images cyst and hemangiomas show signal drop, whereas on ADC maps these lesions return high signal and high ADC values.

The ADC value of the liver can be calculated by drawing a region of interest (ROIs) on the ADC maps. ADC value is usually expressed in ($\times 10^{-3}$) mm^2/s and is strongly depends on the b-value chosen for its calculation. With mono-exponential fitting, two b-values are chosen for ADC calculation. The ADC value is overestimated when $b = 0$ s/mm^2 is chosen as the first value, because of the effect of microperfusion [2]. ADC calculated with $b > 50$ s/mm^2 as the first value (not $b = 0$) is more reproducible and represents pure diffusion [2]. ADC is more reproducible and represent pure diffusion when b-values >50 s/mm^2 are used, but a substantial variations in ADC exist even when these b-values are used. The greater the b-value, the greater the noise and the lower the SNR.

Bi-exponential fitting requires 8 or more b-values and produce IVIM DWI. In addition to ADC, other diffusion parameters can be calculated with IVIM DWI including perfusion-related diffusion (D* or D$_{fast}$), pure diffusion (D or D$_{slow}$), and perfusion fraction (f). For more accurate and reproducible calculation of D* very low b-values (between 0 and 20 s/mm^2) are necessary [2].

Applications of Liver DWI

DWI proved to be useful for liver lesion detection and characterization. DWI has the potential for the diagnosis of liver cirrhosis and for staging of fibrosis. Further-more, it can be used for assessment of tumor treatment response.

Liver Lesion Detection and Characterization

DWI for Characterization of Focal Liver Lesions

Both direct visual assessment of DWI and ADC calculation could be used for lesion characterization. Visual assessment using low and high b-values and ADC map images could distinguish solid from cystic lesions (Table 2). Cystic lesions display significant signal drop on high b-values, whereas solid lesions usually retain high signal on high b-values (Figs. 1 and 2).

Table 2 Characterization of focal liver lesions by visual assessment of low *b*-value, high *b*-value, and ADC maps

	Low *b*-value	High *b*-value	ADC map
Simple cyst	Hyperintense	Hypointense	Iso- to hyperintense
Malignant lesions (HCCs, metastases)	Hyperintense	Iso- to hyperintense	Hypointense
Hemangioma, FNH, adenoma	Hyperintense	Iso- to hyperintense	Iso- to hyperintense
Necrotic HCC or metastasis	Hyperintense	Peripheral hyperintensity	Peripheral hypointensity

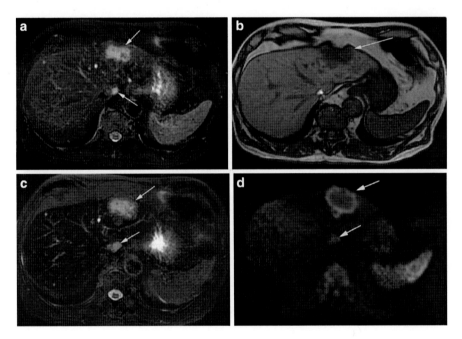

Fig. 1 A 71 years old male patient with metastases from colon cancer at left lobe of liver (*arrows*). (a) Axial fat-saturated T2WI shows tumors as heterogeneous intermediate signal intensity. Small cysts were noted as bright lesions in left and right lobes of liver. (b) Tumors and cysts display low signal intensity compared to liver on axial T1WI. (c) The tumors show heterogeneous intermediate signal and the cysts show high signal intensity on axial SPIO-enhanced T2WI. (d) Axial DWI ($b = 1,000$ s/mm^2) shows tumors as hyperintense relative to the liver, whereas cysts display isointense signal

Several publications used ADC measurement for discriminating malignant from benign lesions with acceptable diagnostic accuracy (Table 3) [3–15]. Most malignant tumors show high signal intensity on DWI (both low and high *b*-values) and low signal on ADC map (Figs. 3, 4, and 5). This finding may be due to increase cellular density, complex histological architecture, or increased nuclear/cytoplasmic ratio of malignant tumors which impair the diffusion of protons.

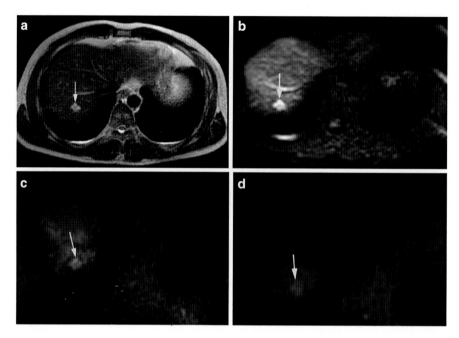

Fig. 2 A 31 years old male with hepatic hemangioma (*arrow*). (**a**) Axial T2-weighted images shows high signal intensity lesion at the right lobe liver. (**b**) The lesion appears hyperintense on axial DWI ($b = 0$ s/mm^2). (**c, d**) The lesion shows decrease signal on moderate and high b-values ($b = 400$ and $b = 800$ s/mm^2) consistent with benign lesion

However, considerable overlap in ADC exists between malignant lesions and benign lesions, particularly solid benign lesions such as adenoma or FNH (Fig. 6) [14, 16]. The decrease in ADC in solid benign lesions may be related to increase cellularity that restricts diffusion.

Benign lesions such as hemangiomas or simple cysts which are the most common lesions observed in clinical practice appear high signal on low b-value DWI and usually return iso to low signal on high b-values. These benign lesions usually return high ADC (Fig. 7). On the other hand cystic (mucinous) or necrotic tumor tends to return high ADC, and could be falsely diagnosed as benign.

Haradome et al. reported that combined interpretation of T2WI and DWI yielded better diagnostic accuracy for discrimination benign from malignant focal liver lesions than each sequence alone [17]. DWI was superior to T2-weighted images for the detection of malignant hepatic lesions; however no difference was observed for characterization of focal hepatic lesions or for detection of benign lesions [18]. DWI, especially with a low b-value 20 s/mm^2, was superior to T2-weighted images for detection of hepatic metastases, particularly for small lesions less than 10 mm [12].

Inan et al. reported that DWI could help in the differential diagnosis of hydatid and simple cysts of the liver. Most hydatid cysts (95 %) were hyperintense, whereas most simple cysts (93 %) were isointense with the liver. ADC was 2.9 for hydatid

Table 3 Mean apparent diffusion coefficients (ADCs) of focal liver lesions, ADC cutoff, sensitivity and specificity for diagnosing malignant lesions

	Cieszanowski	Miller	Namimoto	Battal	Parikh	Bruegel	Gourtsoyianni	Kim	Holzapfel	Taouli
Number of lesions	215	542	59	143	211	204	37	79	185	52
b-Values (s/mm²)	50,400,800	0,500	30,1200	0,800	0,50,500	50,300,600	0,50,500,1000	≤846	50,300,600	≤500
ADC (mm²/s)										
Metastasis	1.05	1.50	1.15		1.50	1.22	0.99	1.06–1.11	1.08	0.94
HCCs	0.94	1.54	0.99		1.31	1.05	1.38	0.97–1.28	1.12	1.33
Hemangiomas	1.55	2.26	1.95		2.04	1.92	1.90	2.04–2.10	1.69	2.95
Cysts	2.45	3.40	3.05		2.54	3.02	2.55	2.91–3.03	2.61	3.63
FNH-Adenomas	1.18	1.79		1.20	1.49	1.40			1.43	1.75
Benign lesions		2.50	1.95	1.94	2.19		2.55	2.49	2.36	2.45
Malignant lesions		1.52	1.04	0.86	1.39		1.04	1.01	1.09	1.08
Abscess	1.50	1.97		1.20						
Cutoff ADC for differentiating of malignant lesions	1.25	1.5		1.21	1.60	1.63	1.47	1.60	1.41	1.50
Sensitivity	79	57		100	74	90	100	98	91	84
Specificity	83	91		89	77	86	100	80	90	89

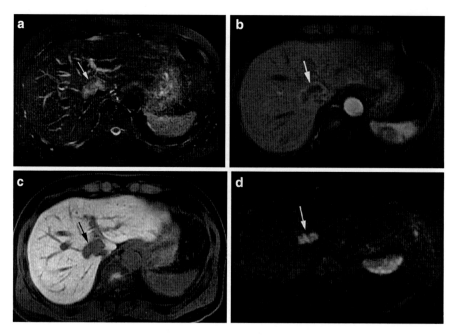

Fig. 3 A 61 years old male with peripheral cholangiocarcinoma at the right lobe of liver anterior to IVC (*arrows*). (**a**) Axial T2-weighted images well-circumscribed lobulated mass with intermediate signal intensity. (**b**) Axial arterial phase of gadoxetic acid-enhanced MRI shows moderate rim enhancement with central heterogeneous poor enhancement. (**c**) Axial hepatobiliary phase image at 20 min shows tumor as hypointense mass. (**d**) The tumor displays high signal intensity on axial DWI ($b = 1,000$ s/mm^2)

cyst vs. 3.5 ($\times 10^{-3}$ mm^2/s) for simple cyst [19]. Fruehwald-Pallamar et al. suggested that DWI could be added to the conventional MRI to increase diagnostic confidence for differentiation between pseudolesions and other focal hepatic lesions. In this study, all hepatic pseudolesions were invisible on DWI [20].

In conclusion, a substantial overlap exist in ADC between malignant and solid benign lesions particularly adenomas and FNH. This overlap in the reported ADC may be due to difference in *b*-value used or type of acquisition technique (breath hold, free-breathing, or respiratory-triggered technique). DWI and ADC should be used as ancillary to conventional MRI (i.e., unenhanced conventional MRI or dynamic contrast-enhanced MRI) for lesion characterization.

Diagnosis and Detection of HCC

HCCs tend to develop in patients with cirrhosis or chronic liver disease. The diagnosis of HCC depends on observation of increased vascularity (hypervascular) on arterial phase and washout on portal venous or equilibrium phase (AASLD

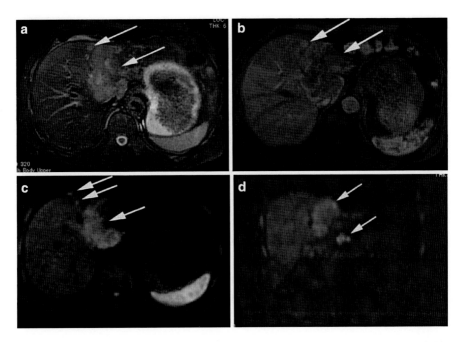

Fig. 4 A 74 years old male with pathologically proved peripheral cholangiocarcinoma with LN metastases (*arrows*). (**a**) Axial T2-weighted images show large well-circumscribed lobulated mass with intermediate signal intensity at the left lobe of liver with satellite lesion around the lesion. (**b**) Axial arterial phase of CE-MRI shows moderate rim enhancement with central heterogeneous minimal enhancement. (**c, d**) The tumor displays high signal intensity on axial and coronal DWI ($b = 1,000$ s/mm^2). Note satellite lesions around the tumor on axial image and lymph nodes metastases inferior to the left lobe of liver on coronal images

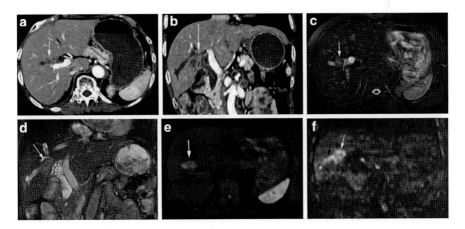

Fig. 5 A 76 years old female with periductal-infiltrating cholangiocarcinoma of right lobe of liver. (**a, b**) Axial and coronal T2WI show poorly defined mass with intermediate signal intensity with dilatation of bile duct due to obstruction by tumor. (**c, d**) Axial and coronal arterial phase of CECT shows minimal enhancement. (**e, f**) Axial and coronal DWI ($b = 1,000$ s/mm^2) shows the tumor as hyperintense with tumor growth along bile duct appears as speculation or branch-like on coronal DWI (*arrow*)

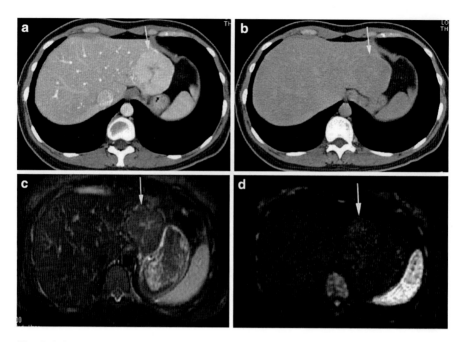

Fig. 6 A 31 years old female patient with hepatic FNH (*arrow*). (**a**) Axial arterial phase CECT shows a bright homogeneous enhancement of the mass with a central scar. (**b**) Axial delayed phase CECT shows the mass as isodense to the liver. (**c**) Axial T2WI shows the mass as slightly hyperintense with hyperintense central scar. (**d**) Axial DWI (*b* = 1,000 s/mm^2) shows the mass as slightly hyperintense

criteria). Dynamic contrast-enhanced CT or MRI has reached a high standard for diagnosis of HCC. With the introduction of liver-specific contrast agent (such as gadoxetic acid), MRI proved to be the best imaging modality for the detection of HCC and for characterization of hepatic nodules in cirrhosis and is superior to CT. Most HCCs show high signal intensity on DWI (both low and high *b*-values) and low signal on ADC map (Figs. 8, 9, 10, 11, and 12).

In a study of 91 patients with 109 HCCs, using lesional hyperintensity with DWI or hypervascularity on arterial phase and washout on portal/delayed phase with dynamic contrast-enhanced MRI (DCE-MRI) as diagnostic criteria for diagnosis of HCC, sensitivity of 84 or 85 % were reported compared to 60 % for hypervascularity on arterial phase and washout on portal/equilibrium phase with DCE-MRI alone [21].

DWI could be helpful to differentiate between HCC and benign hepatocellular nodules (regenerative or dysplastic nodules) or benign pseudolesion in cirrhotic liver. In a study of 98 hepatocellular lesions, including 12 dysplastic nodules, none of the dysplastic nodules were visible (i.e., isointense) on DWI whereas 63 (73 %) out of 86 HCCs were visible on DWI [22]. In another study, hypervascular pseudolesions caused by small arterioportal shunts were invisible on DWI [23].

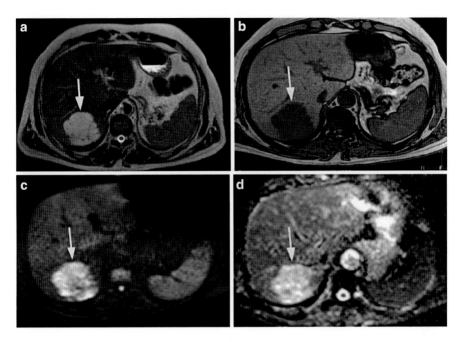

Fig. 7 A 47 years old male patient with colon cancer and hepatic hemangioma (*arrow*). (**a**) Axial T2-weighted images show a high signal intensity lesion at the right lobe of liver. (**b**) Axial T1WI shows the lesion as low signal. (**c, d**) The lesion shows high signal intensity relative to the liver parenchyma on both DWI ($b = 400$ s/mm^2) and ADC map, respectively. The tumor showed peripheral nodular enhancement with centripetal filling on dynamic CT images (not shown)

Lee et al. (AJR 2011) reported that hypointensity on gadoxetic acid-enhanced hepatobiliary phase images and hyperintensity on high b-value DWI suggest well-differentiated HCCs rather than benign hepatocellular nodules (regenerative and dysplastic nodules) in chronic liver disease [24]. When hyperintensity on DWI was used as a criteria for diagnosis of HCC a sensitivity of 81 % and specificity of 73 % were yielded [24]. In the same study, ADC was not significantly different between well-differentiated HCC and benign hepatocellular nodule. The use of visibility with DWI to differentiate HCCs from dysplastic nodules yielded AUC of 0.88, sensitivity of 97.5 % and specificity of 78.95 % [25]. Combination of contrast-enhanced MRI with DWI improved characterization of nodules in cirrhotic liver and yielded AUC of 0.91, sensitivity of 97.5 %, and specificity of 93.22 % [25].

The ADC value has an inverse correlation with the degree of histopathological differentiation of HCCs. The ADC tends to decrease with increase the histopathological grade HCCs. This can help to predict the differentiation of HCC noninvasively [22, 26]. Other study indicated that ADC has no correlation with histopathologic grade of HCC, but the signal of HCC tended to increase as the histopathological grade increased [27].

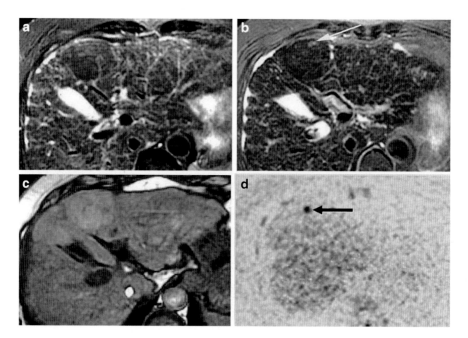

Fig. 8 A 66 years old female with a small HCC within large dysplastic nodule at the left lobe of liver (Nodule-in-nodule pattern). (**a**) Axial T2WI shows dysplastic nodule as large mass with low signal intensity. (**b**) HCC appears as small focus of increased signal intensity within hypointense dysplastic nodule on axial superparamagnetic iron oxide (SPIO)-enhanced T2WI. (**c**) Axial T1WI shows dysplastic nodule as slightly hyperintense mass relative to the liver. (**d**) Axial DWI ($b = 1,000$ s/mm^2) with black and white inversion shows HCC as small focus of increased signal intensity within isointense dysplastic nodule

Le Moigne et al. reported that adding DWI to conventional MRI significantly increased the accuracy and sensitivity from 0.76 and 75.7 % to 0.86 and 87.8 % for the diagnosis of small HCCs in the cirrhotic liver [28]. Combined use of DWI with conventional DCE-MRI helped to provide higher sensitivities than conventional DCE-MRI alone in the detection of small HCC lesions in patients with chronic liver disease [29]. The sensitivity increased to 98 % for the combined approach compared to 85 % for DCE-MRI alone [29].

The diagnostic performance of combined DWI with DCE-MRI was comparable or slightly better than that of combined DCE-MRI and SPIO-enhanced MRI for the assessment of hypervascular lesions in patients with liver cirrhosis [30].

Kim et al. found no additive value of DWI to gadoxetic acid-enhanced MRI for detection of HCC [31]. The diagnostic performance of combined DWI and gadoxetic acid-enhanced MRI was equal to that of gadoxetic acid-enhanced MRI alone.

In conclusion, DWI is useful adjunct to conventional or DCE-MRI for detection of HCC, particularly for small nodules adjacent to vessels or nodules at the periphery of the liver. It could help to distinguish between HCC and other benign

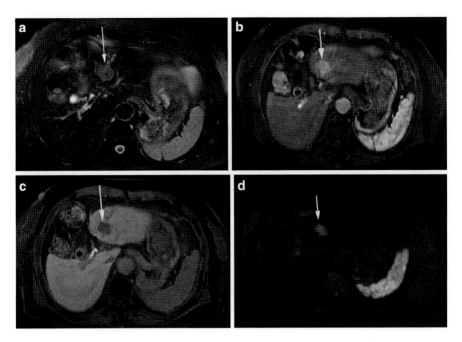

Fig. 9 A 63 years old female with moderately differentiated HCC at left lobe of liver (*arrow*). (**a**) Axial fat-saturated T2WI shows tumor as heterogeneous intermediate signal intensity mass. (**b, c**) Tumor displays hypervascularity on arterial phase and washout on delayed phase of dynamic CE-MRI. (**d**) The tumor appears as hyperintense on axial DWI ($b = 1,000$ s/mm^2)

hepatic nodules or pseudolesions. Significant overlap in the ADC value exists between different grades of HCC and other benign hepatocellular nodules in cirrhotic liver.

Detection of Liver Metastases

Metastases are the commonest malignant tumors of the liver and second most commonly involved organ by metastasis in the body after lymph node. Liver could be involved by metastases from any primary malignant neoplasm in the body. The most common primary tumors include colon, breast, lung, stomach, and pancreas. Liver metastases are usually multiple and generally are divided into hypervascular and hypovascular metastases. MRI proved to be the most accurate modality for detection of hepatic metastases particularly for small lesions ≤1 cm. The introduction of liver-specific contrast agents (hepatocyte-specific and reticulo-endothelial cell-specific agents) increased the accuracy of MRI for detection of liver metastases.

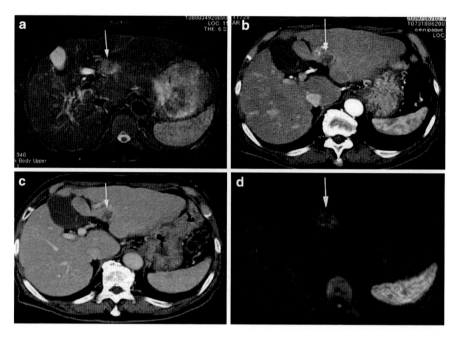

Fig. 10 A76 years old male with NBNC liver cirrhosis and poorly differentiated HCC at left lobe of liver (*arrow*). (**a**) Axial fat-saturated T2WI shows tumor as heterogeneous intermediate signal intensity mass. (**b, c**) Tumor displays hypovascularity on arterial phase and delayed phase of dynamic CECT. (**d**) The tumor appears as hyperintense on axial DWI ($b = 1,000$ s/mm^2)

Combining diffusion-weighted images (DWI) with conventional MRI or with liver-specific contrast-enhanced MRI has the potential to improve sensitivity or accuracy for detection of liver metastasis (Fig. 13). Combination of MnDPDP MR imaging and DWI resulted in the highest diagnostic accuracy for detection of colorectal hepatic metastases [32]. Combination of DWI and gadoxetic acid-enhanced MRI resulted in better diagnostic accuracy for the detection of small hepatic metastases than each imaging sequence alone [33]. Other studies indicated that combined DWI and gadoxetic acid-enhanced MRI has the potential to increase accuracy and sensitivity but not significantly different from that of gadoxetic acid-enhanced MRI [31, 34]. Other reports show no additional value of DWI to hepatobiliary phase of gadoxetic acid-enhanced MRI for detection of liver metastases; however addition of DWI and unenhanced MRI was useful for lesion characterization particularly for lesions ≤1 cm [35, 36].

Eiber et al. indicated that in patients with colorectal cancer DWI alone has a significantly higher detection rate for liver lesions compared to dynamic contrast-enhanced CT, especially in lesions with a diameter less than 10 mm [37].

Combination of SPIO-MRI with DWI was more reliable than contrast-enhanced CT and contrast-enhanced US for detection of liver metastasis particularly for lesions ≤1 cm [38].

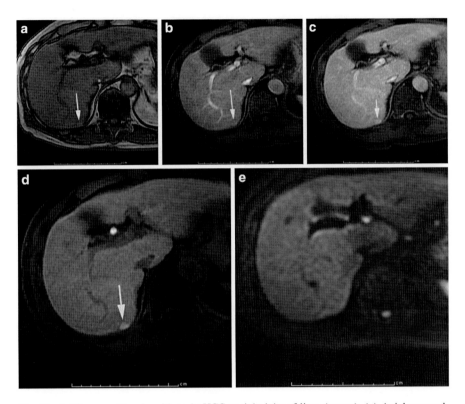

Fig. 11 A 60 years old male with early HCC at right lobe of liver (*arrow*). (**a**) Axial opposed-phase T1WI shows tumor as hyperintense nodule. (**b, c**) Tumor displays subtle hyperintensity on arterial phase and delayed phases of dynamic CE-MRI. (**d**) Tumor shows hyperintensity on hepatobiliary phase image (20 min) of gadoxetic acid-enhanced T1WI. (**e**) The tumor appears as isointense on axial DWI ($b = 1,000$ s/mm^2). Tumor shows no enhancement on dynamic CECT (not shown)

In conclusion DWI is useful adjunct to conventional or DCE-MRI for detection of liver metastases, particularly for small metastases. In patients with impaired renal function with risk of nephrogenic systemic fibrosis, DWI could substitute contrast-enhanced images for the detection of liver metastases.

Diagnosis of Liver Fibrosis and Cirrhosis with DWI

Cirrhosis has been defined as chronic liver disease characterized by diffuse parenchymal necrosis with fibrosis and formation of regenerative nodules. The etiology includes a variety of disorders including viral hepatitis, alcoholic liver disease, biliary diseases (e.g., sclerosing cholangitis and primary biliary cirrhosis), Wilson disease, hemochromatosis, autoimmune disease, congestive heart failure,

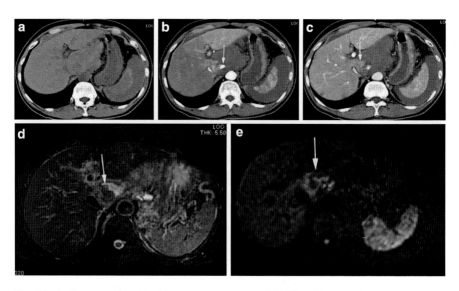

Fig. 12 A 64 years old male with spontaneous ruptured HCC and hemoperitoneum at caudate lobe of liver (*arrow*). (**a**) Axial unenhanced CT shows a hyperdense collection around the caudate lobe of the liver. (**b**) Arterial phase of CECT shows heterogenous enhancement with extravasation of contrast (*arrow*). (**c**) Delayed phase of CECT shows tumor as slightly hypodense to the liver. (**d**) Axial fat-saturated T2WI performed 1 month after CECT shows tumor as heterogeneous intermediate signal intensity mass with small fluid collection adjacent to tumor. (**e**) The tumor appears as hyperintense on axial DWI ($b = 1,000$ s/mm^2)

nonalcoholic steatohepatitis (NASH), glycogen storage disease, Budd-Chiari syndrome, toxic substances, and cryptogenic. Chronic viral hepatitis is the leading cause of liver fibrosis and cirrhosis which can eventually lead to end-stage liver disease and hepatocellular carcinoma HCC.

The disease severity is described by the degree of fibrosis (stage) and necroinflammation (grade). Liver fibrosis is classified into four stages including: F0, no fibrosis; F1, mild fibrosis; F2, moderate fibrosis; F3, advanced fibrosis; and F4, cirrhosis. Grades of activity of hepatic necroinflammation are classified into four grades including: A0, no activity; A1, mild activity; A2, moderate activity; and A3, severe activity. The gold standard for diagnosis of fibrosis/inflammation is liver biopsy. However, liver biopsy is invasive procedure with associated morbidity. Furthermore, it is prone to sampling error and inter-observer variability. Several noninvasive techniques including blood tests, Fibroscan (elastography using ultrasound), MR elastography are used to assess liver fibrosis with relatively good sensitivities and specificities. The role of any noninvasive technique should not be limited to distinguish cirrhosis from normal but also to differentiate between various stages of fibrosis since treatment is administered to patients with liver fibrosis stage F2 and greater.

Conventional MRI (without and with contrast material) is excellent for the evaluation of focal liver lesions associated with cirrhosis; however its role for evaluation of liver fibrosis/inflammation is limited.

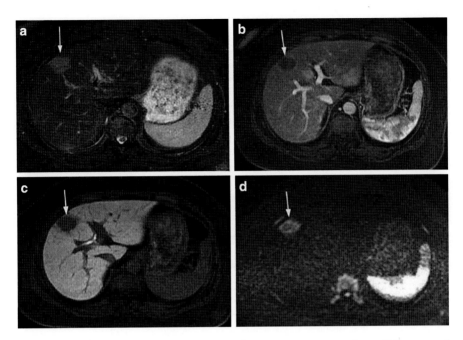

Fig. 13 A 61 years old male with solitary metastasis from colon cancer at the medial segment of left lobe of liver (*arrow*). (**a**) Axial fat-saturated T2WI shows tumor appeared as heterogeneous intermediate signal intensity. (**b**) The tumor displayed ring-like enhancement on arterial phase of gadoxetic acid-enhanced T1WI. (**c**) The tumor appears hypointense on hepatobiliary phase image (20 min) of gadoxetic acid-enhanced T1WI. (**d**) Axial DWI ($b = 1{,}000$ s/mm^2) shows the tumor as high signal intensity relative to the liver

Cirrhotic liver showed increased signal intensity on DWI and restricted diffusion on ADC map compared to normal liver (Fig. 14). Several previous studies described a lower ADC value of cirrhotic liver compared to that of normal liver (Tables 4 and 5) [39–51].

Several reports indicated inverse correlation between liver fibrosis and ADC values. ADC was useful for distinguishing cirrhosis from normal liver; however, the ADC values in each fibrosis group overlapped substantially except between no or early stage of fibrosis (F0 and F1) and advanced fibrosis (F3 or F4) [39, 45, 46]. Do et al. suggested that normalizing liver ADC with spleen ADC improves diagnostic accuracy for detection of liver fibrosis and cirrhosis when using breath-hold DWI [46]. Normalized liver ADC was superior to liver ADC for distinguishing individual stages of fibrosis and for detection of stage $\geq$F2 (AUC = 0.864).

Other reports indicated that ADC could predict individual stages of fibrosis with moderate to good accuracy [40–42, 47, 48, 51]. However, it was inferior to MR elastography and transient elastography (Fibroscan) for predicting stages of fibrosis [40, 47, 51]. Lewin et al. compared DWI to Fibroscan and serum markers for predicting fibrosis in patients with chronic hepatitis and healthy volunteers [40].

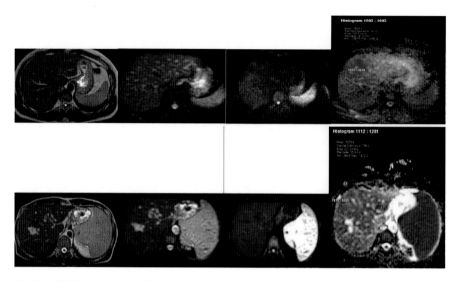

Fig. 14 DWI for diagnosis of liver cirrhosis. A 30 years old male with normal liver (*top row*) and 64 years old male with cirrhosis secondary to chronic hepatitis C (*bottom row*), portal vein occlusion and cavernous transformation of portal vein. T2WI, DWI for $b = 0$ and $b = 400$ mm^2/s, and ADC map (using $b = 0$, $b = 400$ and $b = 800$ mm^2/s). Normal liver shows ADC within normal range measuring about 1.7×10^{-3} s/mm^2. In the cirrhotic patient, T2WI shows minimal morphological changes; however ADC map shows decrease in ADC measuring 1.2×10^{-3} s/mm^2

ADC was favorable for predicting moderate to severe fibrosis compared with other noninvasive tests. Patients with moderate-to-severe fibrosis (F2-F3-F4) had hepatic ADC values ($1.10 \pm 0.11 \times 10^{-3}$ mm^2/s) lower than those without or with mild fibrosis (F0-F1; $1.30 \pm 0.12 \times 10^{-3}$ mm^2/s) and healthy volunteers (mean: $1.44 \pm 0.02 \times 10^{-3}$ mm^2/s). The AUC for ADC were 0.79 and 0.92 for fibrosis stage $\geq$F2 and $\geq$F3, respectively compared to AUC of 0.87 and 0.92 with Fibroscan [40]. Wang et al. reported an inverse correlation between ADCs and stage of fibrosis, but the median ADC values did not consistently decrease with increasing stages of fibrosis. Liver ADC was able to predict stages of fibrosis. However, the ability to predict fibrosis was inferior to that of MR elastography [47]. Kovač et al. founded that DWI is useful for predicting moderate to severe fibrosis in patients with cholestatic hepatitis (primary biliary cirrhosis and primary sclerosing cholangitis). However, transient elastography using Fibroscan provided higher diagnostic accuracy than DWI for predicting the stage of fibrosis. DWI was useful to show the distribution of fibrosis [51].

The initial studies using IVIM suggested that perfusion-related diffusion coefficient (D*) or perfusion parameters played a more important role than pure diffusion coefficient (D) in differentiating cirrhotic from normal livers. Luciani et al. acquired DWI with 10 b-values to calculate pure diffusion (D), perfusion-related diffusion (D*), and perfusion fraction (f), on the basis of the IVIM theory. They found that in cirrhotic livers perfusion-related diffusion (D*) is significantly

Table 4 Mean apparent diffusion coefficients (ADCs) of normal liver and cirrhotic liver

Author	b-Value	Mean ADC for normal liver or fibrosis stage F0 ($\times 10^{-3}$ mm^2/s)	Mean ADC for Cirrhosis or advanced fibrosis ($\times 10^{-3}$ mm^2/s)
Aube, J radiol 2004	200, 400, 600, 800	1.54	1.14
Koinuma, JMRI 2005	0, 128	3.45	1.98
Lewin, Hepatology 2007	0–800	1.44	1.1
Taouli, AJR 2007	0, 500	1.60	1.22
	0, 700	1.42	1.14
	0, 1,000	1.19	1.01
Girometti, Radiol Med. 2007	0, 150, 250, 400	1.54	1.11
Girometti, JMRI 2008	0, 150, 250, 400	1.54	1.14
	0, 150, 250, 400, 600, 800	1.04	0.91
Luciani, Radiology 2008	0, 10, 20, 30, 50, 80, 100, 200, 400, 800	1.39	1.23
Sandrasegaran, AJR 2009	50, 400	1.26	0.99
Do, AJR 2010	0, 50, 500	1.79	1.55
Patel, JMRI 2010	0, 50, 100, 150, 200, 300, 500, 700, 1,000	1.73	1.41
Wang, AJR 2011	50, 500, 1,000	1.00	0.88
Watanabe, Radiology 2011	0, 500	1.38	1.08
Bakan, Eur Radiol 2012	0, 500, 1,000	1.75	1.32
Kovač, Eur J Radiol 2011	0–800	2.01	1.46
Bonekamp, J Clin Gastroenterol 2011	0, 750	1.61	1.33
Taouli, JMRI 2008	0, 500	1.49	1.26

reduced [52]. Patel et al. compared IVIM DWI with dynamic contrast-enhanced MRI (DCE-MRI). They found that D, D*, F, and ADC were significantly reduced in cirrhotic patients. The highest area AUC was observed for ADC measuring (0.808). The perfusion parameters calculated with DCE-MRI were significantly increased. No correlation existed between IVIM and DCE-MRI parameters. The combination of ADC with DCE-MRI parameters provided 84.6 % sensitivity and 100 % specificity for diagnosis of cirrhosis [53].

In conclusion, DWI is useful for predicting liver cirrhosis from normal liver. However, substantial overlap in ADC exists between individual stages of fibrosis and DWI should be used with other MRI-based techniques such as MR elastography or gadoxetic acid-enhanced MRI for evaluation fibrosis/cirrhosis.

Table 5 Mean apparent diffusion coefficients (ADCs) of liver parenchyma for predicting stage of fibrosis

Fibrosis stage	Do, AJR 2010		Sandrasegaran, AJR 2009	Wang, AJR 2011	Lewin, Hepatology 2007	Taouli, JMRI 2008	Kovač Eur J Radiol, 2011	Bonekamp J Clin Gastroenterol, 2011
	ADC ($\times 10^{-3}$ mm²/s)							
F0	1.79	1.54[a]	1.26	1.00	1.44	1.49	2.01	1.61
F1	1.60	1.28[a]	1.05	0.91	1.30	–	1.80	1.43
F2	1.65	1.31[a]	1.04	0.89	–	–	1.64	1.36
F3	1.75	1.17[a]	1.03	0.88	1.21	–	1.63	1.44
F4	1.55	1.20[a]	0.99	0.88	1.10	–	1.46	1.33
≥F1	–	–	–	0.91	–	1.40	–	1.33
AUC	–	–	–	0.88	–	0.848	–	0.77
≥F2	1.68	1.41[a]	≤1.03	0.91	1.10	1.30	1.63	1.31
AUC	0.655	0.864	0.686	0.86	0.79	0.783	0.868	0.77
≥F3	1.53	1.41[a]	≤0.98	0.91	1.21	1.27	1.60	–
AUC	0.689	0.805	0.656	0.84	0.92	0.717	0.906	–
F4	1.68	1.4[a]	≤1.15	0.91	–	–	–	≤1.3
AUC	0.720	0.935	0.919	0.78	–	–	–	0.78

[a]Normalized liver ADC was calculated as the ratio of liver ADC to spleen ADC

Evaluation of Treatment Response

Tumor response to treatment including chemotherapy, radiotherapy, and ablation therapy could be assessed with DWI. An increase in ADC after treatment correlates with positive tumor response to treatment. Changes in ADC after treatment occur earlier than changes in size.

Regarding HCCs, the correlation between ADC and tumor response to treatment was studied after transarterial chemoembolization (TAE) or radiofrequency ablation (RFA). An increase in ADC of HCC was observed in necrotic portion of tumor following TAE compared to viable tumor [54, 55]. In a recent study, increased ADC at day 3 following TAE showed the highest correlation to tumor necrosis compared to FDG-PET and DCE-MRI parameters [56]. Following RFA, the tumor shows low signal intensity on DWI and increase in ADC correlating with tumor necrosis [57]. A rim of high signal is usually observed at the tumor periphery which is likely represents hyperemia due to thermal injury of the surrounding tissue.

High b-value DWI and ADC maps can be used to evaluate early recurrence or local progression of tumor following TAE or RFA (Fig. 15) [57, 58].

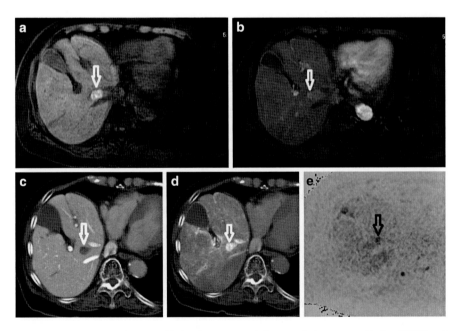

Fig. 15 A 79 years old female with local recurrence follows radiofrequency ablation (RFA) and transarterial chemoembolization for HCC. (**a**) Axial fat-saturated T1WI shows high signal intensity suggestive of hemorrhagic necrosis following RFA. (**b**) Local recurrence appears as an enhancing focus at the periphery of the ablated lesion on arterial phase of dynamic CE-MRI. (**c**, **b**) CT during arterioportography (CTAP) and CT during hepatic angiography show tumor as hypovascular on CTAP and hypervascular on CTHA. (**e**) The tumor appears as hyperintense on axial DWI with black and white inversion ($b = 1,000$ s/mm^2)

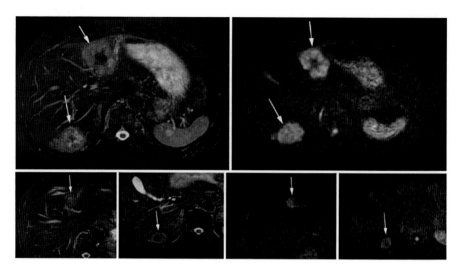

Fig. 16 A 70 years old male with liver metastases from colon before and after chemotherapy. *Upper row* is before chemotherapy, *below row* is after chemotherapy. Axial fat-saturated T2WI and Axial DWI ($b = 1,000$ s/mm^2) shows the tumors as high signal intensity relative to the liver. Tumors show reduction in size following chemotherapy with reduction in signal on high b-value DWI

However, DWI had lower sensitivity to DCE-MRI for the detection of local HCC recurrence [59]. Following TAE, iodized-oil (lipiodol) accumulation in tumor demonstrated as high density on CT obscure visualization of local recurrence. Local recurrence usually demonstrated as focal high signal intensity at the periphery of tumor on DWI and restricted diffusion on ADC map [57–59]. DWI should be evaluated with other conventional MRI sequences and dynamic images to evaluate local recurrence following TAE or RFA.

Regarding liver metastases, a decrease in signal intensity on DWI and increase in ADC following chemotherapy were observed in responding metastastic tumors (Fig. 16) [60, 62, 63]. No significant change in ADC was noticed in non-responding metastatic tumors [60]. Tumoral ADC showed increase at 3–7 days among responders to chemotherapy [61]. Necrotic colorectal metastases with high ADC prior to treatment showed poor response to chemotherapy [60, 61].

Limitations

DWI used for evaluation of focal liver lesions suffers from limited image quality due to poor SNR and limited spatial resolution. Respiratory and cardiac motion and EPI-related artifacts are a challenge. Other challenges include reproducibility of ADC measurements and establishing uniform parameters across different vendors.

References

1. Kwee TC, Takahara T, Niwa T, Ivancevic MK, Herigault G, Van Cauteren M, Luijten PR (2009) Influence of cardiac motion on diffusion-weighted magnetic resonance imaging of the liver. MAGMA 22(5):319–325
2. Guiu B, Cercueil JP (2011) Liver diffusion-weighted MR imaging: the tower of Babel? Eur Radiol 21(3):463–467
3. Gourtsoyianni S, Papanikolaou N, Yarmenitis S, Maris T, Karantanas A, Gourtsoyiannis N (2008) Respiratory gated diffusion-weighted imaging of the liver: value of apparent diffusion coefficient measurements in the differentiation between most commonly encountered benign and malignant focal liver lesions. Eur Radiol 18:486–492
4. Bruegel M, Holzapfel K, Gaa J et al (2008) Characterization of focal liver lesions by ADC measurements using a respiratory triggered diffusion-weighted single-shot echoplanar MR imaging technique. Eur Radiol 18:477–485
5. Kandpal H, Sharma R, Madhusudhan KS, Kapoor KS (2009) Respiratory-triggered versus breath-hold diffusion-weighted MRI of liver lesions: comparison of image quality and apparent diffusion coefficient values. AJR Am J Roentgenol 192:915–922
6. Feuerlein S, Pauls S, Juchems MS et al (2009) Pitfalls in abdominal diffusion weighted imaging: how predictive is restricted water diffusion for malignancy. AJR Am J Roentgenol 193:1070–1076
7. Goshima S, Kanematsu M, Kondo H et al (2008) Diffusion-weighted imaging of the liver: optimizing b value for the detection and characterization of benign and malignant hepatic lesions. J Magn Reson Imaging 28:691–697
8. Low RN, Gurney J (2007) Diffusion-weighted MRI (DWI) in the oncology patient: value of breathhold DWI compared to unenhanced and gadolinium-enhanced MRI. J Magn Reson Imaging 25:848–858
9. Lichy MP, Aschoff P, Plathow C et al (2007) Tumor detection by diffusion-weighted MRI and ADC mapping: initial clinical experiences in comparison to PETCT. Invest Radiol 42:605–613
10. Coenegrachts K, Matos C, Ter Beek L et al (2009) Focal liver lesion detection and characterization: comparison of non-contrast enhanced and SPIO-enhanced diffusion-weighted single-shot spin echo echo planar and turbo spin echo T2-weighted imaging. Eur J Radiol 72:432–439
11. Holzapfel K, Bruegel M, Eiber M et al (2010) Characterization of small (</=10mm) focal liver lesions: value of respiratory triggered echo-planar diffusion-weighted MR imaging. Eur J Radiol 76:89–95
12. Coenegrachts K, Delanote J, Ter Beek L et al (2007) Improved focal liver lesion detection: comparison of single-shot diffusion-weighted echoplanar and single-shot T2 weighted turbo spin echo techniques. Br J Radiol 80:524–531
13. Asbach P, Hein PA, Stemmer A et al (2008) Free-breathing echo-planar imaging based diffusion-weighted magnetic resonance imaging of the liver with prospective acquisition correction. J Comput Assist Tomogr 32:372–378
14. Sandrasegaran K, Akisik FM, Lin C, Tahir B, Rajan J, Aisen AM (2009) The value of diffusion-weighted imaging in characterizing focal liver masses. Acad Radiol 16:1208–1214
15. Demir OI, Obuz F, Sağol O, Dicle O (2007) Contribution of diffusion-weighted MRI to the differential diagnosis of hepatic masses. Diagn Interv Radiol 13:81–86
16. Miller FH, Hammond N, Siddiqi AJ et al (2010) Utility of diffusion-weighted MRI in distinguishing benign and malignant hepatic lesions. J Magn Reson Imaging 32(1):138–147
17. Haradome H, Grazioli L, Morone M et al (2012) T2-weighted and diffusion-weighted MRI for discriminating benign from malignant focal liver lesions: diagnostic abilities of single versus combined interpretations. J Magn Reson Imaging 35(6):1388–1396
18. Yang DM, Jahng GH, Kim HC et al (2011) The detection and discrimination of malignant and benign focal hepatic lesions: T2 weighted vs diffusion-weighted MRI. Br J Radiol 84 (1000):319–326

19. Inan N, Arslan A, Akansel G et al (2007) Diffusion-weighted imaging in the differential diagnosis of simple and hydatid cysts of the liver. AJR Am J Roentgenol 189(5):1031–1036
20. Fruehwald-Pallamar J, Bastati-Huber N, Fakhrai N et al (2012) Confident non-invasive diagnosis of pseudolesions of the liver using diffusion-weighted imaging at 3T MRI. Eur J Radiol 81(6):1353–1359
21. Piana G, Trinquart L, Meskine N, Barrau V, Beers BV, Vilgrain V (2011) New MR imaging criteria with a diffusion-weighted sequence for the diagnosis of hepatocellular carcinoma in chronic liver diseases. J Hepatol 55(1):126–132
22. Muhi A, Ichikawa T, Motosugi U et al (2009) High-b-value diffusion-weighted MR imaging of hepatocellular lesions: estimation of grade of malignancy of hepatocellular carcinoma. J Magn Reson Imaging 30(5):1005–1011
23. Ahn JH, Yu JS, Hwang SH, Chung JJ, Kim JH, Kim KW (2010) Nontumorous arterioportal shunts in the liver: CT and MRI findings considering mechanisms and fate. Eur Radiol 20(2):385–394
24. Lee MH, Kim SH, Park MJ, Park CK, Rhim H (2011) Gadoxetic acid-enhanced hepatobiliary phase MRI and high-b-value diffusion-weighted imaging to distinguish well-differentiated hepatocellular carcinomas from benign nodules in patients with chronic liver disease. AJR Am J Roentgenol 197(5):W868–W875
25. Xu PJ, Yan FH, Wang JH, Shan Y, Ji Y, Chen CZ (2010) Contribution of diffusion-weighted magnetic resonance imaging in the characterization of hepatocellular carcinomas and dysplastic nodules in cirrhotic liver. J Comput Assist Tomogr 34(4):506–512
26. Heo SH, Jeong YY, Shin SS et al (2010) Apparent diffusion coefficient value of diffusion-weighted imaging for hepatocellular carcinoma: correlation with the histologic differentiation and the expression of vascular endothelial growth factor. Korean J Radiol 11(3):295–303
27. Nasu K, Kuroki Y, Tsukamoto T, Nakajima H, Mori K, Minami M (2009) Diffusion-weighted imaging of surgically resected hepatocellular carcinoma: imaging characteristics and relationship among signal intensity, apparent diffusion coefficient, and histopathologic grade. AJR Am J Roentgenol 193(2):438–444
28. Le Moigne F, Durieux M, Bancel B et al (2012) Impact of diffusion-weighted MR imaging on the characterization of small hepatocellular carcinoma in the cirrhotic liver. Magn Reson Imaging 30(5):656–665
29. Xu PJ, Yan FH, Wang JH, Lin J, Ji Y (2009) Added value of breathhold diffusion-weighted MRI in detection of small hepatocellular carcinoma lesions compared with dynamic contrast-enhanced MRI alone using receiver operating characteristic curve analysis. J Magn Reson Imaging 29(2):341–349
30. Chung J, Yu JS, Kim DJ, Chung JJ, Kim JH, Kim KW (2011) Hypervascular hepatocellular carcinoma in the cirrhotic liver: diffusion-weighted imaging versus superparamagnetic iron oxide-enhanced MRI. Magn Reson Imaging 29(9):1235–1243
31. Kim YK, Kim CS, Han YM, Lee YH (2011 Jun) Detection of liver malignancy with gadoxeticacid-enhanced MRI: is addition of diffusion-weighted MRI beneficial? Clin Radiol 66(6):489–496
32. Koh DM, Brown G, Riddell AM et al (2008) Detection of colorectal hepatic metastases using MnDPDP MR imaging and diffusion-weighted imaging (DWI) alone and in combination. Eur Radiol 18(5):903–910
33. Kim YK, Lee MW, Lee WJ, Kim SH, Rhim H, Lim JH, Choi D, Kim YS, Jang KM, Lee SJ, Lim HK (2012) Diagnostic accuracy and sensitivity of diffusion-weighted and of gadoxetic acid-enhanced 3-T MR imaging alone or in combination in the detection of small liver metastasis ($\leq$ 1.5 cm in diameter). Invest Radiol 47(3):159–166
34. Chung WS, Kim MJ, Chung YE et al (2011) Comparison of gadoxetic acid-enhanced dynamic imaging and diffusion-weighted imaging for the preoperative evaluation of colorectal liver metastases. J Magn Reson Imaging 34(2):345–353
35. Löwenthal D, Zeile M, Lim WY et al (2011) Detection and characterisation of focal liver lesions in colorectal carcinoma patients: comparison of diffusion-weighted and Gd-EOB-DTPA enhanced MR imaging. Eur Radiol 21(4):832–840

36. Shimada K, Isoda H, Hirokawa Y, Arizono S, Shibata T, Togashi K (2010) Comparison of gadolinium-EOB-DTPA-enhanced and diffusion-weighted liver MRI for detection of small hepatic metastases. Eur Radiol 20(11):2690–2698

37. Eiber M, Fingerle AA, Brügel M, Gaa J, Rummeny EJ, Holzapfel K (2012) Detection and classification of focal liver lesions in patients with colorectal cancer: retrospective comparison of diffusion-weighted MR imaging and multi-slice CT. Eur J Radiol 81(4):683–691

38. Muhi A, Ichikawa T, Motosugi U et al (2010) Diagnosis of colorectal hepatic metastases: contrast-enhanced ultrasonography versus contrast-enhanced computed tomography versus superparamagnetic iron oxide-enhanced magnetic resonance imaging with diffusion-weighted imaging. J Magn Reson Imaging 32(5):1132–1140

39. Koinuma M, Ohashi I, Hanafusa K, Shibuya H (2005) Apparent diffusion coefficient measurements with diffusion-weighted magnetic resonance imaging for evaluation of hepatic fibrosis. J Magn Reson Imaging 22:80–85

40. Lewin M, Poujol-Robert A, Boelle PY et al (2007) Diffusion-weighted magnetic resonance imaging for the assessment of fibrosis in chronic hepatitis C. Hepatology 46:658–665

41. Taouli B, Tolia AJ, Losada M et al (2007) Diffusion-weighted MRI for quantification of liver fibrosis: preliminary experience. AJR Am J Roentgenol 189:799–806

42. Taouli B, Chouli M, Martin AJ, Qayyum A, Coakley FV, Vilgrain V (2008) Chronic hepatitis: role of diffusion-weighted imaging and diffusion tensor imaging for the diagnosis of liver fibrosis and inflammation. J Magn Reson Imaging 28:89–95

43. Girometti R, Furlan A, Bazzocchi M et al (2007) Diffusion-weighted MRI in evaluating liver fibrosis: a feasibility study in cirrhotic patients. Radiol Med 112:394–408

44. Girometti R, Furlan A, Esposito G et al (2008) Relevance of b-values in evaluating liver fibrosis: a study in healthy and cirrhotic subjects using two single-shot spin-echo echo-planar diffusion-weighted sequences. J Magn Reson Imaging 28:411–419

45. Sandrasegaran K, Akisik FM, Lin C et al (2009) Value of diffusion-weighted MRI for assessing liver fibrosis and cirrhosis. AJR Am J Roentgenol 193(6):1556–1560

46. Do RK, Chandarana H, Felker E et al (2010) Diagnosis of liver fibrosis and cirrhosis with diffusion-weighted imaging: value of normalized apparent diffusion coefficient using the spleen as reference organ. AJR Am J Roentgenol 195(3):671–676

47. Wang Y, Ganger DR, Levitsky J et al (2011) Assessment of chronic hepatitis and fibrosis: comparison of MR elastography and diffusion-weighted imaging. AJR Am J Roentgenol 196(3):553–561

48. Bonekamp S, Torbenson MS, Kamel IR (2011) Diffusion-weighted magnetic resonance imaging for the staging of liver fibrosis. J Clin Gastroenterol 45(10):885–892

49. Watanabe H, Kanematsu M, Goshima S et al (2011) Staging hepatic fibrosis: comparison of gadoxetate disodium-enhanced and diffusion-weighted MR imaging–preliminary observations. Radiology 259(1):142–150

50. Bakan AA, Inci E, Bakan S, Gokturk S, Cimilli T (2012) Utility of diffusion-weighted imaging in the evaluation of liver fibrosis. Eur Radiol 22(3):682–687

51. Kovač JD, Daković M, Stanisavljević D et al (2012) Diffusion-weighted MRI versus transient elastography in quantification of liver fibrosis in patients with chronic cholestatic liver diseases. Eur J Radiol 81(10):2500–2506

52. Luciani A, Vignaud A, Cavet M et al (2008) Liver cirrhosis: intravoxel incoherent motion MR imaging–pilot study. Radiology 249(3):891–899

53. Patel J, Sigmund EE, Rusinek H, Oei M, Babb JS, Taouli B (2010) Diagnosis of cirrhosis with intravoxel incoherent motion diffusion MRI and dynamic contrast-enhanced MRI alone and in combination: preliminary experience. J Magn Reson Imaging 31(3):589–600

54. Kamel IR, Bluemke DA, Ramsey D et al (2003) Role of diffusion-weighted imaging in estimating tumor necrosis after chemoembolization of hepatocellular carcinoma. AJR Am J Roentgenol 181(3):708–710

55. Mannelli L, Kim S, Hajdu CH, Babb JS, Clark TW, Taouli B (2009) Assessment of tumor necrosis of hepatocellular carcinoma after chemoembolization: diffusion-weighted and

contrast-enhanced MRI with histopathologic correlation of the explanted liver. AJR Am J Roentgenol 193(4):1044–1052

56. Braren R, Altomonte J, Settles M et al (2011) Validation of preclinical multiparametric imaging for prediction of necrosis in hepatocellular carcinoma after embolization. J Hepatol 55(5):1034–1040

57. Schraml C, Schwenzer NF, Clasen S et al (2009) Navigator respiratory-triggered diffusion-weighted imaging in the follow-up after hepatic radiofrequency ablation-initial results. J Magn Reson Imaging 29(6):1308–1316

58. Kubota K, Yamanishi T, Itoh S et al (2010) Role of diffusion-weighted imaging in evaluating therapeutic efficacy after transcatheter arterial chemoembolization for hepatocellular carcinoma. Oncol Rep 24:727–732

59. Goshima S, Kanematsu M, Kondo H et al (2008) Evaluating local hepatocellular carcinoma recurrence post-transcatheter arterial chemoembolization: is diffusion-weighted MRI reliable as an indicator? J Magn Reson Imaging 27(4):834–839

60. Koh DM, Scurr E, Collins D et al (2007) Predicting response of colorectal hepatic metastasis: value of pretreatment apparent diffusion coefficients. AJR Am J Roentgenol 188 (4):1001–1008

61. Cui Y, Zhang XP, Sun YS, Tang L, Shen L (2008) Apparent diffusion coefficient: potential imaging biomarker for prediction and early detection of response to chemotherapy in hepatic metastases. Radiology 248(3):894–900

62. Anzidei M, Napoli A, Zaccagna F et al (2011) Liver metastases from colorectal cancer treated with conventional and antiangiogenetic chemotherapy: evaluation with liver computed tomography perfusion and magnetic resonance diffusion-weighted imaging. J Comput Assist Tomogr 35(6):690–696

63. Marugami N, Tanaka T, Kitano S et al (2009) Early detection of therapeutic response to hepatic arterial infusion chemotherapy of liver metastases from colorectal cancer using diffusion-weighted MR imaging. Cardiovasc Intervent Radiol 32(4):638–646

Shape-Based Liver Segmentation Without Prior Statistical Models

Ahmed Afifi and Toshiya Nakaguchi

Abstract In this work, we introduce a shape-based liver segmentation approach. However, unlike the other shape-based approaches, this approach is model-free, and it does not require prior shape or intensity model construction. In contrary, we exploit the relation between consequent slices in multi-slice CT images to estimate and propagate shape and intensity constrains. Then, these constrains are integrated with a shape-based graph cut algorithm to extract the liver object in each slice. This approach needs a simple user interaction and it eliminates the burdens associated with model building like data collection, manual segmentation, registration, and landmark correspondence. Moreover, it is talented to deal with complex shape and intensity variations. This model-free approach was evaluated on 50 CT images from three different datasets with several liver abnormalities, including tumors and cysts, and it achieved high average gauged scores of 80.4, 79.2, and 81.7 for these datasets.

Introduction

Liver tumors are one of the most common causes of death over the world [1], and the accurate diagnosis of these tumors helps to reduce their burden. It has shown that the utilization of computer-aided diagnosis (CAD) systems can greatly improve tumor diagnosis [2, 3], and it is useful for treatment planning, especially for liver transplantation and tumor ablation. In liver CAD systems, the liver segmentation is

A. Afifi (✉)
Faculty of Computers and Information, Menofia University, Shibin Al-Kawm, Menofia, Egypt
e-mail: afifi@ci.menofia.edu; ah.z.afifi@gmail.com

T. Nakaguchi
Graduate School of Engineering, Chiba University, Japan, 1-33, Yayoi-cho, Inage-ku,
Chiba 263-8522, Japan
e-mail: nakaguchi@faculty.chiba-u.jp

A.S. El-Baz et al. (eds.), *Abdomen and Thoracic Imaging: An Engineering & Clinical Perspective*, DOI 10.1007/978-1-4614-8498-1_11,
© Springer Science+Business Media New York 2014

the first and essential process, and its accuracy is of special significance. However, this process is difficult because of low contrast between the liver and surrounding tissues, great differences in liver shape and intensity, and the existence of liver abnormalities. Hence, the conventional segmentation methods cannot produce adequate results.

In literature, there are many attempts to solve the liver segmentation problem and various approaches have been proposed, including intensity- or texture-based approaches, deformable and statistical model-based approaches, and probabilistic atlases-based approaches. In the intensity-based approaches, one or multiple intensity thresholds, region growing, or watershed methods are applied to extract an initial binary volume which consequently refined using morphological filters or knowledge-based approaches. In [4], a predefined threshold was utilized on a simplified image to determine the initial liver area, and then it was refined using morphological filters and deformable contours with gradient information. Although this method showed accurate volume measurement results for the used dataset, it did not consider the change in CT images orientation and variations in liver intensity. Additionally, due to high variations between the intensity of the liver and abnormal tissues, it can miss these tissues in the case of liver abnormality. Rusko et al. [5] proposed a method for liver segmentation in single and multiphase CT images. In this method, thresholding of a single or joint histogram was applied to determine the initial liver volume, and then it was adjusted using a region growing method and a set of anatomical constrains. It has shown that the single-phase method was failed in the case of dense tumors, and the results can be enhanced using multiphase method. However, the latter one added a burden of multiphase acquiring and registration. In [6], the authors applied a region growing method to a smoothed image to define the liver region that was refined in a slice-by-slice manner using morphological filters. The seed for region growing was determined manually for the first slice, and then it is defined from the segmentation of the previous slice. In this method, the intensity of the liver is considered as a single Gaussian distribution and the shape as a single connected object and that is not always true. Therefore, it can miss the small parts of the liver and the dense abnormal tissues inside the liver. R. Beichel et al. [7] proposed an interactive liver segmentation approach by utilizing a hybrid desktop/virtual reality user interface. In their approach, the liver was initially segmented using graph cut approach initialized from user-defined regions. Consequently, the resulted liver volume was corrected and refined interactively using several virtual reality tools. Although this refinement approach achieved accurate segmentation results, it requires high interaction (about 6.5 min) from a medical expert. Another interactive approach based on liver intensity information has been proposed by A. Beck in [8]. In this approach, the operator selects any liver voxel and a 3D fill algorithm starts to flood-fill the volume from there until a defined stop condition is satisfied. The problematic parts in this filled volume are then corrected by recursive filling of missing parts and touching up the results in 3D view. This technique also requires a high interaction to correct the problematic parts founded in the initial volume. In an attempt to overcome the limitations of the intensity-based method,

Foruzan et al. [9, 10] proposed a split thresholding method. In this method, two overlapping ranges are defined to split the original image and then morphological filters and rule-based classification approaches were applied to refine the results. Additionally, they applied anatomical constrains determined from the segmentation of the previous slice as well as the determination of the ribs to control the thresholding method. However, their proposed method considers the intensity information alone, and it cannot detect the abnormal tissues at the boundary of the liver. A texture region growing method was proposed in [11]. In this method, the texture features extracted from the 3D co-occurrence matrix were used for a region growing from a determined seed. This method was evaluated using CT images of healthy volunteers, and it could detect the healthy liver tissues only. In [12], the texture features extracted from the co-occurrence matrix were used for voxel classification and then a 2D region growing method was applied to segment the liver in each CT slice. While this method could give reasonable segmentation for easy cases, it greatly failed in average and difficult cases.

In the deformable model-based approaches, an initial contour or surface is deformed to minimize a predefined energy function. Tibamoso et al. [13] used a predefined shape model to initialize a deformable surface, which iteratively deformed in function of the image intensity and edges. The evaluation results showed that this method could be trapped in the front of liver abnormal tissues. Furthermore, it requires the nontrivial process of 3D prior shape construction. Masutani [14] employed the radial basis function to interpolate a set of interactively defined control points. Wimmer et al. [15] also utilized the radial basis function to interpolate a set of user-defined 2D contours to generate a smooth surface passing through all contours. Then, the final segmentation was obtained using the level set method initialized by the interpolated surface. In these methods depending on the radial basis function interpolation, the placement of the control points greatly affects the segmentation accuracy; however, this procedure is too complex because a large number of control points have to be defined on the 3D volume. In [16], a snake algorithm was introduced to refine the preliminary liver boundary obtained from coarse segmentation. This segmentation was carried out by intensity thresholding and a modified split-and-merge algorithm [17]. The control points used for this snake algorithm were determined from a preliminary determined liver boundary, and they were sampled nonuniformly by a recursive algorithm according to the curvature of the boundary. Although this method produced better results than the conventional deformable model, it highly depends on the threshold value of the coarse segmentation, and it is still computationally expensive. Massoptier et al. [18] use the gradient vector flow (GVF) active contour [19] to adjust the initial liver boundary obtained using a threshold value determined according to automatically estimated liver statistics. Additionally, in [20–22], the GVF active contour is used for liver boundary refinement. However, the accuracy of these methods is greatly affected by the preliminary segmentation, which usually misses the abnormal tissues at the liver boundary. The implicit deformable models, also called implicit active contours or level sets [23], have been utilized for liver segmentation as well. Furukawa et al. [24] applied maximum a posteriori probability (MAP) estimation to extract a rough liver area, and then a modified level set method was applied to get the final segmentation. In this method, the MAP estimation was performed according to a predefined probabilistic atlas as well as the image intensity model. However, this method highly relies on the training data, and it seems to fail in the front of dense tumors. In [25], authors modified the Chan-Vese model [26] to consider multiple objects in the background. Then they applied their modified model to segment the liver in three different resolutions of the input CT volume. In their model, they consider the liver or foreground as a single object and that leads to a missing segmentation of liver lesions and large vessels. In [27, 28], the level set method is also applied to refine an initial segmentation of the liver. Nevertheless, the performance of level set methods is greatly affected by the initial estimation of the liver.

The statistical models have been received high interest from the investigators of liver segmentation approaches. They construct linear or nonlinear models to represent the variation in liver shape and appearance. The method proposed by Kainmuller et al. [29] employed the principal component analysis (PCA) to a very large CT images dataset to construct a statistical shape model (SSM) of the liver. Then, this shape model was matched to the image data, and the segmentation was refined using a deformable mesh. Heimann et al. [30] employed a deformable mesh with internal forces based on an SSM and external forces based on image data. The initialization of the SSM was performed using an evolutionary algorithm [31] to determine the pose and shape parameters of the SSM. Afifi et al. [32, 33] utilized the PCA and kernel PCA to build linear and nonlinear SSM. Then, the SSM was fitted to a preliminary segmentation obtained by textural feature-based classification. In these methods, the shapes were represented as signed distance function and aligned by direct optimization [34]. In [35–37], the SSM was also applied for liver segmentation in CT images. In addition to SSMs, probabilistic atlases were integrated into different liver segmentation approaches [24, 37–39]. In [40], CT enhancement information and priori constraints on shape and location were utilized in 4D graph cuts to segment liver, spleen, and kidneys. A common challenge of the statistical model- and probabilistic atlas-based approaches is the model or atlas construction. It requires a proper collection of a large training dataset to capture all the possible variations, which is a very hard task. Moreover, these algorithms might fail when detecting not standard liver shapes, or they might require too much time to get reasonable results.

In summary, we can conclude that the intensity- and deformable model-based approaches were highly affected by the liver abnormalities. The statistical model- and probabilistic atlas-based approaches could enhance the results; however, they added a burden of model construction and matching. In this chapter, we introduce a model-free shape-based liver segmentation approach. In this approach, we benefit from the high correlation between consequent slices of the same patient to define the shape constrains and to estimate the statistical parameters of the liver and non-liver tissues. A set of points selected on only one slice is utilized to initialize shape and intensity constrains, and consequently, they automatically updated from nearby slices. A graph cut algorithm based on these defined constrains is applied in a slice-by-slice manner to automatically segment the whole volume. Additionally, to reduce the computational time, we build the graph in a narrow band area defined automatically from the adjacent slice.

The rest of this chapter is organized as follows: In section "The Model-Free Segmentation Approach," the model-free segmentation approach is described. Datasets, evaluation metric, and experimental setup are introduced in section "Data and Experimental Setup." In section "Results," the evaluation results of the segmentation approach on 50 CT images are presented. These results are discussed in section "Discussion." Finally, the work is concluded in section "Conclusion."

The Model-Free Segmentation Approach

In this work, the segmentation approach mimics the physician's methodology in determining the boundary of liver. In this methodology, the correspondence between adjacent slices in CT image helps in alleviating the ambiguity of the liver boundary and in detecting the liver abnormalities. In the introduced approach, this information is encoded in the form of shape constrains propagated from one slice to the adjacent slice. These constrains are integrated in a shape-based graph cut algorithm to accurately segment the current slice. Furthermore, to consider inter- and intra-variations of the liver intensity, the intensity model of the liver is atomically estimated in a patient-oriented manner, and it is updated from one slice to another. A simple user interaction is required at first to determine the suitable intensity range for image normalization and to segment one starting slice. The whole procedure of this model-free approach is introduced in Algorithm 1.

Preprocessing

The raw CT data is encoded in either 12 or 16 bits; hence, we have a very large number of gray levels. The first aim of the preprocessing step is to map this raw data to a grayscale data encoded in eight bits. However, the direct mapping of the raw data to grayscale data increases the effect of under-sampling and the effect of non-useful intensity ranges. Windowing the raw data around the soft tissue of abdomen before mapping it enhances the produced image [41]. In this preprocessing step therefore, we perform image normalization in the soft tissue window.

Algorithm 1: The model-free segmentation approach

Input: Contrast enhanced CT volume and the set of fixed parameters.

Output: Binary volume, liver is the foreground.

Procedure:

Step-1: Performing image normalization in soft tissue window and then applying nonlinear diffusion filter to each slice.

Step-2: Selecting one slice as the start slice and then define the liver landmarks on it.

Step-3: Estimating initial shape, intensity, and graph cuts constrains from the start slice.

for all lower slices, starting from the start slice to the last one. **do**

Step-4: Define a narrow band around the liver object.

Step-5: Performing slice segmentation using shape-based graph cuts algorithm.

Step-6: Adding the segmentation results of this slice to the output volume.

Step-7: Updating shape, intensity, and graph cuts constrains according to current slice segmentation.

end for

for all upper slices, starting from the start slice to the first one. **do**

Repeat Step-4 and Step-5.

if the segmented object contains multiple parts **then**

Step-8: Selecting the left most one as the liver object.

end if

Repeat Step-6 and Step-7.

end for

Step-9: Applying the post-processing procedure to the output volume.

return output volume.

This window is determined by plotting the histogram of the raw data and selecting the lower and upper bounds of the right distribution in the histogram as shown in Fig. 1. Then, these lower and upper bounds are used to map the original raw data to a grayscale data according to (1). The original image and the produced gray scale one are shown in Fig. 2:

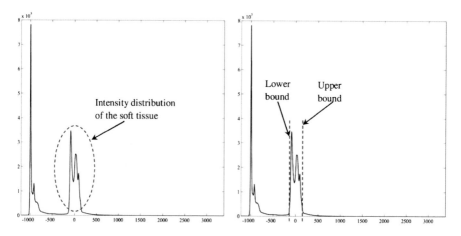

Fig. 1 Determination of the lower and upper bounds used for intensity mapping

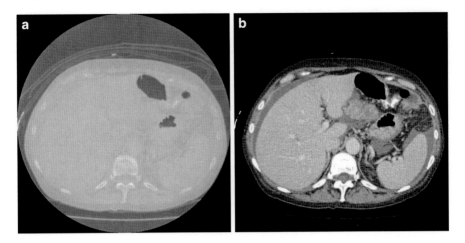

Fig. 2 Mapping the raw CT data to grayscale image, (**a**) original data, and (**b**) the produced gray image

$$
I_g(x,y) = \begin{cases} 0 & \text{if} \quad I_o(x,y) \le \text{Lo} \\ \dfrac{255(I_o(x,y) - \text{Lo})}{\text{Hi} - \text{Lo}} & \text{if} \quad \text{Lo} < I_o(x,y) < \text{Hi} \\ 255 & \text{if} \quad I_o(x,y) \ge \text{Hi} \end{cases} , \tag{1}
$$

where I_o is the raw CT image, I_g is the produced gray level image, Lo is the selected lower intensity bound, and Hi is the selected upper intensity bound.

After mapping the whole CT volume to a grayscale volume, a nonlinear diffusion filter [42, 43] is applied to each 2D slice in the volume to reduce the noise and to increase the liver homogeneity. In contrast to the convolution and rank filters (median filter, mean filter, etc.), the nonlinear diffusion filter can remove the noise from homogenous areas while keeping clear and sharp edges as shown in Fig. 3. The nonlinear diffusion filter is obtained by the time solution of (2):

$$
\begin{aligned}
\frac{\partial I_g(x,y,t)}{\partial t} &= \operatorname{div}\left(C\left(\left|\nabla I_{\sigma_g}(x,y,t)\right|^2\right)\nabla I_g(x,y,t)\right) \\
&= \nabla C \cdot \left(\left|\nabla I_{\sigma_g}(x,y,t)\right|^2\right)\nabla I_g(x,y,t)
\end{aligned} \tag{2}
$$

where $I_g(x,y,0)$ is the original gray image, t refers to the iteration steps, and C is a diffusivity function that depends on the gradient magnitude of the image. $I_{\sigma_g}(x,y)$ is a smoothed version of $I(x,y)$ which is obtained by convolving it with a Gaussian of standard deviation σ_g. In this work, a rapidly decreasing diffusivity function suggested in [44] is implemented as

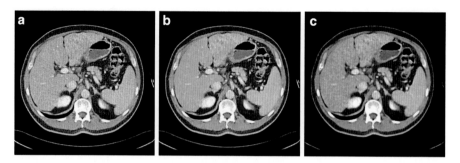

Fig. 3 Output of the preprocessing step, (**a**) input image, (**b**) smoothed image using a nonlinear diffusion filter, and (**c**) smoothed image using the median filter

$$C = \begin{cases} 1 & \text{if} \quad g \leq 0 \\ 1 - e^{-\dfrac{3.315}{(g/K)^4}} & \text{if} \quad g > 0 \end{cases}. \tag{3}$$

The conductance parameter, K, determines the contrast of edges that will have significant effect on the smoothing.

Initialization

A simple user interaction is required to determine and segment one slice in the CT volume. The segmentation result of this slice, represented as a binary template, is used to define the initial shape constrains as well as the initial intensity model of the corresponding case. Consequently, these constrains are automatically propagated in a slice-by-slice manner.

From the anatomical knowledge of the liver, we can divide the whole CT volume into two main parts: the upper part and the lower part. In the upper part, the liver starts as a single small object behind the heart, and it grows up to be a single large object at the end of this part. In the lower part, the liver starts as a single large object, and it is divided into two or more segments and then ends as a single small object behind the colon and the kidney as shown in Fig. 4. These two parts are separated by a slice containing nearly the largest cross section of the liver, which is selected as the starting slice for segmentation. In this slice, the liver object is very clear and its boundary can be distinguished from the other objects visually. Therefore, the initial liver segmentation is performed in less than 1 min according to the following procedure:

1. The user selects from 20 to 30 landmarks on the liver boundary as shown in Fig. 5a.
2. The liver boundary is then estimated using the cubic spline interpolation [45] as shown in Fig. 5b.
3. The liver object is defined as the object inside the liver boundary as shown in Fig. 5c.

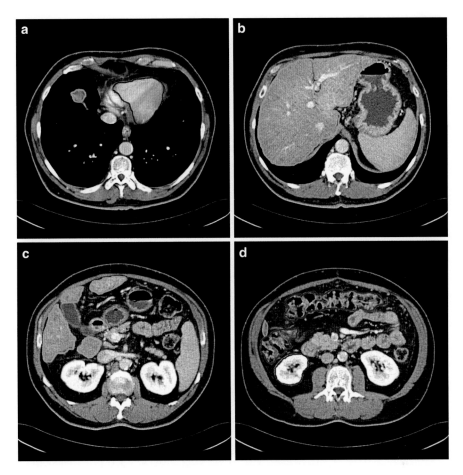

Fig. 4 The main anatomical structure of the liver, (**a**) start slice of the liver (liver in *green* and cardiac in *red*), (**b**) end of the upper part, (**c**) a slice in the lower part with a liver divided to four segments, and (**d**) the end slice of the liver (liver in *green*, kidney in *red,* and colon in *blue*)

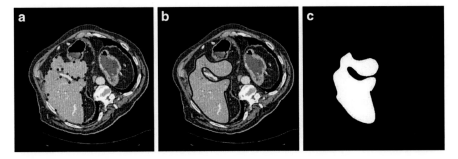

Fig. 5 Start slice segmentation, (**a**) selected landmarks, (**b**) estimated liver boundary, and (**c**) corresponding shape template

Estimation of the Shape and Intensity Constrains

The shape constrains are applied as a prior probability of the liver location, and the intensity constrains are defined as the probability of the liver intensity model at each pixel. These constrains are automatically determined for each slice according to the segmented liver object in the previous slice. The estimation process is performed according to the following procedure:

1. Define the binary liver template in the start slice as $Temp_{str}$, the binary liver object in this slice as $object_{str}$, the binary liver template in the previous slice as $Temp_{prv}$, the binary liver object in this slice as $object_{prv}$, the pixels belonging to the liver in the previous slice as $Liver_{prv}$, and the pixels not belonging to the liver in the previous slice as non - $Liver_{prv}$.
2. Determine the minor axis of the ellipse that fit the object in $Temp_{prv}$ and denote it as m_{ax} (Fig. 6a).
3. Erode the $Temp_{prv}$ with a disk structuring element of radius $round(0.02 \times m_{ax})$ and consider the result as the shape template of the current slice (Fig. 6b). This erosion value has been decided after studying the average change of the minor liver axes in different cases.
4. *If* Area($object_{prv}$) $\geq 0.1 \times$ Area($object_{str}$), calculate the histogram of $Liver_{prv}$ and non - $Liver_{prv}$ as the intensity model; *else*, use the previously used intensity model.
5. Erode $Temp_{prv}$ with a disk structuring element of radius $round(0.1 \times m_{ax})$ and the result is considered as the object hard constrains in the graph cut algorithm (Fig. 6c).
6. Dilate the $Temp_{prv}$ with a disk structuring element of radius $max(2, round(0.1 \times m_{ax}))$. Then, the edge of the resulting binary template is determined and dilated with a disk structuring element of radius 1. The result of this step is considered as the background hard constrains in the graph cut algorithm (Fig. 6c).
7. Define a narrow band window surrounding the liver object as the smallest rectangle fitting the dilated object calculated in step 5 (Fig. 6d).

Segmentation Using Graph Cuts

Introduction to Graph Cuts

An image segmentation problem can be considered as a binary labeling problem. In which, a unique label $A_p \in$ "obj", "bkg" is assigned to each pixel in the image. A good labeling or segmentation A, $A = A_1, A_2, \ldots, A_{|P|}$: $|P|$ is the number of image pixel, has to minimize a predefined energy function. Boykov et al. [46] introduced a solution for this problem using a graph cut algorithm. In the graph cuts, a graph $G = \langle V, \varepsilon \rangle$ is defined as a set of nodes V and a set of edges ε. The nodes of

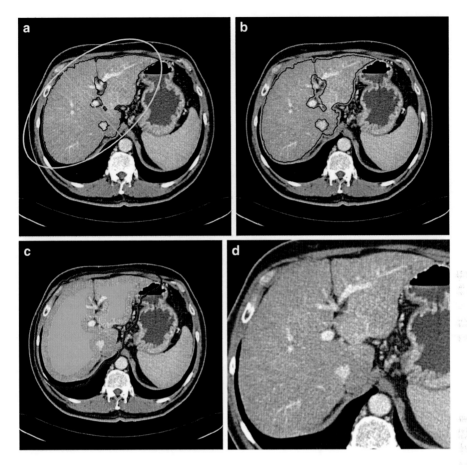

Fig. 6 Constrain estimation, (**a**) sample previous slice (liver contour in *red* and the minor axis in *green*), (**b**) the contour of the estimated shape template shown on the current slice, (**c**) the estimated constrains for graph cut (object in *green* and background in *red*), and (**d**) the slice after applying the narrow band constrain

the graph represent the image pixels in addition to two specially designated terminal nodes S (source) and T (sink), which represent the object and background labels. The set of edges ε in the graph includes two types of edges: edges between neighboring pixels, which are defined as n-links, and edges connecting all pixels to the terminal nodes, which are defined as t-links. All graph edges $e \in \varepsilon$, including n-links and t-links, are assigned some nonnegative weight/cost w_e. An example of a simple 2D graph of 3×3 image is shown in Fig. 7a.

A binary label A_p that partition the underlying image into object and background segments can be obtained by determining an $s - t$ cut on the graph. The $s - t$ cut is a subset of edges $C \in \varepsilon$ such that the terminals S and T become completely separated by removing these edges as shown in Fig. 7b. The cost of a cut is defined as the sum of the weights/costs of all edges included in that cut, $|C| = \sum_{e \in C} w_e$. The cut with a

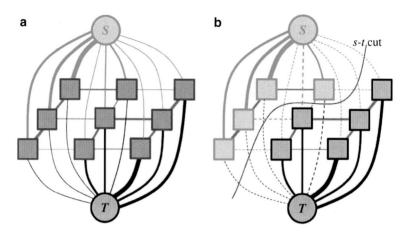

Fig. 7 An undirected graph of 3×3 image (**a**) and (**b**) $s - t$ cut. The thickness of the edges represents their costs. Figure based on [41]

minimal cost gives the optimal segmentation according to the designated energy function. It is important to formulate a precise energy function that can be encoded via n-links and t-links. In addition, a set of hard constrains for object and background, similar to these introduced in [47], can be imposed using infinity cost t-links. The graph cut algorithm has been successfully applied to liver vessels segmentation in [48] and to interactive 2D and 3D images segmentation in [49–52].

The goal of energy minimization is to find a labeling $A = \{A_1, A_2, \ldots, A_{|p|}\}$, which minimize the Gibbs energy function $E(A)$ defined in (4):

$$E(A) = R(A) + \mu B(A), \tag{4}$$

where

$$R(A) = \sum_{p \in P} R_p A(p), \tag{5}$$

$$B(A) = \sum_{p \in P, q \in \aleph_p} B_{pq}(A_p, A_q).\delta(A_p, A_q), \tag{6}$$

and

$$\delta(A_p, A_q) = \begin{cases} 1 & \text{if} \quad A_p \neq A_q \\ 0 & \text{if} \quad A_p = A_q \end{cases} . \tag{7}$$

The parameter μ in (4) determines the relative importance of the boundary term, $B(A)$, versus the regional term, $R(A)$, and $\aleph_p$ defines the neighborhood of pixel p. $R_p(A_p)$ is the penalty of assigning a label A_p to a pixel p, and $B_{pq}(A_p, A_q)$ is the penalty of labeling the pair of pixels p and q with labels A_p and A_q, respectively. In the presented approach, this energy function is adjusted to include the shape constrains as a penalty added to the regional term. Hence, the regional term $R(A)$ is computed by adding two penalties: the data penalty $R_D(A_p)$ and the shape penalty $R_s(A_p)$. The data penalty reflects on how the intensity of pixel p fits into the intensity model of the object (liver) and background (non-liver tissues). The shape penalty is encoded as the prior probability of a pixel to be inside or outside the liver object. The data, shape, and boundary penalties are calculated as in (8), (9), and (10), respectively:

$$
R_D(A_p) = \begin{cases} \dfrac{\log\left(\mathrm{pr}\left(I_p \in \text{``obj''}\right)\right)}{\log\left(\mathrm{pr}\left(I_p \in \text{``obj''}\right)\right) + \log\left(\mathrm{pr}\left(I_p \in \text{``bkg''}\right)\right)} & \text{if} \quad A_p = 1 \\[3mm] \dfrac{\log\left(\mathrm{pr}\left(I_p \in \text{``bkg''}\right)\right)}{\log\left(\mathrm{pr}\left(I_p \in \text{``obj''}\right)\right) + \log\left(\mathrm{pr}\left(I_p \in \text{``bkg''}\right)\right)} & \text{if} \quad A_p = 0 \end{cases}, \tag{8}
$$

$$
R_s(A_p) = \begin{cases} 1 - shape_{temp} & \text{if} \quad A_p = 1 \\ shape_{temp} & \text{if} \quad A_p = 0 \end{cases}, \tag{9}
$$

$$
B_{pq} = e^{-\frac{|I_p - I_q|^2}{2\sigma^2}} \times \frac{1}{d(p,q)}, \tag{10}
$$

where $shape_{temp}$ is the estimated shape template of the objected (liver) in the current slice, I_p is the intensity value of a pixel p, $\mathrm{pr}(I_p \in \text{" obj "} (\text{" bkg "}))$ is the probability of p to be an object (" obj ") or background (" bkg ") pixel, and $d(p,q)$ is the Euclidian distance between pixels p and q. The total energy function can be obtained by including the shape penalty into the Gibbs energy function as shown in (11):

$$
E_T(A) = (1 - \lambda)R_D(A) + \lambda R_s(A) + \mu B(A). \tag{11}
$$

The parameter λ determines the relative importance of the data penalty versus the shape penalty. This total energy function can be minimized efficiently using the graph cut algorithm. To achieve this goal, a graph with cut cost equaling the value of $E_T(A)$ is constructed using the edge weights defined in (12), (13), and (14). Furthermore, the hard constrains defined in section "Estimation of the Shape and Intensity Constrains" are implemented via infinity cost edges:

$$
w_{sp} = \begin{cases} \infty & \text{if} \quad p \in \text{``obj''} \\ 0 & \text{if} \quad p \in \text{``bkg''} \\ (1 - \lambda)R_D(A_p = 0) + \lambda R_s(A_p = 0) & \text{otherwise} \end{cases}. \tag{12}
$$

$$
w_{pt} = \begin{cases} 0 & \text{if} \quad p \in \text{``obj''} \\ \infty & \text{if} \quad p \in \text{``bkg''} \\ (1 - \lambda)R_D(A_p = 1) + \lambda R_s(A_p = 1) & \text{otherwise} \end{cases}. \tag{13}
$$

$$w_{pq} = B_{pq}(A_p, A_q).$$ (14)

Post-processing

In this stage, any tissue surrounded completely by the segmented liver tissue is added to the final segmentation, which smoothed using a 3D filter. To achieve this goal, the following procedure is applied:

1. Perform a hole filling to each 2D slice.
2. Perform binary image closing to the 3D volume using a ball-structuring element of radius 3.
3. Perform a hole filling to each 2D slice again.
4. Smooth the final volume by applying a binary median filter of $3 \times 3 \times 3$ size.

Data and Experimental Setup

In this work, we perform a qualitative evaluation of the model-free segmentation approach using three datasets: both training and testing datasets of MICCAI2007 [53] and JAMIT contest dataset [54]. In this section, data description, evaluation metrics, and the parameter setting of the introduced segmentation approach will be introduced.

Datasets

The first dataset used for evaluation is the MICCAI2007 training dataset. This dataset contains 20 CT images acquired using a variety of CT scanners, including 4, 16, and 64 detector rows. All of these images were acquired contrast-dye-enhanced in the central venous phase. According to the machine and protocol used, pixel spacing is varied from 0.55 to 0.8 mm in x/y direction, and the slice spacing is varied from 1 to 5 mm. In some cases, the entire anatomy is rotated around the z-axes. Most images in this dataset have liver abnormalities, including tumors, metastasis, and cysts of different sizes. The second dataset is the MICCAI2007 testing dataset, which contains 10 CT images and has the same characteristic of the previous dataset. The third dataset is the dataset used in JAMIT contest for liver tumor detection. This dataset contains 20 CT images acquired contrast-dye-enhanced in portal venous phase. The pixel spacing is varied from 0.5 to 1 mm in x/y direction, and the slice spacing is varied from 0.8 to 1 mm. This data is used at the contest for liver tumor detection, and it has different kinds of liver abnormalities, including tumors and cysts.

Parameter Setting

The number of iteration of the nonlinear diffusion filter influences the quality of the smoothing process and then affects the homogeneity of the liver. A large number of iterations make the object more smooth; however, it greatly increases the processing time. From numerous experiments on randomly selected cases from MICCAI2007 training dataset, we set the number of iterations to 10. This value is optimal for keeping the balance between the object smoothing and the processing time. The other parameters of the nonlinear diffusion filter, time step, and K were set to 0.125, 1.5, and 3, respectively. Graph cut parameters have been adjusted using 5 CT images having different characteristics: 3 from MICCAI2007 training dataset and 2 from JAMIT dataset. Parameter μ, which determines the influence of the boundary penalty, was set to 2. The parameter λ, which determines the influence of the shape penalty in the regional term, was set to 0.2. These parameters were fixed for all images in all datasets. The parameter σ in the boundary term was dynamically selected from each slice as the average absolute intensity difference between the neighboring pixels (15):

$$\sigma = \frac{1}{|P|} \sum_{p \in P, q \in \aleph_p} |I_p - I_q| \tag{15}$$

Evaluation Metrics

$$\text{Sensitivity} = \frac{\text{True Positive}}{\text{True Positive} + \text{False Negative}} \tag{16}$$

$$\text{Specificity} = \frac{\text{True Negative}}{\text{False Positive} + \text{True Negative}} \tag{17}$$

$$\text{Precision} = \frac{\text{True Positive}}{\text{True Positive} + \text{False Positive}} \tag{18}$$

$$\text{Accuracy} = \frac{\text{True Positive} + \text{True Negative}}{\text{Number of Voxels}} \tag{19}$$

$$\text{Error Rate} = \frac{\text{False Positive} + \text{False Negative}}{\text{Number of Voxels}} \times 100 \tag{20}$$

Evaluation was performed using two sets of evaluation metrics. The first set of metrics contains five general segmentation metrics of sensitivity (16), specificity (17), precision (18), accuracy (19), and the error rate (20).

The second set of metrics, which was used in MICCAI2007 Grand Challenge workshop [55], includes five metrics. Two of these metrics are volume based and the other three are surface based. These five metrics are calculated for a segmented liver volume A and a reference liver volume B as the following:

1. Volumetric overlap error (VOE), in percent: it is 0 for a perfect segmentation and 100 if the two volumes A and B do not overlap at all:

$$\text{VOE} = \left(1 - \left(\frac{|A \cap B|}{|A \cup B|}\right)\right). \tag{21}$$

2. Relative volume difference (RVD), in percent: a positive value refers to over-segmentation and a negative value refers to under-segmentation. The value of 0 means that both A and B have the same volume; however, it does not imply that they are identical [55]:

$$\text{RVD} = \left(\frac{|A| - |B|}{|B|}\right) \times 100. \tag{22}$$

3. Average symmetric surface distance (ASD), in mm: the value of 0 refers to a perfect segmentation: for each surface voxel of A, the Euclidian distance from the closest surface voxel of B is calculated. This distance is also calculated from B to A. The ASD is computed as the average of these distances.
4. Root mean square symmetric surface distance (RMD), in mm: it is similar to the ASD; however, instead of Euclidian distance, the squared distance is calculated. The RMD is computed as the square root of the average squared distance.
5. Maximum symmetric surface distance (MSD), in mm: it is similar to ASD; however, instead of the average, the maximal Euclidian distance is calculated.

Heimann et al. [55] provide a methodology for combining these different measures in one precision score. They transform the result ρ_i of each error measure i to a gauged score $\varphi_i \in [0,100]$ and the final score is then computed as the average of all scores. To perform this transformation, they use a manual segmentation of non-expert to get the average user errors ρ'_i for each measure. Considering the performance of the manual segmentation as 75 out of 100, they calculate the corresponding score for measure i as

$$\varphi_i = \max\left(0, \left(100 - 25\frac{\rho_i}{\rho'_i}\right)\right). \tag{23}$$

The score of 100 points represents a perfect segmentation, and a score of 75 can be regarded as equivalent to non-expert segmentation. They also reported that the error measures of the non-expert are equivalent to 6.4 %, 4.7 %, 1, 1.8, and 19 mm for VOD, the absolute value of RVD, ASD, RMD, and MSD, respectively.

Results

The segmentation approach was applied to 50 CT images described in section "Datasets." We implemented the approach using Matlab® environment on Windows®-based personal computer with a Corei7 (2.8 GHz) processor and 6GB of memory. In order to reduce the processing time required for the smoothing stage, it was performed in parallel on the eight cores of the Corei7 processor using the Matlab® parallel computing toolbox.

Experiments on Clinical Data

The shape constrains play an essential role in the introduced model-free segmentation approach. The estimation of these constrains from the adjacent slice is assessed by computing the Jaccard coefficient (24), between the estimated shape and the manually segmented liver object at each slice. Figure 8 shows the computed coefficient between the true liver object and the estimated shape template and between the true liver object and the segmented one. From this figure, we can prove that the estimated template provides a good knowledge about the position and the shape of the true liver objects at each slice even in the case of large slice spacing:

$$J_{\text{coeff}} = \frac{|L \cap M|}{|L \cup M|}, \tag{24}$$

where L is the estimated shape template and M is the manually segmented object.

The evaluation results of the proposed approach using the first set of metrics are shown in Table 1 for the MICCAI2007 training dataset and in Table 2 for the JAMIT dataset. The evaluation of the MICCAI2007 testing dataset using this set of metrics is not available because the ground truth of this dataset is not publicly available.

Tables 3 and 4 show the accuracy of the proposed approach using the second set of metrics for the MICCAI2007 training dataset and the JAMIT dataset. The evaluation results of the MICCAI2007 testing dataset using this set of metrics which were calculated by the committee of the "3D Segmentation in the Clinic: A Grand Challenge" workshop of MICCAI2007 are shown in Table 5. The best, moderate, and worst segmentation results in MICCAI2007 training dataset and JAMIT dataset are shown in Figs. 9, 10, 11, 12, 13, and 14 in 2D view.

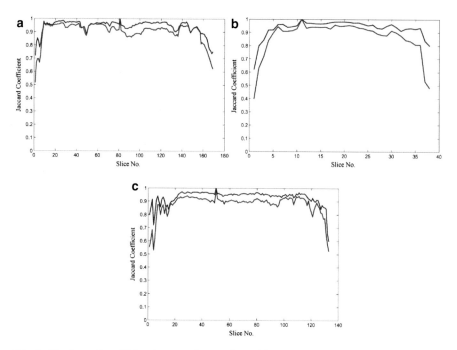

Fig. 8 The Jaccard coefficient between the true liver object and the estimated shape template in *blue*, and the coefficient between the true liver objected and the segmented one in *red*: (**a**) sample from the MICCAI2007 training dataset with slice spacing of 1 mm, (**b**) sample from the MICCAI2007 training dataset with slice spacing of 5 mm, and (**c**) sample from JAMIT dataset with slice spacing of 1 mm

Comparative Results

In this section, the comparative results of the proposed approach on both MICCAI2007 datasets are reported. The results of MICCAI2007 training dataset are compared to the methods introduced in [5, 10] and the final scores are shown in Table 6. In [10], the authors combine split thresholding and anatomical knowledge to segment the liver in contrast-enhanced CT images. Although they utilize the anatomical knowledge to roughly estimate the liver location, the final segmentation depends on the intensity information alone. Accordingly, their segmentation results, which were considered as an initial estimation of the liver boundary, were greatly affected by the liver abnormalities. Ruska et al. in [5] applied the anatomical knowledge to refine an initial segmentation estimated using intensity thresholding. However, their proposed method for single-phase CT images was highly relying on the intensity model of the liver, and it could not extract the liver in the cases containing large and dense tumors.

Table 1 Evaluation of the results for the MICCAI2007 training dataset based on general segmentation metrics

Case	Sensitivity	Specificity	Precision	Accuracy	Error rate %
#1	0.9790	0.9971	0.9467	0.9962	0.3799
#2	0.9815	0.9940	0.9472	0.9927	0.7282
#3	0.9838	0.9966	0.9472	0.9958	0.4177
#4	0.9686	0.9983	0.9698	0.9967	0.3266
#5	0.9803	0.9988	0.9732	0.9981	0.1922
#6	0.9854	0.9973	0.9486	0.9968	0.3235
#7	0.9318	0.9993	0.9832	0.9964	0.3581
#8	0.9436	0.9972	0.9686	0.9928	0.7187
#9	0.9583	0.9991	0.9828	0.9969	0.3095
#10	0.9754	0.9963	0.9560	0.9947	0.5290
#11	0.9849	0.9985	0.9715	0.9978	0.2224
#12	0.9855	0.9980	0.9645	0.9973	0.2694
#13	0.9434	0.9984	0.9693	0.9957	0.4310
#14	0.9788	0.9992	0.9677	0.9987	0.1263
#15	0.9806	0.9993	0.9793	0.9987	0.1334
#16	0.9715	0.9966	0.9662	0.9942	0.5758
#17	0.9840	0.9976	0.9559	0.9970	0.3030
#18	0.9707	0.9972	0.9495	0.9959	0.4134
#19	0.9655	0.9973	0.9628	0.9952	0.4828
#20	0.9618	0.9986	0.9551	0.9975	0.2490
Average	0.9707	0.9977	0.9633	0.9963	0.3745
Std. dev.	0.0157	0.0013	0.0119	0.0017	0.1692

The results of MICCAI2007 testing dataset have been compared to the best automatic method (Kainmüller et al. [29]) and all interactive methods reported by T. Heimann et al. in [55]. Averaged results for individual measures of all methods are summarized in Table 7. As done in [55], all scores are rounded down to the nearest integer, and runtime is given as the average time to segment one image volume and it includes interaction time and computation time. Additionally, all approaches have been classified according to the time required for interaction. Less than 1 min was regarded as low interaction, less than 5 min as medium interaction, and more than 5 min as high interaction. Referring to Table 7, the proposed approach shares the best position with Beichel et al. MBR; however, the proposed approach is significantly faster, requires less amount of interaction, and does not require extensive manual refinement. The automatic method of Kainmuller et al. achieved these results by using an extensive training set of 112 liver shapes to build an SSM consists of around 7,000 landmarks. The total score of the same method was 73 when the number of training shapes used to build the SSM was 43 [29].

Table 2 Evaluation of the results for the JAMIT dataset based on general segmentation metrics

Case	Sensitivity	Specificity	Precision	Accuracy	Error rate %
#1	0.9776	0.9993	0.9767	0.9986	0.1422
#2	0.9745	0.9993	0.9583	0.9988	0.1169
#3	0.9667	0.9993	0.9757	0.9983	0.1732
#4	0.9672	0.9991	0.9752	0.9980	0.2023
#5	0.9699	0.9989	0.9785	0.9975	0.2489
#6	0.9708	0.9987	0.9753	0.9974	0.2611
#7	0.9212	0.9981	0.9487	0.9952	0.4818
#8	0.9653	0.9993	0.9650	0.9987	0.1337
#9	0.9733	0.9995	0.9747	0.9990	0.0994
#10	0.9614	0.9990	0.9604	0.9981	0.1948
#11	0.9604	0.9997	0.9836	0.9989	0.1076
#12	0.9673	0.9977	0.9708	0.9955	0.4529
#13	0.9542	0.9989	0.9611	0.9978	0.2240
#14	0.9591	0.9995	0.9809	0.9985	0.1469
#15	0.9647	0.9991	0.9806	0.9975	0.2545
#16	0.9592	0.9995	0.9786	0.9987	0.1327
#17	0.9744	0.9991	0.9662	0.9985	0.1531
#18	0.9719	0.9996	0.9766	0.9991	0.0883
#19	0.9745	0.9996	0.9827	0.9991	0.0901
#20	0.9687	0.9995	0.9762	0.9988	0.1229
Average	0.9651	0.9991	0.9723	0.9981	0.1914
Std. dev.	0.0121	0.0005	0.0093	0.0011	0.1090

Discussion

The proposed approach provides efficient solutions for the liver segmentation challenges. The shape constrains are utilized to alleviate the ambiguity of the liver boundary and to reduce the effect of liver abnormalities. These shape constrains are estimated in a slice-by-slice manner to transfer the anatomical knowledge from clear liver cross sections to the ambiguous cross sections. Since these constrains are estimated in a case-specific manner, the proposed approach is robust for liver shape variations. The statistical model of the liver is also constructed in a same manner to consider liver intensity variations. Figures 15 and 16 show that the presented model-free approach can efficiently extract the liver in different cases containing large and dense tumors. Successful segmentation of complex and atypical liver shapes is illustrated in Fig. 17.

Referring to Tables 1 and 2, very high level of sensitivity and specificity indicates that the proposed approach alleviates over- and under-segmentation. A minimum accuracy, a precision, and a maximum segmentation error of 0.9927, 0.9467, and 0.7282 % reflect the efficiency of the proposed approach. Additionally,

Table 3 Evaluation of the results for the MICCAI2007 training dataset based on the metrics of Heimann et al. [55]

Case	VOE [%]	Score	RVD [%]	Score	ASD mm	Score	RMD mm	Score	MSD mm	Score	Total score	Time (s) Initial	Time (s) Total
#1	7.21	72	2.41	87	1.00	75	1.83	75	21.34	72	76	46	162
#2	6.95	73	3.62	81	0.64	84	1.29	82	10.95	86	81	40	112
#3	6.71	74	3.83	80	0.56	86	1.22	83	11.18	86	82	40	112
#4	5.98	77	0.12	99	0.84	79	2.08	71	19.12	75	80	39	190
#5	4.29	83	1.01	95	0.57	86	1.56	78	20.83	73	83	35	197
#6	6.46	75	3.87	79	0.68	83	1.46	80	16.48	79	79	39	111
#7	8.28	68	5.22	72	1.14	71	2.65	63	25.89	66	68	38	184
#8	8.44	67	2.58	86	1.52	62	3.07	57	26.57	66	68	37	210
#9	5.76	78	2.49	87	0.75	81	1.49	79	14.80	81	81	38	190
#10	6.65	74	2.03	89	0.82	80	1.64	77	15.89	79	80	39	200
#11	4.27	83	1.38	93	0.75	81	1.80	75	21.84	72	81	35	193
#12	4.89	81	2.18	88	0.66	84	1.46	80	18.48	76	82	37	187
#13	8.40	67	2.67	86	0.97	76	1.80	75	20.04	74	76	38	134
#14	5.22	80	1.14	94	0.38	91	0.78	89	10.41	87	88	36	82
#15	3.94	85	0.13	99	0.59	85	1.59	78	18.22	76	85	37	197
#16	6.04	76	0.54	97	0.86	78	1.67	77	17.73	77	81	40	180
#17	5.88	77	2.94	84	0.59	85	1.30	82	12.07	84	82	38	131
#18	7.69	70	2.23	88	0.96	76	2.31	68	18.39	76	76	39	221
#19	6.92	73	0.28	99	1.40	65	3.08	57	23.03	70	73	38	268
#20	7.09	72	0.70	96	0.75	81	1.57	78	13.36	83	82	40	111
Average	6.35	75	2.06	89	0.80	80	1.78	75	17.83	77	79.2	38.5	168.6
Std. dev.	1.4	5.3	1.4	7.5	0.3	7.2	0.6	8.3	4.7	6.3	5.1	2.4	47.2

Table 4 Evaluation of the results for the JAMIT dataset based on the metrics of Heimann et al. [55]

Case	VOE [%]	Score	RVD [%]	Score	ASD mm	Score	RMD mm	Score	MSD mm	Score	Total score	Time (s) Initial	Time (s) Total
#1	4.47	83	0.10	99	0.66	83	1.44	80	14.51	81	85	35	185
#2	6.51	75	1.69	91	0.72	82	1.37	81	13.20	83	82	38	179
#3	5.61	78	0.92	95	0.91	77	2.20	70	25.44	67	77	40	196
#4	5.61	78	0.82	96	0.69	83	1.39	81	19.36	75	83	38	185
#5	5.04	80	0.88	95	0.94	77	1.97	73	20.03	74	80	36	290
#6	5.24	80	0.46	98	0.66	83	1.40	80	21.49	72	83	37	301
#7	12.2	52	2.90	85	1.62	60	4.13	43	33.66	56	59	37	202
#8	6.74	74	0.03	100	1.04	74	2.41	67	32.65	58	75	38	188
#9	5.07	80	0.14	99	0.51	87	0.99	86	11.00	86	88	39	164
#10	7.52	71	0.10	99	0.90	78	1.81	75	17.40	77	80	40	221
#11	5.47	79	2.36	87	0.60	85	0.99	86	9.30	88	85	36	160
#12	6.01	77	0.35	98	0.80	80	1.87	74	24.85	68	79	34	196
#13	8.13	68	0.73	96	1.24	69	2.60	64	21.47	72	74	36	181
#14	5.85	77	2.23	88	0.96	76	2.53	65	32.07	58	73	37	205
#15	5.34	79	1.62	91	0.59	85	1.07	85	10.33	87	85	38	231
#16	6.05	76	1.98	89	0.66	84	1.51	79	15.95	79	81	35	174
#17	5.78	77	0.85	95	0.83	79	1.79	75	17.90	77	81	37	175
#18	5.02	80	0.48	97	0.73	82	1.66	77	18.54	76	82	36	197
#19	4.19	84	0.84	96	0.41	90	0.76	89	7.27	91	90	40	172
#20	5.37	79	0.76	96	0.62	84	1.09	85	9.12	88	86	38	164
Average	6.06	76	1.01	95	0.80	80	1.75	76	18.78	76	80.4	37.25	198.3
Std. dev.	1.7	6.8	0.8	4.4	0.3	6.7	0.8	10.5	7.9	10.4	6.7	1.7	38

Table 5 Evaluation of the results for the MICCAI2007 testing dataset based on the metrics of Heimann et al. [55]

Case	VOE [%]	VOE Score	RVD [%]	RVD Score	ASD mm	ASD Score	RMD mm	RMD Score	MSD mm	MSD Score	Total score	Time (s) Initial	Time (s) Total
#1	5.2	80	2.4	87	0.7	82	1.4	81	14.7	81	82	35	221
#2	5.9	77	5.0	74	0.8	80	1.7	76	19.4	74	76	40	223
#3	3.9	85	2.2	88	0.7	83	1.1	84	14.0	82	84	37	218
#4	5.0	80	2.5	86	0.7	81	1.4	80	10.4	86	83	36	122
#5	6.1	76	1.2	94	1.0	76	1.9	74	21.5	72	78	36	118
#6	5.8	78	0.7	96	0.8	79	1.8	74	20.1	74	80	37	204
#7	3.8	85	1.5	92	0.5	87	1.2	84	16.0	79	85	38	170
#8	6.2	76	1.1	94	1.0	75	2.3	68	22.2	71	77	35	113
#9	4.2	84	1.2	94	0.5	87	1.2	83	16.0	79	85	37	284
#10	4.5	82	0.5	98	0.6	86	1.2	84	11.5	85	87	36	108
Average	5	80	1.8	90	0.7	82	1.5	79	16.6	78	81.7	36.7	178.1
Std. dev.	0.9	3.6	1.3	7.0	0.18	4.3	0.4	5.5	4.1	5.3	3.8	1.5	60.8

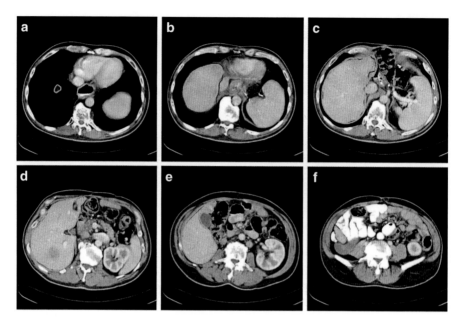

Fig. 9 2D visualization of the best case in MICCAI2007 dataset according to the scores in Table 3. (**a–f**) Case #14 slices 83, 80, 76, 67, 57, and 45. The *green* contour represents the manual reference and the *red* one represents the segmentation result

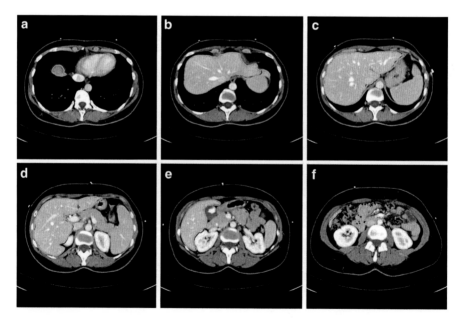

Fig. 10 2D visualization of the moderate segmented case in MICCAI2007 dataset according to the scores in Table 3. (**a–f**) Case #6 slices 96, 85, 72, 56, 40, and 20. The *green* contour represents the manual reference and the *red* one represents the segmentation result

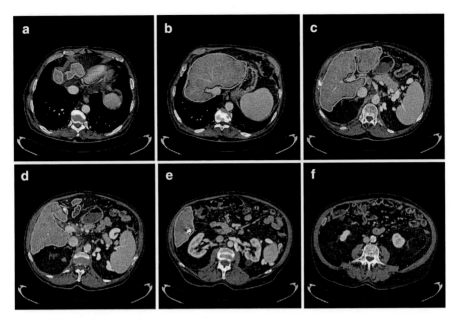

Fig. 11 2D visualization of the worst segmented case in MICCAI2007 data set according to the scores in Table 3, (**a–f**) case #7 slices 229, 206, 154, 140, 104, 57. The *green* contour represents the manual reference and the *red* one represents the segmentation result

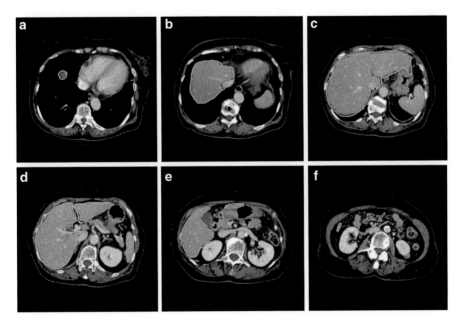

Fig. 12 2D visualization of the best case in JAMIT dataset according to the scores in Table 4. (**a–f**) Case #19 slices 18, 35, 57, 75, 105, and 151. The *green* contour represents the manual reference and the *red* one represents the segmentation result

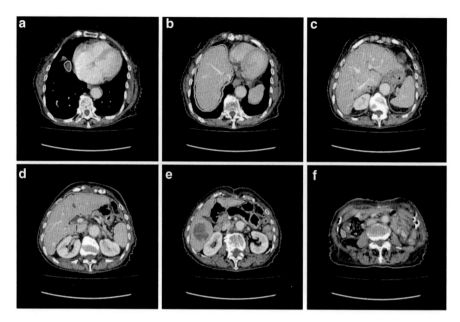

Fig. 13 2D visualization of the moderate segmented case in JAMIT dataset according to the scores in Table 4. (**a–f**) Case #16 slices 10, 31, 53, 77, 109, and 155. The *green* contour represents the manual reference and the *red* one represents the segmentation result

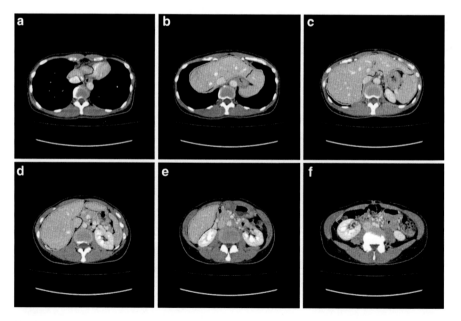

Fig. 14 2D visualization of the worst segmented case in JAMIT dataset according to the scores in Table 4. (**a–f**) Case #7 slices 16, 45, 76, 109, 144, and 184. The *green* contour represents the manual reference and the *red* one represents the segmentation result

Table 6 Scores of the proposed approach on MICCAI2007 training dataset compared to the scores of Ruska et al. [5] and Foruzan et al. [10]

Case	Proposed	Ruska et al. [5]	Foruzan et al. [10]
#1	76	59	32
#2	81	78	47
#3	82	71	33
#4	80	81	44
#5	83	77	21
#6	79	78	53
#7	68	73	8
#8	58	73	40
#9	81	70	39
#10	80	75	31
#11	81	70	34
#12	82	70	23
#13	76	74	0
#14	88	70	76
#15	85	83	0
#16	81	8	12
#17	82	79	52
#18	76	78	23
#19	73	85	34
#20	82	71	70
Average	79.2	71	34
Std. dev.	5.1	16	21

based on the scores shown in the last column of Tables 3, 4, and 5, the average performance of the proposed approach (80.4 for JAMIT dataset, 79.2 and 81.7 for MICCAI2007 datasets) can be regarded as closer to the reference manual segmentation than the average human performance [55]. Small deviation of these scores shows the ability of the proposed approach to deal with extreme cases as well as easy and moderate cases. The processing time required to segment a CT volume on a personal computer with the specification described in section "Results" ranges from 2 to 5 min. This time is significantly less than the manual or other conventional segmentation methods.

In general, the proposed approach can efficiently utilize the anatomical knowledge of the liver to achieve accurate segmentation results. The precision of this approach is high for all parts of the liver with a small degradation at the most top and the most bottom parts as shown in Fig. 18a. However, in some cases, having extremely ambiguous boundaries between the liver and the heart, this degradation increases at the top part of the liver due to false segmentation of heart parts as a liver as shown in Fig. 18b. This problem can be solved by applying more advanced heart–liver separation methodology. Additionally, to check the effect of start slice selection and initialization, two additional segmentations have been performed and reported in Table 8. These results show that all segmentations have roughly the same or slightly different scores.

Table 7 Comparative results of MICCAI2007

Method	VOE [%]	Score	RVD [%]	Score	ASD mm	Score	RMD mm	Score	MSD mm	Score	Total score	Runtime [min]
#1	5.2 ± 0.9	80	1.0 ± 1.7	91	0.8 ± 0.2	80	1.4 ± 0.4	80	15.7 ± 3.5	79	82 ± 2	36
#2	5.0 ± 0.9	**80**	1.8 ± 1.3	**90**	0.7 ± 0.17	**82**	1.5 ± 0.4	**79**	16.6 ± 4.1	**78**	82 ± 5	**3**
#3	6.1 ± 2.1	76	− 2.9 ± 2.9	85	0.9 ± 0.3	76	1.9 ± 0.8	74	18.7 ± 8.5	75	77 ± 9	15
#4	6.6 ± 1.6	74	1.8 ± 2.5	88	1.0 ± 0.3	74	1.9 ± 0.4	73	18.5 ± 4.1	76	77 ± 4	7
#5	7.2 ± 1.2	72	2.5 ± 2.3	86	1.1 ± 0.2	73	1.9 ± 0.5	71	17.1 ± 5.4	77	76 ± 5	20
#6	6.4 ± 1.0	75	4.7 ± 1.8	75	1.0 ± 0.2	75	1.8 ± 0.5	75	19.3 ± 5.6	75	75 ± 4	
#7	6.9 ± 1.4	73	1.3 ± 2.9	88	1.1 ± 0.3	73	2.1 ± 0.5	71	21.3 ± 4.0	72	75 ± 5	7
#8	6.5 ± 1.1	74	1.1 ± 1.9	90	1.1 ± 0.4	72	2.5 ± 1.2	66	23.4 ± 10.5	69	74 ± 9	31
#9	8.1 ± 1.1	68	6.1 ± 2.6	68	1.3 ± 0.2	67	2.2 ± 0.4	69	18.7 ± 4.5	75	69 ± 5	4–7
#10	10.4 ± 3.1	59	3.7 ± 6.2	70	2.0 ± 0.7	50	5.0 ± 2.4	34	40.5 ± 18.2	47	52 ± 19	60
#11	14.3 ± 9.4	48	3.1 ± 10.7	62	3.6 ± 3.1	34	7.9 ± 5.9	24	49.2 ± 20.4	38	41 ± 27	30

As done in [55], results for each measure are reported as mean and standard deviation over all test images, together with mean score. All scores are averaged to a final score given as mean and standard deviation over all images. The methods are #1: Beichel et al. MBR (high), #2: our approach (low), #3: Kainmüller et al. (automatic), #4: Beck and Aurich (high), #5: Dawant et al. (med), #6: second rater, #7: Lee et al. (low), #8: Beichel et al. CBR (med), #9 Wimmer et al. (med), #10: Slagmolen et al. (med), and #11: Beichel et al. (low)

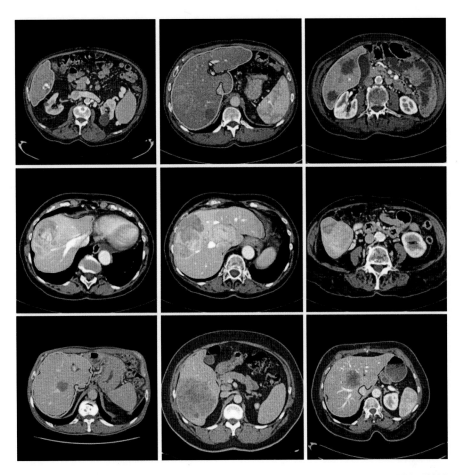

Fig. 15 Segmentation results of cases containing dense liver abnormalities (MICCAI2007 dataset). The *green* contour represents the manual reference and the *red* one represents the segmentation result

Conclusion

The portal venous CT images are the most important and the most common tool for diagnosis of liver diseases. The vasculature and lesions are most visible in this phase; however, the extraction of the liver is challenging due to the contrast of the normal and abnormal liver tissues and the existence of noise. In this work, we introduce a novel model-free shape-based approach for liver segmentation in portal venous CT images using a case-specific knowledge. In which, the relation between consequent slices of the same image is exploited to estimate the shape and intensity information of the liver. Then, this information is integrated into the graph cut

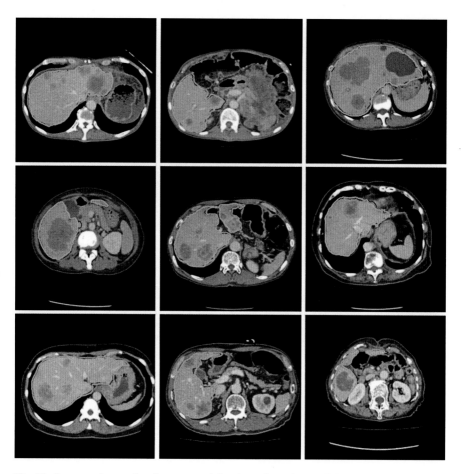

Fig. 16 Segmentation results of cases containing dense liver abnormalities (JAMIT dataset). The *green* contour represents the manual reference and the *red* one represents the segmentation result

algorithm to segment the whole CT image. Unlike the other shape-based segmentation approaches, which use training data to build a statistical model, this approach does not require any prior training for model construction. Accordingly, it is not restricted to the trained model, and it can be applied when there is no enough training data available. The evaluation results demonstrated the high precision of the proposed approach. It efficiently estimates the liver boundary even with the existence of large and dense liver abnormalities. The utilization of a case-specific knowledge increases the ability of the proposed approach to deal with difficult and atypical liver shapes. Additionally, it removes the burden of model construction and matching. A low processing time required by the proposed approach makes it suitable for clinical application.

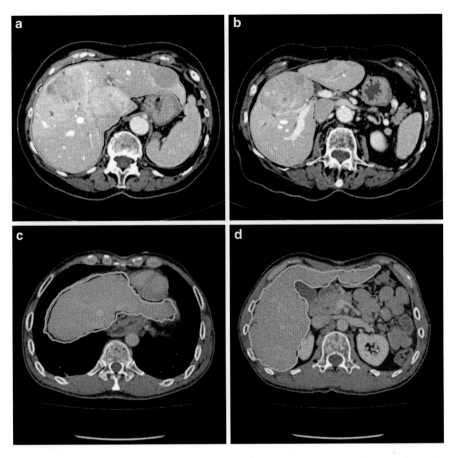

Fig. 17 Segmentation results of cases containing atypical liver shapes, (**a, b**) 2D view of case#11 in MICCAI2007 dataset and (**c, d**) 2D view of case#12 in JAMIT dataset. The *green* contour represents the manual reference and the *red* one represents the segmentation result

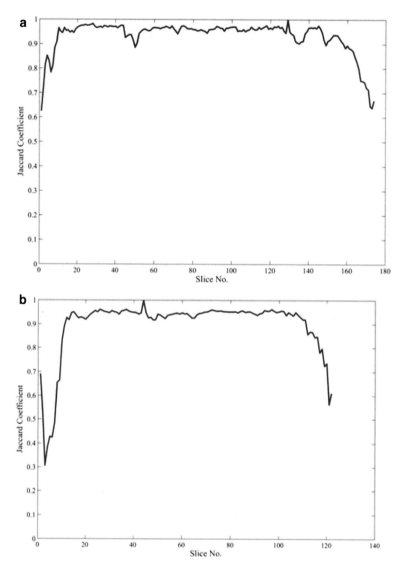

Fig. 18 Jaccard coefficient between manual segmentation and the results of the proposed approach at different slices, (**a**) typical case and (**b**) case with false-positive at the top part of the liver

Table 8 Evaluation results of the proposed approach using different initializations, MICCAI2007 training dataset

Segmentation method	VOE [%]	Score	RVD [%]	Score	ASD mm	Score	RMD mm	Score	MSD mm	Score	Total score
Original	6.35 ± 1.48	75	2.06 ± 1.49	89	0.8 ± 0.3	80	1.78 ± 0.6	75	17.83 ± 4.7	77	79.2 ± 5.1
Additional #1	6.5 ± 1.3	75	2.1 ± 1.4	89	0.8 ± 0.3	80	1.8 ± 0.6	75	18.2 ± 4.7	76	79 ± 4.9
Additional #2	6.34 ± 1.3	75	2.0 ± 1.3	89	0.8 ± 0.2	81	1.8 ± 0.6	75	18.2 ± 4.8	77	79.5 ± 4.7

References

1. Ferlay J, Shin HR, Bray F, Forman D, Mathers C, Parkin DM (2010) GLOBOCAN 2008 v1.2, Cancer Incidence and Mortality Worldwide: IARC CancerBase No. 10 [Internet]. International Agency for Research on Cancer, Lyon, France. http://globocan.iarc.fr. Accessed 15/03/2013
2. Doi K (2005) Current status and future potential of computer-aided diagnosis in medical imaging. Br J Radiol 75:S3–S19
3. Fujita H, Zhang1 X, Kido S, Hara T, Zhou X, Hatanaka Y, Xu R (2010) An introduction and survey of computer-aided detection/diagnosis (CAD). In: 2010 international conference on future computer, control and communication (FCCC2010), pp 200–205
4. Lim SJ, Jeong YY, Ho YS (2006) Automatic liver segmentation for volume measurement in CT images. J Vis Commun Image Represent 17:860–875
5. Rusko L, Bekes G, Fidrich M (2009) Automatic segmentation of the liver from multi- and single-phase contrast-enhanced CT images. Med Image Anal 13:871–882
6. Chen Y, Wang Z, Zhao W, Yang X (2009) Liver segmentation from CT images based on region growing method. In: Proc. 3rd international conference on bioinformatics and biomedical engineering (ICBBE), pp 1–4
7. Beichel R, Bauer C, Bornik A, Sorantin E, Bischof H (2007) Liver segmentation in CT data: a segmentation refinement approach. In Proc. of MICCAI 2007 Workshop: 3D Segmentation in the Clinic-A Grand Challenge. pp 235–245
8. Beck A, Aurich V (2007) HepaTux A semiautomatic liver segmentation system. In Proc. of MICCAI 2007 Workshop: 3D Segmentation in the Clinic-A Grand Challenge. pp 225–233
9. Foruzana AH, Zoroofia RA, Horib M, Satoc Y (2009) A knowledge-based technique for liver segmentation in CT data. Comput Med Imaging Graph 33:567–587
10. Foruzana AH, Zoroofia RA, Horib M, Satoc Y (2009) Liver segmentation by intensity analysis and anatomical information in multi-slice CT images. Int J Comput Assist Radiol Surg 4 (3):287–297
11. Gambino O, Vitabile S, Re GL, Tona GL, Librizzi S, Pirrone R, Ardizzone E, Midiri M (2010) Automatic volumetric liver segmentation using texture based region growing. In: Proc. of international conference on complex, intelligent and software intensive systems, pp 146–152
12. Susomboon R, Raicu DS, Furst J (2007) A hybrid approach for liver segmentation. In: Proc. MICCAI workshop on 3-D segmentation in clinic: a grand challenge, pp 151–160
13. Tibamoso G, Rueda A (2009) Semi-automatic liver segmentation from computed tomography (CT) scans based on deformable surfaces. SLIVER07 Results [Online]. http://sliver07.isi.uu. nl/results/20091022201318/description.pdf
14. Masutani Y (2002) RBF-based representation of volumetric data: application in visualization and segmentation. In: Proc. medical image computing and computer-assisted intervention (MICCAI), pp 300–307
15. Wimmer A, Soza G, Hornegger J (2007) Two-stage semi-automatic organ segmentation framework using radial basis functions and level sets. In: Proc. MICCAI workshop on 3-D segmentation in clinic: a grand challenge, pp 179–188
16. Gao J, Kosaka A, Kak A (2005) A deformable model for automatic CT liver extraction. Acad Radiol 12(9):1178–1189
17. Rahardja K, Kosaka A (1996) Vision-based bin picking: recognition and localization of multiple complex objects using simple visual cues. In: Proc. IEEE/RSJ international conference on intelligent robots and systems, pp 1448–1457
18. Massoptier L, Casciaro S (2008) A new fully automatic and robust algorithm for fast segmentation of liver tissue and tumors from CT scans. Eur Radiol 18:1658–1665
19. Xu C, Prince J (1998) Snakes, shapes, and gradient vector flow. IEEE Trans Image Process 7 (3):359–369
20. Alomari RS, Kompalli S, Chaudhary V (2008) Segmentation of the liver from abdominal CT using Markov random field model and GVF snakes. In: Proc. international conference on complex, intelligent and software intensive systems, pp 293–298

21. Liu F, Zhao B, Kijewski P, Ginsberg MS, Wang L, Schwartz LH (2004) Automatic liver contour segmentation using GVF snake. In: Proc. SPIE medical imaging: image processing, vol 5370, pp 1466–1473

22. Liu F, Zhao B, Kijewski PK, Wang L, Schwartz LH (2005) Liver segmentation for CT images using GVF snake. Med Phys 32(12):3699–3706

23. Sethian JA (1996) Level set methods and fast marching methods, 2nd edn. Cambridge University Press, Cambridge

24. Furukawa D, Shimizu A, Kobatake H (2007) Automatic liver segmentation method based on maximum a posterior probability estimation and level set method. In: Proc. MICCAI workshop on 3-D segmentation in clinic: a grand challenge, pp 117–124

25. Manuel LF, Rubio JL, Ledesma-Carbayo MJ, Pascau J, Tellado JM, Ramn E, Desco M, Santos A (2009) 3D liver segmentation in preoperative CT images using a level-sets active surface method. In: Proc. 31st annual international conference of the IEEE EMBS, pp 3625–3628

26. Chan TF, Vese LA (2001) Active contours without edges. IEEE Trans Image Process 10 (2):266–277

27. Lee J, Kim N, Lee H, Seo JB, Won HJ, Shin YM, Shin YG (2007) Efficient liver segmentation exploiting level-set speed images with 2.5D shape propagation. In: Proc. MICCAI workshop on 3-D segmentation in clinic: a grand challenge, pp 189–196

28. Freiman M, Eliassaf O, Taieb Y, Joskowicz L, Azraq Y, Sosna J (2008) An iterative Bayesian approach for nearly automatic liver segmentation: algorithm and validation. Int J Comput Assist Radiol Surg 3(5):439–446

29. Kainmuller D, Lange T, Lamecker H (2007) Shape constrained automatic segmentation of the liver based on a heuristic intensity model. In: Proc. MICCAI workshop on 3-D segmentation in clinic: a grand challenge, pp 109–116

30. Heimann T, Meinzer H, Wolf I (2007) A statistical deformable model for the segmentation of liver CT volumes. In: Proc. MICCAI workshop on 3-D segmentation in clinic: a grand challenge, pp 161–166

31. Schwefel H-P (1995) Evolution and optimum seeking. Wiley, New York

32. Afifi A, Nakaguchi T, Tsumura N, Miyake Y (2010) Shape and texture priors for liver segmentation in abdominal computed tomography scans using the particle swarm optimization algorithm. Med Imaging Technol 28(1):53–62

33. Afifi A, Nakaguchi T, Tsumura N, Miyake Y (2010) A model optimization approach to the automatic segmentation of medical images. IEICE Trans Inform Syst E93-D(4):882–889

34. Poli R, Kennedy J, Blackwell T (2007) Particle swarm optimization: an overview. Swarm Intell 1:33–57

35. Saddi KA, Rousson M, Chefd'hotel C, Cheriet F (2007) Global-to-local shape matching for liver segmentation in CT imaging. In: Proc. MICCAI workshop on 3-D segmentation in clinic: a grand challenge, pp 207–2014

36. Lamecker H, Lange T, Seebass M (2004) Segmentation of the liver using a 3D statistical shape model. Technical report, Zuse Institute, Berlin, Germany

37. Okada T, Shimada R, Hori M, Nakamoto M, Chen Y-W, Nakamura H, Sato Y (2008) Automated segmentation of the liver from 3D CT images using probabilistic atlas and multilevel statistical shape model. Acad Radiol 15(11):1390–1399

38. Linguraru MG, Li Z, Shah F, Chin S, Summers RM (2009) Automated liver segmentation using a normalized probabilistic atlas. In: Proc. SPIE medical imaging: biomedical applications in molecular, structural, and functional imaging, vol 7262, pp 72622R72622R-8

39. Park H, Bland PH, Meyer CR (2003) Construction of an abdominal probabilistic atlas and its application in segmentation. IEEE Trans Med Imaging 22(4):483–492

40. Linguraru MG, Pura JA, Chowdhury AS, Summers RM (2010) Multi-organ segmentation from multi-phase abdominal CT via 4D graphs using enhancement, shape and location optimization. Medical image computing and computer-assisted intervention MICCAI2010, lecture notes in computer science, vol 6363

41. Bidaut L (2000) Data and image processing for abdominal imaging. Abdom Imaging 25:341–360
42. Weickert J (1997) A review of nonlinear diffusion filtering. Scale-Space Theory Comput Vis 1552:1–28
43. Lamecker H, Lange T, Seebass M (2004) Segmentation of the liver using a 3D statistical shape model. ZIB-Report 04–09 [Online]. http://opus.kobv.de/zib/volltexte/2004/785/pdf/ZR04-09. pdf
44. Weickert J, Romeny BM, Viergever MA (1998) Efficient and reliable schemes for nonlinear diffusion filtering. IEEE Trans Image Process 7(3):398–410
45. de Boor C (1978) A practical guide to splines. Springer, New York
46. Boykov Y, Veksler O, Zabih R (2001) Fast approximate energy minimization via graph cuts. IEEE Trans Pattern Anal Mach Intell 23(11):1222–1239
47. Griffin LD, Colchester ACF, Roll SA, Studholme CS (1994) Hierarchical segmentation satisfying constraints. In: Proc. of British machine vision conference (BMVC94), pp 135–144
48. Esneault S, Lafon C (2010) Liver vessels segmentation using a hybrid geometrical moments/ graph cuts method. IEEE Trans Biomed Eng 57(2):276–283
49. Boykov Y, Lea GF (2006) Graph cuts and efficient N-D image segmentation. Int J Comput Vis 70(2):109–131
50. Nagahashi T, Fujiyoshi H, Kanade T (2007) Image segmentation using iterated graph cuts based on multi-scale smoothing. In: Proc. 8th Asian conference on computer vision (ACCV), part II, pp 806–816
51. Boykov Y, Jolly M-P (2000) Interactive organ segmentation using graph cuts. In: Proc. medical image computing and computer-assisted intervention (MICCAI), pp 276–286
52. Freedman D, Zhang T (2005) Interactive graph cut based segmentation with shape priors. In: Proc. IEEE computer society conference on computer vision and pattern recognition (CVPR), vol 1, pp 755–762
53. Segmentation of the Liver 2007 (SLIVER07). http://sliver07.isi.uu.nl/. Last visited: Accessed 10 Apr 2013
54. The Japanese Society of Medical Imaging Technology, JAMIT Computer-aided Diagnosis (CAD). http://www.jamit.jp/english/. Overview, last visited: Accessed 10 Apr 2013
55. Heimann T, Ginneken BV, Styner MA, Arzhaeva Y, Aurich V, Bauer C, Beck A, Becker C, Beichel R, Bekes G, Bello F, Binnig G, Bischof H, Bornik A, Cashman PMM, Chi Y, Cordova A, Dawant BM, Fidrich M, Furst JD, Furukawa D, Grenacher L, Hornegger J, Kainmu ̈ller D, Kitney RI, Kobatake H, Lamecker H, Lange T, Lee J, Lennon B, Li R, Li S, Meinzer H-P, Nemeth G, Raicu DS, Rau A-M, van Rikxoort EM, Rousson M, Rusko L, Saddi KA, Schmidt G, Seghers D, Shimizu A, Slagmolen P, Sorantin E, Soza G, Susomboon R, Waite JM, Wimmer A, Wolf I (2009) Comparison and evaluation of methods for liver segmentation from CT datasets. IEEE Trans Med Imaging 28(8):1251–1265

Biography

Ahmed Afifi was born in Menofia, Egypt, in January 1980. He received BSc and MSc degrees from Menofia University, Menofia, Egypt, in 2000 and 2005, respectively, and PhD degree from Chiba University, Japan, in 2011. He is currently a lecturer in Computer Science Department, Faculty of Computers and Information, Menofia University, Egypt, since 2011. His research interests include medical image processing, pattern recognition, and computer vision.

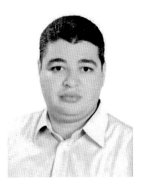

Toshiya Nakaguchi was born in Hyogo Prefecture, Japan, in April 1975. He received B.E., M.E., and Ph.D. degrees from Sophia University, Tokyo, Japan, in 1998, 2000, and 2003, respectively. He was a research fellow supported by Japan Society for the Promotion of Science from April 2001 to March 2003. He moved to the Department of Information and Image Sciences, Chiba University, in April 2003, as an assistant professor. From 2006 to 2007, he was a research fellow in Center of Excellence in Visceral Biomechanics and Pain, in Aalborg, Denmark, supported by CIRIUS, Danish Ministry of Education. He is currently an associate professor in the Department of Medical System Engineering, Chiba University, Japan, since 2010. His research interests include medical engineering, color image processing, and computer vision and computer graphics. Dr. Nakaguchi is a member of the IEEE; IS&T; the Japanese Society of Medical Imaging Technology (JAMIT); the Institute of Electronics, Information and Communication Engineers (IEICE), Japan; and Society of Photographic Science and Technology of Japan.

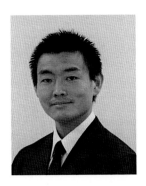

CT Imaging Characteristics
of Hepatocellular Carcinoma

Masahiro Okada and Takamichi Murakami

Abstract Computed tomography (CT) is essential for the diagnosis of liver tumors. In the CT criteria of hypervascular hepatocellular carcinoma (HCC), the diagnosis is based on hemodynamic findings, such as arterial enhancement, followed by washout in the portal-venous and/or equilibrium phase. In this chapter, typical and atypical findings (HCC mimickers) of HCC on CT and current diagnostic techniques to image HCC were stated.

Focus Points

1. Dynamic CT with an intravenous bolus injection of contrast medium is essential to diagnose HCC.
2. Four-phase imaging (unenhanced, arterial, portal-venous, and equilibrium phases) on liver dynamic CT is usually performed to diagnose HCC.
3. A characteristic enhancement pattern consisting of arterial enhancement and the corresponding washout at portal-venous and equilibrium phases are very important for the diagnosis of HCC.

Introduction

Hepatocellular carcinoma (HCC) is the fifth most common tumor in the world, and the incidence of HCC is rising [1, 2]. The majority of HCCs develop in cirrhotic livers, and the early detection and characterization of this entity is important for decisions on therapeutic strategy. Several therapeutic methods are currently used for patients with HCC. Patients diagnosed with HCC are candidates for curative

M. Okada, M.D., Ph.D. (✉) • T. Murakami, M.D., Ph.D.
Department of Radiology, Kinki University Faculty of Medicine, 377-2 Ohno-Higashi,
Osaka-Sayama, Osaka 589-8511, Japan
e-mail: mokada@gaia.eonet.ne.jp

A.S. El-Baz et al. (eds.), *Abdomen and Thoracic Imaging: An Engineering & Clinical Perspective*, DOI 10.1007/978-1-4614-8498-1_12,
© Springer Science+Business Media New York 2014

treatment options, such as surgical resection and liver transplantation. Radio-frequency ablation (RFA) has become one of the most widely used procedures for the treatment of HCC. In the cases of many or large hypervascular lesions in the liver, transcatheter arterial chemoembolization (TACE) is a useful procedure. Molecular-targeted drug, such as sorafenib, is a new therapy of active multikinase inhibitor with effects on tumor-cell proliferation and tumor angiogenesis and allows to demonstrate superior survival in patients with advanced HCCs.

Sonography is frequently the first examination and can be sensitive in detecting HCC but depending on the operator. MRI has superior contrast resolution and may better detect lesions, but CT is a convenient examination and frequently employed initially because of high throughput of CT examination (short examination time). Nuclear medicine imaging and conventional angiography are less useful for the detection of HCC because of low spatial and contrast resolution.

Multidetector-row computed tomography (MDCT) plays an important role on HCC imaging, because it provides several advantages, such as volumetric study (with higher spatial and time resolution), reduced scan time, reduced motion artifact, and reduced radiation exposure. Moreover, recently advanced CT technology of dual-energy CT has a high potential for liver imaging, including monochromatic image and CT dose reduction.

The diagnostic criteria for HCC are based on the typical hemodynamic pattern of dynamic CT (arterial hypervascularity and washout at portal-venous and/or equilibrium phase), although there are some atypically enhancing HCCs. According to the American Association for the Study of Liver Diseases (AASLD), a liver nodule larger than 1 cm in size in a cirrhotic liver that demonstrates the typical hemodynamic pattern on CT and MRI can be diagnosed as HCC without biopsy. We should follow this international guideline when HCC diagnosis is made on imaging modalities.

Most importantly, we should understand HCC findings of CT on the basis of multistep hepatocarcinogenesis and multistep change of intranodular blood supply of hepatic nodules. Therefore, the balance between arterial flow and portal flow in the nodule is important to diagnose HCC. In this chapter, CT imagings of HCC including atypical findings of HCC and HCC mimickers are discussed. Moreover, we should know optimal scan methods of the liver CT in this article and make diagnosis of HCC correctly.

Etiology of Hepatocellular Carcinoma

There are multiple factors involved in the etiology of HCC. HCC most commonly appears in a patient with chronic viral hepatitis (hepatitis B or hepatitis C) and/or with cirrhosis. Especially, in East Asia, it is related often to viral hepatitis, such as hepatitis C and B, whereas, in western countries, alcohol is the main cause, although virus-related hepatitis increases.

There are some other important factors that contribute to the international burden of HCC. Obesity [3], diabetes [4], heavy use of alcohol [5], and nonalcoholic steatohepatitis [6] are linked with carcinogenesis from non-B non-C liver cirrhosis.

Multistep Hepatocarcinogenesis of Hepatocellular Carcinoma

Increased arterial neovascularization combined with decreased portal blood flow is seen within the hepatic nodules on multistep carcinogenesis from regeneration to HCC. This fact has been reported by using CT during hepatic arteriography (CTHA) and CT during arterial portography (CTAP) [7, 8].

Normal hepatic artery decreased in accordance with increasing grade of malignancy, but abnormal arteries due to tumor angiogenesis developed in high-grade dysplastic nodule (DN) and increased in well-, moderately and poorly differentiated HCCs (Fig. 1). The change of intranodular blood supply occurs during hepatocarcinogenesis.

Microscopic invasion of stroma and portal tracts is important to differentiate HCC from DN [9]. On the multistep carcinogenesis, high-grade DN develops foci of malignancy [9]. Hypervascularity of HCC is a characteristic on imaging, because of progressive sinusoidal capillarization and unpaired artery on pathology [10, 11].

Modern CT Imaging of the Liver

In patients with a suspicion of HCC (such as rising alpha-fetoprotein and protein induced by vitamin K absence or antagonist-II levels), one of the best methods of diagnosis involves a CT scan of the liver using intravenous (IV) contrast agent and a four-phase scanning (unenhanced, arterial phase, portal-venous phase and equilibrium phase) to increase the ability of the diagnostic radiologists to detect small or subtle HCCs.

CT is now widely available and represents an important method for the diagnostics of liver lesions and planning of therapy. Dynamic MDCT with an intravenous bolus injection of contrast medium (CM) is essential to diagnose liver tumor [12, 13]. Diagnostic accuracy of the liver tumors has improved, because MDCT has higher spatial and temporal resolutions by the increase of both gantry rotation speed and the number of detector rows. But rapid scan speed with a MDCT scanner sometimes increases the difficulty to image hypervascular HCC during the arterial phase after CM injection. The optimal technique for IV injection of CM is very important to diagnose HCC. Therefore, we should know the optimal scanning protocol to start in the arterial phase after IV injection of CM.

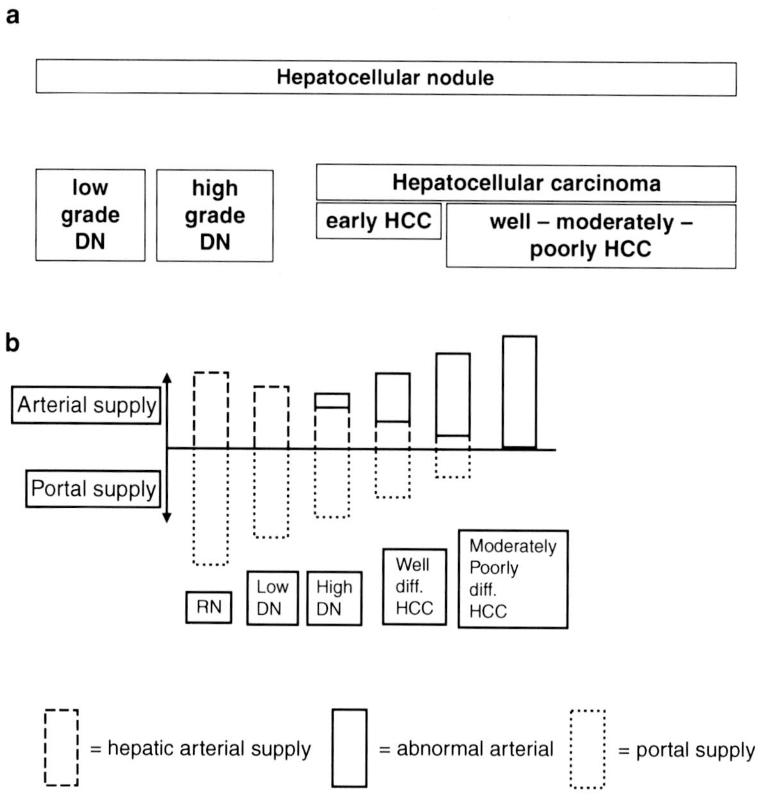

a

b

Fig. 1 (**a**) Terminology of nodular hepatocellular lesions. International Working Party. Hepatology 1995. DN = dysplastic nodule; well-moderately-poorly HCC = well-moderately-poorly differentiated hepatocellular carcinoma (HCC). (**b**) Change of intranodular blood supply on multistep carcinogenesis from regeneration to HCC. RN = regenerative nodule, low DN = low-grade dysplastic nodule, high DN = high-grade dysplastic nodule, well-diff. HCC = well-differentiated HCC, and moderately poorly diff. HCC = moderately or poorly differentiated HCC. Arterial supply is decreasing from RN to high-grade DN and is increasing from well-differentiated HCC to moderately and poorly differentiated HCC because of the proliferation of unpaired (abnormal) arteries, whereas portal supply is gradually decreasing from RN to moderately and poorly differentiated HCC

The arterial phase imaging is useful to detect hypervascular HCC. On arterial phase of liver dynamic CT, there is a good correlation between tumor vascularity on CT and angiography. The portal-venous and equilibrium phases imaging are useful for the differential diagnosis of HCC, because the washout of CM from the tumor in these phases is a typical finding of hypervascular HCC (Fig. 2). On portal-venous and equilibrium phases, a minimum enhancement of 50 Hounsfield units (HU) should be achieved as adequate liver enhancement to obtain high conspicuity of low-attenuated hepatic lesions at the portal-venous and equilibrium phases [14–16].

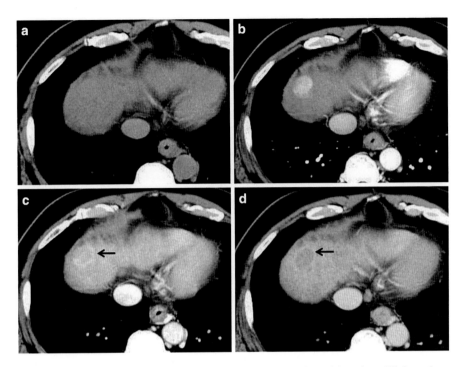

Fig. 2 Unenhanced CT (**a**), arterial phase (**b**), portal-venous phase (**c**), and equilibrium phase (**d**) of the CT show iso-density, hyper-density, washout with hyper-density ring (corona; *arrow*) enhancement, and washout with hyper-density capsule (*arrow*), respectively

However, arterial parenchyma enhancement due to arterioportal venous (AP) shunt may become a false-positive lesion (mimic HCC) on dynamic MDCT that evaluates hemodynamics of liver tumor, and it may sometimes reduce specificity. The finding of washout pattern is useful to distinguish non-tumorous AP shunt from hypervascular HCC, because AP shunt substantially showed no washout of the liver at the portal-venous and equilibrium phases. In other words, HCC shows both focal arterial enhancement and the corresponding washout in the portal and equilibrium phases, but AP shunt shows arterial enhancement alone and wedge-shaped appearance. However, the differentiation between HCC and AP shunt is sometimes difficult because some HCCs (especially small HCCs) do not demonstrate washout.

Scanning through the upper abdomen can be performed in less than 2–3 s by using state-of-the-art MDCT scanners with more than 64 channels, even though a spatial resolution of 0.6 mm is employed for both longitudinal and short axis of the body (transverse slice thickness), so-called isotropic voxel volume imaging. Three-dimensional (3D) images can be reconstructed from the isotropic voxel imaging data by using multiplanar reconstruction (MPR), volume rendering (VR) (Fig. 3), and maximum intensity projection techniques. These 3D images are useful for preoperative anatomical evaluation for surgeons and preoperative explanations for patients [17].

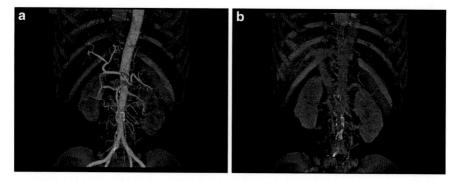

Fig. 3 (**a**) Volume rendering of hepatic arterial phase. Detailed depiction of hepatic arteries (right hepatic artery, left hepatic artery, proper hepatic artery, common hepatic artery) and superior mesenteric artery is obtained during early arterial phase by using CT angiography with intravenous injection of CM. (**b**) Volume rendering of portal-venous phase. Detailed depiction of portal vein system (portal vein, splenic vein, superior mesenteric vein) is obtained during portal-venous phase by using CT angiography with intravenous injection of CM

Scanning Protocol of Liver Dynamic CT to Detect Hepatocellular Carcinoma (Table 1)

A. *Four-phase liver dynamic CT.*

Dynamic CT of the liver is performed by using bolus injection of iodine CM [18–20]. A four-phase (unenhanced CT, arterial phase, portal-venous phase, and equilibrium phase) examination protocol of liver dynamic CT should be employed for the diagnosis of HCC. By the use of different dynamic CT phases, good characterization of hepatic space-occupying lesions can be achieved.

B. *CM injection parameters in the liver dynamic CT.*

It is important to optimize the parameters of the CT examination. There are several important technical factors for the injection of CM, such as volume and concentration of CM, injection rate, injection duration, *body weight* (*BW*), and scan delay time in the hepatic arterial phase. The volume and concentration of CM and the injection rate are directly related to maximum liver enhancement [21–24], whereas patients' BWs are inversely related [25]. A rapid injection of CM is effective for the depiction of hypervascular HCC, when using the same volume and concentration of CM [26, 27]. The concentration and injection rate of CM are important for determining the amplitude of contrast enhancement in artery and hypervascular HCCs during arterial phase. And, the injection duration of CM is also important to predict peak enhancement time in the liver, because it may be the only factor to restrict temporal changes in contrast enhancement. When the alternative of injection rate or injection duration of CM is fixed, the other factor should be variable depending on the patients' BW.

Table 1 Optimal imaging parameters of liver dynamic CT for hypervascular HCC

Total volume and concentration of CM
600 mgI/kg (i.e., 300 mgI/mL, 2 mL/kg) in patients with liver damage
Injection duration of CM
30 s
Injection rate of CM
Total volume of CM/30 s (i.e., 120 mL/30 s = 4 mL/s)
Phases of liver dynamic CT
Arterial phase of dynamic CT
Fixed scan timing, approximately 40 s postinjection of CM
Bolus tracking, approximately 20-s delay after achievement of 100-HU attenuation of the aorta
Portal-venous phase of dynamic CT
Fixed scan timing, approximately 70–90 s postinjection of CM
Bolus tracking, approximately 30-s delay after arterial scanning
Equilibrium phase of dynamic CT
Fixed scan timing, approximately 180–300 s postinjection of CM

Note. HCC Hepatocellular carcinoma, *CM* contrast medium

C. *Scan timing after CM injection for arterial, portal-venous, and equilibrium phases of dynamic CT.*

The injection duration of CM is important to predict peak enhancement time in the liver, because the injection duration of CM is equal to the time of peak aortic enhancement after an arrival of CM to the abdominal aorta; in other words, it may be the only factor to restrict temporal changes in contrast enhancement. When injection duration of 30 s is employed, scanning is substantially made at arterial (approximately 40 s postinjection), portal-venous (approximately 70–90 s postinjection), and equilibrium phases (approximately 180–300 s postinjection) at whole liver containing the tumor. Ichikawa et al. stated that the peak enhancement time of the aorta, portal vein, and liver constantly appears approximately 10, 20, and 30 s after any fixed injection durations (completion of CM injection), respectively [28].

D. *Computer-assisted bolus-tracking technique.*

It is important to predict the peak time of aortic enhancement to achieve optimal detection of HCC at the arterial phase for patients with hypervascular HCC, because blood is supplied to tumors from the hepatic artery (which is a branch of the abdominal aorta). The routine use of computer-assisted bolus-tracking techniques (i.e., SmartPrep®) for hepatic arterial phase scanning is recommended to detect hypervascular HCC [29], because the imaging by bolus-tracking technique is useful to catch the optimal scan timing during hepatic arterial phase in patients with severe cardiac dysfunction.

The scan delay for the arterial phase is about 20 s (i.e., optimal scan delay after a 30-s contrast injection of the hepatic arterial phase ranges from 5 to 10 s for the detection of hypervascular HCCs [30]) for the 16- or 64-MDCT scanner after achievement of 100-HU attenuation of the descending aorta measured with bolus-tracking technique. A certain scan delay after arterial phase acquisition was used for the portal-venous phase acquisition (optimal scan delay after a 30 s contrast injection of the portal venous phase is 35 s after the completion of contrast injection or somewhat longer [30]).

E. *Body weight (BW)-tailored dose (volume x concentration of CM)*.

To achieve adequate liver enhancement for all patients with a wide variety of BW on CT, recent clinical studies have suggested that the dose of CM should be tailored according to patients' BWs, because a fixed dose of CM does not allow the same effects for the contrast enhancement of liver in patients with different BWs [31–33]. The variation in liver enhancement among patients with different BWs is cancelled by using the BW-tailored dose of CM [31]. When a tailored dose of CM according to patients' BW is injected in the liver CT, a fixed injection duration method allows the minimization of the variation in aortic peak enhancement time for each patient [28, 34]. In patients with lighter BW, the injection rate can be reduced without reducing the degree of enhancement in the liver [31]. For the liver dynamic CT, 600 mgI/mL of CM is recommended [35].

American Association for the Study of Liver Diseases

The diagnostic algorithm for suspected HCC by the AASLD guideline states that an imaging diagnosis of HCC should be made if a lesion larger than 1 cm shows a typical vascular enhancement pattern on a single dynamic imaging study (Fig. 4) [36]. For hepatic nodules smaller than 1 cm, repeated sonography at 3 months is recommended to investigate the nodular size. Four-phase MDCT and dynamic contrast-enhanced MRI are recommended in this algorithm as imaging modalities to detect arterial hypervascularity and washout at portal-venous and/or equilibrium phase for hepatic nodules larger than 1 cm. Therefore, confirmation of arterial enhancement and the corresponding washout in the portal and equilibrium phases on dynamic CT is important to diagnose HCC after sonographic detection of hepatic nodule on the screening program. A biopsy is not needed to confirm the diagnosis of HCC if certain imaging criteria are met. When typical findings of HCC, such as arterial hypervascularity and washout at portal-venous and/or equilibrium phase on liver dynamic CT, could not be obtained, other contrast-enhanced imagings or biopsy of hepatic nodules are recommended.

Classification of Nodules in Multistep Hepatocarcinogenesis

1. Regenerative nodule (RN).

Regenerative nodules (RNs) represent a region of parenchyma enlarged in response to necrosis, altered circulation, or other stimuli. In chronic

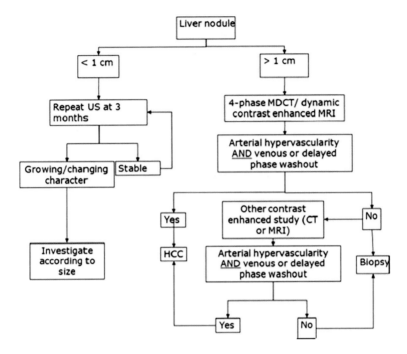

Fig. 4 American Association for the Study of Liver Diseases (AASLD) guideline

hepatitis B, macronodular hepatic nodules (>3 mm in diameter) are substantially seen, although micronodular nodules (<3 mm in diameter) are seen in other causes of cirrhosis. When RNs contain iron, they are substantially hyperattenuation or isoattenuation to the liver on unenhanced CT. Most RNs are difficult to depict on enhanced CT, because they show similar enhancement pattern compared to the surrounding liver parenchyma [37], but RNs may show early enhancement in comparison to or less than the surrounding liver [38]. And on the equilibrium phase, RN may show multiple hypoattenuation nodules which are separated by hyperenhancing fibrous tissue in the liver.

2. *Dysplastic nodule (DN)*.

Dysplastic nodules (DNs) are subclassified on the basis of cellular abnormalities, such as low-grade DN, containing hepatocytes with mild atypia, and high-grade DN, containing hepatocytes with moderate atypia, but insufficient for the diagnosis of malignancy. Low-grade DNs are difficult to distinguish histologically from RNs [9]. High-grade DN is most likely to progress to HCC than is low-grade DN. High-grade DN has pathologic features of increased cell density of this lesion, mild thickened cell plates, and foci of increased cell proliferation. The differentiation between high-grade DN and well-differentiated HCC in the liver cirrhosis can be difficult, because of overlap on imaging. However, rapid interval growth is one of the criteria of malignancy on imaging. DNs containing foci of HCC are considered to be premalignant lesions.

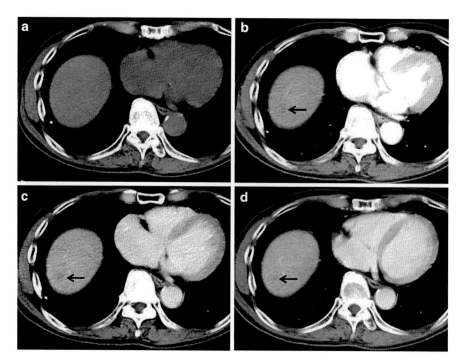

Fig. 5 Low-grade dysplastic nodule. Unenhanced CT (**a**), arterial phase (**b**), portal-venous phase (**c**), and equilibrium phase (**d**) of the CT show iso-density, hypodensity (*arrow*), washout with hypodensity (*arrow*), and washout with hypodensity (*arrow*), respectively

DNs may be detected as hypoattenuation in the arterial and/or portal-venous phase, because of normal or slightly decreased portal-venous supply to the DNs (Fig. 5), although DNs are not seen on imaging as frequently [39]. DNs are usually isoattenuation to the surrounding liver [40]. Lim et al. stated that helical dynamic triple-phase CT including arterial, portal-venous, and delayed phases depicted 14 % of high-grade DNs and 7 % of low-grade DNs [41].

3. *Hepatocellular carcinoma (HCC)*.
   MDCT provides detailed information about tumor vascularization and can also help differentiate its pathological grade noninvasively.

   (a) *Early hepatocellular carcinoma (early HCC)*.
       Tumor cells of early HCC grow in a replacing fashion. And portal tracts may be present in these lesions. The invasion into intralesional portal tracts is seen, and this invasion is called as "stromal invasion." And early HCC does not show distal metastasis. Decrease or disappearance of ductular reaction is important to differentiate early HCC from fibrosis with chronic hepatitis [42]. Stromal invasion of early HCC has the active matrix metalloproteinase-1 (MMP-1) [43].

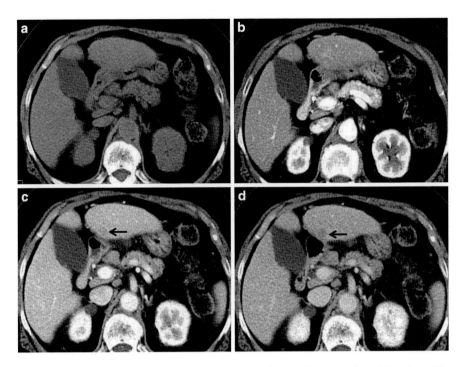

Fig. 6 Early HCC. Unenhanced CT (**a**), arterial phase (**b**), portal-venous phase (**c**), and equilibrium phase (**d**) of the CT show iso-density, iso-density, washout with hypodensity (*arrow*) and washout with hypodensity (*arrow*), respectively

Early detection of early HCC may permit effective treatment and achieve long-term cure, although the natural history of early HCC is not well known. Treatment of early-stage HCC is potentially curative therapy with 5-year survival rates of 50–70 % [44, 45]. Early HCC substantially shows hypovascular tumor and slightly washout on liver dynamic CT (Fig. 6).

It may be difficult to differentiate early HCC from other benign lesions, such as RN and DN. US-assisted biopsy of the lesion can be used to differentiate neoplastic lesions from non-neoplastic lesions.

(b) *Well-differentiated hepatocellular carcinoma (well-differentiated HCC).*

On pathology, microscopic invasion of stroma and portal tracts is the primary diagnostic feature to differentiate well-differentiated HCC from DNs [46]. The diagnosis of well-differentiated HCC can be difficult, commonly requiring examination by several imaging modalities [47, 48]. Well-differentiated HCC has relatively low malignant potential and rarely invades vessels or metastasis to other sites [49]. Fatty changes of tumor tissue were occasionally observed (Fig. 7). Minimal enhancement of the tumor is substantially seen in well-differentiated HCC. Even though HCC is usually considered to be a hypervascular tumor, well-differentiated tumors can be hypovascular tumor.

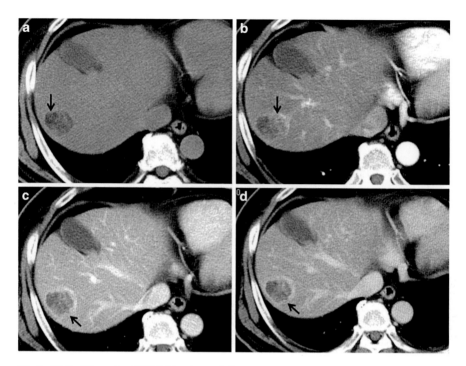

Fig. 7 Well-differentiated HCC. Unenhanced CT (**a**), arterial phase (**b**), portal-venous phase (**c**), and equilibrium phase (**d**) of the CT show hypodensity with fat deposit (*arrow*), hyper-density (arterial enhancement; *arrow*) with hypodensity (fat component), washout with ring enhancement (capsule; *arrow*) and washout with ring enhancement (capsule; *arrow*), respectively

(c) *Moderately   differentiated   hepatocellular   carcinoma   (moderately differentiated HCC).*

Dynamic CT substantially reveals a basket pattern which means hypervascularity of moderately differentiated HCCs (Fig. 8). A peak of enhancement is usually seen at the arterial phase followed by a rapid decrease of enhancement at the portal-venous and equilibrium phases, because moderately differentiated HCC has greater arterial blood supply. Lesions larger than 3 cm are often heterogeneous, with mosaic or mixed pattern arising from intratumoral necrosis, hemorrhage, fatty deposit, and interstitial fibrosis. The appearance of HCC on CT depends on tumor size and histologic tumor grades.

(d) *Poorly differentiated hepatocellular carcinoma (poorly differentiated HCC).*

In poorly differentiated HCC, gradually increasing enhancement over time is substantially seen (Fig. 9). Asayama et al. state that the arterial blood supply of poorly differentiated HCC is lower than that of moderately

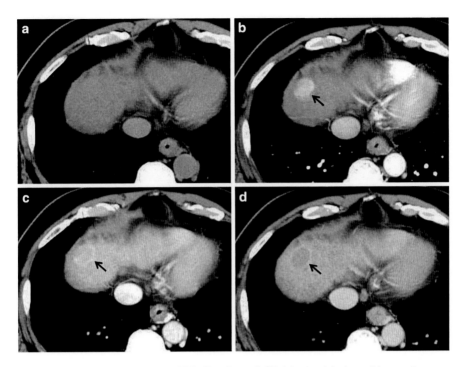

Fig. 8 Moderately differentiated HCC. Unenhanced CT (**a**), arterial phase (**b**), portal-venous phase (**c**), and equilibrium phase (**d**) of the CT show iso-density, hyper-density (arterial enhancement; *arrow*), slight washout with ring enhancement (capsule; *arrow*) and clear washout with ring enhancement (capsule; *arrow*), respectively

differentiated HCC by CT during hepatic angiography. Therefore, the arterial blood supply decreases as the histologic grade progresses in the late stage of HCC development. The enhancement of poorly differentiated HCC shows greater arterial vascularization than that of well-differentiated HCC. The presence of arterial hypervascularization of the poorly differentiated HCCs and some of the moderately differentiated HCCs indicates that lesions with this contrast enhancement pattern are most likely an advanced-to-late stage.

Cirrhosis

CT Features of Liver Cirrhosis

Liver cirrhosis (LC) is one of the most important factors in hepatocarcinogenesis. Liver cirrhosis demonstrates less contrast enhancement of the liver than normal liver and sometimes shows inhomogeneous enhancement because of

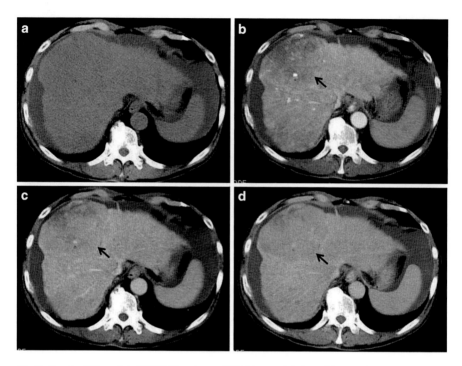

Fig. 9 Poorly differentiated HCC. Unenhanced CT (**a**), arterial phase (**b**), portal-venous phase (**c**), and equilibrium phase (**d**) of the CT show almost iso-density, indistinct hypodensity (hypovascular enhancement; *arrow*), washout (*arrow*) without ring enhancement and washout (*arrow*) without ring enhancement, respectively. Ascites is seen at the subphrenic space

regeneration, fibrosis, and the altered portal-venous flow (Fig. 10). In addition, collateral vessels, such as paraumbilical vein, splenorenal shunt, and esophageal varices, are seen due to portal hypertension. Ascites is also seen in patients with liver cirrhosis.

MDCT Findings of Hepatocellular Carcinoma

The CT appearance of HCC depends on tumor size and histologic grade. Small HCC is defined as nodules smaller than 2–3 cm in size, whereas lesions larger than 3 cm in size are often heterogeneous with a mosaic or mixed pattern arising from a necrosis, fibrosis, fatty degeneration, and hemorrhage [50].

A characteristic enhancement pattern consisting of hyperenhancement in the arterial phase and washout in the portal-venous or equilibrium phase is associated

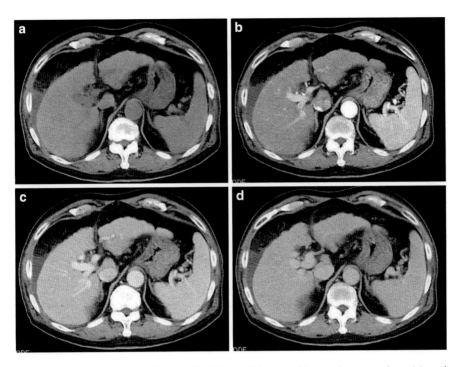

Fig. 10 Liver cirrhosis. Unenhanced CT (**a**), arterial phase (**b**), portal-venous phase (**c**), and equilibrium phase (**d**) of the CT show peripheral irregularity of the liver, splenomegaly, and ascites at the subphrenic space. No tumor is seen in the liver

with high specificity (nearly 100 %) for the diagnosis of HCC. But dynamic CT with extracellular CM has some diagnostic limitations related to tumor size. Hepatic nodules larger than 1 cm in diameter show high accuracy of hypervascular HCCs in a cirrhotic liver, although it is difficult to diagnose subcentimeter HCCs [36]. Therefore, the confirmation by biopsy is sometimes required for questionable hepatic nodules to determine the diagnosis. Thus, the key characteristics of HCC on CT are hypervascularity in the arterial phase scans, washout in the portal and equilibrium phase studies, a pseudocapsule, and a mosaic pattern. Both calcifications and intralesional fat may be appreciated.

There is insufficient diagnostic performance for the early detection of both small and early HCCs even with state-of-the-art CT. Gadoxetic acid disodium (gadolinium ethoxybenzyl diethylenetriaminepentaacetic acid, Gd-EOB-DTPA; PRIMOVIST® Bayer Schering Pharma AG, Berlin, Germany) is a hepatocyte-specific MR contrast agent. Gd-EOB-DTPA-enhanced MRI is a promising examination to diagnose small HCC [51] and depicts early HCCs, such as well-differentiated HCC, in the early stage of hepatocarcinogenesis, because Gd-EOB-DTPA has the properties of an extracellular gadolinium chelate, as well as being a hepatocyte-targeting agent. Gd-EOB-DTPA-enhanced MRI enables hepatocyte-phase imaging to start 10–20 min postinjection. Therefore, additional dynamic imaging modality, such as Gd-EOB-DTPA-enhanced MRI, is recommended, when liver dynamic CT shows indeterminable result in the diagnostic process of HCCs [36].

Characteristic Features of Hepatocellular Carcinoma on Dynamic CT

Unenhanced CT substantially shows a hypodense nodule. Arterial phase of dynamic CT reveals arterial hypervascularity, because hypervascular HCC has greater arterial blood supply. Arterial hypervascularity of HCC is followed by washout at the portal-venous and equilibrium phases (Figs. 2 and 8). And fibrous capsule around tumor is sometimes seen in the case of large (>2 cm in size) HCC (Table 2) (Figs. 2 and 8). This fibrous capsule is enhanced at portal-venous phase and equilibrium phase, because fibrous tissue substantially shows delayed enhancement.

On liver dynamic multiphase CT, unenhanced image acquisitions are carried out at baseline and then after intravenous bolus administration of iodinated CM. According to the clinical query, the most appropriate injection protocol should be chosen. In many countries including Japan, four-phase liver dynamic CT is substantially used for the examination of hypervascular HCC. And the higher tumor-to-liver contrast in the dynamic CT is required for the detection and characterization of HCC. It is believed that the minimum difference of approximately 10 HU between hepatic nodules and surrounding liver is needed to detect the nodules.

Mosaic pattern is composed of the variable tissue composition of HCC. Enhancing nodules in HCC indicate viable tumor cells, and low attenuation areas represent necrosis, fibrosis, or hemorrhage [52].

Nodule-in-nodule appearance is consisted of histologically different components, such as moderately differentiated HCC and well-differentiated HCC or dysplastic nodule with malignant focus. Thus, these mosaic pattern and nodule-in-nodule appearance are often used in conjunction with hypervascularity at arterial phase, washout at portal-venous and equilibrium phases, and fibrous capsule around tumor as characteristic features of HCC (Table 3).

Table 2 Important findings of liver dynamic CT for hypervascular HCC

- Early enhancement during the arterial phase and washout (lower attenuation than surrounding liver parenchyma) during the portal-venous and/or equilibrium phases in contrast-enhanced CT
- Persistent enhancing fibrous capsule around tumor during the portal-venous and/or equilibrium phases

Table 3 Characteristic features of HCC

• Arterial enhancement (washin) and washout
• Mosaic appearance
• Nodule-in-nodule appearance
• Capsule or pseudocapsule

Vascular Invasion

Vascular invasion and histopathologic grading are identified as prognostic parameters. Vascular invasion is found to be more common in poorly differentiated HCC and diffuse type HCC. This is thought to be related to the portal-venous drainage of HCC. The rates of vascular invasion are reported as significantly lower in patients with well-differentiated tumors when compared with moderately and poorly differentiated tumors [53].

Relatively high rate of HCC invasion into the portal vein is found in patients with advanced HCCs, and this portal invasion is classified as Vp0 (none), Vp1 (microscopic), Vp2 (into the segmental branch), and Vp3 (into the lobar vein or the main trunk) in Japan [54].

Uncommon Features

Hepatocellular Carcinoma Mimics

1. Arterial portal shunting.
   Shunts rarely show delayed washout on post-contrast image (Fig. 11), although chronic shunts give damage in the shunting area and may show slightly washout. And shunts may demonstrate vessels through them and wedge-shaped appearance.
2. Focal nodular hyperplasia (FNH) or FNH-like nodule.
   FNH-like nodule is seen in the chronic liver disease and disorder of intrahepatic blood flow [55], although FNH is seen in non-cirrhotic liver. FNH is a benign and generally asymptomatic hepatic tumor, whereas focal nodular hyperplasia-like nodules (FNH-like nodules) are focal lesions occurring in liver cirrhosis and are morphologically very similar to classical FNH in an otherwise normal liver. They are sometimes misdiagnosed as HCC on CT imaging because both types of lesions show arterial phase enhancement. FNH and FNH-like nodule usually appear homogeneous, well defined, and hypoattenuating or isoattenuating relative to the liver at unenhanced CT (Fig. 12), and they classically demonstrate intense early enhancement and may show isoattenuating relative to the liver at

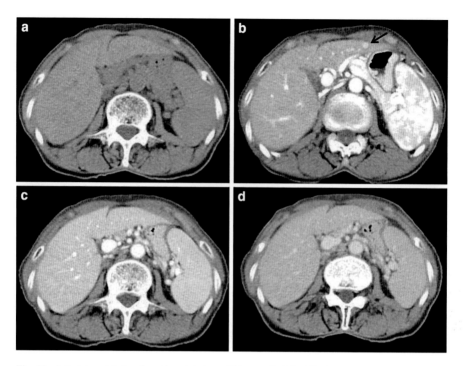

Fig. 11 Arterial portal shunting. Arterial phase ((**b**) *arrow*) of the CT shows small enhancement in the lateral segment of the left lobe, although other phases ((**a**) unenhanced CT, (**c**) portal-venous phase, and (**d**) equilibrium phase) have iso-density of the region

delayed scans. A central scar (if present) may demonstrate delayed enhancement.

3. Liver hemangioma.

   Liver hemangioma shows peripheral globular enhancement, progression of enhancement toward the center of the nodule at arterial phase and portal-venous phase (filling in phenomenon), and persistence of enhancement at equilibrium phase in contrast-enhanced CT (Fig. 13). This is the key point of the differential diagnosis between liver hemangioma and HCC, because HCC shows washout at equilibrium phase. It is rarely difficult to differentiate small hemangiomas (especially high-flow hemangioma) and small HCC on liver dynamic CT.

4. Hypervascular liver metastasis.

   Hypervascular liver metastases include primary tumors such as neuroendocrine/islet cell tumor, carcinoid, renal cell carcinoma, melanoma, and thyroid carcinoma. Most metastases appear hypoattenuating at unenhanced CT, although neuroendocrine tumor metastases may appear hyperattenuating at unenhanced CT. Most hypervascular metastases show early enhancement of viable tumor at arterial phase and become mild hyper- to mild hypoattenuation to the liver in portal-venous phase (Fig. 14).

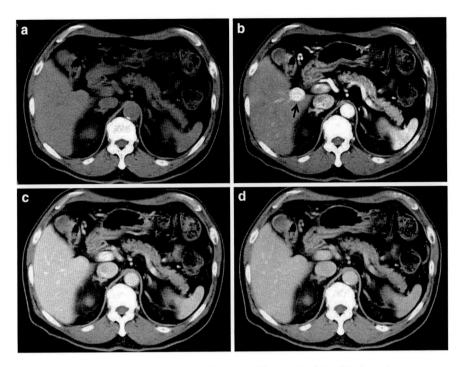

Fig. 12 Focal nodular hyperplasia. Arterial phase ((**b**) *arrow*) of the CT shows homogeneous enhancement in the segment 5/6 of the right lobe, although other phases [(**a**) unenhanced CT, (**c**) portal-venous phase, and (**d**) equilibrium phase] have iso-density of the tumor

Hepatic Perfusion CT

CT can be used not only to image anatomical structure but also to analyze liver function. CT perfusion is performed by serial images after the administration of a bolus of iodinated contrast agent, enabling detailed analysis of liver hemodynamics. The impulse residue function (IRF) of a localized bolus in hepatic blood flow is fundamental to perfusion CT. The passage of contrast agent enables the calculation of a TDC and is shown as the IRF. Mathematically, IRF is calculated as a tissue curve. CT perfusion is obtained by monitoring the first pass through the vasculature after bolus injection of an iodinated contrast agent. Perfusion technique with dynamic contrast enhancement can enable the quantitative analysis of not only liver tissue vascularity but also HCC vascularity (Fig. 15). As an example, perfusion CT is performed by the acquisition of serial images of the same slice level after a bolus administration of 30–40 mL of iodinated contrast medium [56]. Patients with hypervascular HCC show the high blood volume and blood flow and short transit time [57].

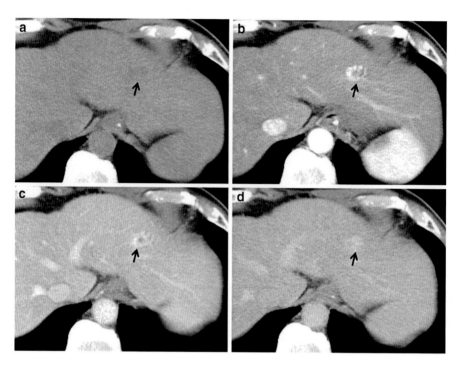

Fig. 13 Liver hemangioma. Unenhanced CT (**a**), arterial phase (**b**), portal-venous phase (**c**), and equilibrium phase (**d**) of the CT show slightly low-density, peripheral globular enhancement, progression of enhancement toward the center of the nodule, and persistence of enhancement, respectively. *Arrows* show liver hemangioma in the lateral segment of the left lobe

CT perfusion is employed to calculate hepatic blood flow by using a color-encoded display of parameters from the liver time–density curve (TDC), with iodine contrast agent. Hepatic perfusion CT enables analysis of the measurement of following: tissue blood flow (TBF, mL/min/100 g); tissue blood volume (TBV, mL/100 g); mean transit time (MTT, sec), which is the average time for blood elements to traverse the vasculature from arterial inlet to venous outlet (proportional to perfusion pressure); and hepatic arterial fraction (HAF; %), which is the ratio of arterial perfusion to total liver perfusion. Thus, liver functional maps are calculated by the input function based on regions of interest (ROIs) set on the aorta and portal vein. The passage of contrast material through blood vessels enables the calculation of the TDC. In postprocessing software of CT perfusion, a deconvolution-based method has become widely used for liver perfusion CT imaging [56, 58]. Enhancement of the abdominal aorta is used as a substitute for hepatic artery input.

CT perfusion is a feasible technique for quantifying tumor vascularity and angiogenesis in advanced HCC [59] and depicts tumor vascular physiology in patients with HCC. Thus CT perfusion can be used for detection of tumor

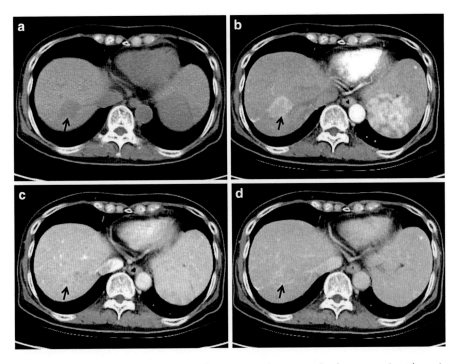

Fig. 14 Hypervascular liver metastases from pancreatic neuroendocrine tumor (gastrinoma). Unenhanced CT ((**a**) *arrow*) of the CT shows irregular low-density tumor in the segment 8 of the right lobe. Arterial phase ((**b**) *arrow*) of the CT shows heterogeneous enhancement in the segment 8 of the right lobe. Portal-venous phase (**c**) and equilibrium phase (**d**) of the CT show heterogeneous enhancement (slightly high-density; *arrows*) in the segment 8 of the right lobe

angiogenesis and in assessing response to antiangiogenic treatment for various cancers [60]. Great impact of perfusion CT has been shown in the assessment of patients with HCC, especially that of tumor response to antiangiogenic drugs, such as sorafenib (Nexavar, Bayer Schering Pharma AG, Berlin, Germany) [61, 62].

Iterative Reconstruction

Iterative reconstruction (IR) is a statistical reconstruction method that may be influenced by high background activity such as in the liver. IR technique, such as Adaptive Statistical iterative Reconstruction (ASiR) of GE healthcare, solves this by subtracting noise, not merely masking it [63].

CT image quality is strongly proportional to radiation dose. Several parameters, such as milliamperage (mA), exposure time, peak kilovoltage (kVp), and pitch, are

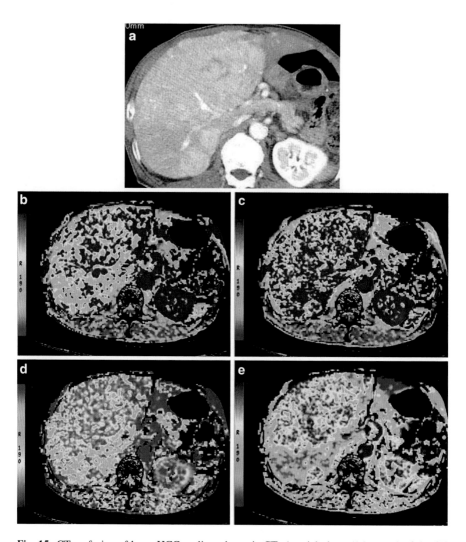

Fig. 15 CT perfusion of large HCC on liver dynamic CT. Arterial phase ((**a**) arrow) of the CT shows huge enhancement of hypervascular HCC in the entire right lobe. Tissue blood flow (**b**), tissue blood volume (**c**), mean transit time (**d**), and hepatic arterial fraction (**e**) show hepatic perfusion parameters as liver imaging function

adjusted based on the relation between the benefit and risk to patients. In general, CT characteristics are largely determined by peak tube voltage (kVp), which determines the upper limit of X-ray energy, and tube current (mA). Images obtained with low-voltage X-rays contain a high degree of noise, although this is alleviated by increasing the tube current. IR technique enables a reduction in radiation dose compared with the usual filtered back-projection algorithm, alternatively, enables a reduction in image noise when employed at the same radiation dose as that for the filtered back-projection. Generally, dose reduction causes an increase in noise and image artifacts. But, IR delivers enhance image quality by improved low contrast detectability whilst preserving anatomical detail.

Volume Helical Shuttle

The volume helical shuttle (VHS) is a breakthrough technique for liver imaging. Hypervascular HCC can be analyzed by using several whole liver scans, such as 12 phases in the arterial phase of dynamic CT (Fig. 16). We performed the world's first VHS CT scan for dynamic CT angiography and also for liver- and brain-perfusion studies, with high temporal resolution. VHS scan technique that we have developed with GE healthcare can provide almost real-time hemodynamic change by shuttling the CT scanning cradle back and forth during scanning, and also enables wider coverage for complete organ imaging: >120 mm longitudinally [64]. Thus, VHS offers dynamic blood flow studies, leading to a new concept termed "four-dimensional (4D) CT."

Dual-Energy CT

Dual-energy CT is a promising technique used to obtain material-specific images, because it makes possible the differentiation of materials and tissues in images obtained based on the differences in iodine and water densities. Dual-energy CT has been shown to have improved ability to detect contrast agent and to distinguish high-density substances created by iodine from those created by calcium or other substances. Postprocessing algorithms enable subtraction of iodine maps from dual-energy CT data (e.g., subtraction of calcification) to create a virtual noncontrast image. Dual-energy CT can be used with multidetector CT as current clinical settings, and the technology is based on the simultaneous acquisition of two data sets (high and low energy). Finally dual-energy CT allows to create accurate material decomposition images and monochromatic spectral images with energy from 40 to 140 k-electron voltage (keV). CT images at 80 kVp or the equivalent 55 keV monochromatic images may show a higher contrast-to-noise ratio for hypervascular HCCs because the attenuation value of iodine increases with the use of low-voltage X-rays [65]. Monochromatic images reconstructed from dual-energy CT data may provide some improvement of detection of hypervascular HCCs.

Several previous studies have employed dual-energy CT for clinical use in the abdominal region [66–68] and thus are useful for the detection and characterization of renal stones [69]. Dual-energy CT allows to increase the sensitivity of imaging of hypervascularized and hypovascularized liver lesions, and by the use of virtual native imaging, it has become possible to avoid additional native imaging which

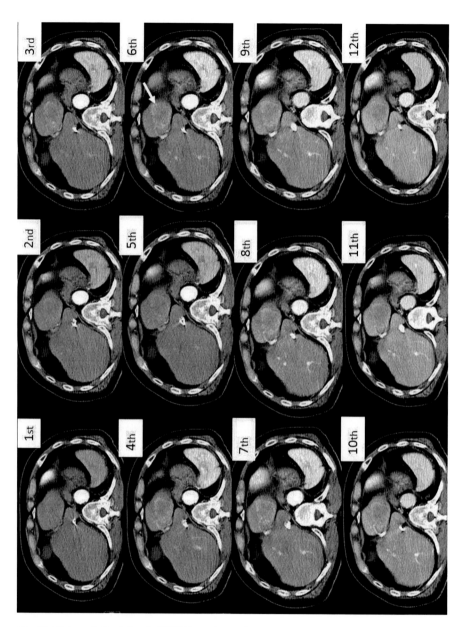

Fig. 16 Volume helical shuttle (VHS) in patients with small HCC. 1st, 1st phase; 2nd, 2nd phase; 3rd, 3rd phase; 4th, 4th phase; 5th, 5th phase; 6th, 6th phase; 7th, 7th phase; 8th, 8th phase; 9th, 9th phase; 10th, 10th phase; 11th, 11th phase; 12th, 12th phase. A HCC located in segment 2 of the liver shows arterial enhancement of tumor, and the enhancement gradually increased from 1st phase to 9th phase of VHS in this case. At 6th phase of VHS shows the peak tumor-to-liver contrast (*arrow*)

reduces the X-ray exposition of patients. Moreover, dual-energy CT provides an accurate method of quantitating liver iron [70], offers more specific tissue characterization, and can improve the assessment of vascular disease [71].

Low-Tube Voltage CT

The standard CT setting for liver imaging includes multiphase CT scans at 120 kVp with bolus injection of contrast media. Low-tube voltage CT is a promising method for obtaining higher contrast of HCCs in the dynamic CT (Fig. 17), because iodinated contrast media provide greater X-ray attenuation (higher conspicuity of hepatic lesions) with low-tube voltage through an increased photoelectric effect [72, 73]. When low-voltage X-rays (such as 80 kVp) are used, iodine contrast agents are more conspicuous at low- than at high-tube voltage settings, although there is high image noise in large patients [74]. The increased noise of low-voltage X-ray scanning may be a problem, because the density of the liver is relatively homogeneous. Therefore, maintaining an appropriate signal-to-noise ratio (SNR) in low-voltage raw data is an important factor in dual-energy scanning. Beam hardening artifact is greater on low-voltage than on 120 kVp X-ray images, so a technique with reduced beam hardening in the images is desirable, such as monochromatic images made by dual-energy scanning. ASiR can improve SNR and reduce beam hardening in the low-tube voltage CT.

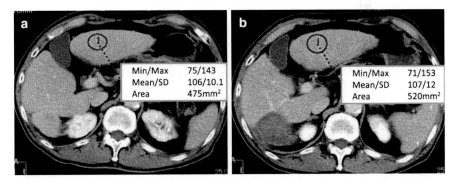

Fig. 17 Comparison between 100 and 120 kVp of CT tube voltage on the equilibrium phase of liver dynamic CT. This is a case of HCC before and post RFA. Liver parenchymal enhancement after injection of contrast agent (600 mgI/kg), with 120 kVp of CT setting. Because ASIR was used for the lower KVp CT, CT value of the liver with 100 kVp and low amount of contrast medium (480 mgI/kg) is similar to that with 120 kVp and high amount of contrast medium. By using ASIR, 100 kV CT shows the same noise level (SD) as 120 kVp CT. Mean/SD of CT value for 120 kVp (a) and 100 kVp (b) is 106/12 and 107/12 HU

Conclusion

We described typical and atypical findings of HCC on liver dynamic CT and introduced new CT technologies to image and analyze HCC. It is important to understand liver dynamic CT examinations for the strategy of HCC therapy.

References

1. Bosch FX, Ribes J, Diaz M, Cleries R (2004) Primary liver cancer: worldwide incidence and trends. Gastroenterology 127(5 Suppl 1):S5–S16
2. Marrero JA, Welling T (2009) Modern diagnosis and management of hepatocellular carcinoma. Clin Liver Dis 13:233–247
3. Calle EE, Rodriguez C, Walker-Thurmond K, Thun MJ (2003) Overweight, obesity, and mortality from cancer in a prospectively studied cohort of U.S. adults. N Engl J Med 348:1625–1638
4. El-Serag HB, Tran T, Everhart JE (2004) Diabetes increases the risk of chronic liver disease and hepatocellular carcinoma. Gastroenterology 126:460–468
5. Chen CJ, Yu MW, Liaw YF (1997) Epidemiological characteristics and risk factors of hepatocellular carcinoma. J Gastroenterol Hepatol 12:S294–S308
6. Marrero JA, Fontana RJ, Su GL, Conjeevaram HS, Emick DM, Lok AS (2002) NAFLD may be a common underlying liver disease in patients with hepatocellular carcinoma in the United States. Hepatology 36:1349–1354
7. Matsui O (2004) Imaging of multistep human hepatocarcinogenesis by CT during intra-arterial contrast injection. Intervirology 47:271–276
8. Hayashi M, Matsui O, Ueda K et al (1999) Correlation between the blood supply and grade of malignancy of hepatocellular nodules associated with liver cirrhosis: evaluation by CT during intraarterial injection of contrast medium. AJR Am J Roentgenol 172:969–976
9. Hanna RF, Aguirre DA, Kased N, Emery SC, Peterson MR, Sirlin CB (2008) Cirrhosis-associated hepatocellular nodules: correlation of histopathologic and MR imaging features. Radiographics 28:747–769
10. Park YN, Yang CP, Fernandez GJ, Cubukcu O, Thung SN, Theise ND (1998) Neoangiogenesis and sinusoidal "capillarization" in dysplastic nodules of the liver. Am J Surg Pathol 22:656–662
11. Roncalli M, Roz E, Coggi G et al (1999) The vascular profile of regenerative and dysplastic nodules of the cirrhotic liver: implications for diagnosis and classification. Hepatology 30:1174–1178
12. Murakami T, Onishi H, Mikami K et al (2006) Determining the optimal timing for early arterial phase hepatic CT imaging by measuring abdominal aortic enhancement in variable contrast injection protocols. J Comput Assist Tomogr 30:206–211
13. Noguchi Y, Murakami T, Kim T et al (2003) Detection of hepatocellular carcinoma: comparison of dynamic MR imaging with dynamic double arterial phase helical CT. AJR Am J Roentgenol 180:455–460
14. Walkey MM (1991) Dynamic hepatic CT: how many years will it take 'til we learn? Radiology 181:17–18
15. Brink JA, Heiken JP, Forman HP, Sagel SS, Molina PL, Brown PC (1995) Hepatic spiral CT: reduction of dose of intravenous contrast material. Radiology 197:83–88
16. Heiken JP, Brink JA, McClennan BL, Sagel SS, Crowe TM, Gaines MV (1995) Dynamic incremental CT: effect of volume and concentration of contrast material and patient weight on hepatic enhancement. Radiology 195:353–357

17. Takahashi S, Murakami T, Takamura M et al (2002) Multi-detector row helical CT angiography of hepatic vessels: depiction with dual-arterial phase acquisition during single breath hold. Radiology 222:81–88
18. Tada S, Fukud K, Aoyagi Y, Harada J (1980) CT of abdominal malignancies: dynamic approach. AJR Am J Roentgenol 135:455–461
19. Young SW, Turner RJ, Castellino RA (1980) A strategy for the contrast enhancement of malignant tumors using dynamic computed tomography and intravascular pharmacokinetics. Radiology 137:137–147
20. Araki T, Itai Y, Furui S, Tasaka A (1980) Dynamic CT densitometry of hepatic tumors. AJR Am J Roentgenol 135:1037–1043
21. Dean PB, Violante MR, Mahoney JA (1980) Hepatic CT contrast enhancement: effect of dose, duration of infusion, and time elapsed following infusion. Invest Radiol 15:158–161
22. Berland LL, Lee JY (1988) Comparison of contrast media injection rates and volumes for hepatic dynamic incremented computed tomography. Invest Radiol 23:918–922
23. Claussen CD, Banzer D, Pfretzschner C, Kalender WA, Schorner W (1984) Bolus geometry and dynamics after intravenous contrast medium injection. Radiology 153:365–368
24. Yagyu Y, Awai K, Inoue M et al (2005) MDCT of hypervascular hepatocellular carcinomas: a prospective study using contrast materials with different iodine concentrations. Am J Roentgenol 184:1535–1540
25. Kormano M, Partanen K, Soimakallio S, Kivimaki T (1983) Dynamic contrast enhancement of the upper abdomen: effect of contrast medium and body weight. Invest Radiol 18:364–367
26. Awai K, Inoue M, Yagyu Y et al (2004) Moderate versus high concentration of contrast material for aortic and hepatic enhancement and tumor-to-liver contrast at multi-detector row CT. Radiology 233:682–688
27. Han JK, Kim AY, Lee KY et al (2000) Factors influencing vascular and hepatic enhancement at CT: experimental study on injection protocol using a canine model. J Comput Assist Tomogr 24:400–406
28. Ichikawa T, Erturk SM, Araki T (2006) Multiphasic contrast-enhanced multidetector-row CT of liver: contrast-enhancement theory and practical scan protocol with a combination of fixed injection duration and patients' body-weight-tailored dose of contrast material. Eur J Radiol 58:165–176
29. Tomemori T, Yamakado K, Nakatsuka A, Sakuma H, Matsumura K, Takeda K (2001) Fast 3D dynamic MR imaging of the liver with MR SmartPrep: comparison with helical CT in detecting hypervascular hepatocellular carcinoma. Clin Imaging 25:355–361
30. Kanematsu M, Goshima S, Kondo H et al (2005) Optimizing scan delays of fixed duration contrast injection in contrast-enhanced biphasic multidetector-row CT for the liver and the detection of hypervascular hepatocellular carcinoma. J Comput Assist Tomogr 29:195–201
31. Awai K, Hiraishi K, Hori S (2004) Effect of contrast material injection duration and rate on aortic peak time and peak enhancement at dynamic CT involving injection protocol with dose tailored to patient weight. Radiology 230:142–150
32. Awai K, Hori S (2003) Effect of contrast injection protocol with dose tailored to patient weight and fixed injection duration on aortic and hepatic enhancement at multidetector-row helical CT. Eur Radiol 13:2155–2160
33. Kondo H, Kanematsu M, Goshima S et al (2008) Abdominal multidetector CT in patients with varying body fat percentages: estimation of optimal contrast material dose. Radiology 249:872–877
34. Erturk SM, Ichikawa T, Sou H, Tsukamoto T, Motosugi U, Araki T (2008) Effect of duration of contrast material injection on peak enhancement times and values of the aorta, main portal vein, and liver at dynamic MDCT with the dose of contrast medium tailored to patient weight. Clin Radiol 63:263–271
35. Yamashita Y, Komohara Y, Takahashi M et al (2000) Abdominal helical CT: evaluation of optimal doses of intravenous contrast material—a prospective randomized study. Radiology 216:718–723

36. Bruix J, Sherman M (2011) Management of hepatocellular carcinoma: an update. Hepatology 53:1020–1022
37. Brancatelli G, Federle MP, Ambrosini R et al (2007) Cirrhosis: CT and MR imaging evaluation. Eur J Radiol 61:57–69
38. Krinsky GA, Lee VS (2000) MR imaging of cirrhotic nodules. Abdom Imaging 25:471–482
39. Baron RL, Peterson MS (2001) From the RSNA refresher courses: screening the cirrhotic liver for hepatocellular carcinoma with CT and MR imaging: opportunities and pitfalls. Radiographics 21(Spec No(32)):S117–S132
40. Lim JH, Cho JM, Kim EY, Park CK (2000) Dysplastic nodules in liver cirrhosis: evaluation of hemodynamics with CT during arterial portography and CT hepatic arteriography. Radiology 214:869–874
41. Lim JH, Kim MJ, Park CK, Kang SS, Lee WJ, Lim HK (2004) Dysplastic nodules in liver cirrhosis: detection with triple phase helical dynamic CT. Br J Radiol 77:911–916
42. Park YN, Kojiro M, Di Tommaso L et al (2007) Ductular reaction is helpful in defining early stromal invasion, small hepatocellular carcinomas, and dysplastic nodules. Cancer 109:915–923
43. Okazaki I, Wada N, Nakano M et al (1997) Difference in gene expression for matrix metalloproteinase-1 between early and advanced hepatocellular carcinomas. Hepatology 25:580–584
44. Llovet JM, Schwartz M, Mazzaferro V (2005) Resection and liver transplantation for hepatocellular carcinoma. Semin Liver Dis 25:181–200
45. Llovet JM, Burroughs A, Bruix J (2003) Hepatocellular carcinoma. Lancet 362:1907–1917
46. International Consensus Group for Hepatocellular Neoplasia (2009) Pathologic diagnosis of early hepatocellular carcinoma: a report of the international consensus group for hepatocellular neoplasia. Hepatology 49:658–664
47. Kim MJ, Choi JY, Chung YE, Choi SY (2008) Magnetic resonance imaging of hepatocellular carcinoma using contrast media. Oncology 75(Suppl 1):72–82
48. Imai Y, Murakami T, Yoshida S et al (2000) Superparamagnetic iron oxide-enhanced magnetic resonance images of hepatocellular carcinoma: correlation with histological grading. Hepatology 32:205–212
49. Sugihara S, Nakashima O, Kojiro M, Majima Y, Tanaka M, Tanikawa K (1992) The morphologic transition in hepatocellular carcinoma. A comparison of the individual histologic features disclosed by ultrasound-guided fine-needle biopsy with those of autopsy. Cancer 70:1488–1492
50. Choi BI, Kim CW, Han MC et al (1989) Sonographic characteristics of small hepatocellular carcinoma. Gastrointest Radiol 14:255–261
51. Onishi H, Kim T, Imai Y et al (2012) Hypervascular hepatocellular carcinomas: detection with gadoxetate disodium-enhanced MR imaging and multiphasic multidetector CT. Eur Radiol 845–854
52. Stevens WR, Gulino SP, Batts KP, Stephens DH, Johnson CD (1996) Mosaic pattern of hepatocellular carcinoma: histologic basis for a characteristic CT appearance. J Comput Assist Tomogr 20:337–342
53. Jonas S, Bechstein WO, Steinmuller T et al (2001) Vascular invasion and histopathologic grading determine outcome after liver transplantation for hepatocellular carcinoma in cirrhosis. Hepatology 33:1080–1086
54. Todo S, Furukawa H (2004) Living donor liver transplantation for adult patients with hepatocellular carcinoma: experience in Japan. Ann Surg 240:451–459
55. Quaglia A, Tibballs J, Grasso A et al (2003) Focal nodular hyperplasia-like areas in cirrhosis. Histopathology 42:14–21
56. Cuenod C, Leconte I, Siauve N et al (2001) Early changes in liver perfusion caused by occult metastases in rats: detection with quantitative CT. Radiology 218:556–561

57. Hashimoto K, Murakami T, Dono K et al (2007) Quantitative tissue blood flow measurement of the liver parenchyma: comparison between xenon CT and perfusion CT. Dig Dis Sci 52:943–949

58. Cenic A, Nabavi DG, Craen RA, Gelb AW, Lee TY (1999) Dynamic CT measurement of cerebral blood flow: a validation study. Am J Neuroradiol 20:63–73

59. Sahani DV, Holalkere NS, Mueller PR, Zhu AX (2007) Advanced hepatocellular carcinoma: CT perfusion of liver and tumor tissue—initial experience. Radiology 243:736–743

60. Ma SH, Le HB, Jia BH et al (2008) Peripheral pulmonary nodules: relationship between multi-slice spiral CT perfusion imaging and tumor angiogenesis and VEGF expression. BMC Cancer 8:186

61. Llovet JM, Ricci S, Mazzaferro V et al (2008) Sorafenib in advanced hepatocellular carcinoma. N Engl J Med 359:378–390

62. Ippolito D, Sironi S, Pozzi M et al (2008) Hepatocellular carcinoma in cirrhotic liver disease: functional computed tomography with perfusion imaging in the assessment of tumor vascularization. Acad Radiol 15:919–927

63. Yanagawa M, Tomiyama N, Honda O et al (2010) Multidetector CT of the lung: image quality with garnet-based detectors. Radiology 255:944–954

64. Okada M, Kim T, Murakami T (2011) Hepatocellular nodules in liver cirrhosis: state of the art CT evaluation (perfusion CT/volume helical shuttle scan/dual-energy CT, etc.). Abdom Imaging 36:273–281

65. Schindera ST, Nelson RC, Mukundan S Jr et al (2008) Hypervascular liver tumors: low tube voltage, high tube current multi-detector row CT for enhanced detection—phantom study. Radiology 246:125–132

66. Graser A, Johnson TR, Bader M et al (2008) Dual energy CT characterization of urinary calculi: initial in vitro and clinical experience. Invest Radiol 43:112–119

67. Grosjean R, Sauer B, Guerra RM et al (2008) Characterization of human renal stones with MDCT: advantage of dual energy and limitations due to respiratory motion. Am J Roentgenol 190:720–728

68. Scheffel H, Stolzmann P, Frauenfelder T et al (2007) Dual-energy contrast-enhanced computed tomography for the detection of urinary stone disease. Invest Radiol 42:823–829

69. Primak AN, Fletcher JG, Vrtiska TJ et al (2007) Noninvasive differentiation of uric acid versus non-uric acid kidney stones using dual-energy CT. Acad Radiol 14:1441–1447

70. Goldberg HI, Cann CE, Moss AA, Ohto M, Brito A, Federle M (1982) Noninvasive quantitation of liver iron in dogs with hemochromatosis using dual-energy CT scanning. Invest Radiol 17:375–380

71. Johnson TR, Krauss B, Sedlmair M et al (2007) Material differentiation by dual energy CT: initial experience. Eur Radiol 17:1510–1517

72. Brooks RA (1977) A quantitative theory of the Hounsfield unit and its application to dual energy scanning. J Comput Assist Tomogr 1:487–493

73. Nakayama Y, Awai K, Funama Y et al (2005) Abdominal CT with low tube voltage: preliminary observations about radiation dose, contrast enhancement, image quality, and noise. Radiology 237:945–951

74. Yeh BM, Shepherd JA, Wang ZJ, Teh HS, Hartman RP, Prevrhal S (2009) Dual-energy and low-kVp CT in the abdomen. Am J Roentgenol 193:47–54

Biography

Dr. Okada graduated from Keio University School of Medicine in 1993, and he became Fellow and Assistant Professor in Keio University. He is currently a lecturer of radiology, Kinki University Faculty of Medicine. His main scientific interests include abdominal diagnostic imaging, and he has published more than 50 papers.

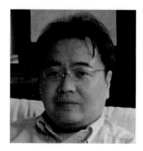

Clinical Applications of Hepatobiliary MR Contrast Agents

Antoine Wadih and Sebastian Feuerlein

Abstract Modern hepatocellular-specific MR contrast agents such as gadoxetic acid are an important adjunct to conventional extracellular contrast material in MRI examinations of the liver. They allow not only evaluation of vascular structures and early dynamic contrast kinetics but are also able to determine the presence or absence of functioning hepatocytes. In addition, the high biliary excretion rate of 50% allows a true T1 cholangiopancreatography phase with improved characterization of biliary abnormalities and leaks.

Introduction

The ability of hepatic MRI to characterize focal and diffuse liver disease has been greatly improved by the introduction of hepatocyte-specific contrast agents. Historically, this group included gadolinium-based agents (gadobenate dimeglumine), manganese-based agents (mangafodipir trisodium), and reticuloendothelial agents (iron oxide particles, SPIO). The latter two agents are no longer commercially available and suffered from inherent problems such as unsuitability for bolus injection and consecutive inability to evaluate hepatic vascular structures. Recently, gadolinium-ethoxybenzyl-diethylenetriamine pentaacetic acid (gadoxetic acid disodium, Eovist®, Bayer HealthCare) was introduced to the US market after being used under the brand name Primovist® in the European Union and Australia for many years. Gadoxetic acid is characterized by rapid and specific hepatocellular uptake, resulting in approximately 50 % biliary excretion in patients with normal hepatic function [1]. This results in a hepatocellular phase about 20 min after

A. Wadih, M.D. • S. Feuerlein, M.D. (✉)
Department of Radiology and Medical Imaging, University of Virginia Medical Center, Charlottesville, VA, P.O. Box 800170 22908, USA
e-mail: AW4WN@hscmail.mcc.virginia.edu; sfeuerlein@yahoo.com

A.S. El-Baz et al. (eds.), *Abdomen and Thoracic Imaging: An Engineering & Clinical Perspective*, DOI 10.1007/978-1-4614-8498-1_13,
© Springer Science+Business Media New York 2014

contrast administration, allowing for a single exam imaging strategy. In addition, gadoxetic acid is suitable for bolus injection and therefore not only facilitates evaluation in hepatocellular imaging phases that target parenchymal and biliary lesions but also enables MRI in the arterial and portal venous distribution phases for assessment of tissue perfusion and the intrahepatic vasculature itself. Gadobenate dimeglumine (Multihance®, Bracco) is a gadolinium-based contrast agent that is approved for bolus injection and most commonly used as extracellular agent. Due to a biliary excretion rate of 2 %, a hepatobiliary phase can be acquired about 2 h after intravenous contrast administration. However, this usually necessitates the patient being taken off the scanner between dynamic and hepatobiliary imaging and is therefore undesirable both from a patient and workflow perspective. This chapter mainly focuses on the application of gadoxetic acid; however, most of the general principles of image interpretation also apply to hepatobiliary imaging using gadobenate dimeglumine. The physiology of hepatobiliary contrast agents will be described followed by the MRI techniques typically used. Clinical applications of the agent will then be presented with discussion of focal liver lesions and the evaluation of biliary pathologies.

Hepatobiliary Contrast Agents: Properties and Mechanism

Gadoxetic acid is a derivative of Gd-DTPA (Magnevist®) to which a lipophilic ethoxybenzyl moiety has been added (Fig. 1). This chemical change results in an increased protein binding which does not only allow for specific uptake of the contrast agent into liver cells but also achieves a higher T1 relaxivity compared to other gadolinium-based contrast materials [2]. The increased relaxivity however cannot fully compensate for the fact that the recommended dose of gadoxetic acid of 0.025 mmol/kg only represents 25 % of the gadolinium molecules given with other extracellular contrast agents commonly used for liver MRI (recommended dose 0.1 mmol/kg). During the initial trials performed in 1996, a dose of 0.0125 mmol/kg was shown to be sufficient for the detection of hepatic metastases [3]. Hence, a double dose of 0.025 mmol/kg was chosen somewhat randomly to enable proper parenchymal enhancement and detection and character-ization of liver lesions with little regard to the evaluation of arterially enhancing lesions or the vasculature itself.

Molecular Properties

At the level of the hepatocytes, gadoxetic acid is actively transported into the cell through the "organic anion transporting polypeptide 8" (OATP8), which belongs to the solute carrier transporter superfamily of the OATPs, located at the sinusoidal membranes of the cells (Fig. 2). The uptake of gadoxetic acid can be limited by

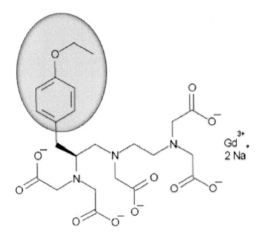

Fig. 1 Chemical structure of gadoxetic acid. Note the lipophilic ethoxybenzyl group (*red circle*) that has been added to the Gd-DTPA (Magnevist®) molecule to increase protein-binding capabilities

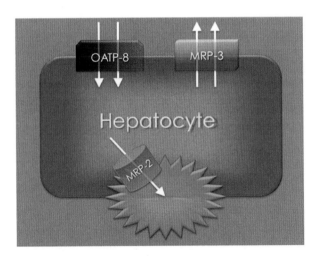

Fig. 2 Model of a hepatocyte showing the different membrane transporter proteins. Gadoxetic acid is actively transported from the bloodstream into the hepatocyte by the "organic anion transporting polypeptide 8" (OATP8) located at the sinusoidal membranes. The molecules can then be excreted into the biliary canaliculi via the "multidrug resistance-associated protein 2" (MRP2) or back into the bloodstream via MRP3. The function of all membrane proteins can be altered by up- or downregulation

competition with other endogenous compounds such as bilirubin and therapeutic drugs. In functional liver cells, gadoxetic acid can then be excreted into the biliary canaliculi via the "multidrug resistance-associated protein 2" (MRP2) located at the canalicular membrane of the cell or back into the bloodstream via MRP3 located at

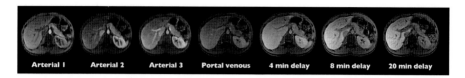

Fig. 3 Different contrast phases after injection of 0.025 mmol/kg gadoxetic acid. Note the reversal of portal vein-to-liver contrast between arterial and delayed imaging and the absence of a true equilibrium phase due to progressive enhancement of the hepatic parenchyma

the sinusoidal membrane (Fig. 2). It is important to note that the function of all membrane proteins involved with the transport of gadoxetic acid can be altered by up- or downregulation, most commonly by retrieval from or insertion into the cell membrane [3]. A large number of factors can have an influence on the regulation of the membrane proteins such as oxidative stress or cholestasis [3]. The resulting alterations in uptake and excretion of gadoxetic acid at the level of the hepatocytes can affect the enhancement pattern of the liver rendering characterization of certain atypical liver lesions more complex and challenging.

Pharmacokinetics

When gadoxetic acid is injected intravenously, it is initially distributed in the extracellular fluid compartment just as the extracellular agents. Despite its significantly lower dose, it can be used for dynamic imaging of the liver similar to extracellular contrast agents; however, detection rate for subtle hyperenhancing lesions might be limited. Since gadoxetic acid is competing with other molecules such as bilirubin at the membrane transporter proteins, the degree of hepatic excretion is dependent on the liver function. In patients without significant liver disease, approximately 50 % of gadoxetic acid is excreted through the biliary system as described above and 50 % through the kidneys. Hepatic-specific enhancement is detectable as early as 1–2 min after contrast administration (Fig. 3) [4]. The high biliary excretion rate allows for a new hepatobiliary phase that becomes significant for imaging at about 10 min and is unique to this class of agents. Enhancement in the hepatobiliary phase depends on the constellation of molecular transporters (Fig. 2) and typically reflects the presence of functioning hepatocytes and biliary canaliculi. The unique contrast kinetics with a steady background increase of hepatic parenchymal signal intensity over the first 20–30 min after contrast administration prohibits a true equilibrium phase with gadoxetic acid (Fig. 3) [4]. This change in background signal intensity has the potential to complicate evaluation of vascular structures and vascular lesions.

Protocol Optimization

The recommended time frame for hepatobiliary phase acquisition is within a relatively broad window of 10–120 min, with a delay of 20 min being most commonly used. In order to minimize the scanning time, some of the standard sequences can safely be acquired during the "wait time" between the early contrast phases and the hepatobiliary phase. It has been shown that ADC values of most organs are not different if acquired after contrast injection [5, 6] so diffusion-weighted imaging can be moved into the time slot between dynamic and hepatobiliary imaging. Similar holds true for standard T2-weighted turbo spin-echo (TSE) sequences. By using this strategy, total imaging time can be as low as 25 min. There is conflicting evidence regarding the quality of post-contrast acquisition of high-resolution respiratory-triggered 3D MR cholangiopancrea-tography (MRCP) sequences [7, 8]. Assuming a slow increase of intrabiliary concentration of the T2 shortening gadolinium-based contrast agent and a long image acquisition time secondary to the necessary respiratory triggering technique, it can reasonably be speculated that reduced intrabiliary T2 signal is a potential problem as confirmed by Ringe et al. [7]. It is therefore currently recommended that 3D MRCP sequences be performed prior to contrast administration.

While most institutions use a delay of about 20 min after contrast injection for the hepatobiliary phase, more delayed imaging can offer better opacification of the biliary tree allowing for noninvasive contrast-enhanced MR cholangiography [9]. These extra sequences can be acquired after 30 and if needed 40 min, but given this substantial amount of extra time necessary, they are mostly reserved for specific clinical indications such as evaluation for suspected postoperative bile leakage. Since acquisition speed is not of critical importance for the delayed T1-weighted gradient echo sequences, respiratory triggering can be used to reduce respiratory motion artifacts and also increase spatial resolution [10].

Imaging Appearance of Focal Liver Lesions

The characterization of focal liver lesions is a common clinical request for abdominal radiologists, partly due to the widespread use of cross-sectional imaging and the associated discovery of incidental liver lesions. Accurate classification of these lesions is crucial to enable selection of the most appropriate treatment strategy. Despite the high tissue contrast and fast dynamic imaging with MRI, some focal liver lesions are difficult to confidently characterize with extracellular contrast agents alone. Gadoxetic acid with its hepatobiliary properties is a very important adjunct to conventional MR imaging providing further information about the properties of the lesion, improving diagnostic confidence and accuracy [11].

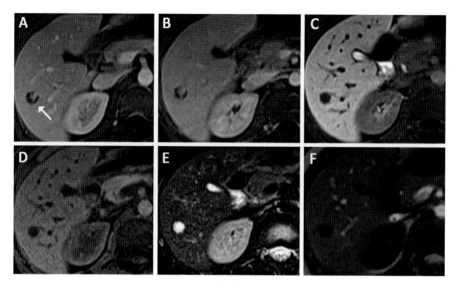

Fig. 4 Hemangioma in 39 year-old female (*white arrow* in (**a**)). Axial post-gadoxetic acid series ((**a**) arterial, (**b**) portal venous, (**c**) delayed 20 min) demonstrate peripheral nodular enhancement in the early phases followed by hypointensity on hepatobiliary phase imaging. Blood pool signal intensity was confirmed using the main portal vein on a different slice position (not shown). The lesion is hypointense on T1 non-contrast (**d**) and markedly hyperintense on fat-saturated T2 turbo spin-echo (**e**) also consistent with a hemangioma. Magnetization-prepared T1 GRE sequence (**f**) is an inversion recovery technique with the inversion time optimized for hemangioma; therefore the significant signal suppression on this sequence can serve as additional confirmation

Cavernous Hemangioma

Hepatic hemangiomas (Figs. 4 and 5) are the most common benign hepatic tumors and are frequently found incidentally at routine examinations. Using CT or MRI extracellular contrast agents, hemangioma typically shows peripheral nodular arterial enhancement with progressive centripetal filling on the portal venous and equilibrium phase. This enhancement pattern is highly specific for hemangioma. However, high-flow or "flash-filling" hemangiomas, which account for about 20 % of all hemangiomas and 40 % of hemangiomas less than 1 cm in diameter [12, 13], show immediate homogenous enhancement in the arterial phase. With extracellular agents, the enhancement characteristics of hemangiomas usually follow the blood pool in the later imaging phases, so lesions will be iso- or mildly hyperintense to the liver parenchyma in the portal venous and equilibrium phases, depending on the variable degree and speed of filling. However, this hyperintensity allows confident diagnosis of hemangioma. Due to the absence of a true equilibrium phase and the increasing enhancement of the liver parenchyma with gadoxetic acid, hemangiomas are typically hypointense compared to background liver starting a few minutes after contrast administration [13]. This hypointensity of

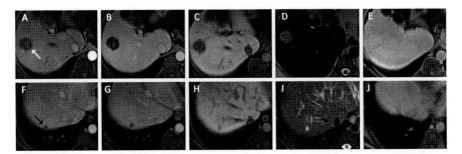

Fig. 5 Multiple focal liver lesions detected on CT in a 37 year-old female with history of colon cancer. The *upper* row shows one of the larger lesions (*white arrow*), the *lower* row one of the smaller subcentimeter lesions (*black arrow*) ((**a/f**) arterial, (**b/g**) portal venous, (**c/h**) hepatobiliary phase, (**d/i**) T2 turbo spin-echo, (**e/j**) 30 min post-gadobenate dimeglumine). Based on the initial gadoxetic acid exam ((**a–d**) and (**f–i**)) confident characterization was not possible due to atypical arterial enhancement pattern, and despite some features suggesting hemangioma such as very high T2 signal intensity and blood pool signal intensity on hepatobiliary phase images. The patient was brought back for additional gadobenate dimeglumine (Multihance®) series, which on the 30-min delayed series demonstrated hyperintensity compared to background liver confirming the suspected diagnosis of hemangioma for not only the large but also the smallest lesions

hemangiomas in the later phases makes its differentiation form hepatocellular carcinoma (HCC) and hypervascular metastases more challenging, in particular for high-flow hemangiomas lacking the classic peripheral nodular enhancement with progressive filling or lesions smaller than 1 cm (Fig. 5). This differentiation of small and/or atypical hemangioma from metastasis is a common pitfall with the use of gadoxetic acid [14, 15]. While comparison of lesion signal intensity with that of the portal vein as representative of the blood pool could be very helpful to establish the diagnosis of a hemangioma, accurate measurements of signal intensity can be challenging in small lesions. Combination with other signal characteristics such as high T2 signal intensity and ringlike arterial enhancement will also help increasing diagnostic accuracy for hemangioma versus metastasis [14]. In selected cases, it might ultimately be necessary to bring patients back and add delayed sequences after administration of a conventional extracellular contrast agent, where the blood pool remains hyperintense compared to the hepatic parenchyma, allowing the confident diagnosis of hemangioma if lesions are iso- or hyperintense (Fig. 5).

Focal Nodular Hyperplasia

Focal nodular hyperplasia (FNH) are the second-most commonly encountered benign liver lesions after hemangioma with a prevalence of about 1 % [16]. In contrast to hepatic adenoma, they are classified as a regenerative lesion rather than a true neoplastic lesion [16]. FNHs have a strong female predilection of about eight to one and are believed to be a hyperplastic response of the hepatic parenchyma to a

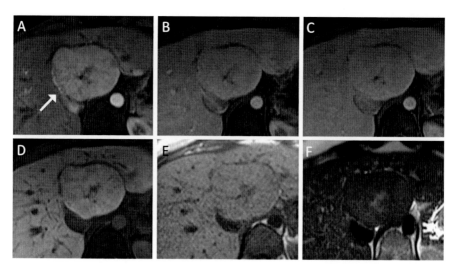

Fig. 6 Liver lesion in a 37 year-old female representing a typical FNH with central T2-hyperintense scar and multiple fibrous septa with spoke wheel pattern ((**a**) arterial, (**b**) portal venous, (**c**) 4-min delay, (**d**) hepatobiliary phase, (**e**) T1 non-contrast, (**f**) T2 turbo spin-echo). The lesion demonstrates typical arterial hyperenhancement and isointensity on the 20-min post-gadoxetic acid images highly suggestive of FNH

preexisting vascular malformation [16]. They are asymptomatic in most patients with none of the known complication inherent to other focal lesions such as spontaneous hemorrhage or malignant transformation. FNHs are often incidental findings and no usually no treatment is required. Currently, FNHs are classified as classic (80 %) or nonclassic (20 %). The latter group may lack the nodular abnormal architecture or malformed vessels, but always show bile duct proliferation. At gross pathology, FNHs demonstrate lobulated contours and nodular hyperplastic parenchyma with normal-appearing hepatocytes but a thickened plate architecture characteristic of regeneration. The parenchyma is surrounded by radiating fibrous septa originating from a central scar that contains large arterial vessels and is seen in about 50 % of cases [17]. The arterial blood in FNH, as opposed to that in adenomas flows centrifugally from the anomalous central arteries to the periphery of the lesion. FNHs contain abnormal bile ducts that have no connection to the hepatic biliary tree.

Typically, FNHs are iso- or slightly hypointense on T1-weighted images and slightly hyper- or isointense on T2-weighted images (Figs. 6 and 7). When the central scar is visible, it is hypointense to the lesion on the T1-weighted images and hyperintense on T2-weighted images. FNHs do not have a true capsule, although a pseudocapsule resulting from compression of the surrounding liver parenchyma by the lesion can be seen. On the dynamic contrast-enhanced images, FNHs show intense homogeneous enhancement in the arterial phase and become isointense to the liver in the portal venous phase. On delayed phase imaging, FNHs are iso- or hyperintense compared to the surrounding liver parenchyma, likely secondary to the

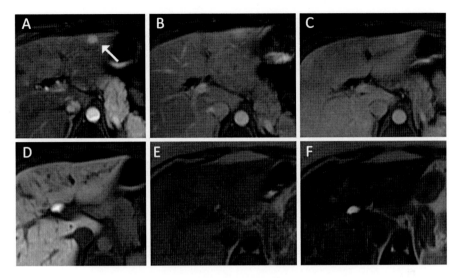

Fig. 7 FNH with similar imaging features as lesion in Fig. 6 (*white arrow*), however due to smaller size much less classical appearance ((**a**) arterial, (**b**) portal venous, (**c**) 4-min delay, (**d**) hepatobiliary phase, (**e**) T1 non-contrast, (**f**) T2 turbo spin-echo). Diagnosis here is mostly based on isointensity of the lesion on delayed images

combination of functioning hepatocytes and reduced or absent biliary drainage [18]. The central scar, while hyperintense on delayed images when an extracellular contrast agent is given, appears hypointense compared to the background liver due to the intense specific hepatic enhancement.

Hepatic Adenoma

Hepatic adenomas are benign neoplasm of the liver often associated with the use of oral contraceptives and consecutive strong female predilection [19]. Growth of adenomas is driven by both the dose and duration of estrogen use. Other risk groups for hepatocellular adenoma are patients with type I glycogen storage disease and patients on anabolic/androgenic steroids. Many or most patients with no more than a few adenomas are asymptomatic and almost invariably have normal liver function and no elevation of serum "tumor markers" such as AFP. Large adenomas may cause a sensation of right upper quadrant fullness or discomfort. However, a possible clinical manifestation of hepatic adenoma if not discovered incidentally is spontaneous rupture or hemorrhage, leading to acute abdominal pain or even signs of hypovolemia [20]. Liver adenomatosis appears to be a distinct entity characterized by ten or more hepatic adenomas. Although the adenomas in liver adenomatosis are histologically similar to other adenomas, they are not steroid dependent and more likely to lead to symptoms, impaired liver function, hemorrhage, and perhaps malignant degeneration [20].

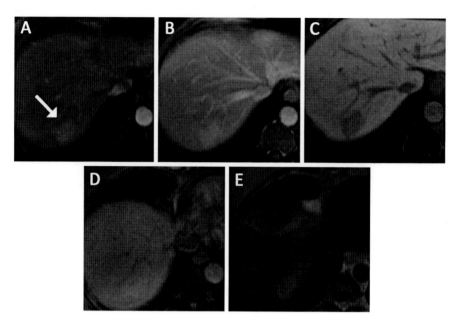

Fig. 8 Liver lesion found in a 42 year-old female with vague abdominal pain (*white arrow*). Lesion is hyperenhancing on arterial phase (**a**) and portal venous phase (**b**), however hypointense on hepatobiliary phase (**c**) suggestive of hepatic adenoma (in the absence of cirrhosis). The lesion also demonstrates T1 hyperintensity (**d**) suggestive of fat or glycogen content and T2 hyperintensity (**e**), both in keeping with the suspected adenoma

Hepatocellular adenoma (Fig. 8) varies in size from 1 to 15 cm and consists of cells resembling normal hepatocytes separated by dilated sinusoids. These sinusoids are perfused by arterial pressure because the adenomas lack portal venous supply [20]. This contributes to the hypervascular nature of the hepatic adenoma and explains the increased predilection for hemorrhage particularly in the presence of poor connective tissue support. Because a capsule is usually absent or incomplete, hemorrhage may spread into the liver or abdominal cavity. Bile ductules are notably absent from adenomas, a key histologic feature that helps distinguish hepatocellular adenoma from FNH when using hepatocellular contrast agents. Adenoma cells are larger than normal hepatocytes and contain large amounts of glycogen and lipid. Adenomas can undergo malignant transformation to HCC, even after years of maintaining a stable appearance [21].

Large hepatocellular adenomas typically appear heterogeneous on T1- and T2-weighted imaging due to hemorrhage and necrosis. On T1-weighted images, they are usually hypointense to the liver parenchyma. Areas of increased signal intensity can be present reflecting intralesional hemorrhage, glycogen, or fat. Intratumoral fat can be confirmed by chemical shift artifact on T1-weighted GRE opposed-phase images or with fat suppression. On T2-weighted images, heterogeneously increased signal intensity relative to the liver parenchyma is typically seen. On dynamic enhanced images using extracellular contrast agents,

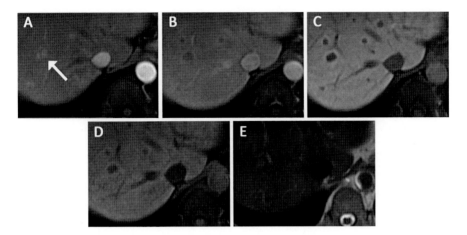

Fig. 9 Seventy-two year-old male with carcinoid metastasis to the liver (*white arrow*). The lesion is hyperenhancing on arterial phase (**a**) with washout and ringlike enhancement on the portal venous and 4-min delayed phases (**b, c**) and hypointensity on the hepatobiliary phase (**d**). A flash-filling hemangioma would have been difficult to exclude; however, only minimal T2 hyperintensity (**e**) and ringlike enhancement make metastasis the more likely option

heterogeneous arterial enhancement is present, though often to a lesser degree than with FNH. With gadoxetic acid, HCA show similar hemodynamics in the arterial, portal venous, and equilibrium phases as with extracellular contrast agents. However, in the hepatobiliary phase, HCA are typically hypointense to the rest of the liver parenchyma, reflecting the absence of functioning bile ducts and dysfunctional intralesional bilirubin excretion. This feature allows reliable differentiation of FNH and HCA in most cases. However, approximately 5–10 % of hepatic adenoma can demonstrate iso- or even hyperintensity compared to the surrounding liver on delayed imaging after gadoxetic acid [22, 23]. In these cases, the clinical history as well as secondary imaging findings such as the central scar and pseudocapsule of FNH and hemorrhage, necrosis, and T1 shorting contents of HCA should be used for lesion characterization.

Hepatic Metastasis

Metastatic disease to the liver is much more common than primary liver tumors. The most common sites of primary malignancy are the gastrointestinal tract, in particular colorectal cancer, followed by breast cancer, lung cancer, genitourinary malignancies, and melanoma. MRI has proven to be the most effective method for evaluation of metastatic liver disease owing to its ability to acquire multiple phases of contrast enhancement without ionizing radiation as well as to use inherent tissue contrast to both detect and characterize lesions. Hepatic metastases from extrahepatic malignancies (Fig. 9) do not contain functioning hepatocytes or bile ducts and therefore do not retain contrast in the hepatocellular phase [24]. As a consequence, all metastatic lesions typically appear uniformly hypointense in comparison with surrounding liver tissue in the hepatobiliary phase. Due to the improved lesion-to-liver contrast with clearly demarcated margins in a strongly enhancing background, liver parenchyma imaging with gadoxetic acid in the hepatobiliary phase is particularly useful for detection of hypovascular metastases, which are often more difficult to perceive on dynamic imaging with extracellular agents [25]. Using gadoxetic acid in the hepatobiliary phase in addition to the dynamic phases has been shown to increase the sensitivity for detection of liver metastasis. It was shown that hepatobiliary phase images showed a significantly better detection rate over precontrast and dynamic imaging with an improved sensitivity from 87 to 96 %, in particular for lesions smaller than 1 cm (71–90 %) [25].

Liver metastases often show some degree of enhancement in the hepatobiliary phase. Metastatic lesions from colorectal cancer showing more than 50 % enhancement compared to that of the adjacent liver on hepatobiliary phase images accounted for around 80 % of lesions [26]. In another study [27], 62 % of liver metastasis from breast cancer showed a central, round hyperintense portion surrounded by a relatively hypointense rim, resulting in a "target" appearance on 20-min delayed hepatobiliary phase. This "target" appearance was pathologically confirmed to originate from an internal central component of desmoplastic reaction with large interstitial space and fibrosis retaining the extracellular component of gadoxetic acid.

If lesion detection is requested rather than lesion characterization in particular in patients with known GI malignancy, the delayed hepatobiliary phase can be acquired after 10 min instead of 20 min to reduce overall imaging time. A recent study found that the hepatobiliary phase obtained at 10 min provided similar diagnostic performance for detection of liver metastasis from colorectal carcinoma compared with the images obtained after 20 min despite a lower tumor to liver CNR and overall image quality [28].

Hepatocellular Carcinoma

The natural history of liver cirrhosis has extensively been studied starting with increasing fibrosis secondary to a certain insult, whether chemical, infectious, inflammatory, or metabolic and progressing to cirrhosis. Reactive proliferation of normal hepatocytes within the surrounding fibrous stroma produces regenerative nodules. With persistent insult, increase in size and cellularity with changes of atypia occur leading to the formation of dysplastic nodules. A focus of small HCC may then develop within a dysplastic nodule which can grow into progressed HCC (Fig. 10) [29]. A major challenge in the classification of cirrhosis-associated nodules is the distinction between dysplastic nodules (DN) and early HCC due to the lack of reliable objective imaging criteria. The International Consensus Group of Hepatocellular Neoplasia (ICGHN) established objective criteria for the

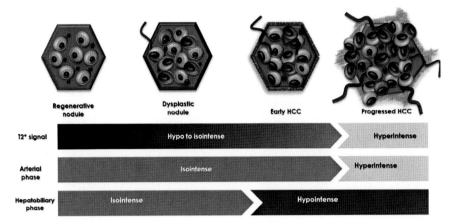

Fig. 10 Development of HCC from cirrhosis-associated nodules. Conventional imaging features usually do not allow differentiation of dysplastic nodules and early HCC; however, hypointensity on hepatobiliary phase imaging in a nodule that otherwise appears like a dysplastic nodule has been shown to be highly suggestive of early HCC [30]

distinction between DN and early HCC [30]. "Stromal invasion" which is defined as growth of tumor tissue into the portal tracts, fibrous septa, and/or blood vessels was recognized as the most important pathologic finding for differentiating these two entities [31]. However, making this distinction based on imaging alone remains challenging.

Dysplastic nodules are hypovascular lesions. This hypovascularity is attributed to a relative decrease of density of preexisting portal tracts as the parenchymal component increases within the nodule. Transition from dysplastic nodule to early HCC is represented by stromal invasion on histology. After DN transform into early HCC, vascularity decreases more severely because of decrease in preexisting arterial and portal venous blood supply caused by stromal invasion. However, while cirrhosis-associated nodules usually express normal membrane protein pattern and therefore demonstrate isointensity on hepatobiliary phase imaging, early HCC is characterized by a reduced expression of OATP8 and therefore appears hypointense on hepatobiliary imaging. Development of progressed HCC is characterized by proliferation of abnormal arteries (neovascularization) [31] and consequent hyperintensity on arterial phase imaging [29] as well as T2 hyperintensity, which makes this stage of the process relatively easy to diagnose, also owed to the usually larger size of these lesions. A tumor capsule is a characteristic sign of HCC and is present in 60–82 % of cases. Vascular and biliary invasion occurs frequently in HCC and can affect both the portal and hepatic veins [29].

While the diagnosis of progressed HCC is usually based on arterial hyperenhancement, portal venous washout, and T2 hyperintensity, the main challenge remains in the differentiation of dysplastic nodules and early HCC, especially given the much better prognosis and potential for curative treatment options with early stage lesions. A recent study could demonstrate that hypointensity on hepatocellular phase imaging has 97 % sensitivity and 100 % specificity for the detection of early HCC [30], much higher numbers than fat content on T1-weighted sequences or low unenhanced CT attenuation. This is underscoring the tremendous value of hepatobiliary contrast agents for imaging of HCC.

Since introduction of hepatocellular contrast agents, hypointensity in the hepatobiliary phase has been used as one of the main elements to diagnose progressed HCC. However, there is a certain subset of well- or moderately differentiated HCC, typically 10–20 % according to most studies that show isointensity or even hyperintensity on hepatocellular phase imaging compared to the background liver [32, 33]. It has been suggested that this could be secondary to varying degrees of residual hepatobiliary function, reflective of different stages of tumor differentiation [34]. It could be shown that while hypointensity is associated with reduced expression of the membrane protein responsible for taking up gadoxetic acid into the liver cell (OATP8, Fig. 2), the hyperintense lesions demonstrate upregulation of both OATP8 and the protein exporting gadoxetic acid back into the hepatic sinusoids, MRP3 [35]. As mentioned, these lesions are well or moderately differentiated; there have been no reported cases of poorly differentiated hyperenhancing HCC [32, 33].

Focal Fatty Sparing

Focal fatty changes in the liver are usually easily confirmed with a variety of modalities based on chemical shift properties on T1-weighted imaging, echotexture on ultrasound, the absence of mass effect on the vessels, and just general morphology. In few situations, focal fatty sparing in the background of diffuse hepatic steatosis can pose a diagnostic challenge particularly when the focal area has a mass-like appearance. In fact, since hepatic metastases usually contain no fat, they could be thought of as regions of focal sparing within the fatty liver (Fig. 11). The only difference of an area of focal fatty sparing and a metastatic lesion is the enhancement curve which for focal fatty sparing should parallel the one of surrounding liver parenchyma, while metastatic tissue usually enhances less than liver. Use of gadoxetic acid contrast agent for dynamic imaging can be helpful for better characterization of an area of focal fatty sparing. Using signal enhancement ratios of all dynamic phases, including the hepatobiliary phase, it was demonstrated that there was no significant difference in contrast enhancement effects of the liver parenchyma between areas of fatty change and area of nonfatty change, suggesting the preserved function of hepatocytes for the uptake of gadoxetic acid in the area of fatty change of the liver [36]. This means that although an area of focal fatty sparing containing normal liver parenchyma shows low signal intensity compared to the liver parenchyma in the hepatobiliary phase similar to a metastatic lesion, if the enhancement of the area parallels that of the liver parenchyma, a metastatic lesion is rather unlikely.

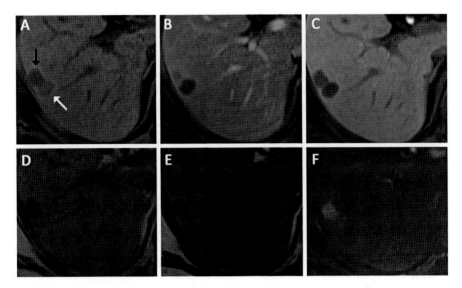

Fig. 11 Seventy-two year-old female with gastric adenocarcinoma and two liver lesions. Lesion 1 (*black arrow*) demonstrates hypointensity on arterial phase (**a**), progressive filling on portal venous phase (**b**) and hypointensity on hepatobiliary phase (**c**). In-phase (**d**) and opposed-phase (**e**) imaging show a significantly fatty liver with relative sparing of the lesion. These imaging findings along with the marked T2 hyperintensity (**f**) were highly suggestive of a hemangioma. Lesion 2 (*white arrow*) shows no significant enhancement, but similar fatty sparing as lesion 1 (although with higher T1 signal intensity) and only minimal T2 hyperintensity. This lesion proved to be a metastasis on follow-up imaging. It is noteworthy that lesion 2 in isolation would have been difficult to differentiate from an atypical hemangioma. The fact that the lesion appears hypointense compared to the blood pool (portal vein) might have helped

Evaluation of the Biliary Tree

Gadoxetic acid does not only cause T1 shortening within the bloodstream and the liver cells but also within the biliary tree, a characteristic that can be used for T1-weighted MR cholangiography as addition to the classic T2-weighted MRCP. The use of T1-weighted gradient echo sequences has advantages over the T2 turbo spin-echo technique that is most commonly used, namely, higher spatial resolution, shorter acquisition time, and insensitivity to other fluid-filled structures [37]. Accurate depiction of the biliary tree is crucial in patients undergoing preoperative evaluation for liver transplant, or other complex liver surgery to avoid inadvertent injury to variant or aberrant bile ducts. Regarding the evaluation of postoperative patients, T1-weighted biliary tree imaging adds a functional component to T2-MRCP, which is particularly helpful in the assessment of potential biliary leakages and/or perihepatic fluid collections after gallbladder or liver surgery (Fig. 12).

Analysis of biliary opacification also allows semiquantitative assessment of excretory liver function; however, this is of only minimal practical value.

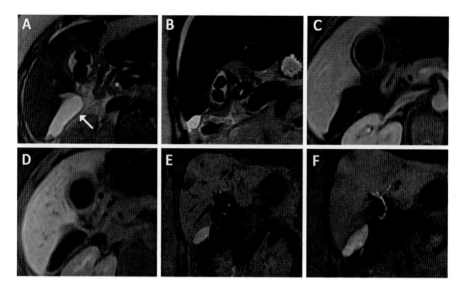

Fig. 12 Twenty-nine year-old female with history of attempted cholecystectomy 3 days prior at outside hospital and concern for bile duct injury. T2-weighted turbo spin-echo sequences (**a, b**) show signs of cholecystitis with gallbladder wall thickening and gallstones as well as a subhepatic fluid collection (*white arrow*). Portalvenous (**c**) and hepatobiliary phase (**d**) images neither demonstrate filling of the gallbladder nor contrast within the fluid collection. Two hour delayed images (**e, f**) clearly show contrast accumulation within the subhepatic fluid collection confirming the suspected bile leak

More relevance could be attributed to the ability of gadoxetic acid-based T1 cholangiography to evaluate gallbladder filling and cystic duct obstruction similar to scintigraphic methods. Limited data suggests that T1-weighted cholangiography has a very high positive predictive value for acute and to a lesser degree chronic cholecystitis based on filling of the gallbladder [37].

Due to the fact that gadoxetic acid competes at the OATP8 membrane transporter protein with bilirubin, T1-weighted cholangiography is often not feasible in cases of high-grade biliary obstruction due to lack of excretion. At our institution, gadoxetic acid is not used if the total serum bilirubin is 5 mg/dL or higher. If gadoxetic acid is used with elevated bilirubin levels below 5 mg/dL, longer delay times should be anticipated to allow for full biliary opacification.

References

1. Vogl TJ, Kummel S, Hammerstingl R et al (1996) Liver tumors: comparison of MR imaging with Gd-EOB-DTPA and Gd-DTPA. Radiology 200(1):59–67
2. Rohrer M, Bauer H, Mintorovitch J, Requardt M, Weinmann HJ (2005) Comparison of magnetic properties of MRI contrast media solutions at different magnetic field strengths. Invest Radiol 40(11):715–724
3. Van Beers BE, Pastor CM, Hussain HK (2012) Primovist, Eovist: what to expect? J Hepatol 57 (2):421–429

4. Feuerlein S, Boll DT, Gupta RT, Ringe KI, Marin D, Merkle EM (2011) Gadoxetate disodium-enhanced hepatic MRI: dose-dependent contrast dynamics of hepatic parenchyma and portal vein. AJR Am J Roentgenol 196(1):W18–W24

5. Colagrande S, Mazzoni LN, Mazzoni E, Pradella S (2012) Effects of gadoxetic acid on quantitative diffusion-weighted imaging of the liver. J Magn Reson Imaging 2013 Aug; 38(2):365–70. doi: 10.1002/jmri.23978. Epub 2012 Dec 13

6. Choi JS, Kim MJ, Choi JY, Park MS, Lim JS, Kim KW (2010) Diffusion-weighted MR imaging of liver on 3.0-Tesla system: effect of intravenous administration of gadoxetic acid disodium. Eur Radiol 20(5):1052–1060

7. Ringe KI, Gupta RT, Brady CM et al (2010) Respiratory-triggered three-dimensional T2-weighted MR cholangiography after injection of gadoxetate disodium: is it still reliable? Radiology 255(2):451–458

8. Kim KA, Kim MJ, Park MS et al (2010) Optimal T2-weighted MR cholangiopancreatographic images can be obtained after administration of gadoxetic acid. Radiology 256(2):475–484

9. Seale MK, Catalano OA, Saini S, Hahn PF, Sahani DV (2009) Hepatobiliary-specific MR contrast agents: role in imaging the liver and biliary tree. Radiographics 29(6):1725–1748

10. Asbach P, Warmuth C, Stemmer A et al (2008) High spatial resolution T1-weighted MR imaging of liver and biliary tract during uptake phase of a hepatocyte-specific contrast medium. Invest Radiol 43(11):809–815

11. Huppertz A, Balzer T, Blakeborough A et al (2004) Improved detection of focal liver lesions at MR imaging: multicenter comparison of gadoxetic acid-enhanced MR images with intraoperative findings. Radiology 230(1):266–275

12. Tamada T, Ito K, Yamamoto A et al (2011) Hepatic hemangiomas: evaluation of enhancement patterns at dynamic MRI with gadoxetate disodium. AJR Am J Roentgenol 196(4):824–830

13. Gupta RT, Marin D, Boll DT et al (2012) Hepatic hemangiomas: difference in enhancement pattern on 3T MR imaging with gadobenate dimeglumine versus gadoxetate disodium. Eur J Radiol 81(10):2457–2462

14. Motosugi U, Ichikawa T, Onohara K et al (2011) Distinguishing hepatic metastasis from hemangioma using gadoxetic acid-enhanced magnetic resonance imaging. Invest Radiol 46 (6):359–365

15. Goshima S, Kanematsu M, Watanabe H et al (2010) Hepatic hemangioma and metastasis: differentiation with gadoxetate disodium-enhanced 3-T MRI. AJR Am J Roentgenol 195 (4):941–946

16. Hussain SM, Terkivatan T, Zondervan PE et al (2004) Focal nodular hyperplasia: findings at state-of-the-art MR imaging, US, CT, and pathologic analysis. Radiographics 24(1):3–17; discussion 8–9

17. Nguyen BN, Flejou JF, Terris B, Belghiti J, Degott C (1999) Focal nodular hyperplasia of the liver: a comprehensive pathologic study of 305 lesions and recognition of new histologic forms. Am J Surg Pathol 23(12):1441–1454

18. Zech CJ, Grazioli L, Breuer J, Reiser MF, Schoenberg SO (2008) Diagnostic performance and description of morphological features of focal nodular hyperplasia in Gd-EOB-DTPA-enhanced liver magnetic resonance imaging: results of a multicenter trial. Invest Radiol 43 (7):504–511

19. Trotter JF, Everson GT (2001) Benign focal lesions of the liver. Clin Liver Dis 5(1):17–42, v

20. Grazioli L, Federle MP, Brancatelli G, Ichikawa T, Olivetti L, Blachar A (2001) Hepatic adenomas: imaging and pathologic findings. Radiographics 21(4):877–892; discussion 92–4

21. Colli A, Fraquelli M, Massironi S, Colucci A, Paggi S, Conte D (2007) Elective surgery for benign liver tumours. Cochrane Database Syst Rev 1, CD005164

22. Denecke T, Steffen IG, Agarwal S et al (2012) Appearance of hepatocellular adenomas on gadoxetic acid-enhanced MRI. Eur Radiol 22(8):1769–1775

23. Grazioli L, Bondioni MP, Haradome H et al (2012) Hepatocellular adenoma and focal nodular hyperplasia: value of gadoxetic acid-enhanced MR imaging in differential diagnosis. Radiology 262(2):520–529

24. Goodwin MD, Dobson JE, Sirlin CB, Lim BG, Stella DL (2011) Diagnostic challenges and pitfalls in MR imaging with hepatocyte-specific contrast agents. Radiographics 31 (6):1547–1568

25. Choi JY, Choi JS, Kim MJ et al (2010) Detection of hepatic hypovascular metastases: 3D gradient echo MRI using a hepatobiliary contrast agent. J Magn Reson Imaging 31(3):571–578

26. Kim A, Lee CH, Kim BH et al (2012) Gadoxetic acid-enhanced 3.0T MRI for the evaluation of hepatic metastasis from colorectal cancer: metastasis is not always seen as a "defect" on the hepatobiliary phase. Eur J Radiol 81(12):3998–4004

27. Ha S, Lee CH, Kim BH et al (2012) Paradoxical uptake of Gd-EOB-DTPA on the hepatobiliary phase in the evaluation of hepatic metastasis from breast cancer: is the "target sign" a common finding? Magn Reson Imaging 30(8):1083–1090

28. Sofue K, Tsurusaki M, Tokue H, Arai Y, Sugimura K (2011) Gd-EOB-DTPA-enhanced 3.0 T MR imaging: quantitative and qualitative comparison of hepatocyte-phase images obtained 10 min and 20 min after injection for the detection of liver metastases from colorectal carcinoma. Eur Radiol 21(11):2336–2343

29. Hussain SM, Reinhold C, Mitchell DG (2009) Cirrhosis and lesion characterization at MR imaging. Radiographics 29(6):1637–1652

30. Sano K, Ichikawa T, Motosugi U et al (2011) Imaging study of early hepatocellular carcinoma: usefulness of gadoxetic acid-enhanced MR imaging. Radiology 261(3):834–844

31. Kondo F (2011) Assessment of stromal invasion for correct histological diagnosis of early hepatocellular carcinoma. Int J Hepatol 2011:241652

32. Huppertz A, Haraida S, Kraus A et al (2005) Enhancement of focal liver lesions at gadoxetic acid-enhanced MR imaging: correlation with histopathologic findings and spiral CT—initial observations. Radiology 234(2):468–478

33. Saito K, Kotake F, Ito N et al (2005) Gd-EOB-DTPA enhanced MRI for hepatocellular carcinoma: quantitative evaluation of tumor enhancement in hepatobiliary phase. Magn Reson Med Sci 4(1):1–9

34. Bartolozzi C, Crocetti L, Lencioni R, Cioni D, Della Pina C, Campani D (2007) Biliary and reticuloendothelial impairment in hepatocarcinogenesis: the diagnostic role of tissue-specific MR contrast media. Eur Radiol 17(10):2519–2530

35. Kitao A, Zen Y, Matsui O et al (2010) Hepatocellular carcinoma: signal intensity at gadoxetic acid-enhanced MR Imaging—correlation with molecular transporters and histopathologic features. Radiology 256(3):817–826

36. Yamamoto A, Tamada T, Sone T, Higashi H, Yamashita T, Ito K (2010) Gd-EOB-DTPA-enhanced magnetic resonance imaging findings of nondiffuse fatty change of the liver. J Comput Assist Tomogr 34(6):868–873

37. Fayad LM, Holland GA, Bergin D et al (2003) Functional magnetic resonance cholangiography (fMRC) of the gallbladder and biliary tree with contrast-enhanced magnetic resonance cholangiography. J Magn Reson Imaging 18(4):449–460

Fast Object Detection Using Color Features for Colonoscopy Quality Measurements

Jayantha Muthukudage, JungHwan Oh, Ruwan Nawarathna,
Wallapak Tavanapong, Johnny Wong, and Piet C. de Groen

Abstract The effectiveness of colonoscopy depends on the quality of the inspection of the colon. There was no automated measurement method to evaluate the quality of the inspection. To address this, we have been investigating automated post-procedure quality measurement. The limitation of post-processing quality measurement is that quality measurements become available only long after the procedure was over and the patient was released. A better approach is to inform any suboptimal inspection immediately so that the endoscopist can improve the quality of the inspection in real-time during the procedure. Both post-processing and real-time quality measurements require a number of analysis tasks such as detecting a bite-block region as an indicator that a procedure is an upper endoscopy, not colonoscopy, detecting a blood region as an indicator for inflammation or bleeding, and detecting a stool region as an indicator of quality of the colon preparation. Color is the most distinguishable characteristic for differentiation among these object classes and normal pixels. In this paper, we propose a method to detect these object classes using color features. The main idea is to partition very large positive examples of these objects into a number of groups. Each group is called a "positive plane" and is modeled using a convex hull enclosing feature points of

J. Muthukudage (✉) • J. Oh (✉) • R. Nawarathna
Department of Computer Science and Engineering, University of North Texas,
Denton, TX 76203, USA
e-mail: MuthukudageKumara@my.unt.edu; Junghwan.Oh@unt.edu;
RuwanNawarathna@my.unt.edu

W. Tavanapong • J. Wong
Department of Computer Science, Iowa State University, Ames, IA 50011, USA
e-mail: tavanapo@cs.iastate.edu; wong@cs.iastate.edu

P.C. de Groen
Mayo Clinic College of Medicine, Rochester, MN 55905, USA

A.S. El-Baz et al. (eds.), *Abdomen and Thoracic Imaging: An Engineering
& Clinical Perspective*, DOI 10.1007/978-1-4614-8498-1_14,

that particular group. Comparisons with traditional classifiers such as K-nearest neighbor (K-NN) and Support Vector Machines (SVM) prove the effectiveness of the proposed method in terms of accuracy and execution time that is critical in the targeted real-time quality measurement system.

Introduction

Advances in video technology are being incorporated into today's healthcare practices. Endoscopy is introduced to inspect a human body cavity to locate abnormal lesions. Examples of endoscopic procedures are colonoscopy, upper gastrointestinal endoscopy, enteroscopy, bronchoscopy, cystoscopy, laparoscopy, wireless capsule endoscopy (WCE), and minimally invasive surgeries (e.g., video endoscopic neurosurgery). These endoscopes come in various sizes, but all have a tiny video camera at the tip of the endoscope. During an endoscopic procedure, this tiny video camera generates a video signal of an existing or created space inside the human body, which is displayed on a monitor for analysis by the physician. Colonoscopy is an important screening procedure for colorectal cancer. During a colonoscopy procedure, the colon is inspected for colorectal cancers.

In the US, colorectal cancer is the second leading cause of all cancer deaths behind lung cancer [1]. As the name implies, colorectal cancers are malignant tumors that develop in the colon and rectum. The survival rate is higher if the cancer is found and treated early before metastasis to lymph nodes or other organs occurs. Colonoscopy has contributed to a marked decline in the number of colorectal cancer-related deaths. However, recent data suggest that there is a significant (4–12 %) miss-rate for the detection of even large polyps and cancers [2–4]. The miss-rate may be related to the experience of the endoscopist and the location of the lesion in the colon, but no prospective studies related to this have been done thus far.

The effectiveness of colonoscopy in prevention of colorectal cancers depends on the quality of the inspection of the colon, which generally can be evaluated in terms of the withdrawal time (time spent during the withdrawal phase when the endoscope is gradually withdrawn) and the thoroughness of the inspection of the colon mucosa. Current American Society for Gastrointestinal Endoscopy (ASGE) guidelines suggest that (1) on average the withdrawal phase during a screening colonoscopy should last a minimum of 6 min and (2) the visualization of cecum anatomical landmarks such as the appendiceal orifice and the ileocecal valve should be documented [5].

There was no automated measurement method to evaluate the endoscopist's skills and the quality of colonoscopy procedures. To address this critical need, we have investigated an automated post-procedure quality measurement system [6, 7] to process de-identified videos of colonoscopy in MPEG-2 format [8]. The limitation of post-processing quality measurement is that quality measurements become

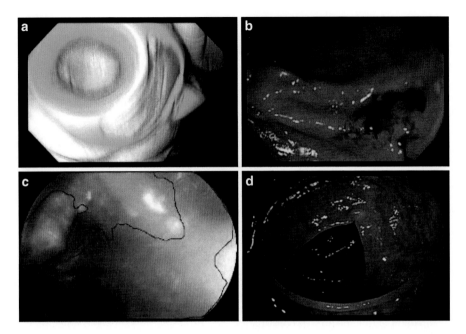

Fig. 1 Sample frames of (**a**) Green Bite-block, (**b**) Blood, (**c**) Stool areas marked with *blue lines*, and (**d**) Normal colonoscopy frame

available only long after the procedure was done and the patient was released. The endoscopist can only improve the quality of the next colonoscopy procedures. However, a better approach is to inform any suboptimal inspection immediately so that the endoscopist can improve the quality in real-time during the procedure. This system has been placed at Mayo Clinic Rochester for a clinical trial since the beginning of 2011 [9]. The goal of this new system is to achieve real-time analysis and feedback to aid the endoscopist towards optimal inspection to improve overall quality of colonoscopy during the procedure. Since our system captures colonoscopy videos in MPEG-2 format at about 30 frames per second, to achieve real-time analysis and feedback, all analysis tasks must be completed within 33 ms. We call this requirement the "real-time requirement."

For both post-processing and real-time quality measurements, the system needs to run a number of software modules for various processing. Modules detecting the objects such as bite-block, blood, and stool (see Fig. 1) are essential for generating various quality metrics due to the following reasons.

- Typically, upper endoscopy and colonoscopy procedures are performed in the same room at different times. It is necessary to distinguish the type of a procedure prior to execution of any quality measurement method to evaluate the procedure. For instance, stool detection generates useful information only for colonoscopy, but not for upper endoscopy. We need to develop a method to detect the procedure type at the beginning of the procedure so that only colonoscopy-related modules run on the procedure. In upper endoscopy, a bite-block (see Fig. 1a) is inserted for patient protection. By detecting a bite-block appearance, we can distinguish colonoscopy from upper endoscopy

- Blood detection plays several important roles in various endoscopies, for example, blood detection in wireless capsule endoscopy (WCE) aims to find abnormal regions in the small bowel. On the other hand, blood detection in colonoscopy has two applications: detection of bleeding and erythema and estimation of whether polypectomies [1] are performed during the procedure. We propose a method to detect blood regions in colonoscopy videos

- The diagnostic accuracy of colonoscopy depends on the quality of bowel preparation [10]. Without adequate bowel preparation, missed lesions may be covered by stool. The quality of bowel cleansing is generally assessed by the quantity of solid or liquid stool in the lumen. Despite a large body of published data on methods that could optimize cleansing, a substantial level of inadequate cleansing occurs in 10–75 % of patients in randomized controlled trials [11]. Poor bowel preparation has been associated with patient characteristics, such as inpatient status, history of constipation, use of antidepressants, and noncompliance with cleansing instructions. To assess the quality of bowel preparation, we propose a method to compute the amount of mucosa covered by stool

Since all these objects do not pose any other distinguishable characteristics (i.e., shape or texture) other than color, we use color feature. In our previous work [12], we developed a method detecting stool regions in colonoscopy frames. This method was developed solely for post-processing quality measurement. Consequently, it does not meet the real-time requirement for the real-time quality measurement system. In this proposed study, we extend the previous method to detect regions of bite-blocks and blood with good accuracy in addition to stool and to reduce detection time to satisfy the real-time requirement. The main idea is to partition very large positive examples (pixel values) of each object into a number of groups, in which each group is called "positive plane." Each positive plane is modeled as a separate entity for that group of positive examples. Our previous method for modeling each plane is very time-consuming. As a result, it does not meet the real-time requirement. To overcome this drawback, we propose to use a "convex hull" to represent a positive plane. The convex hull representation enables real-time object detection. Our experimental results show that the proposed method is more accurate, faster, and more robust.

The rest of the paper is organized as follows. Section "Related Work" discusses the related work. Section "Proposed Methodology" describes the proposed methodology and the three applications for detecting stool, bite-block, and blood. Section "Experimental Method and Results" shows our experimental results. Finally, Section "Conclusion and Future Work" summarizes our concluding remarks.

Related Work

Color-based classification plays a major role in the field of medical image analysis. A significant number of studies on object detection based on color features can be found in the literature. Some of them are briefly summarized in this section.

In [13], we proposed a method to classify stool images in colonoscopy videos using a Support Vector Machine (SVM) classifier. The colonoscopy video frame is down-sampled into equal-sized blocks in order to reduce the size of the feature vector. Some pixel-based values such as average color and a color-histogram of each block are used to form a feature vector for the SVM classifier. Then, a stool mask is made for each video frame using the trained SVM classifier, and some post-processing methods are applied to improve the detection accuracy. The post-processing methods include a majority filter and a morphological opening filter. Finally, the frames having more than 5 % of stool area (pixels) are classified as stool frames. A disadvantage of this SVM-based method is the detection time, which is not fast enough to be used in the real-time environment.

In our previous method [12], we proposed a method to detect stool regions for post-processing quality measurement. First, we partition the data (stool pixel values) set into a number of groups, and model each group as a separate data set. The separate data set is called "positive plane." For the modeling of each positive plane, it is divided into a number of blocks using a thresholding mechanism. The block division including the number of blocks significantly affects the detection time. Hence, we need to find a replacement of the block division to meet the real-time requirements.

Most related works on blood detection are conducted on wireless capsule endoscopy (WCE) videos. In [14], a methodology was proposed aiming at the detection of bleeding patterns in WCE videos. In this study, the features used are the histograms of hue, saturation, and value [15], and co-occurrence matrix of the dominant colors. These features are then used with a SVM ensemble to detect bleeding patterns in WCE videos. Another method to detect bleeding and other blood-based abnormalities in WCE images was presented in [16]. This work was based on a previously published method in [17]. The segmentation is carried out on smoothed and de-correlated *RGB* (Red, Green, and Blue) color channels using a fuzzy segmentation algorithm. The segmentation result is then transformed to a Local Global graph, which mathematically describes the local and global relationships between the segmented regions in terms of a graph. This graph is used for merging similar segmented regions. In [18], the detection of bleeding patterns is done in two steps. First, the detection of frames with potential bleeding areas is performed based on the assumption that blocks representing bleeding areas are more saturated than the others. Pre-classification detects a frame as a bleeding frame if at least one block represents a bleeding area. In the second step, the initial classification is verified and refined based on pixel-based multi-thresholding of the saturation and intensity. Finally, a bleeding level is assigned to that particular frame based on the pixel values. The work in [19] uses a Neural Network classifier with chromaticity moments for the classification of bleeding and ulcer regions. All the blood detection methods mentioned above suffer from very slow detection time. Thus, they are not applicable to our real-time environment. To the best of our knowledge, there is no methodology for the detection of a bite-block appearance in the literature.

Proposed Methodology

This section explains the proposed method in detail. The method consists of three stages: Training (Section "Training Stage"), Modeling (Section "Convex Hull Models of Green Bite-Block, Blood, and Stool"), and Detecting (Section "Detecting Stage").

Training Stage

It consists of eight steps as shown in Fig. 2. They are described in the following subsections.

Training Dataset Generation

In this subsection, we explain Steps 1, 2, and 3 in the training stage (Fig. 2). The domain expert marked and annotated the contents of colonoscopy frames into four classes: bite-block, blood, stool, and normal frames. They are used as training data. Figure 1 shows some sample frames of the four classes used in this study. We extract and store the pixels values from these marked and annotated areas. These pixels contain some duplicate values, which are removed to create a unique set of training examples (pixel values) in *RGB* color space. As per the property of high discriminative power [20], we transform these pixels in *RGB* color space into those in *HSV* (Hue, Saturation and Value) color space.

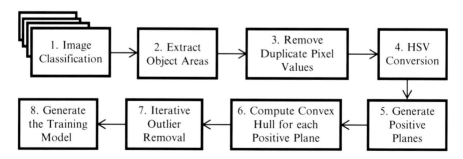

Fig. 2 Steps in training stage

HSV Conversion

This subsection explains Step 4 in the training stage (Fig. 2). *RGB* color space is defined by the three chromaticities of the red, green, and blue and represented as a three-dimensional Cartesian coordinate system. *RGB* is a device-dependent color model. That is, different devices produce given *RGB* values differently. Thus, an *RGB* value does not define the same colors across different devices [20]. Also, *RGB* color channels are strongly correlated. This characteristic makes the *RGB* color space less discriminative.

HSV color space describes colors in terms of their color (Hue), shade (Satura-tion), and brightness (Value) [20]. Hue is typically expressed as an angle value from 0 to $360°$ representing hues of various colors. In this study, Hue is expressed as a number from 0 to 1 instead of an angle from $0°$ to $360°$ as seen in (1). Saturation is an amount of grayness in a color and represented as a number in the range of 0 and 1. Value (brightness or intensity) of a color is represented as a number from 0 to 255. In the proposed method, *RGB* color values of a pixel are converted to *HSV* values of the same pixel using (1).

$$H = \begin{cases} \left(\dfrac{G-B}{\Delta}\right), C_{max}=R \\ \left(\dfrac{B-R}{\Delta}\right), C_{max}=G \\ \left(\dfrac{R-G}{\Delta}\right), C_{max}=B \end{cases} \quad S = \begin{cases} 0, & \Delta=0 \\ \dfrac{\Delta}{C_{max}}, & \Delta <> 0 \end{cases} \quad V = C_{max} \quad (1)$$

where $C_{max} = max(R,G,B)$, $C_{min} = min(R,G,B)$, and $\Delta = C_{max} - C_{min}$.

Positive Plane Generation

This subsection explains Step 5 in the training stage (Fig. 2). Now we have the positive examples of the three object classes (bite-block, blood, and stool) in *HSV* color space. We project all these examples into *HSV* color cube in which each channel (H, S, and V) is represented as an axis in the 3D Cartesian coordinate system. This step is illustrated in Fig. 3 in which *HSV* color cube is shown in the *XYZ* coordinate system. Z-values are in a different range than the X and Y values, but the same scales are used for illustration purpose.

In the next step, we create 256 planes in the *HSV* color cube along Value (Z) axis so that each integer location of Value axis has a plane parallel to *HS* planes as seen in Fig. 3. Only a small number of positive planes are shown in the figure. Either H or S axis can be selected as the index axis. Based on our experiments, usage of Value

Fig. 3 Placement
of planes along value axis

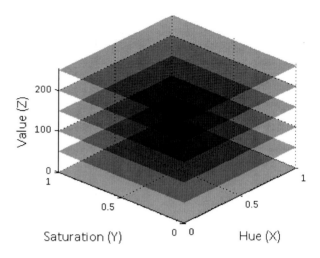

axis as the index axis offers the best detection accuracy. Then, we assign a number
(from 0 to 255) to each plane (i.e., Plane#0, Plane#1 ... Plane#255). Some planes
contain a very small number of positive class examples. Among these 256 planes,
hence, we keep the planes in which its positive class examples are greater than or
equal to a certain threshold. In our study, we use three for the threshold value which
was decided experimentally. Each selected plane is called a "Positive Plane." Each
positive plane contains a subset of positive examples (pixels) and is later modeled
as a 2D classifier. For instance, Plane#0 (at $V = 0$) is treated as a classifier for
positive class examples on Plane#0.

Computation of a Convex Hull for Each Positive Plane

This subsection explains Step 6 in the training stage (Fig. 2). For each positive plane
selected in Section "Positive Plane Generation", we generate a convex hull.
Algebraically, a convex hull of a dataset X can be characterized as the set of all
of the convex combinations of finite subsets of points from X: that is a set of points
in the form of $\sum_{j=1}^{n} \alpha_i x_j$, where n is an arbitrary nonzero positive integer,
the numbers, α_i, are nonnegative and sum to 1, and the point x_j is in X. So, the
convex hull, $H_{\text{convex}}(X)$ of set X is given in (2), where α_i is a fraction between
0 and 1 in $\mathbb{R}$ (real numbers). The maximum value of k can be the number of data
points in the dataset, which contribute to the convex hull.

$$H_{\text{convex}}(X) = \left\{ \sum_{i=1}^{k} \alpha_i x_i \middle| x_i \in X, \alpha_i \in \mathbb{R}, \alpha_i \geq 0, \sum_{i=1}^{k} \alpha_i = 1, k = 1, 2, \ldots \right\} \quad (2)$$

To generate a convex hull that adheres to the constraints given in (2), we use the
quick hull algorithm introduced in [21]. The basic steps of the quick hull algorithm
are given below, and its graphical representation is given in Fig. 4.

Fig. 4 Convex hull
generation using
the quick hull algorithm

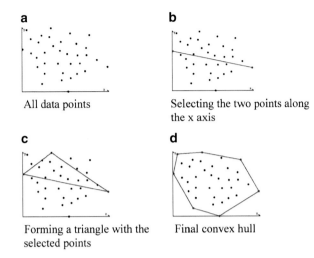

a

All data points

b

Selecting the two points along
the x axis

c

Forming a triangle with the
selected points

d

Final convex hull

1. Find the furthest and closest points from the origin along the x-axis; these two points will be the vertices of the convex hull. Partition the points into two halves using the line drawn between the two points selected (Fig. 4b)
2. Select a point from one side of the line drawn in Step 1, which is the furthest point from the line. This point along with the two points selected in the above step creates a triangle. The points lying inside of that triangle will be discarded since they cannot be any vertices of the convex hull (Fig. 4c)
3. Repeat Step 2 for the other side of the line drawn in Step 1
4. Repeat Steps 2 and 3 on the two new lines formed by the triangle
5. Iterate until no more points are left

Iterative Outlier Removal

This subsection explains Steps 7 and 8 in the training stage (Fig. 2). After obtaining the convex hull as described in Section "Computation of a Convex Hull for each Positive Plane", we perform a procedure for outlier removal, in which we remove outliers in several stages in order to improve the overall accuracy of the proposed method. For the outlier removal we use (3). The reason why we are using this equation instead of a typical outlier removal method like "Box plot" is that it is easy to be applied to our convex hulls. Using (3), we remove convex hull vertices from the original data points and recalculate convex hull on reduced data points. The subscript i in the equation represents the number of iterations, which is determined experimentally (i.e., in our study, $i = 1$) and provided in the beginning of the outlier removal procedure. Outlier removal procedure stops when it iterates i time(s).

$$H_{\text{Convex}(i)}(X) = H_{\text{Convex}}\left(X - \sum_{n=0}^{i-1} H_{\text{convex}(n)}(X)\right) \tag{3}$$

As mentioned in Section "Positive Plane Generation", a positive plane has at least three vertices (positive examples), so this outlier removal is applied to a convex hull with four or more vertices. After performing the outlier removal, we store the positive plane number along with the coordinate values of convex hull vertices for that particular positive plane. This procedure is done for all the positive planes. We then combine all the positive convex hulls in a model. We call this "convex hull model." This convex hull model is used for the detecting stage.

Convex Hull Models of Green bite-block, Blood, and Stool

In this section, we present three different applications of the proposed method. We use the algorithm mentioned in Section "Training Stage" to generate convex hull models for three different classes of objects: green bite-block, blood, and stool. Although a bite-block could be of any color, the most commonly used bite-blocks in our data set are green. Thus, we design our method to detect green bite-blocks. However, our method can be easily extended to detect a different bite-block color. The selection of positive planes is depicted in Figs. 5a and 6b for each object class. For ease of illustration, we only present a small number of positive planes in this figure.

An example of a positive plane (plane #200) for each application can be seen in Fig. 6. In this figure, the positive examples at the corresponding positive plane and $H_{\text{convex}(1)}$ along with $H_{\text{convex}(0)}$ are shown. Please note that the Hue (X) axis is shown in different scales for each class to capture the dataset clearly.

Detecting Stage

In this section, we explain how to use the convex hull model generated in Section "Training Stage" to detect the three classes of objects from an unseen colonoscopy frame. First, we convert the pixel values in a video frame from RGB to HSV. Each pixel in the video frame is evaluated using the convex hull model. This evaluation is performed by selecting the corresponding positive plane. The Value (Z) of a pixel is obtained and used as an index to choose the corresponding positive plane. For example, if the Value (Z) of a pixel in an unseen video frame is 5, then Plane #5 in the corresponding model is selected and examined if it is a positive plane. This will dramatically reduce the number of comparisons so that the searching time is significantly reduced. In other words, the detecting time of the

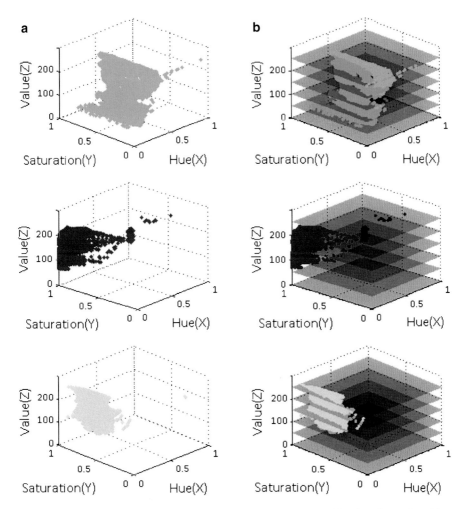

Fig. 5 Selection of positive planes. (**a**) *HSV* cubes and corresponding locations of positive example pixels, and (**b**) Several planes inserted into the *HSV* cube of (**a**). First row: Green bite-block, second row: Blood, and third row: Stool

proposed technique is dependent on neither the number of positive planes nor how many positive examples in the corresponding plane. By comparing the *HS* (*XY*) values of the pixel with the convex hull generated in the training stage, we label the pixel as positive or negative. Pixels that are either on or inside the convex polygon (formed by convex hull vertices) are labeled as positive examples. As mentioned above, three different convex hull models are generated from the training examples for green bite-blocks, blood, and stool. The corresponding convex hull model is used for detection of each class of objects.

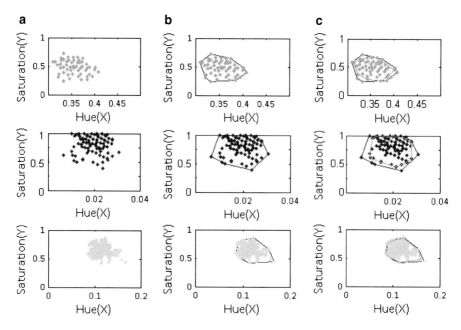

Fig. 6 Examples of convex hulls. (**a**) Positive class examples projected on a positive plane (plane #200) as looking into the *HSV* cube in Fig. 5(b) from *top*. (**b**) Convex hull (*red polygon*) for the positive plane and (**c**) Convex hull (*green polygon*) after first level outlier removal. First row: Green bite-block, second row: Blood, and third row: Stool

Experimental Method and Results

In this section, we first provide a brief background on SVM and k-nearest neighbor (K-NN) classifiers that were used to compare with our proposed method in Section "Classification Algorithms". We describe the result of the comparison in terms of detection accuracy in Section "Accuracy Evaluation" and computation time in Section "Evaluation of Computation Time". Next, we present the evaluation result that our proposed method works better with the *HSV* color space than with the *RGB* color space in terms of detection accuracy in Section "Accuracy Comparison Between *RGB* and *HSV* Color Spaces". Next, we present an accuracy comparison when selecting different color planes as an index plane in Section "Accuracy Comparison of the Proposed Method with Different Index Axes". We provide some sample results in Section "Evaluation Examples". Finally, Section "Computer-aided Quality-Assisted Colonoscopy System" describes a real application that uses the proposed method in a clinical trial.

For our experiments, we used a set of 68 real colonoscopy and upper endoscopy videos. This video set contains 20 videos recorded from Fujinon scope, and 48 videos recorded from Olympus scope to make it scope-independent. The average

Table 1 Number of frames used for the experiment

Object class	Fujinon	Olympus	Total frames
Bite-block	0	700	700
Blood	100	400	500
Stool	300	500	800
Total	400	1,600	2,000

Table 2 Number of examples (pixels) used for the experiment

Object class	Positive examples
Bite-block	140,000
Blood	44,000
Stool	106,000
Total	290,000

length of the videos is around 20 min, and their frame size is 720×480 pixels. These frames have a black boundary around the edges of the frame as seen in Fig. 1. We ignore all the black boundaries. From this video set, we extracted a total of 2,000 video frames showing positive regions of each object as summarized in Table 1. Our domain expert confirmed the ground truth classification. From these frames, we obtained only unique positive examples of a total of 290,000 pixels for this experiment as seen in Table 2. For the evaluation of bite-block detection, currently we have only Olympus video frames. All the computations in our experiments were performed on a PC-compatible workstation with an Intel Core i7 quad core CPU, 8GB RAM, and Windows 7 operating system.

Classification Algorithms

We compare the proposed method with two most popular classifiers: SVM and k-Nearest Neighbor (K-NN). We explain each classification algorithm in brief in the followings.

Support Vector Machine

SVM is a supervised learning model for classification and regression analysis [22]. From a given set of labels and corresponding training data, SVM builds support vectors, which are points in space. SVM takes a training data set D given in (4) as input. The set D is a set of n points (i.e., x_i, in $\mathbb{R}^p$, a set of real numbers in p-dimensional space and the corresponding y_i which is a class label of either 1 (positive) or -1 (negative)). The aim is to find a hyper plane that clearly separates the two classes into two regions while maximizing the margin between the two classes. Any hyper plane can be written as a set of points (i.e., x_i) satisfying the condition given in the (5).

$$D = \left\{ (x_i, y_i) \,\middle|\, x_i \in \mathbb{R}^p, \quad y_i \in \{-1, 1\} \right\}_{i=1}^n \tag{4}$$

$$wx - b = 0 \tag{5}$$

Here, w is the normal vector of the hyper plane; $w \cdot x$ is the dot product of the vectors x and w. The offset of the hyper plane relative to the origin along the normal vector is b/w. If the data set is linearly separable, the two hyper planes that form the margin between two classes can be written as given in (6) and (7). The distance between these two hyper planes is $2/w$. By minimizing the $\|w\|$, one can maximize the margin between the two hyper planes.

$$wx - b = 1 \tag{6}$$

$$wx - b = -1 \tag{7}$$

If the data set is not linearly separable, we need a kernel function, which maps the points in the data set into a higher dimensional data space where the data set can be linearly separable. Radial basis function (RBF) [22], which is one of the recently used kernel functions, was used in this study.

K-Nearest Neighbor

K-NN (k-nearest-neighbor) [23] has been widely used for classification problems. It is based on a distance function that measures the difference or similarity between two instances. The standard Euclidean distance $d(x, y)$ between two instances x and y is often used as the distance function as defined in (8).

$$d(x, y) = \sqrt[2]{\sum_{i=1}^n \left(a_i(x) - a_i(y) \right)^2} \tag{8}$$

Where $a_i(x)$ is the value of the ith attribute of x, and $a_i(y)$ is the value of the ith attribute of y.

Given an instance x, K-NN assigns the most common class of x's k nearest neighbors to x, as shown in (9). We use C and c to denote the class variable and its value, respectively. The class of the instance x is denoted by $c(x)$.

$$c(x) = \arg \max_{c \in C} \sum_{i=1}^k \delta(c, c(y_i)) \tag{9}$$

where $y_1, y_2, \ldots, y_k$ are the k nearest neighbors of x, k is the number of the neighbors, and $\delta(c, c(y_i)) = 1$ if $c = c(y_i)$, and $\delta(c, c(y_i)) = 0$ otherwise.

Table 3 Accuracy metric

		Predicted class	
		Positive	Negative
Actual Class	Positive	TP	FN
	Negative	FP	TN

Accuracy Evaluation

We compare the proposed method with the K-NN and SVM classifiers using a commonly used performance metric *accuracy*. As seen in Table 3, Actual Class is the class to which a particular example belongs (*positive* or *negative*), and the Predicted Class is the result from the classifier, which can be categorized into TP—True Positive, TN—True Negative, FP—False Positive, and FN—False Negative. *Accuracy* is defined as (TP+TN)/(TP+FP+FN+TN), and it represents the number of correctly classified instances.

We partitioned the testing dataset of pixels (shown in Table 2) into 90 partitions, each having 10,000 data points by adding appropriate numbers of negative pixels to capture the computation time of the three techniques more accurately. We named these partitions as partition 1, partition 2, ... and partition 90. The tests were performed on these partitions in incremental manner. For instance, the first test was done on the data points from partition 1, and the second test was done on the data points from both partition 1 and partition 2, and so on. For each test, a tenfold cross-validation [24] was conducted to achieve a better estimation. Accuracy comparisons for three object detections are given in Fig. 7. The proposed method's accuracy is very close to the accuracy of SVM, and far better than that of the KNN in the bite-block detection (Fig. 7a) and that of the blood detection (Fig. 7b). For the stool detection, the accuracy of the proposed method is better than those of both classifiers (Fig. 7c). This is due to the fact that the hue range for the stool examples is much larger than that for the bite-block and blood examples, and the proposed method is more robust than SVM and KNN in handling variations in our applications. The hue range is getting larger when more data points are included and causes the accuracies of SVM and KNN to be lower with the increasing size of the data set as shown in Fig. 7c.

Evaluation of Computation Time

We compare the computation time of the proposed method and the K-NN and the SVM classifiers. Figure 8 shows the comparison of execution times for detection of the three object classes. The *x*-axis represents the number of data points in the

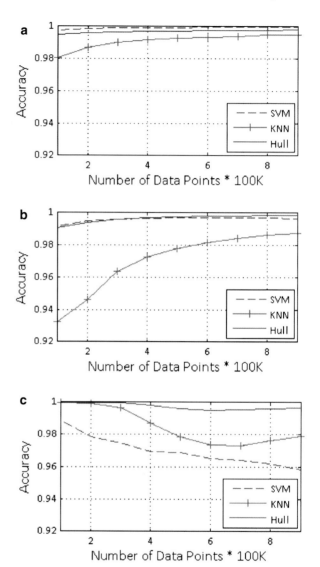

Fig. 7 Accuracy comparisons of proposed (Hull) with SVM and K-NN for (**a**) Bite-block, (**b**) Blood, and (**c**) Stool detections

testing set and the y-axis represents the time taken to classify all the points in the testing set (positive and negative), which was only the detecting time excluding the training time. Figure 8 shows that the proposed method is one or two times faster than the other two techniques.

Fig. 8 Execution time comparisons of the proposed method (Hull), SVM, and K-NN for (**a**) Bite-block, (**b**) Blood, and (**c**) Stool detections

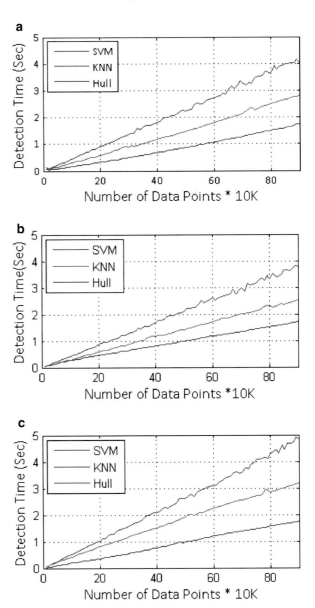

Accuracy Comparison between *RGB and* HSV *color spaces*

For this comparison, the red axis was used as the index axis for the *RGB* color space and the value axis was used as the index axis in the *HSV* color space. The accuracy calculation was done in the same way in Section "Accuracy Evaluation". Table 4 shows that the *HSV* color space outperforms the *RGB* color space in all three classes of object detection.

Table 4 Accuracy comparison between *RGB* and *HSV* color spaces

Number of data points (* 100 K)	Bite-block		Blood		Stool	
	RGB	*HSV*	*RGB*	*HSV*	*RGB*	*HSV*
1	0.97	0.99	0.99	0.99	0.99	0.99
2	0.98	0.99	0.96	0.99	0.99	0.99
3	0.98	0.99	0.96	0.99	0.99	0.99
4	0.98	0.99	0.96	0.99	0.98	0.99
5	0.98	0.99	0.95	0.99	0.98	0.99
6	0.98	0.99	0.95	0.99	0.98	0.99
7	0.98	0.99	0.95	0.99	0.98	0.99
8	0.98	0.99	0.96	0.99	0.98	0.99
9	0.98	0.99	0.96	0.99	0.98	0.99
Average	0.98	0.99	0.96	0.99	0.98	0.99

Table 5 Accuracy of the proposed method with different index axes

Data points (*100 K)	Green bite-block			Blood			Stool		
	Hue	Sat	Val	Hue	Sat	Val	Hue	Sat	Val
1	0.99	0.99	0.99	0.71	0.88	0.99	0.99	0.99	0.99
2	0.99	0.99	0.99	0.76	0.85	0.99	0.99	0.99	0.99
3	0.99	0.99	0.99	0.83	0.86	0.99	0.96	0.98	0.99
4	0.99	0.99	0.99	0.86	0.87	0.99	0.93	0.95	0.99
5	0.99	0.99	0.99	0.89	0.87	0.99	0.91	0.94	0.99
6	0.99	0.99	0.99	0.91	0.88	0.99	0.9	0.93	0.99
7	0.99	0.99	0.99	0.92	0.89	0.99	0.9	0.93	0.99
8	0.98	0.98	0.99	0.93	0.91	0.99	0.92	0.94	0.99
9	0.97	0.97	0.99	0.94	0.92	0.99	0.92	0.94	0.99
Average	0.99	0.99	0.99	0.86	0.88	0.99	0.94	0.95	0.99

Accuracy Comparison of the Proposed Method with Different Index Axes

Experiments were conducted using the proposed method with different index axes (selecting Hue or Saturation axis instead of Value axis). The results are shown in Table 5, where Hue, Saturation (Sat), and Value (Val) were each used as an index axis. Testing was carried out in the same way as in Section "Accuracy Evaluation". As seen in the table, when the index axis is Value, the accuracy for detection of all three classes of objects is better.

Evaluation Examples

Figure 9 shows some example frames detected by the proposed method. The numbers (i.e., 1, 2, and 3) on each frame of the first column represent the regions

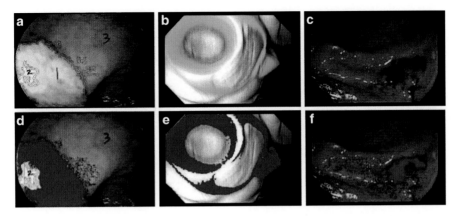

Fig. 9 Detected examples. (**a**) Frame with a stool region, (**b**) Frame with a green bite-block region, (**c**) Frame with a blood region, (**d**) Detected regions (with *blue markings*) from (**a**) using the stool model, (**e**) Detected regions (with *blue markings*) from (**b**) using the green bite-block model, and (**f**) Detected regions (with *blue markings*) from (**c**) using the blood model. ((**a**) and (**d**) are frames from Fujinon scope, and (**b**), (**c**), (**e**), and (**f**) are frames from Olympus scope)

manually segmented and annotated for the ground truth. For instance, Region 1 in Fig. 9a was labeled as stool by the domain expert. The first row of Fig. 9 consists of the original frames with the ground truth marked for stool, green bite-block, and blood. The second row contains the results (blue-colored areas) from the proposed method for each frame in the first row.

Computer-aided Quality-Assisted Colonoscopy System

We placed our novel computer-aided quality assist colonoscopy system at Mayo Clinic Rochester to conduct a clinical trial to evaluate its impact in improving inspection quality of the colon. This new system based on a real-time video processing framework and middleware called SAPPHIRE [9] accepts video signals from a colonoscope and processes the information in each video frame for quality metric generation in real-time using a set of software modules. The proposed stool and bite-block detection modules were implemented as dynamic-linked libraries and integrated with SAPPHIRE. The stool module estimates the amount of stool debris in the colon when a colonoscopy procedure is performed. The bite-block module detects a procedure type (either colonoscopy or upper endoscopy) at the beginning of the procedure so that only colonoscopy-related modules run on that colonoscopy procedures. Figure 10 shows a sample snapshot of the output of this system; stool-related metric is marked in a red box shown on a head up display (HUD).

Fig. 10 A snapshot of a
head up display on a frame
captured using Olympus
scope; some information
generated from Stool is
manually outlined in a *red
box*

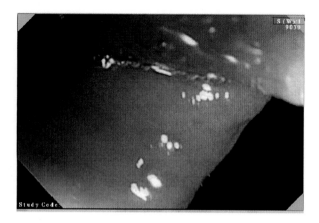

Conclusion and Future Work

Detecting objects from colonoscopy videos is very essential for both post-processing and real-time quality measurements. We propose a method to detect a bite-block, blood, and stool pixels using color features. Our method provides an acceptable accuracy and very fast detection time. Our proposed method offers a significant reduction in execution time when compared to K-NN and SVM, which is essential for real-time environments. In addition, our method is an incremental learning method to learn new positive class examples without running the entire training process from beginning as we can recompute each positive plane separately. This adds the valuable ability of incremental learning to our method. The proposed method is applicable everywhere that needs a color-based region or object detection. As future work, we will work on a method to create a combination of a concave hull and a convex hull to model positive examples in a given positive plane. This would improve the overall detection accuracy even more.

Acknowledgment This work is partially supported by NSF STTR-Grant No. 0740596, 0956847, National Institute of Diabetes and Digestive and Kidney Diseases (NIDDK DK083745), and the Mayo Clinic. Any opinions, findings, conclusions, or recommendations expressed in this paper are those of authors. They do not necessarily reflect the views of the funding agencies. Johnny Wong, Wallapak Tavanapong, and JungHwan Oh hold positions at EndoMetric Corporation, Ames, IA 50014, U.S.A, a for profit company that markets endoscopy-related software. Johnny Wong, Wallapak Tavanapong, JungHwan Oh, and Mayo Clinic own stocks in EndoMetric. Johnny Wong, Wallapak Tavanapong, and JungHwan Oh have received royalty payments from EndoMetric.

References

1. American Cancer Society (2011) Colorectal cancer facts & figures 2011–2013. American Cancer Society, Atlanta
2. Johnson DD, Fletcher JG, MacCarty RL et al (2007) Effect of slice thickness and primary 2D versus 3D virtual dissection on colorectal lesion detection at CT colonography in 452 asymptomatic adults. AJR Am J Roentgenol 189(3):672–680
3. Pabby A, Schoen RE, Weissfeld JL, Burt R, Kikendall JW, Lance P et al (2005) Analysis of colorectal cancer occurrence during surveillance colonoscopy in the dietary prevention trial. Gastrointest Endosc 61(3):385–391
4. Rex DK, Bond JH, Winawer S, Levin TR, Burt RW et al (2002) Quality in the technical performance of colonoscopy and the continuous quality improvement process for colonoscopy: recommendations of the U.S. multi-society task force on colorectal cancer. Am J Gastroenterol 97(6):1296–1308
5. Douglas KR, John LP, Todd HB, Amitabh C, Jonathan C, Stephen ED et al (2006) Quality indicators for colonoscopy. Am J Gastroenterol 101:873–885
6. Oh J, Hwang S, Cao Y, Tavanapong W, Liu D, Wong J et al (2009) Measuring objective quality of colonoscopy. IEEE Trans Biomed Eng 56(9):2190–2196
7. Hwang S, Oh J, Lee J, de Groen PC, Cao Y, Tavanapong W, Wong S, et al (2005) Automatic measurement of quality metrics for colonoscopy videos. In: Proceedings of ACM multimedia 2005, Singapore, pp 912–921, Nov 2005
8. Stanek S, Tavanapong W, Wong J, Oh J, de Groen PC (2008) Automatic real-time capture and segmentation of endoscopy video, PACS and imaging informatics. In: Proceedings of SPIE medical imaging, vol 6919, pp 69190X-69190X-10, Feb 2008
9. Stanek SR, Tavanapong W, Wong J, JungHwan Oh, Nawarathna RD, Muthukudage J, de Groen PC (2011) SAPPHIRE middleware and software development kit for medical video analysis. In: Proceedings of the 24th international symposium on computer-based medical systems (CBMS), pp 1–6, June 2011
10. Cappel MS, Friedel D (2002) The role of sigmoidoscopy and colonoscopy in the diagnosis and management of lower gastrointestinal disorders: endoscopic findings, therapy, and complications. Med Clin North Am 86(6):1253–1288
11. Ness RM, Manam R, Hoen HJ, Chalasani N (2001) Predictors of inadequate bowel preparation for colonoscopy. Am J Gastroenterol 96:1797–1802
12. Muthukudage J, Oh J, Tavanapong W, Wong J, de Groen PC (2011) Color based stool region detection in colonoscopy videos for quality measurements. Lecture Notes in Computer Science, vol 7087/2011, pp 61–72
13. Hwang S, Oh J, Tavanapong W, Wong J, de Groen PC (2008) Stool detection in colonoscopy videos. In: Proceedings of international conference of the IEEE engineering in medicine and biology society (EMBC), Vancouver, British Columbia, pp 3004–3007, Aug 2008
14. Giritharan B, Yuan X, Liu J, Buckles B, Oh J, Tang SJ (2008) Bleeding detection from capsule endoscopy videos. In: Proceedings of the 30th annual international conference of the IEEE engineering in medicine and biology society, 2008 (EMBS' 08), Vancouver, British Columbia, pp 4780–4783
15. Manjunath BS, Ohm J, Vasudevan VV, Yamada A (2011) Color and texture descriptors. IEEE Trans Circ Syst Video Techn 11(6):703–715
16. Karargyris A, Bourbakis N (2008) A methodology for detecting blood-based abnormalities in wireless capsule endoscopy videos. In: Proceedings of the 8th IEEE international conference on bioinformatics and bioengineering, 2008 (BIBE'08), Athens, Greece, pp 1–6
17. Bourbakis N (2005) Detecting abnormal patterns in WCE images. In: Proceedings of the 5th IEEE symposium on bioinformatics and bioengineering, 2005 (BIBE'05), Minneapolis, Minnesota, pp 232–238

18. Lau PY, Correia P (2007) Detection of bleeding patterns in WCE video using multiple features. In: Proceedings of the 29th annual international conference of the IEEE engineering in medicine and biology society (EMBS'07), Vancouver, British Columbia, pp 5601–5604
19. Li B, Meng MQ (2009) Computer-based detection of bleeding and ulcer in wireless capsule endoscopy images by chromaticity moments. Comput Biol Med 39(2):141–147
20. Tkalcic M, Tasic JF (2003) Colour spaces: perceptual, historical and applicational background, EUROCON 2003. Computer as a Tool. The IEEE Region 8, vol 1, pp 304–308, Sept 2003
21. Barber CB, Dobkin DP, Huhdanpaa H (1996) The quickhull algorithm for convex hulls. ACM Trans Math Softw 2(4):469–483
22. Cortes C, Vladimir V (1995) "Support-vector networks" machine learning. vol 20
23. Aha DW, Kibler D, Albert MK (1991) Instance-based learning algorithms. Mach Learn 6:37–66
24. Rodriguez JD, Perez A, Lozano JA (2010) Sensitivity analysis of k-fold cross validation in prediction error estimation. IEEE Trans Pattern Anal Mach Intell 32(3):569–575

Biography

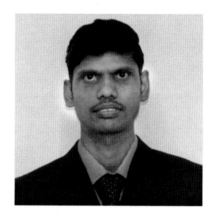

Jayantha Muthukudage received his Master's Degree in Computer Science from the University of North Texas in 2012 and his Bachelor's degree in Computer Science from the University of Peradeniya, Sri Lanka in 2006. Now, he is a PhD student in the department of Computer Science and Engineering, University of North Texas. He is expected to complete his PhD in the summer of 2013. His major research interests are endoscopy image analysis, objects detections, and quality analysis of endoscopy videos.

JungHwan Oh received M.S. and Ph.D. degrees in computer science from the University of Central Florida in 1997 and 2000, respectively. Dr. Oh worked with the Department of Computer Science and Engineering at University of Texas, Arlington from 2001 to 2006. In 2006, he joined the Department of Computer Science and Engineering at University of North Texas. He has established a medical video research with the collaboration of Iowa State University and Mayo Clinic in 2003. This research focuses on the medical video (colonoscopy, endoscopy, broncoscopy, minimal access surgery, etc.) analyses and mining. As results of these researches, a number of proposals have been granted from National Science Foundation and National Institute of Health. He has organized a number of workshops and Special Sessions on multimedia data processing and served as a member of program committee and an editor of various international conferences on imaging science, systems, and information technology. He is the author or coauthor of more than 90 journal articles, book chapters, and conference papers.

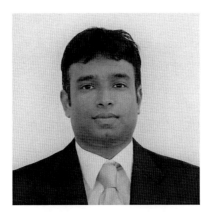

Ruwan Nawarthna received his Master's Degree in Computer Science from the University of North Texas in 2011 and his Bachelor's degree in Computer Science from the University of Peradeniya, Sri Lanka in 2005. Now, he is a PhD student in the department of Computer Science and Engineering, University of North Texas. He is expected to complete his PhD in the summer of 2013. His major research interests are endoscopy image analysis, camera motion analysis, and multi-class image texture analysis.

Wallapak Tavanapong received the B.S. degree in Computer Science from Thammasat University, Thailand, in 1992 and the M.S. and Ph.D. degrees in Computer Science from the University of Central Florida in 1995 and 1999, respectively. She joined Iowa State University in 1999 and is currently an Associate Professor of Computer Science. She is a co-founder and a Chief Technology Officer of EndoMetric, a software company that offers computer-aided technology for endoscopy procedures. Her current research interests include high performance multimedia computing in healthcare, multimedia content analysis and mining, multimedia databases, multimedia systems and communications, electronic medical records, and high performance databases. Her research has been supported by funding agencies such as the U.S. National Science Foundation, Agency for Healthcare Research and Quality, and Mayo Clinic in Rochester. She has served as an editorial board member for ACM SIGMOD Digital Symposium Collection, an NSF panel reviewer, a program committee member for international conferences, and a referee for reputable conferences and journals.

Johnny Wong is a Professor & Associate Chair of the Computer Science Department and Information Assurance Program at Iowa State University. His research interests include Software Systems & Networking, Security & Medical Informatics. Most of his research projects are funded by government agencies and industries. He is the President/CEO of a startup company EndoMetric, with products for Medical Informatics. He has served as a member of program committee of various international conferences on intelligent systems and computer networking. He was the program co-Chair of the COMPSAC 2006 and General co-Chair of the COMPSAC 2008 conference. He has published over 100 papers in peer-reviewed journals and conferences.

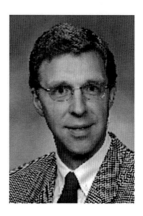

Dr. Piet C. de Groen, M.D., is a Consultant in Gastroenterology and Hepatology at Mayo Clinic, Professor of Medicine at Mayo Clinic College of Medicine, and former Program Director of the Mayo Clinic/IBM Computational Biology Collaboration. He is an NIH-funded clinical investigator and international expert in medical informatics, primary liver cancers, and colonoscopy. His endoscopic research is focused on measuring what happens during colonoscopy. Together with collaborators at Iowa State University and the University of North Texas, he has created a first-of-a-kind new software system that automatically captures and analyzes "inside-the-patient" video information of medical procedures performed via endoscopy. At present he is studying patient- and endoscopist-specific features, including quality of the colon preparation and effort of the endoscopist to visualize mucosa, remove remaining fecal material, and adequately distend the colon. The ultimate goal of his endoscopic research related to colonoscopy is a fully automated quality control system that provides real-time feedback to the endoscopist and insures individualized healthcare by virtually guaranteeing a high quality examination for each patient. Another goal is to extend the technology to other organs examined using endoscopy equipment such as esophagus, stomach, small bowel, bronchi, bladder, and joints and combine the information obtained from the optical signal with information derived from molecular tests and other imaging modalities.

Colon Surface Registration Using Ricci Flow

Wei Zeng, Rui Shi, Zhengyu Su, and David Xianfeng Gu

Abstract Shape registration is very fundamental for shape analysis problems, especially for abnormality detection in medical applications. In virtual colonoscopy, CT scans are typically acquired with the patient in both supine and prone positions. The registration of these two scans is desirable so that the user can clarify situations or confirm polyp findings at a location in one scan with the same location in the other, thereby improving polyp detection rates and reducing false positives. However, this supine-prone registration is challenging because of the substantial distortions in the colon shape due to the patient's change in position. In this work, we present an efficient algorithm and framework for performing this registration through the use of conformal geometry and Ricci flow to guarantee that the registration is a diffeomorphism (a one-to-one and onto mapping). The taeniae coli and colon flexures are automatically extracted for each supine and prone surface, employing the colon geometry. The two colon surfaces are then divided into several segments using flexures, and each segment is cut along a taenia coli and conformally flattened to the rectangular domain using Ricci flow. Corresponding feature points between supine and prone are found and used to adjust the conformal flattening to be quasi-conformal, such that the features become aligned. We present multiple methods of visualizing our results, including 2D flattened rendering, corresponding 3D endoluminal views, and rendering of distortion measurements. We demonstrate the efficiency and efficacy of our registration method by illustrating matched views on both the 2D flattened colon images and in the 3D volume rendered colon endoluminal view. We analytically evaluate the correctness of the results by measuring the distance between features on the registered colons.

W. Zeng (✉)
Florida International University, 11200 SW 8th St, Miami, FL 33199, USA
e-mail: wzeng@cs.fiu.edu

R. Shi • Z. Su • D.X. Gu
Stony Brook University, 100 Nicolls Rd, Stony Brook, NY 11790, USA
e-mail: rshi@cs.stonybrook.edu; zysu@cs.stonybrook.edu; gu@cs.stonybrook.edu

A.S. El-Baz et al. (eds.), *Abdomen and Thoracic Imaging: An Engineering & Clinical Perspective*, DOI 10.1007/978-1-4614-8498-1_15,
© Springer Science+Business Media New York 2014

Keywords Ricci flow • Conformal mapping • Quasi-conformal mapping • Diffeomorphism • Surface matching • Surface registration

Introduction

Colorectal cancer is the third most incident cancer and the second leading cause of cancer-related mortality in the USA [1]. Optical colonoscopy (OC), whereby precancerous polyps can be located and removed, has been recommended for screening and has helped to greatly reduce the mortality rate of colorectal cancer [2]. Virtual colonoscopy (VC) techniques have been developed as viable noninvasive alternatives to OC for screening purposes [3, 4]. For a VC procedure, computed tomography (CT) scans of the abdomen are commonly acquired with the patient in both supine (facing up) and prone (facing down) positions. From these scans, the colon wall can be extracted as in Fig. 1 and visualized by the VC user as a volume rendered endoluminal view, mimicking the endoscopic view of an OC.

The use of computer-aided detection (CAD) of colonic polyps has also been suggested [5–7]. A CAD scheme can help to reduce the necessary reading and interpretation time of the user and can act as a second reader to improve detection rates in VC. Though various CAD methods can achieve different accuracies, a common problem among them is the presence of false positives in the results. A reduction of these false positives would help the user to focus on true suspicious areas and not waste time on unimportant regions.

In addition to the general VC and CAD techniques, researchers have worked to find new ways of visualizing the data to aid the user in identifying polyps or assisting with interventional needs. Volumetric curved planar reformation has been used to aid the viewer in locating polyps with a 3D surface superimposed over the standard CT slices [8]. For simulating intestinal surgery, a system has been developed to visualize the colon and provide collision processing [9]. There has also been work in creating a correlation between the VC navigation view and the OC view based upon the different view paths [10]. In this work, we aim to add another visualization tool to the doctor's toolbelt. The main goal of our work is to allow the user to view one location on the colon (whether in a 2D flattened view or a 3D endoluminal view) in one scan, and then jump to and view the identical region in the other scan. We also show how the user can visualize the deformation of the colon surface if such a utility is desired.

Throughout the development of VC, the registration of the supine and prone scans has remained a constant and challenging problem [11–13]. Being able to register these two scans is useful for both a routine VC system and a CAD system. In the case of a VC system, providing the user the ability to jump from one area in one scan to the same area in the other scan would allow for the easy comparison of these areas when something might be unclear in one of the scans, or for confirming a finding. For a CAD system, a proper registration could help achieve greater accuracy while at the same time reducing false positive results. We are presently

Fig. 1 A colon reconstructed from its (**a**) supine and (**b**) prone scans

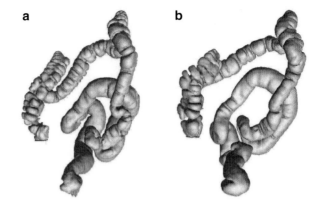

interested in performing supine-prone registration due to the visualization possibilities that it presents, both for viewing corresponding regions of the colon surface and for visualizing the elastic deformation of the colon.

In this paper, we present a method of supine-prone registration using conformal colon flattening. Conformal colon flattening has been introduced as an enhancement for VC navigation [14] and has been utilized successfully for CAD [5]. According to conformal geometry theory, there exists an angle preserving map which periodically flattens the colon surface onto a planar rectangle. This mapping minimizes the total stretching energy. Because the conformal mapping is locally shape preserving, it offers an effective way to visualize the entire colon surface and exposes all of the geometric structures hidden in the original shape embedded in 3D.

The characteristics of the deformation between supine and prone are determined by the elasticity properties of the tissues and muscles. The strain-stress relations for different types of tissues or muscles are different. If the strain-stress relation deformation is independent of the orientation, then local deformation is practically a scaling, and the global deformation is conformal. In that case, we can flatten each supine and prone surface to a planar rectangle conformally, and those two rectangles should be similar. By aligning the planar rectangles, we can get a one-to-one and onto mapping and obtain the registration between them. In this work, we introduce this registration approach and carefully design experiments to test whether the deformation between supine and prone is conformal or not. Our experimental results show that the deformation is not conformal, but close to conformal.

An elastic deformation with bounded angle distortion is called a quasi-conformal map. The angle distortion for a quasi-conformal map can be represented as a complex valued function, the so-called Beltrami coefficient. The Beltrami coefficient fully controls the quasi-conformal map, which is determined by the elasticity of the underlying material. By better understanding the deformation between supine and prone, we can understand the elasticity of the tissues and muscles and vice versa.

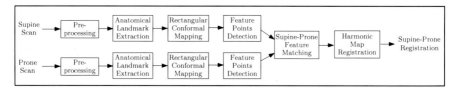

Fig. 2 The pipeline for supine-prone colon registration

The nonrigid elastic deformation between supine and prone colons poses a great challenge for shape registration. In this work, we locate and match the anatomical landmarks [15], including flexures and taeniae coli, and internal features on conformally flattened supine and prone surfaces [16], and compute the registration by harmonic maps with these feature constraints. The resulting supine-prone registration is a quasi-conformal map (diffeomorphism), which reflects the elastic deformation of the muscle and tissue. The distortion is evaluated by the Beltrami coefficients. Our experiments on 6 pairs of supine-prone colons obtained an average $\mathbb{R}^3$ distance error of 7.85 mm for the feature points and polyps evaluated. To the best of our knowledge, this is the first work to apply geometric mapping for supine-prone colon registration by converting the 3D registration problem to a 2D image matching problem. The whole process is efficient and automatic, and our registration method performs better than other existing methods (see section "Analytic Registration Evaluation").

Figure 2 shows our registration pipeline, which primarily consists of five stages. As the input, the supine and prone CT scans are subjected to the pre-processing steps, including cleansing, segmentation with topological simplification, and surface mesh reconstruction, which have been studied previously and are outside the scope of this paper. Given the supine and prone surfaces, anatomical landmarks are extracted (see section "Taeniae Coli and Flexures Extraction" and [15]). Using these landmarks, the colon surfaces of both supine and prone are decomposed to segments. For each segment, a flat rectangular conformal mapping is obtained (see section "Conformal Colon Flattening"). Based on these flat images, feature points are detected and their correspondences between supine and prone are obtained (see [15]). With the feature correspondence constraints, the supine-prone registration is performed using harmonic maps (see sections "Quasi-Conformal Map" and "Surface Registration Framework").

Given the completed supine-prone registration, we present the methods in which we visualize the results of our registration algorithm. We first demonstrate flattened rendering of the colon in the native 2D registration format (see section "Flattened Colon Rendering"). For the endoluminal views which would be used by a radiologist reading a case, we detail a method to provide correlated views between supine and prone (see section "Visualization of Quasi-Conformality"). To better understand where the deformation occurs most on the colon surface, we show the visualization of the Beltrami coefficient both in 2D and 3D (see section "Visualization of Quasi-Conformality"). The results of our registration are analyzed and discussed in section "Experimental Results". We verify the efficacy of our work using both objective analytic and subjective visual methods. We present the related work in the next section and brief background information on conformal mapping and quasi-conformal mapping in section "Conformal Geometry Theory" to familiarize the reader with the terms.

Related Work

Early work on supine-prone registration for VC applications focused on using the centerlines and various landmarks. A basic method applies linear stretching and shrinking operations to the centerline, where local extrema are matched and used to drive the deformations [11]. Improved methods of centerline correlation were also investigated for use in reducing false positive results [13]. Correlating individual points along the centerline through the use of dynamic programming has also been suggested [12, 17].

More recently, the taeniae coli (three bands of smooth muscle along the colon surface) have been used as features which can be correlated between the two scans [18, 19]. This relies on a manual identification of one of the three taeniae coli, and then an automatic algorithm repeats the line representing the identified taenia coli at equal distances. Further progress has been made where the haustral folds and the points between them can be automatically detected, and the taeniae coli are identified by connecting these points [20]. However, this method is only feasible on the ascending and transverse portions of the colon.

Deformation fields have also been suggested for use in supine-prone registration. Motion vectors can be identified for matched centerline regions, interpolated for non-matched regions, and then propagated to the entire volume [21]. It has also been proposed to use a free-form deformation grid to model the possible changes in the colon shape from supine to prone [22].

Conformal mapping has been successfully used for many medical applications, such as brain cortex surface morphology study [23] and colonic polyp detection [5]. In this work, we perform the supine-prone registration through conformal mapping based on Ricci flow. The colon surface is reconstructed from CT images, represented as a topological cylinder in the discrete form of a triangular mesh, and conformally mapped to a planar rectangle. The subsequent registration is carried out through the 2D conformal mapping images of the supine and prone colons.

Ricci flow was first introduced by Hamilton [24] and later it was generalized to the discrete case [25]. Ricci flow is a powerful tool to compute surface uniformization, deforming any arbitrary surfaces to one of the 3 canonical spaces with different background geometries, the sphere, the Euclidean plane, or the hyperbolic disk. The discrete computational algorithms can be found in [26–29]. Ricci flow can also be generalized to compute general quasi-conformal maps by the auxiliary metric method [30]. Discrete surface Ricci flow method has been successfully used in many applications in both engineering and medical imaging, such as general 3D shape matching, registration and tracking [27, 31, 32], shape indexing and comparison in Teichmüller space [33], homotopy detection [29], vestibular system morphometry [34], brain mapping [35, 36], 3D human facial expression recognition [37], virtual colonoscopy [16, 38], wireless sensor network routing, load balancing and data storage [39–42], and so on.

Because the deformation from supine to prone is not conformal, we generalize the conformal colon flattening method to a quasi-conformal flattening for registration purpose. Most existing colon registration methods cannot guarantee the mapping to be a diffeomorphism (one-to-one and onto mapping). Due to the complicated geometric structure of the colon surface, the existing methods often introduce folding or singularities in the mapping. Our method is based on the biophysical nature of the deformation from supine to prone, which is physically elastic and anisotropic. Due to the material properties of the muscles and tissues, the deformation can be exactly modeled as a quasi-conformal map. Our experimental results validate that the mapping is indeed quasi-conformal.

Conformal Geometry Theory

This section briefly introduces the background knowledge in conformal geometry, necessary for the discussion in the work. For more details, we refer readers to [43] for Riemann surface theory, [44] for Teichmüller theory, [45] for quasi-conformal mapping, and [46] for differential geometry.

Conformal Mapping

Let S_1, S_2 be two metric surfaces, with Riemannian metrics $\mathbf{g}_1$ and $\mathbf{g}_2$, respectively. A map $\varphi : S_1 \rightarrow S_2$ is *angle-preserving* or *conformal*, if and only if the pull back metric induced by ϕ satisfies

$$\phi^* \mathbf{g}_2 = e^{2\lambda} \mathbf{g}_1,$$

where $e^{2\lambda}$ is called the *conformal factor*. The simplest conformal mapping is the complex holomorphic functions $f : \mathbb{C} \rightarrow \mathbb{C}$, satisfying the Cauchy–Riemann equation

$$\partial_{\bar{z}} f(z) = 0,$$

where $z = u + iv$ and the complex differential operators are

$$\partial_z = \frac{1}{2}(\partial_u - i\partial_v), \partial_{\bar{z}} = \frac{1}{2}(\partial_u + i\partial_v).$$

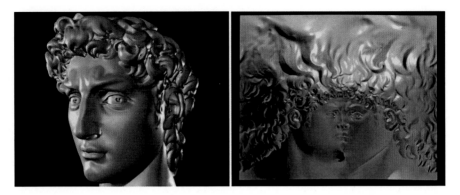

Fig. 3 Conformal mapping preserves local shapes

Locally, a conformal mapping is a scaling transformation; therefore, it preserves local shapes. As shown in Fig. 3, the 3D surface of Michelangelo's David head is conformally mapped to the planar rectangle, although the global shape has been distorted, the local shapes are well preserved. On the planar image, one can still easily locate the main geometric features. This property is valuable for virtual colonoscopy, where the colon wall surface is conformally flattened onto a 2D image. Because the mapping is shape-preserving, the polyps can be detected on the planar image directly.

Given an oriented metric surface $(S, \mathbf{g})$, $U \subset S$ is a neighborhood, then there is a conformal mapping φ from the unit disk $\mathbb{D}$ to U, such that the Riemannian metric is written in a special form

$$\mathbf{g} = e^{2\lambda(u,v)}(du^2 + dv^2) = e^{2\lambda(z)}dzd\bar{z},$$

where $z = u + iv$ are called *isothermal parameters* of the surface. Suppose the surface is covered by an atlas, such that all local coordinates are isothermal parameters, and all the chart transitions are biholomorphic, then the atlas is called a *conformal structure* of the surface, induced by the Riemannian metric. A surface with a conformal structure is called a *Riemann surface*.

Uniformization

The surface uniformization theorem claims that for any metric surface $(S, \mathbf{g})$, there exists a unique conformal factor $e^{2\lambda}$, such that the Riemannian metric $e^{2\lambda}\mathbf{g}$ induces a constant Gaussian curvature, which is one three possible choices $\{+1, 0, -1\}$ depending on the surface topology.

As shown in Fig. 4, for closed surfaces, genus zero surfaces can conformally mapped to the unit sphere $\mathbb{S}^2$, genus one surfaces can conformally deformed to Euclidean metric $\mathbb{E}^2$, high genus surfaces can conformally deformed to hyperbolic

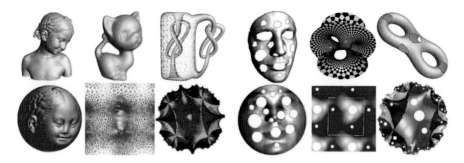

Fig. 4 Uniformization for surfaces, computed by discrete surface Ricci flow

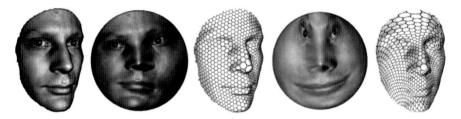

Fig. 5 Comparison between conformal mapping (frame 2 and 3) and a general diffeomorphism (frame 4 and 5)

metric $\mathbb{H}^2$. For compact surfaces with boundaries, all the boundaries are mapped to circles on the canonical domains, as shown in the right half of the figure.

The uniformization theorem allows us to map all types of shapes to one of the three canonical domains, the sphere, the plane, or the hyperbolic disk and register the shapes on the 2D canonical domain. This simplifies the problem of surface matching and registration and has been broadly applied in medical imaging field.

Quasi-Conformal Mapping

Figure 5 shows another characteristic of conformal mappings, it maps infinitesimal circles to infinitesimal circles. In contrast, a general diffeomorphism maps infinitesimal circles to infinitesimal ellipses. The general diffeomorphisms are represented as *quasi-conformal* map.

Given two Riemann surfaces S_1 and S_2 with conformal atlases, choose a local conformal parameter (isothermal parameters) z for S_1 and w for S_2, respectively. Let $f : S \to D$ is a diffeomorphism between the surfaces, then its local representation is $w = f(z)$, the *Beltrami coefficient* of the mapping f is defined as

$$\mu(z) = \frac{\partial_{\bar{z}} f}{\partial_z f}(z). \tag{1}$$

Fig. 6 Geometric
interpretation of Beltrami
coefficient

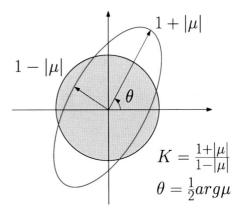

$$K = \frac{1+|\mu|}{1-|\mu|}$$

$$\theta = \frac{1}{2}arg\mu$$

Globally, one can use Beltrami differential $\mu(z)d\bar{z}/dz$ to represent the mapping. At each point z, the eccentricity and the orientation of the infinitesimal ellipse are given by

$$K = \frac{1+|\mu|}{1-|\mu|}, \theta = \frac{1}{2}arg\mu$$

as shown in Fig. 6.

General diffeomorphisms between surfaces (induced by natural deformations) are quasi-conformal mappings. Each quasi-conformal mapping is associated with its Beltrami differential. Inversely, the mapping can be uniquely determined by its Beltrami differential (under certain normalization conditions) by solving the so-called *Beltrami equation*,

$$\partial_{\bar{z}}f(z) = \mu(z)\partial_z f(z). \tag{2}$$

For example, consider all the normalized diffeomorphisms from the unit disk to itself, $f : \mathbb{D} \to \mathbb{D}$, such that $f(0) = 0$ and $f(1) = 1$, then the space of normalized diffeomorphisms and the space of Beltrami coefficients have a one-to-one correspondence.

$$\{Normalized\ Diff\} \sim \{Beltrami\ Coefficient\}.$$

Suppose $(S_1,\mathbf{g}_1)$ and $(S_2,\mathbf{g}_2)$ are two metric surfaces, with local isothermal parameters z and w, respectively. $\varphi : (S_1,\mathbf{g}_1) \to (S_2,\mathbf{g}_2)$ is a quasi-conformal mapping with Beltrami coefficient μ. Then the same mapping $\varphi : (S_1, \mathbf{g}) \to (S_2, \mathbf{g}_2)$ under the auxiliary metric

$$\tilde{\mathbf{g}} = |dz + \mu d\bar{z}|^2, \tag{3}$$

is conformal. Therefore a quasi-conformal mapping can be converted to be a conformal mapping under the auxiliary metric associated with the Beltrami coefficient.

Surface Ricci Flow

Surface Ricci flow is a powerful tool to design Riemannian metrics using prescribed Gaussian curvatures, it can be applied for computing surface conformal mappings and quasi-conformal mappings directly.

Let both $\mathbf{g}$ and $\mathbf{g}$ are Riemannian metrics of a surface S, $\mathbf{g} = e^{2\lambda}\mathbf{g}$, then the Gaussian curvature and geodesic curvature induced by them satisfies the following Yamabe equation:

$$\bar{K} = e^{-2\lambda}(K - \Delta_{\mathbf{g}}\lambda)$$
$$\bar{k}_g = e^{-\lambda}(k_g - \partial_{\mathbf{n},\mathbf{g}}\lambda) \quad.$$

The surface uniformization metric can be obtained by solving the Yamabe equation. Surface Ricci flow is an effective tool for it.

The *normalized surface Ricci flow* is given as

$$\partial_t \mathbf{g}(t) = (\rho - 2K(t))\mathbf{g}(t),$$

where ρ is the mean value of the scalar curvature

$$\rho = \frac{4\pi\chi(S)}{A(0)}$$

where $A(0)$ is the total area of the surface at time $t = 0$, $\chi(S)$ is the Euler characteristic number of the surface. It can be shown that the normalized surface Ricci flow preserves the total area

$$\partial_t A(t) = 0,$$

furthermore, the curvature evolves according to a nonlinear heat diffusion process

$$\partial_t K(t) = \Delta_{\mathbf{g}(t)} K(t) + K(t)(2K(t) - \rho).$$

Hamilton and Chow [24, 47] proved that normalized surface Ricci flow converges to the constant Gaussian curvature metric.

Harmonic Mapping

Suppose $\varphi : (S_1, \mathbf{g}_1) \to (S_2, \mathbf{g}_2)$ is a smooth mapping between two metric surfaces. We choose isothermal parameters of the two surfaces, z for S_1 and w for S_2, respectively, the Riemannian metrics can be represented as

$$\mathbf{g}_1 = \sigma(z)dzd\bar{z}, \mathbf{g}_2 = \rho(z)dwd\bar{w}.$$

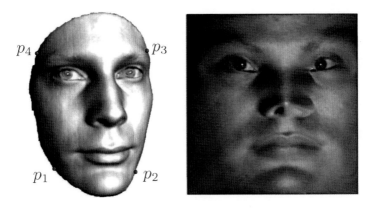

Fig. 7 A harmonic map from a human face surface to a planar rectangle

The *harmonic energy* of the mapping is defined as

$$E(\varphi) = \int_{S_1} \frac{\rho(w(z))}{\sigma(z)} (|w_z|^2 + |w_{\bar{z}}|^2) \sigma(z) \frac{i}{2} dz \wedge d\bar{z} \tag{4}$$

The so-called *harmonic maps* are the minimizers of the harmonic energy. The necessary condition of φ to be a harmonic is the Euler–Lagrange equation

$$w_{z\bar{z}} + \frac{\rho_w}{\rho} w_z w_{\bar{z}} \equiv 0.$$

Given a degree one map, we can use the following nonlinear heat diffusion method to deform it to a harmonic map,

$$\frac{\partial w(z,t)}{\partial t} = -\left(w_{z\bar{z}} + \frac{\rho_w(w)}{\rho(w)} w_z w_{\bar{z}} \right). \tag{5}$$

From the Definition 4, we see the harmonic energy is solely determined by the conformal structure of the source and the Riemannian metric of the target. One can deform the conformal structure by a Beltrami differential μ, then obtain the conformal coordinates $\zeta(z)$, which can be obtained by solving the Beltrami equation.

Harmonic map is the smoothest map in the homotopy class (Fig. 7). If the surfaces are topological disks, the restriction of φ on the boundary is a homeomorphism, then the harmonic map is a diffeomorphism. Furthermore, if the target surface has Riemannian metric with negative Gaussian curvature, then degree one harmonic map must be a diffeomorphism. Harmonic maps have been applied for brain mapping and colon registration in medical imaging.

Computational Strategies

There are many methods for conformal surface mapping in the literature. In the following, we focus on the discrete surface Ricci flow method.

Discrete Surface Ricci Flow

In practice, surfaces are represented as simplicial complex, namely triangle mesh as shown in Fig. 8. We use $M = (V,E,F)$ to denote the mesh with vertex set V, edge set E, and face set F. A *discrete Riemannian metric* on a triangle mesh is a function defined on the edges, $l : E \to \mathbb{R}^+$, satisfies triangular inequality, on each face $[v_i,v_j,v_k]$,

$$l_{ij} + l_{jk} > l_{ki}.$$

The *discrete Gaussian curvature* is defined on the vertices $K : V \to \mathbb{R}$, as angle deficit,

$$K(v) = \begin{cases} 2\pi - \sum_i \alpha_i & v \notin \partial M \\ \pi - \sum_i \alpha_i & v \in \partial M \end{cases}$$

where α_i's are corner angles adjacent to the vertex v, ∂M represents the boundary of the mesh (Fig. 9).

Then the discrete curvatures also satisfy Gauss–Bonnet theorem, namely, the total curvature is a topological invariant

$$\sum_{v \notin \partial M} K(v) + \sum_{v \in \partial M} K(v) = 2\pi\chi(M).$$

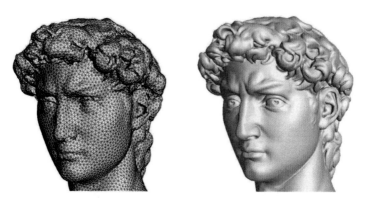

Fig. 8 Smooth surfaces are approximated by triangle meshes

Fig. 9 Discrete curvatures

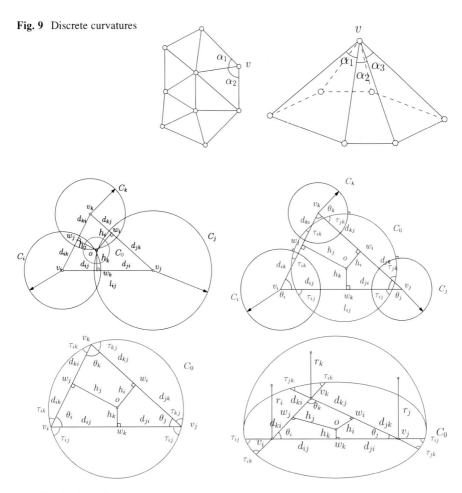

Fig. 10 Configurations

Surface Ricci flow conformally deforms the Riemannian metric, conformal transformation preserves infinitesimal circles. Thurston proposes to replace infinitesimal circles to circles with finite sizes, and by changing the circle radii to approximate the conformal deformation.

Figure 10 shows the common configurations. For the first frame, which is classical Thurston's circle packing, a circle is centered at each vertex v_i, and denoted as (v_i, γ_i), two circles at the end vertices of an edge $[v_i, v_j]$ has an intersection angle $\phi_{i\,j}$, during the deformation, $\phi_{i\,j}$ keeps unchanged. The edge length

$$l_{ij}^2 = \gamma_i^2 + \gamma_j^2 + 2\gamma_i\gamma_j \cos \phi_{ij}.$$

The second frame shows the inversive distance circle packing, where two circles at an edge are disjoint, the edge length is given by

$$l_{ij}^2 = \gamma_i^2 + \gamma_j^2 + 2\gamma_i\gamma_j I_{ij},$$

where $I_{i\,j}$ is called the inversive distance, which is a constant during Ricci flow. The third frame shows the discrete Yamabe flow, where

$$l_{ij}^2 = 2\gamma_i\gamma_j I_{ij}.$$

The last frame shows the circle packing with imaginary radius, the edge length is given by

$$l_{ij}^2 = -\gamma_i^2 - \gamma_j^2 + 2\gamma_i\gamma_j I_{ij}.$$

The power circle is the circle orthogonal to all the three circles centered at the vertices. In Yamabe flow case, the power circle is the circum circle of the triangle; in the case of circle packing with imaginary radius, the power circle is the equator of a hemisphere, which goes through the points (x_i, y_i, γ_i^2), where $v_i = (x_i, y_i)$. The center of the power circle is called the power center. The lines through the power center perpendicular to edge $[v_i, v_j]$ separates the edge to $d_{i\,j}$ and $d_{j\,i}$, the distance from the power center to this edge is h_k. Let $u_i = \log\gamma_i$. By using cosine law, it can be easily shown that

$$\frac{\partial l_{ij}}{\partial u_i} = d_{ij}, \frac{\partial l_{ij}}{\partial u_j} = d_{ji},$$

and

$$\frac{\partial \theta_i}{\partial u_j} = \frac{\partial \theta_j}{\partial u_i} = \frac{h_k}{l_{ij}}.$$

Therefore, differential 1-form

$$\omega = \sum_i K_i du_i,$$

is a closed 1-form, $d\omega = 0$, where K_i is the discrete Gaussian curvature at v_i. We can define the *discrete surface Ricci energy* as

$$E(u_1, \ldots, u_n) = \int^{(u_1, \ldots, u_n)} \sum_i (\bar{K}_i - K_i) du_i,$$

where $\bar{K}_i$ is the desired Gaussian curvature at v_i. We can compute the gradient of the Ricci energy is

$$\nabla E(u_1, \ldots, u_n) = (\bar{K}_1 - K_1, \bar{K}_2 - K_2, \ldots, \bar{K}_n - K_n)^T. \tag{6}$$

Let $[v_i, v_j]$ be an edge, adjacent to two faces $[v_i, v_j, v_k]$ and $[v_j, v_i, v_l]$, then we define the edge weight w_{ij} as

$$w_{ij} = \frac{h_k + h_l}{l_{ij}}.$$

The Hessian matrix is given by

$$\frac{\partial^2 E}{\partial u_i \partial u_j} = \frac{\partial K_i}{\partial u_j} = \begin{cases} -w_{ij} & [v_i, v_j] \in E \\ \sum_k w_{ik} & i = j \\ 0 & \text{otherwise} \end{cases} \tag{7}$$

If the triangulation is Delaunay, namely all the power centers are inside the triangle, then the edge weights are positive. Then the Hessian matrix is diagonal dominant, the energy is convex on the space $\{(u_1, \ldots, u_n) | \sum_i u_i = 0\}$. The metric which produces the target curvature is the unique global minimizer of the Ricci energy. By the convexity of the energy, the metric is unique.

The *discrete surface Ricci flow* is the gradient flow of the Ricci energy,

$$\frac{du_i}{dt} = \bar{K}_i - K_i. \tag{8}$$

Because the Ricci energy is convex, it can be efficiently optimized using Newton's method.

Conformal Colon Flattening

The colon wall surface can be flattened onto a planar rectangle, to expose all the interior geometric features. We use the discrete Yamabe flow method as an example to explain the algorithm in detail. The following symbols are applied: the radius vector $\mathbf{u} = (u_1, \cdots, u_n)^T$, the curvature vector $\mathbf{k} = (K_1, \cdots, K_n)^T$, the target curvature vector $\mathbf{k} = (\bar{K}_1, \cdots, \bar{K}_n)^T$, the Hessian matrix of the Ricci energy H. The input is a triangle mesh, and the target curvature, and a threshold ε. The output is the unique discrete metric, which produces the target curvature

1. Determine the target curvature $\bar{K}_i$ for all vertices.
2. Initialize $u_i = 0$ for all vertices.
3. Compute the edge length using the formula

$$l_{ij} = e^{\frac{u_i}{2}} l_{ij}^0 e^{\frac{u_j}{2}},$$

   where l_{ij}^0 is the initial edge length induced by the Euclidean metric.
4. Compute all the corner angles, vertex curvatures.
5. Compute the circum circles, and the edge weights w_{ij}'s.

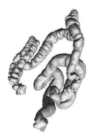
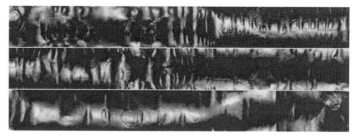

Fig. 11 Colon flattening using Ricci flow

6. Construct the Hessian matrix H, solve the linear system

$$\delta\mathbf{u} = H^{-1}(\mathbf{k} - \mathbf{k}),$$

7. Update the radius vector

$$\mathbf{u} = \mathbf{u} + \delta\mathbf{u}.$$

8. Repeat step 3–7, until $\|\mathbf{k} - \mathbf{k}\| < \epsilon$.

For example, we would like to flatten the colon surface onto the 2D plane. The colon surface is reconstructed from CT images and represented as a triangle mesh M. The colon wall surface is a topological cylinder, the surface is of genus zero with two boundaries, $\partial M = \gamma_0 - \gamma_1$. We set the target curvature to be zero everywhere, and run the above algorithm to compute a flat Euclidean metric. Then we find a shortest path τ connecting γ_0 and γ_1, we slice the surface along τ to get a mesh $\bar{M}$, which is a topological disk. Then we isometrically embed the faces of the mesh $\bar{M}$ using the flat metric, face by face until flatten the whole mesh onto the plan. Figure 11 shows one example of colon flattening.

Quasi-Conformal Map

The quasi-conformal mapping computation is converted to conformal mapping based on auxiliary metric. Suppose M is the input triangle mesh, first we compute a conformal mapping $\varphi : M \to \mathbb{D}$ to map the surface onto the planar domain $\mathbb{D}$, then we compute a quasi-conformal mapping $\tau : \mathbb{D} \to \mathbb{D}$, the composition $\tau \circ \varphi : M \to \mathbb{D}$ gives the quasi-conformal mapping from the surface to the planar domain $\mathbb{D}$, as shown in the following commutative diagram.

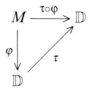

The conformal mapping $\varphi : M \to \mathbb{D}$ can be carried out directly using the Ricci flow method. Therefore, we only need to focus on the quasi-conformal mapping $\tau : \mathbb{D} \to \mathbb{D}$. The key idea is to run Ricci flow on the auxiliary metric. The auxiliary metric is constructed as follows. Assume $\mathbb{D}$ is a domain on the complex plane $\mathbb{C}$. Let $[v_i, v_j]$ be an edge adjacent to two faces $[v_i, v_j, v_k]$ and $[v_j, v_i, v_l]$, the Beltrami coefficient is defined on each face $\mu_{ij}{}^k$ and $\mu_{ji}{}^l$, respectively. The complex coordinates of v_i, v_j are z_i and z_j, respectively. The discrete auxiliary metric on $[v_i, v_j]$ is given by

$$\tilde{l}_{ij} = \frac{1}{2}\left|(z_j - z_i) + \mu_{ij}^k(\bar{z}_j - \bar{z}_i)\right| + \frac{1}{2}\left|(z_j - z_i) + \mu_{ji}^l(\bar{z}_j - \bar{z}_i)\right|. \tag{9}$$

Harmonic Map

Harmonic maps can be computed by minimizing the harmonic energy, or equivalently solving elliptic geometric partial differential equations. Suppose we want to compute a harmonic map from a mesh M to the planar disk $\mathbb{D}$, $\varphi : M \to \mathbb{D}$, the mapping φ is approximated by piecewise linear maps. By using Finite element method, the harmonic energy of mapping has closed form,

$$E(\varphi) = \sum_{[v_i, v_j] \in M} w_{ij} |\varphi(v_i) - \varphi(v_j)|^2,$$

where $w_{i\,j}$ is the cotangent edge weight. Suppose $[v_i, v_j]$ is adjacent to two faces $[v_i, v_j, v_k]$ and $[v_j, v_i, v_l]$, then the edge weight is given by

$$w_{ij} = \frac{1}{2}(\cot \theta_k^{ij} + \cot \theta_l^{ji}),$$

where $\theta_k^{i\,j}$ is the corner angle in $[v_i, v_j, v_k]$ at the vertex v_k. The harmonic map satisfies the following Laplace equation

$$\begin{cases} \Delta\varphi(v_i) = 0 & v_i \notin \partial M \\ \varphi(v_k) = g(v_k) & v_k \in \partial M. \end{cases} \tag{10}$$

where the discrete Laplace–Beltrami operator is given by

$$\Delta\varphi(v_i) = \sum_{[v_i, v_j] \in M} w_{ij}(\varphi(v_j) - \varphi(v_i)).$$

If the triangle mesh is Delaunay, then $\theta_{i\,j}{}^k + \theta_{j\,i}{}^l < \pi$, the Laplace–Beltrami operator Δ is positive definite, so the solution is unique.

The harmonic map can handle hard constraints easily. The landmark constraint can be added in the same way as the boundary vertices. Therefore, it is very flexible to incorporate landmarks. But, the harmonic maps with constraints may not be homeomorphic any more.

In practice, we need to compute harmonic maps under the conformal structure deformed by a Beltrami differential μ. We first use Ricci flow to compute the canonical uniformization Riemannian metric, then construct local conformal coordinate charts. On each chart, for each triangle, we deform it according to auxiliary metric equation (9) and compute the deformed corner angles using cosine law, and update the cotangent edge weight. Then we can solve the Laplace equation (10).

Surface Registration Framework

The framework of *Surface Matching and Registration* can be summarized in diagram (11). Suppose $S_k, k = 1,2$ are the input surfaces. In order to compute the optimal diffeomorphism $\varphi : S_1 \rightarrow S_2$ to register them, we conformally map them onto the plane by $\varphi_k : S_k \rightarrow \mathbb{D}_k$, where $\mathbb{D}_k$ are called *conformal parameter domain*, then construct a planar diffeomorphism $h : \mathbb{D}_1 \rightarrow \mathbb{D}_2$, the registration between two surfaces is given by $f = \varphi_2^{-1} \circ h \circ \varphi_1$. Therefore, 3D matching and registration problems are converted to 2D domains, which simplifies the computation and provides a key to constructing a globally optimal diffeomorphism between surfaces.

$$
\begin{array}{ccc}
S_1 & \xrightarrow{\ f\ } & S_2 \\
\phi_1 \downarrow & & \downarrow \phi_2 \\
D_1 & \xrightarrow{\ h\ } & D_2
\end{array}
\qquad (11)
$$

The quality of the planar diffeomorphism is crucial for the whole mapping quality. We applied the following strategy for finding the optimal mapping,

1. Set the initial Beltrami coefficient to be 0 everywhere, $\mu_0 \equiv 0$.
2. Construct a harmonic map $h_n : \mathbb{D}_1 \rightarrow \mathbb{D}_2$ with respect to the current Beltrami coefficient μ_n, with hard feature constraints.
3. Update the Beltrami coefficient

$$
\mu = \frac{\partial_{\bar{z}} h_n}{\partial_z h_n},
$$

4. Because h_n may not be a homeomorphism, at some points the norm of μ may exceed 1, so we need to truncate it

$$
\mu_{n+1}(p) = \begin{cases} \mu & |\mu(p)| < 1 \\ 1 - \epsilon & |\mu(p)| \geq 1 \end{cases}
$$

5. Repeat steps 2–4, until the process converges.

Visualization

Our method of performing supine-prone registration, whereby the 3D matching problem is reduced to a 2D image registration problem, presents several advantages for the corresponding visualization system. Since the registration is in the form of 2D image maps, a rendering of these flattened colon segments allows for the user to view the entire colon segments, supporting easier verification of the accuracy of the registration and easy navigation. Since these flattened colons also form a one-to-one and onto mapping, it is possible to correlate endoluminal views based on the viewing vector. Lastly, a visualization of the Beltrami coefficient on the colon surface is possible, allowing for the user to view where most of the elastic distortion has occurred.

We introduce a new path through the colon which we call the *flattened center-line*. With a colon segment mapped to a plane such that the segment boundaries are on top and bottom (resulting in a plane taller than it is wide), horizontal line segments then correspond to loop curves on the colon surface. The mass center of a loop is taken to be the central point for that plane of the colon segment. By calculating these mass centers along the entire flattened colon, we generate a path of points which generally mimics that of a centerline. However, since this is calculated from the flattened colons, we refer to it as the flattened centerline. To avoid confusion, we will use the term *skeleton* to refer to the 3D medial axis centerline which is conventionally calculated for VC systems [48].

The flattened centerline can be efficiently calculated as a series of points through the colon lumen using the GPU to render the flattened colon mesh. For a desired number of points in the flattened centerline, the colon mesh is scaled so the longest side of the rectangular mesh is equal to this desired number of points. The mesh is rendered such that the color of each vertex is the original coordinates of the vertex in the volume, with the values interpolated to fill the triangles. Each row of pixels can then be averaged to obtain the mass center for that row, which is the point for that position on the flattened centerline.

Taeniae Coli and Flexures Extraction

The taeniae coli and the flexures (see Fig. 12) are important anatomical landmarks of the colon which do not change despite the change in position of the patient. Corresponding anatomical landmarks in supine and prone colons are automatically extracted in a robust manner, which are then used to cut each colon into its anatomical segments, as well as slicing the colon open for flattening.

The colon contains five segments, which, starting from the cecum, are the ascending colon (A), the transverse colon (T), the descending colon (D), the sigmoid colon (S), and the rectum (R), as shown in Fig. 12a. The first major flexure occurs between the ascending colon and the transverse colon (A-T flexure).

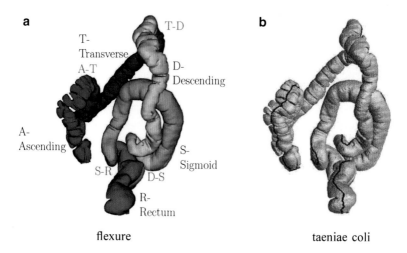

a

T-
Transverse
A-T

T-D

D-
Descending

A-
Ascending

S-R   D-S

S-
Sigmoid

R-
Rectum

flexure

b

taeniae coli

Fig. 12 Anatomical landmarks. (**a**) Flexure and (**b**) Taeniae coli

This is the flexure close to the liver and is called the hepatic flexure. The second major flexure occurs between the transverse colon and the descending colon (T-D flexure). This flexure is close to the spleen and is named the splenic flexure. The third flexure occurs between the descending colon and the sigmoid (D-S flexure), and the final flexure is between the sigmoid and the rectum (S-R flexure). All of these flexures form very sharp bends and are distinguishable from other smaller bends. Theoretically, the A-T flexure forms the topmost point of the ascending colon and the T-D flexure forms the topmost point of the descending colon. Flexures can help in virtual navigation and supine-prone alignment and cutting.

Taeniae coli are three bands of longitudinal muscle on the surface of the colon. They form a triple helix structure from the appendix to the sigmoid colon and are ideal references for virtual navigation. The taeniae coli are named taenia omentalis, taenia mesolica, and taenia libera according to the position on the transverse colon. Taeniae coli can be regarded as ridge breakers for the haustral folds (located between the haustral folds). It is relatively easy to extract the taenia omentalis as it is clearly visible on the transverse and ascending colons. Similar to reported approaches [49, 50], we identify the taeniae coli by detecting the haustral folds, which are computed initially using the heat diffusion and fuzzy C-means clustering algorithms [50]. Using these haustral folds, we extract the taenia omentalis and the other two taeniae coli [18]. Although we extract all three bands of taeniae coli, we mostly use the taenia omentalis for subsequent processing. Figure 12b shows the front view of a taenia coli on the prone colon surface. In our experience, we have been able to extract the taenia coli automatically through the entire colon. However, if fully automatic extraction is impossible in some dataset, a semiautomatic method using a manually placed marker could be employed to improve reliability.

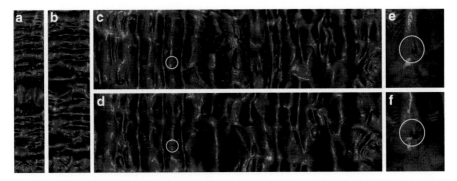

Fig. 13 Visual verification for supine-prone colon registration using volume rendering. (**a**) and (**b**) are the original conformal flattened views of the ascending colon segments (Segment A) of the supine and prone surfaces, respectively. After registration with 16 feature points, a polyp found on the flattened supine surface (*yellow circle* in (**c**)) can be located on the flattened prone surface (*yellow circle* in (**d**)) at nearly the same position. (**e**) and (**f**) are enlargements of the neighborhoods of the same polyp on the supine and prone surfaces, respectively

Flattened Colon Rendering

As our registration results are natively two flat colon meshes with a one-to-one correspondence, our initial visualization is based off of this. Volumetric rendering of flattened colons has been presented and suggested for use in VC naviga-tion [14]. We perform our rendering in much the same way, though we make use of the flattened centerline rather than the skeleton for generating viewpoints, as the flattened centerline is more apt to this task.

With supine and prone placed side by side, it is easy for the user to scan through one colon, and if something suspicious is noted, immediately look at the same location on the neighboring colon. Since the flattened colons are both mapped to planes of the same size, there is a direct one-to-one and onto mapping. This is also trivial to implement in a user interface. We use this view as the basis for our visual inspection of the registration accuracy. An example of this can be seen in Fig. 13, where we compare the flattened, but unregistered, colons against the flattened and registered colons. Using the flattened viewing method, the alignment of the colon anatomy between supine and prone is immediately obvious compared to the unregistered segments.

Visualization of Quasi-Conformality

The elastic deformation between supine and prone is measured by the Beltrami coefficients in Eq. (1) through the resulting registration. In general, this information would likely not be of interest to a radiologist reading a VC study. However, visualizing the amount of distortion in this way may be useful to a doctor seeking to better understand how the colon deforms in certain regions.

Fig. 14 Visualization of
quasi-conformality: (**a**)
circles on the source
(supine) are mapped to (**b**)
ellipses on the target (prone)
by the registration map. The
narrower ellipses
correspond to the larger
deformation

a
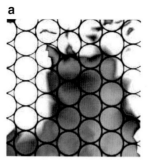

b
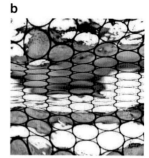

circles on supine   ellipses on supine
                           registered to prone

The quasi-conformal mapping deforms the circles to ellipses. Figure 14 illustrates that the deformation from supine to prone is quasi-conformal. A general fundamental domain is chosen for the supine segment. We use its flat coordinates (as in Fig. 13a) as the texture coordinates and compute the circle-packing texture mapping (zoomed-in view shown in (a)), where the circularity is preserved. After registration to the flattened map of the prone segment, the supine planar image is changed (as in Fig. 13c) and the circles are accordingly deformed to ellipses (zoomed-in view shown in (b)). Using the one-to-one and onto mapping between supine and prone, we can efficiently compute the Beltrami coefficients on the triangular mesh surface. The quasi-conformality of the mapping is evaluated by the local stretching and angle distortion. The maximal local stretching is 11, mathematically called *11-Quasi-Conformal Mapping*.

Based on the diffeomorphism constructed between supine and prone, we simulate the deformation process by a linearly interpolated morphing sequence. Then, we transfer the texture coordinates to each intermediate mesh surface consistently. Through the texture correspondence, we can visually get a better understanding of how the deformation behaves from supine to prone and vice versa. After registration, the supine and prone have the same mesh connectivity, but different geometry. As shown in Figs. 15 and 16, the morphing views sp_1, sp_2, sp_3, sp_4 between supine and prone are generated by the linear interpolation of geometry at each vertex. Directly from the stretching-colored views (a), one can easily comprehend where the main deformation happens. The global surface distortion is mainly affected by the local stretching deformation, valued by the ratio between the long axis and short axis of the ellipse locally. The local angle distortion, however, is intrinsic to the material properties of the organ muscle and tissue. Compared with the stretching, the angle distribution is more uniform through the whole deformation, as shown in (b). Here, the red color denotes the largest stretching (angle distortion), blue color the lowest stretching, and yellow and green in between. The consistent texture mapping of checker-board (c) and circle-packing (d) textures also demonstrates the quasi-conformality of the deformation.

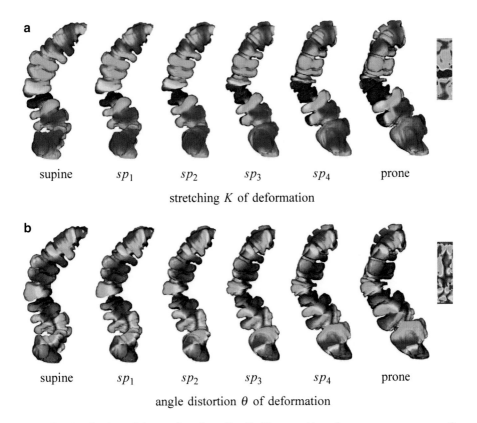

Fig. 15 Visualization of the quasi-conformality (I). The morphing views $s\,p_1, s\,p_2, s\,p_3, s\,p_4$ of geometry between supine and prone are generated by the linear interpolation of the one-to-one registration. The deformation is simulated on the colon segment geometry and four consistent textures are mapped to it to illustrate the corresponding parts of the geometry. In (**a**) and (**b**), *red* indicates the largest stretching (angle distortion) and *blue* indicates the least

Experimental Results

We validate our algorithms using real VC colon data from the publicly available National Institute of Biomedical Imaging and Bioengineering (NIBIB) Image and Clinical Data Repository provided by the National Institute of Health (NIH). We perform electronic colon cleansing incorporating the partial volume effect [51], segmentation with topological simplification [5], and reconstruction of the colon surface via surface nets [52] on the original CT images in a pre-processing step. Though the size and resolution of each CT volume varies from dataset to dataset, the general data size is approximately $512 \times 512 \times 450$ voxels and the general resolution is approximately $0.7 \times 0.7 \times 1.0$ mm. In this paper, the colon surface is modeled as a topological cylinder and discretely represented by a triangular mesh.

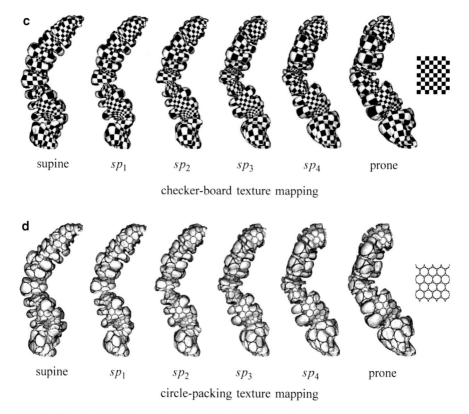

c

supine sp_1 sp_2 sp_3 sp_4 prone

checker-board texture mapping

d

supine sp_1 sp_2 sp_3 sp_4 prone

circle-packing texture mapping

Fig. 16 Visualization of the quasi-conformality (II). The quasi-conformality of the deformation is also visualized by the texture mapping sequences (**c**) and (**d**)

We have developed our algorithms using generic C++ on the Windows XP platform. The linear systems in solving the Laplace equation are solved using the Matlab C++ library. All of the experiments are conducted on a workstation with a Core 2 Quad 2.50GHz CPU with 4GB RAM. The colon surface used for our testing has 200K faces. Our method is efficient and effective. Table 1 shows the statistics for the conformal mapping of each segment. We cut each segment open by the corresponding taeniae coli and map it to a rectangle by the discrete Ricci flow method. Different segments will have different sizes of rectangles, e.g., the ratio between the height and the width of the rectangle, the so-called *conformal module*. Conformal module is a conformal invariant. Surfaces with the same conformal module are conformal to each other. Table 2 shows the conformal modules for 5 corresponding supine and prone segments, respectively, where the different conformal modules verify that the supine and prone colon surfaces are not conformal, but with nonrigid elastic deformations.

We evaluate our registration results using two methods. The first is an objective analytic evaluation, whereby distances between corresponding points on the registered colons are calculated. The second method is a more subjective visual

Table 1 Statistics for conformal mapping

Colon	Segment	# Vertices	# Faces	Time(s)
Supine	Ascending (A)	35,251	70,366	21
	Transverse (T)	43,255	86,364	27
	Descending (D)	44,910	89,659	23
	Sigmoid (S)	37,237	74,296	22
	Rectum (R)	39,712	79,315	23
Prone	Ascending (A)	36,629	73,139	20
	Transverse (T)	42,452	84,781	25
	Descending (D)	44,587	88,981	26
	Sigmoid (S)	38,499	76,823	22
	Rectum (R)	38,177	76,276	23

Table 2 Conformal modulus comparison between the corresponding supine and prone segments

Segment	$M o d$ of Supine	$M o d$ of Prone
Ascending (A)	5.41089	3.85803
Transverse (T)	6.20148	5.87936
Descending (D)	7.77978	6.15164
Sigmoid (S)	3.77068	3.89906
Rectum (R)	3.62033	3.46039

The conformal module for each segment is defined as the ratio of height and width of the flat rectangle map, Mod =height/width. The corresponding segments are not conformally equivalent

verification, whereby we observe the correct alignment of corresponding features in both flattened 2D views and endoluminal views using our consistent view camera mapping.

Analytic Registration Evaluation

Our first evaluation is a distance measurement between corresponding features located on the registered colon surfaces. Since our registration is in the 2D space using the flattened colon surfaces, a point (x,y,z) in $\mathbb{R}^3$ on the original colon surface will be at a location (u,v) in $\mathbb{R}^2$ on the registered surface. Thus, for a point $p_0 = (u_p,v_p)$ on the supine colon surface and its corresponding point $q_0 = (u_q,v_q)$ on the prone colon surface, a perfect registration with zero error is present when $u_p = u_q$ and $v_p = v_q$. For two corresponding points, we compute the L^2 norm of their 2D coordinates with the width of the flattened images fixed to a unit length of 1. Note that the width along the flattened image is equivalent to the colon circumference for that location.

We also compute the 3D distance error in millimeters. For the two corresponding points p_0 and q_0 in $\mathbb{R}^2$, we know their locations r_0 and s_0 in $\mathbb{R}^3$. If we take the supine surface (containing p_0) as the truth and wish to measure the registration error on the prone surface (containing q_0), we can identify the point $p_1 = (u_q,v_q)$ in $\mathbb{R}^2$ on the supine surface and similarly its location r_1 in $\mathbb{R}^3$. The distance error in millimeters is then given to be $|r_1 - r_0|$.

Table 3 Comparison of average distance error between our quasi-conformal registration method and other registration methods

Methods	Dist. Error
Our Quasi-Conformal Mapping	7.85 mm
Centerline registration + statistical analysis (Li et al. [53])	12.66 mm
Linear stretching / shrinking of centerline (Acar et al. [11])	13.20 mm
Centerline feature matching + lumen deformation (Suh and Wyatt. [21])	13.77 mm
Centerline point correlation (de Vries et al. [12])	20.00 mm
Taeniae coli correlation (Huang et al. [18])	23.33 mm

We obtain the corresponding feature points for evaluation in two ways. The first is by manually identifying points of interest (e.g., a polyp) on both colon surfaces. We manually select the center of polyps on the registered flat images. For the polyp shown in Fig. 13, the distance error is 0.0265 in $\mathbb{R}^2$ and 5.31 mm in $\mathbb{R}^3$. We have evaluated our algorithm using a total of 20 pairs on 6 datasets, and the average distance error is 0.0305 in $\mathbb{R}^2$ and 5.65 mm in $\mathbb{R}^3$.

Our second method of finding corresponding points is to use a subset (half) of the whole features. We use these features for evaluation purposes, and only the remaining half are used in the harmonic mapping step. Note that this inherently reduces the quality of the registration, and thus a registration using all feature points will contain less error. We generally computed 16 pairs of feature points for each segment, about 2 feature points along one folding with obvious correspondence. For the registration shown in Fig. 13, the distance error in terms of feature points evaluation is computed to be 0.0325 in $\mathbb{R}^2$ and 7.51 mm in $\mathbb{R}^3$. The average $\mathbb{R}^3$ distance on 6 datasets is 7.85 mm.

A comparison between our method and other methods is performed using our analytic evaluation results in $\mathbb{R}^3$. For those papers that present their distance error, we compare our results with their results in Table 3. Our method produces a registration with significantly smaller distance error between corresponding points than other methods.

Visual Registration Verification

Perhaps a better indicator of the utility of our registration is a visual evaluation of the results, as this mimics most closely how the user of a VC system would use our results. For this, we utilized both the flattened rendering and the 3D correlated endoluminal renderings. In our experience, the correlation between the flattened renderings was good, as was the endoluminal views. In Fig. 13, we show three supine-prone colon segments, flat rendered, both unregistered and registered. The images of the registered segments clearly show very good alignment of the supine and prone colon structures, whereas the unregistered segments show poor alignment.

We have also shown our results to a radiologist who was involved with the early conception of the VC system and thus has over ten years of experience in reading them. He noted that the flat rendering was realistic, and that the anatomy between supine and prone was easily compared and well correlated. He also noted the good correlation between the endoluminal views, and gave his opinion that such views were easier to compare than the flattened views due to his greater familiarity with them (he had not been exposed to flattened rendering prior to viewing this work).

Analysis and Discussion

The deformation between supine and prone scans of the colon surface is elastic, and from physics, elastic deformations are quasi-conformal. Therefore, in principle, our geometric model derives from the real biophysical properties of the muscle. Intuitively, the deformation at each point is determined by the elasticity properties of the colon surface, which are fully represented by the Beltrami coefficients. The physical property is fully encoded in the Beltrami coefficient function.

Previous works have most often focused on centerline alignment. The ground truth for colon deformation is the entire surface deformation, the centerline conveys only very limited information. Since our method uses the surface instead of the centerline, it is expected that we achieve better results than the more crude centerline methods, which has been shown in Table 3.

For the method of registration based on global deformation [22], a deformation field is defined for the whole volume which includes the volume inside the colon surface. Our method focuses on the intrinsic surface deformation itself. In reality, different colon surface parts can touch each other, and this kind of deformation cannot be captured by a method based on global deformation. In addition, volumetric deformation requires much higher storage requirements, and the resolution of the deformation field on the surface is much lower. Our method only considers the surface, and thus it has much more efficient storage and much higher resolution for the conformal field.

We can use the proposed method to register colons as a whole, instead of segmenting them into 5 segments. Then flexure landmarks can be used as internal features in the computation of harmonic map.

Conclusions and Future Work

Shape registration is very fundamental for shape analysis problems, especially for abnormality detection in medical applications. We introduce an efficient framework for the registration of supine and prone colons, through the use of conformal geometry, to improve the accuracy of polyp detection. With the automatically extracted anatomical landmarks, namely the taeniae coli and flexures, we consistently segment the colon surface and conformally flatten the colon surfaces to the rectangular domain using the discrete surface Ricci flow method. Then we align the flattened domains by adjusting the conformal mapping to be quasi-conformal through the harmonic map with feature constraints. We demonstrate the efficiency of our method by both analytic evaluation and the 2D and 3D consistent registration views. The Beltrami coefficient is employed to analyze the physical deformation of the colon muscle and tissue.

With the ability to measure and view the elastic distortion between segments of the supine and prone colons, we are seeking further outlets to which this work can be applied. We are looking at applying this registration to our CAD work to achieve better sensitivity and specificity. Additionally, we are looking to extend our work from 2D surface registration to 3D volumetric registration for colon wall segmentations which contain thickness.

References

1. Horner MJ, Ries LAG, Krapcho M, Neyman N, Aminou R, Howlader N, Altekruse SF, Feuer EJ, Huang L, Mariotto A, Miller BA, Lewis DR, Eisner MP, Stinchcomb DG, Edwards BK (eds.) SEER cancer statistics review, 1975–2006. National Cancer Institute," 2009, http://seer.cancer.gov/csr/1975_2006/
2. Center MM, Jemal A, Smith RA, Ward E (2009) Worldwide variations in colorectal cancer. CA: A Cancer J Clin 59(6):366–378
3. Hong L, Muraki S, Kaufman A, Bartz D, He T (1997) Virtual voyage: Interactive navigation in the human colon. In: Proceedings of SIGGRAPH, ACM, pp 27–34
4. Johnson CD, Dachman AH (2000) CT colography: The next colon screening examination. Radiology 216(2):331–341
5. Hong W, Qiu F, Kaufman A (2006) A pipeline for computer aided polyp detection. IEEE Trans Visualiz Comput Graph 12(5):861–868
6. Zhao L, Botha CP, Bescos JO, Truyen R, Vos FM, Post FH (2006) Lines of curvature for polyp detection in virtual colonoscopy. IEEE Trans Visualiz Comput Graph 12(5):885–892
7. Zhu H, Liang Z, Pickhardt PJ, Barish MA, You J, Fan Y, Lu H, Posniak EJ, Richards RJ, Cohen HL (2010) Increasing computer-aided detection specificity by projection features for CT colonography. Medic Phys 37(4):1468–1481
8. Williams D, Grimm S, Coto E, Roudsari A, Hatzakis H (2008) Volumetric curved planar reformation for virtual endoscopy. IEEE Trans Visualiz Comput Graph 14(1):109–119
9. Raghupathi L, Grisoni L, Faure F, Marchal D, Cani M.-P, Chaillou C (2004) An intestinal surgery simulator: Real-time collision processing and visualization. IEEE Trans Visualiz Comput Graph 10(6):708–718
10. Marino J, Qiu F, Kaufman A (2008) Virtually assisted optical colon-oscopy. Proc. of SPIE Med Imag 6916:69160J
11. Acar B, Napel S, Paik DS, Li P, Yee J, Jeffrey Jr RB, Beaulieu C (2001) Medial axis registration of supine and prone CT colonography data. In: Proceedings of Engineering in Medicine and Biology Society (EMBS), IEEE CS Press, pp 2433–2436
12. de Vries AH, Truyen R, van der Peijl J, Florie J, van Gelder RE, Gerritsen F, Stoker J (2006) Feasibility of automated matching of supine and prone CT-colonography examinations. Br J Radiol 79:740–744
13. Näppi J, Okamura A, Frimmel H, Dachman A, Yoshida H (2005) Region-based supine-prone correspondence of false-positive CAD polyp candidates in CT colonography. Acad Radiol 12:695–707

14. Hong W, Gu X, Qiu F, Jin M, Kaufman A (2006) Conformal virtual colon flattening. In: Proceeings of ACM symposium on solid and physical modeling, ACM, pp 85–93

15. Gurijala KC, Kaufman A, Zeng W, Gu X (2010) Extraction of landmarks and features from virtual colon models. In: The MICCAI'10 workshop on challenges and opportunities in virtual colonoscopy and abdominal imaging (MICCAI'10-VCAI), Beijing, China, 20 Sep 2010

16. Zeng W, Marino J, Gurijala K, Gu X, Kaufman A (2010) Supine and prone colon registration using quasi-conformal mapping. IEEE Trans Visualiz Comput Graph (IEEE TVCG) 16(6):1348–1357

17. Nain D, Haker S, Grimson WEL, Cosman Jr E, Wells WW, Ji H, Kikinis R, Westin CF (2002) Intra-patient prone to supine colon registration for synchronized virtual colonoscop. In: Proceedings of MICCAI, Springer, pp 573–580

18. Huang A, Roy D, Franaszek M, Summers RM (2005) Teniae coli guided navigation and registration for virtual colonoscopy. In: Proceedings of IEEE Visualization, IEEE CS Press, pp 279–285

19. Huang A, Roy DA, Summers RM, Franaszek M, Petrick N, Choi JR, Pickhardt PJ (2007) Teniae coli-based circumferential localization system for CT colonography: Feasability study. Radiology 243(2):551–560

20. Umemoto Y, Oda M, Kitasaka T, Mori K, Hayashi Y, Suenaga Y, Takayama T, Natori H (2008) Extraction of teniae coli from CT volumes for assisting virtual colonoscopy. Proc. SPIE Med Imag 6916:69160D

21. Suh JW, Wyatt CL (2009) Deformable registration of supine and prone colons for computed tomographic colonography. J Comput Assist Tomograp 33(6):902–911

22. Plishker W, Shekhar R (2008) Virtual colonoscopy registration regularization with global chainmil. In: Proceedings of MICCAI workshop on virtual colonoscopy, IEEE CS Press, pp 116–121

23. Gu X, Wang Y, Chan TF, Thompson PM, Yau S-T (2004) Genus zero surface conformal mapping and its application to brain surface mapping. IEEE Trans Med Imag 23(8):949–958

24. Hamilton RS (1998) The Ricci flow on surfaces. Math General Relativ 71:237–262

25. Chow B, Luo F (2003) Combinatorial Ricci flows on surfaces. J Different Geomet 63(1):97–129

26. Jin M, Kim J, Luo F, Gu X (2008) Discrete surface Ricci flow. IEEE Trans Visualiz Comput Graph 14(5):1030–1043

27. Zeng W, Samaras D, Gu XD (2010) Ricci flow for 3D shape analysis. IEEE Trans Patt Anal Mach Intell 32(4):662–677

28. Zhang M, Li Y, Zeng W, Yau S-T, Gu X (2012) Canonical conformal mapping for high genus surfaces with boundaries. Int J Comput Graph 36(5):417–426

29. Zeng W, Jin M, Luo F, Gu X (2009) Computing canonical homotopy class representative using hyperbolic structure. In: IEEE international conference on shape modeling and applications (SMI'09), Beijing, China, 26–28 June 2009

30. Zeng W, Lui LM, Luo F, Chan T, Yau S-T, Gu X (2012) Computing quasiconformal maps using an auxiliary metric with discrete curvature flow. Numeriche Mathematica 121 (4):671–703

31. Zeng W, Yin XT, Zeng Y, Lai YK, Gu X, Samaras D (2008) 3D face matching and registration based on hyperbolic Ricci flow. In: The CVPR Workshop on 3D Face Processing (CVPR'08-3DFP), Anchorage, Alaska, 27 June 2008

32. Zeng W, Gu X (2011) Registration for 3D surfaces with large deformations using quasi-conformal curvature flow. In: IEEE conference on computer vision and pattern recognition (CVPR'11), Colorado Springs, Colorado, 20–25 June 2011

33. Jin M, Zeng W, Luo F, Gu X (2009) Computing Teichmüller shape space. IEEE Trans Visualiz Comput Graph 15(3):504–517

34. Zeng W, Lui L, Shi L, Wang D, Chu WC, Cheng JC, Hua J, Yau S-T, Gu X (2010) Shape analysis of vestibular systems in adolescent idiopathic scoliosis using geodesic spectra.

In: The 13th international conference on medical image computing and computer assisted intervention (MICCAI'10), Beijing, China, 20–24 Sept 2010

35. Wang Y, Shi J, Yin X, Gu X, Chan TF, Yau S-T, Toga AW, Thompson PM (2012) Brain surface conformal parameterization with the Ricci flow. IEEE Trans Med Imag 31(2):251–264

36. Zeng W, Shi R, Wang Y, Yau S-T, Gu X (2013) Teichmüller shape descriptor and its application to Alzheimer's disease study. Int J Comput Vision (IJCV), 105(2):155–170

37. Zeng W, Li H, Chen L, Morvan J-M, Gu X (2013) An automatic 3d expression recognition framework based on sparse representation of conformal images. In: The 10th IEEE international conference on face and gesture recognition (FG'13), Shanghai, China, 22–26 April 2013

38. Qiu F, Fan Z, Yin X, Kauffman A, Gu X (2009) Colon flattening with discrete Ricci flow. In: Proceedings of MICCAI

39. Sarkar R, Yin X, Gao J, Gu X (2009) Greedy routing with guaranteed delivery using ricci flows. In: International conference on information processing in sensor networks (IPSN'09), IEEE CS Press, pp 121–132

40. Zeng W, Sarkar R, Luo F, Gu X, Gao J (2010) Resilient routing for sensor networks using hyperbolic embedding of universal covering space. In: The 29th IEEE conference on computer communications (INFOCOM'10), San Diego, California, 15–19 March 2010

41. Sarkar R, Zeng W, Gao J, Gu X (2010) Covering space for in-network sensor data storag. In: International conference on information processing in sensor networks (IPSN'10), Stockholm, Sweden, 12–16 April 2010

42. Jiang R, Ban X, Goswami M, Zeng W, Gao J, Gu X (2011) Exploration of path space using sensor network geometry. In: International conference on information processing in sensor networks (IPSN'11), Chicago, Illinois, 12–14 April 2011

43. Farkas HM, Kra I (1991) Riemann surfaces (graduate texts in mathematics). Springer, Berlin

44. Papadopoulos A (2007) Handbook of Teichmüller theory. European Mathematical Society

45. Ahlfors L (1966) Lectures in quasiconformal mappings. Van Nostrand Reinhold, New York

46. Schoen R, Yau S-T (1994) Lectures on differential geometry. International Press of Boston, Boston

47. Chow B (1991) The Ricci flow on the 2-sphere. J Different Geom 33(2):325–334

48. Bitter I, Kaufman AE, Sato M (2001) Penalized-distance volumetric skeleton algorithm. IEEE Trans Visualiz Comput Graph 7(3):195–206

49. Chowdhury AS, Yao J, Vanuitert R, Linguraru M, Summers R (2008) Detection of anatomical landmarks in human colon from computed tomographic colonography images. In: Proceedings of the 19th international conference on pattern recognition (ICPR), IEEE CS Press, pp 1–4

50. Lamy J, Summers RM (2007) Teniae coli detection from colon surface: Extraction of anatomical markers for virtual colonoscopy. In: Proceedings of the third annual symposium on visual computing, Springer, pp 199–207

51. Wang Z, Liang Z, Li L, Li B, Eremina D, Lu H (2006) An improved electronic colon cleansing method for detection of colonic polyps by virtual colonoscopy. IEEE Trans Biomed Eng 53(8):1635–1646

52. Gibson SFF (1998) Constrained elastic surface nets: Generating smooth surfaces from binary segmented data. In: Proceedings of MICCAI, Springer, pp 888–898

53. Li P, Napel S, Acar B, Paik DS, Jeffrey Jr RB Beaulieu CF (2004) Registration of central paths and colonic polyps between supine and prone scans in computed tomography colonography: Pilot study. Med Phys 31(10):2912–2923

Biography

Wei Zeng is an assistant professor of the School of Computing and Information Sciences at Florida International University. Dr. Zeng received her Ph.D. from Chinese Academy of Sciences in 2008 and her thesis was titled as "Computational Conformal Geometry Based Shape Analysis." Her research interests include computational conformal geometry, Teichmüller quasiconformal geometry, discrete differential geometry, discrete Ricci flow, geometric analysis, and their applications to surface matching, registration, tracking, recognition, and shape analysis. Her research areas span over medical imaging, computer vision, computer graphics and visualization, wireless sensor network, geometric modeling, and computational topology.

Rui Shi is a Ph.D. candidate in the Department of Computer Science at Stony Brook University. He received his B.S. degree in Automation at University of Science and Technology of China. His research direction towards surface registration and applications of geometric algorithm in Wireless Sensor Network. He has published papers in CVPR, IPMI, InfoCom, IJCV, and so on.

Zhengyu Su is a Ph.D. candidate in the Department of Computer Science at Stony Brook University. He received his B.S. degree in Electrical Engineering at University of Science and Technology of China. His research direction towards area preserving mapping and it's applications in Graphics and Medical Imaging. He has published papers in CVPR, IPMI, and so on.

David Xianfeng Gu received his Ph.D. degree in Computer Science from Harvard University in 2003. He is an associate professor of computer science and the director of the 3D Scanning Laboratory in the Department of Computer Science at Stony Brook University. His research interests include computer vision, graphics, geometric modeling, and medical imaging. His major works include global conformal surface parameterization in graphics, tracking and analysis of facial expression in vision, manifold splines in modeling, brain mapping and virtual colonoscopy in medical imaging and computational conformal geometry. He is the winner of the US National Science Foundation CAREER award in 2004.

Efficient Topological Cleaning for Visual Colon Surface Flattening

Wei Zeng, Rui Shi, Zhengyu Su, and David Xianfeng Gu

Abstract Conformal mapping provides a unique way to flatten the three-dimensional (3D) anatomically complicated colon wall. Visualizing the flattened 2D colon wall supplies an alternative means for the task of detecting abnormality as compared to the conventional endoscopic views. In addition to the visualization, the flattened colon wall carries supplementary geometry and texture information for computer-aided detection of abnormality. It is hypothesized that utilizing both the original 3D and the flattened 2D colon walls shall improve the detection capacity of currently available computed tomography colonography. One of the major challenges for the conformal colon flattening is how to make the input colon wall inner surface to be genus zero, as this is required by the flatten algorithm and will guarantee high flatten quality. This paper describes an efficient topological cleaning algorithm for the conformal colon flattening pipeline. Starting from a segmented colon wall, the Marching Cube algorithm was first applied to generate the surface, then we apply our topological clearance algorithm to remove the topological outliers to guarantee the output surface is exactly genus 0. The cleared or denoised colon surface was then flattened by a Ricci flow. The pipeline was tested by 14 patient datasets with comparison to our previous work.

W. Zeng (✉)
School of Computing and Information Sciences, Florida International University,
11200 SW 8th St, Miami, FL 33199, USA
e-mail: wzeng@cs.fiu.edu

R. Shi • Z. Su • D.X. Gu
Department of Computer Science, Stony Brook University, 100 Nicolls Rd,
Stony Brook, NY 11790, USA
e-mail: rshi@cs.stonybrook.edu; zysu@cs.stonybrook.edu; gu@cs.stonybrook.edu

A.S. El-Baz et al. (eds.), *Abdomen and Thoracic Imaging: An Engineering
& Clinical Perspective*, DOI 10.1007/978-1-4614-8498-1_16,
© Springer Science+Business Media New York 2014

Introduction

Virtual colonoscopy (VC), mimicking the conventional optical colonoscopy (OC), is a medical imaging procedure which uses X-rays or magnetic resonance (MR) signals and computers (1) to produce two- and three-dimensional (3D) images of the colon (large intestine) from the lowest part, i.e., the rectum, all the way toward the lower end (i.e., the cecum) of the small intestine and (2) to visualize the colon mucosal surface by endoscopic views on a screen [1, 2]. The procedure has shown the potential to screen colonic polyps and detect colon diseases, including diverticulosis and cancer [3].

Traditional paradigm in VC employs X-ray computed tomography or computed tomography colonography (CTC) to achieve the tasks of screening and detection due to the high speed of CT scanning and high contrast between colon wall and colon lumen filled by $CO2$ or air in CT images. While MR colonography (MRC) has an attractive point of non-ionization radiation [4], it faces several drawbacks, e.g., lower spatial resolution, prone to motion artifacts, and noticeable susceptibility artifacts on the interface between air and tissue/colon wall. Therefore, MRC remains in the early research development stage, while CTC has been successfully demonstrated to be more convenient and efficient than OC as a screening modality [3]. A combination of VC screening with OC follow-up for therapeutic intervention could be a cost-effective means to prevent the deadly disease of colon cancer.

However, because of the length of the colon with complicated structures, inspecting the entire colon wall is time consuming and prone to errors by current VC technologies. Moreover, because of the complicated colon structure, the field-of-view (FOV) of the VC endoscopic views is limited, resulting in incomplete examinations. Flattening the 3D wall into a 2D image would effectively increase the FOV and provide supplementary information to the VC endoscopic views [5]. Thereafter, various flattening techniques [6–11] have been developed, among which the conformal mapping algorithm [8, 10] showed advantages in generating 2D colon wall image with minimal distortion by preserving the structural angles.

Paik et al. [9] used cartographic projections to project the whole solid angle of the camera. This approach samples the solid angle of the camera and maps it onto a cylinder which is finally mapped to a 2D planar image. However, this method causes distortions in shape. Bartrol et al. [7] moved a camera along the central path of the colon. However, this approach does not provide a complete overview of the colon. Haker et al. [5] employed certain angle-preserving mappings, based on a discretization of the Laplace–Beltrami operator, to flatten a surface onto a plane in a manner which preserves the local geometry. However, the flattened result of their method is not efficient for applications like polyp identification, and it requires a highly accurate and smooth surface mesh to achieve a good mean-curvature calculation. Wang et al. [11] explored a volume-based flattening strategy to visualize the textures of the original 3D colon wall in the flattened 2D image. However, the distance-based mapping may not be accurate enough for detection of small polyps. The associated computation is intensive.

Hong et al. [8, 12] utilized conformal structure to flatten the colon wall onto a planar image. Their method is angle preserving and minimizes the global distortion. First, the colon wall is segmented and extracted from the CTC image dataset. The topology noise (i.e., minute handle) is removed by a volumetric algorithm. The holomorphic 1-form, a pair of orthogonal vector fields, is then computed on the 3D colon surface mesh using the conjugate gradient method. The colon surface is cut along a vertical trajectory traced using the holomorphic 1-form. Consequently, the 3D colon surface is conformal mapped onto a 2D rectangle. The flattened 2D mesh is then rendered using a direct volume rendering method accelerated with the GPU strategy. For applications like polyp detection, the shape of the polyps is well preserved on the flattened colon images, and thus provides an efficient way to enhance the navigation of a virtual colonoscopy system.

Unfortunately, the denoise algorithm in [8, 12] cannot always get genus 0 surface (actually only one case succeeds out of 14). In this paper, topological denoise is solved by our new algorithm, which guarantees the output surface to be genus 0. This efficient denoise algorithm greatly improved the efficiency and accuracy and deliver comparable flattening results.

Topological Denoise Framework

Figure 1 shows the colon flattening pipeline with and without the topological denoise. From acquired CTC datasets, our first task was to segment each image data volume and extract the corresponding colon wall. This was achieved by a statistical maximum a posteriori expectation-maximization (MAP-EM) algorithm [13]. Then a triangle mesh of the colon wall mucosal surface was generated by the standard Marching Cube algorithm. To remove topology handles, we apply a surface-based denoise algorithm. In our present pipeline, the Marching Cube algorithm was applied prior to topological denoising. After denoising, we developed Ricci flow method to perform the conformal flattening task.

Conformal mapping has many unique properties in flattening the colon wall, as shown in [8]. However, as we mentioned, previous denoise methods cannot guarantee the output surface is genus 0. Our contribution: we developed and applied a new topological denoise algorithm, which is very efficient and can guarantee the output surface to be genus 0.

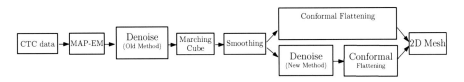

Fig. 1 Pipeline for our previous and current methods

Surface Topology

This section briefly introduces the background knowledge in surface topology, especially algebraic topology theory.

Homotopy

A surface S is a two-dimensional manifold, a *path* is a continuous map from the unit interval to the surface,

$$\gamma : [0, 1] \to S,$$

Two paths γ_0, γ_1 are *homotopic*, if there exists a homotopy between them,

$$F(t, \cdot) : [0, 1] \times [0, 1] \to S,$$

such that

$$F(0, \cdot) = \gamma_0(\cdot), F(1, \cdot) = \gamma_1(\cdot),$$

and denoted as $\gamma_0 \sim \gamma_1$. Intuitively, if two paths can deform from one to the other without leaving the surface, then they are homotopic (Fig. 2).

A path is called a *loop*, if its end point coincides with its starting point $\gamma(0) = \gamma(1)$. A special loop is called a trivial loop,

$$e(t) = p, \forall t \in [0, 1].$$

Consider all the loops through a fixed base point $p \in S$,

$$\mathcal{L} := \{\gamma : [0, 1] \to S | \gamma(0) = \gamma(1) = p\},$$

we use $[\gamma]$ to denote the homotopy class of a loop γ. Then the loop space $\mathcal{L}$ can be classified by the homotopy relation, the quotient space

$$\mathcal{L}/ \sim = \{[\gamma] | \gamma \in \mathcal{L}\}$$

has a natural group structure.

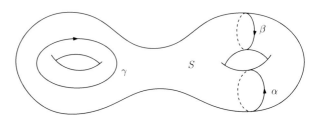

Fig. 2 α is homotopic to β, but not homotopic to γ

We define the *product* of two loops as the concatenation of them, operator $\cdot$: $\mathcal{L} \times \mathcal{L} \to \mathcal{L}$,

$$\gamma_1 \cdot \gamma_2 = \begin{cases} \gamma_1(2t - 0) & 0 \le t \le 1/2 \\ \gamma_2(2t - 1) & 1/2 \le t \le 1 \end{cases} \tag{1}$$

It is obvious that the product of the trivial loop $e(t) \equiv p$ and any loop γ equals to γ itself,

$$\gamma \cdot e = e \cdot \gamma.$$

We reverse the orientation of a loop,

$$\gamma^{-1}(t) := \gamma(1 - t),$$

then γ^{-1} is the inverse of γ,

$$\gamma^{-1} \cdot \gamma = \gamma \cdot \gamma^{-1} = e.$$

It is easy to be verified, if γ_1, γ_2 are homotopic to $\tilde{\gamma}_1, \tilde{\gamma}_2$, respectively, then

$$\gamma_1 \cdot \gamma_2 \sim \tilde{\gamma}_1 \cdot \tilde{\gamma}_2,$$

this means the product can be defined on homotopy classes without any ambiguity,

$$[\gamma_1] \cdot [\gamma_2] = [\gamma_1 \cdot \gamma_2],$$

and

$$[\gamma]^{-1} = [\gamma^{-1}].$$

Therefore all homotopy classes of loops through a base point under the product form a group, which is the so-called *the first fundamental group* of the surface, and denoted as $\pi_1(S,p)$.

Fundamental Group

Definition 1 (Fundamental Group). All the homotopy classes of loops with base point p under the product Eq. (1) form a group, the so-called fundamental group of the surface, denoted as $\pi_1(S,p)$.

Let $p, q \in S$ are two different base points on the surface. Let $\tau : [0,1] \to S$ is a path connecting them, such that $\tau(0) = p$ and $\tau(1) = q$. For each loop $\gamma \in \pi_1(S, p)$, there is a unique loop $\tilde{\gamma} \in \pi_1(S, q)$,

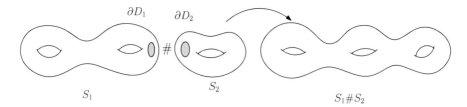

Fig. 3 Connected sum

$$\tilde{\gamma} = \tau \circ \gamma \circ \tau^{-1},$$

this gives an isomorphism between the two fundamental groups $\pi_1(S,p)$ and $\pi_1(S,q)$,

$$\pi_1(S,p) \cong \pi_1(S,q),$$

therefore, the fundamental group is independent of the choice of the base point. So we can omit the base point and simply denote the fundamental group as $\pi_1(S)$.

The fundamental group of a compact surface is finitely generated. Suppose $\{\gamma_1,\gamma_2,\ldots,\gamma_m\}$ are the generators of $\pi_1(S,p)$, then any loop $\gamma \in \pi_1(S,p)$ can be represented as

$$\gamma = \gamma_{i_1}^{n_1}\gamma_{i_k}^{n_k} \cdots \gamma_{i_k}^{n_k},$$

where $1 \le i_1,i_2,\ldots,i_k \le m$, and all powers $n_1,n_2,\ldots,n_k$ are integers. We call such representation of the loop a word. It is possible that some complicated words can shrink to a point, namely, the product of generators may be trivial, we call all such words relations.

Surfaces are connected sum of tori.

Definition 2 (Connected Sum). The connected sum $S_1 \# S_2$ is formed by deleting the interior of disks $D_i \subset S_i$ and attaching the resulting punctured surfaces $S_i - D_i$ to each other by a homeomorphism $h : \partial D_1 \to \partial D_2$, where D_i represents the boundary of D_i. Let $p \in D1$ and $q \in D2$, p is equivalent to q, $p \sim q$ if $q = h(p)$ (Fig. 3). So

$$S_1 \# S_2 := \{(S_1 - D_1) \cup (S_2 - D_2)\}/ \sim .$$

Theorem 3 (Classification for Compact Orientable Surface). *Any closed connected orientable surface is homeomorphic to either a sphere or a finite connected sum of tori,*

$$S = \mathbb{S}^2 \# T_1 \# T_2 \cdots \# T_g,$$

where S_2 is the unit sphere, T_i is a torus, $i = 1, 2,\cdots, g$. g is called the genus of the surface, and each T_i is a handle.

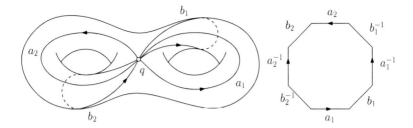

Fig. 4 Canonical fundamental group generator

Intuitively, each handle is a torus T_i, which is the direct product of two circles, $T_i = \mathbb{S}^1 \times \mathbb{S}^1$. We denote the first circle as a_i and the second as b_i, then all such pairs $\{(a_i,b_i)\}$ are the generators of $\pi_1(S,p)$.

Definition 4 (Canonical Fundamental Group Basis). A fundamental group basis $\{a_1,b_1,a_2,b_2,\ldots,a_g,b_g\}$ is canonical, if

(1) a_i and b_i intersect at the same point p.
(2) a_i and a_j, b_i and b_j, a_i and b_j only touch at p.

As shown in Fig. 4, if we slice the surface along the canonical fundamental group generators, we will get a 4g-gon. The boundary is

$$a_1 b_1 a_1^{-1} b_1^{-1} a_2 b_2 a_2^{-1} b_2^{-1} \cdots a_g b_g a_g^{-1} b_g^{-1}$$

which can shrink to a point. For general compact orientable closed surfaces, the following theorem holds:

Theorem 5 (Fundamental Groups of General Surfaces). *The fundamental group of the surface $S = \mathbb{S}^2 \#_g T^2$ is the group with generators $\{a_1,b_1,a_2,b_2,\cdots,a_g,b_g\}$ and one relation $\Pi_{k=1}^{g}[a_k, b_k] = e$, where $[a, b] = aba^{-1}b^{-1}$.*

Covering Spaces

Definition 6 (Covering Space). Let $\pi : \tilde{S} \to M$ be a continuous map and π is onto. Suppose for all $q \in S$, there is an open neighborhood U of q such that

$$\pi^{-1}(U) = \cup_{j \in J} \tilde{U}_j,$$

for some collection $\{\tilde{U}_j, j \in J\}$ of subsets of $\tilde{S}$ satisfying $\tilde{U}_j \cap \tilde{U}_k =$ if $j \neq k$, and with $p|_{\tilde{U}_j} : \tilde{U}_j \to U$ a homeomorphism for each $j \in J$. Then $p : \tilde{S} \to M$ is a *covering*.

The automorphisms of the covering space which are commutative with the projection are called deck transformations.

Definition 7 (Deck Transformation). Suppose $\pi : \tilde{S} \to S$ is a covering. An automorphism $\tau : \tilde{S} \to \tilde{S}$ is called a *deck transformation* if $\pi \circ \tau = \pi$.

All the deck transformations form a group $Deck(\tilde{S})$, the *deck transformation group*. S is homeomorphic to the quotient space

$$\tilde{S}/Deck(\tilde{S}) \cong S.$$

Definition 8 (Fundamental Domain). A closed subset $D \in \tilde{S}$ is called a *fundamental domain* of the $Deck(\tilde{S})$, if

$$\tilde{S} = \bigcup_{\tau \in Deck} \tau D,$$

$\tilde{S}$ is the union of conjugates of D, and the intersection of any two conjugates has no interior.

Among all covering spaces for a given surface, the one with the simplest topology is the so-called universal covering.

Definition 9 (Universal Covering). Suppose $\pi : \tilde{S} \to S$ is a covering. If $\tilde{S}$ is simply connected $(\pi_1(\tilde{M}, \tilde{q}) = \langle e \rangle)$, then the covering is the *universal covering*.

The universal covering space can be constructed explicitly as the follows:

$$\tilde{S} := \{\gamma : [0, 1] \to S | \gamma(0) = p\} / \sim$$

namely, the space of all homotopy classes of paths starting from the base point p is isomorphic to the universal covering space of the surface.

Theorem 10 (Universal Covering Space for Surfaces). *The universal covering spaces of orientable closed surfaces are sphere* $\mathbb{S}^2$ *(genus zero), plane* $\mathbb{E}^2$ *(genus one), and disk* $\mathbb{H}^2$ *(high genus).*

Geodesics and Cut Locus

Suppose the surface is with a Riemannian metric $\mathbf{g} = (g_{ij})$, then it determines the Levi–Civita connection. The connection is represented by the Christoffel symbols

$$\Gamma^i_{kl} = \frac{1}{2} g^{im} \left(\frac{\partial g_{mk}}{\partial x^l} + \frac{\partial g_{ml}}{\partial x^k} - \frac{\partial g_{kl}}{\partial x^m} \right)$$

Suppose $\mathbf{v} = v^i \mathbf{e}_i$ and $\mathbf{u} = u^j \mathbf{e}_j$, then

$$\nabla_{\mathbf{v}} \mathbf{u} = \nabla_{v^i \mathbf{e}_i} u^j \mathbf{e}_j = v^i \nabla_{\mathbf{e}_i} u^j \mathbf{e}_j = v^i u^j \nabla_{\mathbf{e}_i} \mathbf{e}_j + v^i \mathbf{e}_j \nabla_{\mathbf{e}_i} u_j$$

therefore

$$\nabla_{\mathbf{v}}\mathbf{u} = \left(v^i u^j \Gamma_{ij}^k + v^i \frac{\partial u^k}{\partial x^i}\right)\mathbf{e}_k.$$

Definition 11 (Geodesic). Suppose $\gamma : [0,1] \to (S,\mathbf{g})$ is a path on the surface, if it satisfies

$$\nabla_{\dot{\gamma}}\dot{\gamma} \equiv 0,$$

then γ is a geodesic.

The geodesic is fully determined by the starting point $\gamma(0)$ and the initial tangent direction $\dot{\gamma}(0)$. For any point $p \in S$, and tangent direction $\mathbf{v} \in T_pS$, there exists a unique geodesic $\gamma(t) = \gamma(t;p,\mathbf{v})$, such that $\gamma(0) = p$ and $\dot{\gamma}(0) = \mathbf{v}$.

Definition 12 (Exponential map). The exponential map is defined as

$$exp_p : T_pS \to S, \mathbf{v} = \gamma(1;p,\mathbf{v}).$$

We fix the base point p, and issue geodesics from p, until the boundary of the geodesic disk meets itself. The locus where the geodesic front meets is the cut locus.

Definition 13 (Cut locus). Fix a point $p \in S$, the cut locus is the closure of points q, where the exponential map $e\,x\,p_p$ is not diffeomorphic at q.

The cut locus forms a graph, the surface removes the cut locus is a topological disk.

Surface Ricci Flow

Suppose S is a surface in three-dimensional Euclidean space $\mathbb{R}^3$, therefore it has naturally the induced Euclidean metric $\mathbf{g}$. The Gaussian curvature is determined by the Riemannian metric $\mathbf{g}$, and satisfies the following Gauss–Bonnet theorem:

Theorem 14 (Gauss–Bonnet Theorem) *The total Gaussian curvature of a closed metric surface is*

$$\int_S KdA = 2\pi\chi(S),$$

where $\chi(S)$ is the Euler number, which equals to $\chi(S) = 2 - 2g$ for closed surface with genus g.

Ricci flow is a powerful curvature flow method invented by Hamilton [14] for the purpose of proving Poincaré's conjecture. Intuitively, it describes the process to

Fig. 5 Conformal Mapping
preserves angle: the angle
on the texture domain is
well preserved after mapped
to the surface, so the shape
information of colon
surface is well preserved

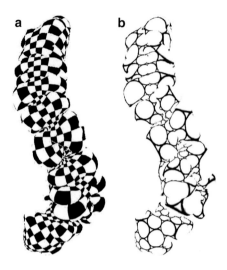

a   b

deform the Riemannian metric according to curvature such that the curvature
evolves like a heat diffusion process:

$$\frac{d\mathbf{g}}{dt} = -2K\mathbf{g}. \tag{2}$$

The convergence of surface Ricci flow was also proved in [14].

Theorem 15 *Suppose S is a closed surface with a Riemannian metric. If the total
area is preserved, the surface Ricci flow will converge to a Riemannian metric of
constant Gaussian curvature* [14].

Figure 5 shows the conformal parameterization of colon surface computed by
Ricci flow, which preserves angle.

Algorithm

Topological Denoise

In previous works like [8], the denoise process started from the segmentation of the
colon incorporated the simple point concept in a region growing based algorithm to
extract a topologically simple segmentation of the colon lumen. However, the denoise
algorithm cannot guarantee the output surface is genus 0 in practice, so we developed
a new efficient surface-based denoise algorithm to remove the topological noise. As
our method find tiny handles based on surface topology and remove them one by one,
the final surface is guaranteed to be genus 0. The pipeline is like the following:

Fig. 6 A typical tiny hole
and the homotopy basis
(labeled by *yellow line*)
goes around it

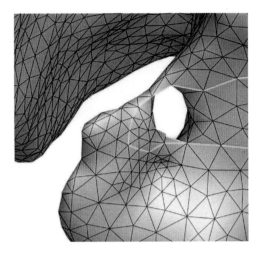

Algorithm 1: Topological Denoise Algorithm

Input: Surfaces M.

   Output: Genus 0 surface $\bar{M}$.

   1. Compute the homotopy basis G of M using Algorithm 2.
   2. For each point p on homotopy basis G, grow a patch P.
   3. Find the shortest homotopy loop p_l starts at p in patch P.
   4. Find the shortest loop $m\,i\,n\{p_l\}$ among all the vertices on G.
   5. Cut M along $m\,i\,n\{p_l\}$ and fill the 2 holes appeared, get $\bar{M}$.
   6. If $\bar{M}$ is not genus 0, goto step 1.

The idea of efficient topological denoise algorithm is like following: we can compute the shortest loop goes though vertex v for all the vertices in mesh M, then find the shortest one among them, it must be the shortest handle loop in M. Furthermore, all the handles of a surface must be "go around" by the homotopy basis. As a result, we just need to compute the shortest loops for vertices on the homotopy basis G instead of all vertices of surface M, which leads to a 10 times speedup. Compared to the old voxel-based denoise algorithm, our surface-based method is much faster and guarantees the output surface to be exactly genus 0. Figure 6 shows a tiny handle went though by the homotopy basis.

A homotopy basis at s can be thought of as a homology basis where all loops meet at a common vertex s, called the basepoint. Erickson and Whittlesey [15] proved that a shortest homotopy basis at a point on a mesh with n vertices can be computed in $O(n\,l\,o\,g\,n)$ time. Figure 7 shows the homotopy basis for genus 1 surface, Algorithm 2 gives the algorithm for computing the homotopy basis:

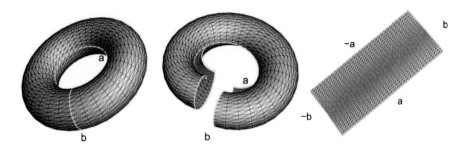

Fig. 7 *Left*: a and b are 2 homotopy basis for a genus 1 surface. *Middle*: The surface becomes a topological disk after cut along the it's homotopy basis. *Right*: Flatten the surface onto the plane

---

Algorithm 2: Homotopy Basis Algorithm

Input: Surfaces M.

    Output: The homotopy basis G of $\bar{M}$.

    1. Find the maximum spanning tree T from a basepoint s.

    2. Find a maximum spanning tree T^* on the edges of the dual graph which do not cross edges in T.

    3. Find all edges $\{e_1, e_2 \ldots e_{2g}\}$ which are neither in T nor are crossed by edges in T^*.

    4. Find the loops containing each e_i (using T), these loops form the homotopy basis.

Discrete Ricci Flow

The computation of the conformal mapping of a triangular mesh is based on the discrete Ricci flow [16, 17], as Algorithm 3 shows.

Algorithm 3: Discrete Ricci Flow

Input: Surface M.

    Output: The metric U of M.

    1. Assign a circle at vertex v_i with radius r_i; For each edge $[v_i, v_j]$, two circles intersect at an angle ϕ_{ij}, called edge weight.

    2. The edge length l_{ij} of $[v_i, v_j]$ is determined by the cosine law:
$$l_{ij}^2 = r_i^2 + r_j^2 - 2r_i r_j \cos\phi_{ij}$$

    3. The angle θ_i^{jk}, related to each corner , is determined by the current edge lengths with the inverse hyperbolic cosine law.

    4. Compute the discrete Gaussian curvature K_i of each vertex v_i:

(continued)

Algorithm 3: Discrete Ricci Flow   (continued)

$$K_i = \begin{cases} 2\pi - \sum_{f_{ijk} \in F} \theta_i^{jk}, interior\ vertex \\ \pi - \sum_{f_{ijk} \in F} \theta_i^{jk}, boundary\ vertex \end{cases} \quad (3)$$

where θ_i^{jk} represents the corner angle attached to vertex v_i in the face f_{ijk}

5. Update the radius r_i of each vertex v_i: $r_i = r_i - \epsilon K_i r_i$
6. Repeat the step 2 through 5, until $\|K_i\|$ of all vertices are less than a specific error tolerance.

Applications and Experimental Results

Colon Flattening

As discussed, the Ricci flow method will deform the Riemannian metric to the uniformization metric, which induces constant curvatures everywhere. This constant is solely determined by the topology of the surface. In our case, the colon wall surface is a topological cylinder. Hence, the uniformization metric induces zero Gaussian curvature for the interior points, and a zero geodesic curvature along the boundaries. However, if there are topological noises on the colon surface, commonly fake handles, then the Ricci flow converges to a negative constant curvature metric and hence the colon surface cannot be conformally flattened onto the Euclidean plane, as shown in Fig. 8a. By running our topological denoise algorithm, the flatten result becomes reasonably good for visualization and geometry processing applications, as shown in Fig. 8b.

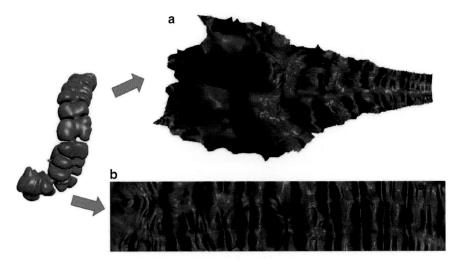

Fig. 8 The flattening of the ascending segment of the colon using (**a**) Run Ricci flow directly, and (**b**) Run our denoise method to clean the topological noise first

Visualization of Polyps

One of the important applications of using colon flattening is to provide a better way for the physicians to visualize and sometimes even detect the polyps. Especially, the polyps present behind the colon folds are hidden and missed during the VC navigation of a 3D model. By using our method, all the shapes on the colon surface are preserved even if the colon surface has many fake handles. Therefore, the shape of the polyps is preserved and hence forms an effective means of polyp visualization. Furthermore, the volume rendering of the flattened colon provides a realistic rendering of the polyps. In addition, the physicians can even zoom-in at the suspicious regions to confirm the location of the polyps. Thus, even relatively smaller polyps can also be seen without any problem.

Figure 10 shows a colon surface flattening result with topology cleaning and the polyp detected. Figure 9 shows a closeup view of some of the polyps observed by navigating along the flattened colon surface that is obtained using our method. As you can see, the shape of all the polyps has been well preserved which is very important for the polyp detection. Figure 9a shows a polyp of larger size, while Fig. 9b shows a polyp of smaller size. Irrespective of their size all the polyps were successfully captured. Figure 9c shows a polyp that is hidden behind a fold. It is difficult to find such polyps by navigating inside the normal colon but by flattening the colon, even the polyps hidden behind the colonic folds can be observed as shown in Fig. 9c. In order to be able to inspect polyps of all sizes, we have rendered the flattened colon using very high resolution of $12,000 \times 1,000$. Some more polyps found by using our method can be seen (shown in the yellow circles) in the top

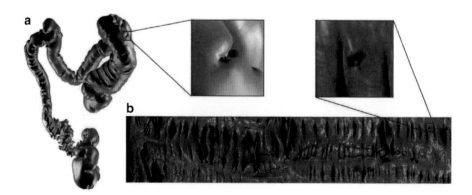

Fig. 9 Closeup view of (**a**) large polyp, (**b**) small polyp, and (**c**) polyp behind a fold on the flattened colon surface

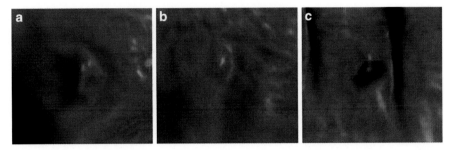

Fig. 10 Topological cleaning. (**a**) The 3D colon model with topological noise such as handles. A close-up of the handle can be seen. (**b**) The corresponding flattening of the 3D colon to 2D rectangle after running our cleaning method. A closeup view of a polyp that is behind a fold on the flattened colon surface can be seen

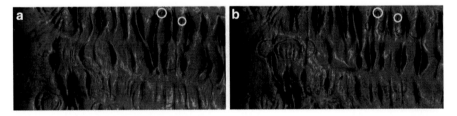

Fig. 11 Visualization of the registration results for the ascending segment of (**a**) supine and (**b**) prone. *Yellow circles* locate the polyps

image of Fig. 11a, b. We have verified the locations of all the polyps by checking with both the OC and VC reports provided by the Walter Reed Army Medical Center for all the colon models. The inspection of the flat colon will only help us to mark the suspicious locations. Not all these locations might be polyps. Hence, note that by providing a flattened colon visualization, we are only providing a better means of navigation to look for the suspicious locations so that no areas of the colon are missed. We do not provide an automatic way of polyp detection. By performing further analysis on this flattened colon such as the size, shape, and density analysis we can detect the polyps automatically which we plan to do in the future.

Table 1 Denoise results and time efficiency

Data Index	#Mesh triangles	# Handles removed by our method	# Handles removed by [8]	# Running time
3033P	830 K	8	5	8.6 min
3033S	1,120 K	26	10	10.3 min
3034P	764 K	24	21	8.1 min
3034S	800 K	7	2	8.2 min
3035S	1,060 K	13	6	10.2 min
3036P	875 K	13	8	8.5 min
3037S	836 K	6	0	8.5 min
3038P	1,167 K	16	10	10.8 min
3039P	920 K	7	5	9.4 min
3039S	1,040 K	9	8	10.0 min
3041P	902 K	15	8	9.7 min
3041S	886 K	4	1	9.1 min
3043P	917 K	11	5	9.4 min
3053S	958 K	4	4	9.6 min

Colon Registration

Our topological noise algorithm can also benefit colon surface registration. We first run our denoise algorithm to remove all fake handles, then run the state-of-the-art flattening and quasi-conformal registration. Hence, we are able to register supine and prone colons, even in the case when the colon surfaces have lots of handles as shown in Fig. 11.

Figure 11 shows the supine and prone colon registration result of the ascending segment of a colon model (with handles) using quasi-conformal mapping. There are two polyps in the colon segment (shown in the yellow circles) of Fig. 11 and we can see a good visual correspondence between the locations of both the polyps in supine and prone. For the analytical evaluation, we followed a similar approach in [18] and computed the distance error in millimeters for all the six registration results. The average distance error is 8.14 mm, which is reasonably good.

Experiment Result

CTC datasets was random selected from a database. The presented algorithm was implemented in a similar manner as the previous algorithm [8] for a fair comparison. These algorithms were executed on a PC platform of Intel Xeon X5450 3.0GHz CPU and 8.00 GB RAM. To get the maximum quality, we use the original un-simplified mesh for conformal mapping. The triangle number of the 14 datasets ranges from 700 to 1,200 k. The method in [8] can only find around half of the handles, while our method can completely remove all the handles. Table 1 shows

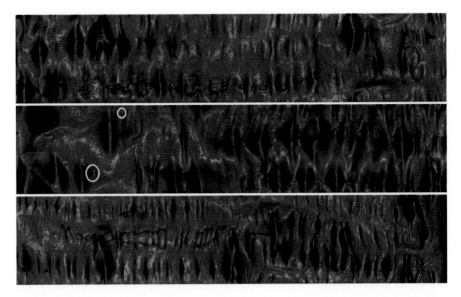

Fig. 12 Whole flattened colon image processed by our denoise algorithm *Yellow circles* locate the polyps

the denoise result comparison between our method and the method in [8], as well as the total running time for denoise and conformal flattening. Notice that only 1 out of 14 case (3053S) reached genus 0 using method in [8], which means most of the data are not qualified as input of the conformal flattening algorithm, while all 14 reached genus 0 using our denoise algorithm.

For the final colon image, Fig. 12 shows a whole flattened colon image processed by our topological denoise algorithm. Figure 13 shows the flattening results for more colons denoised by our algorithm.

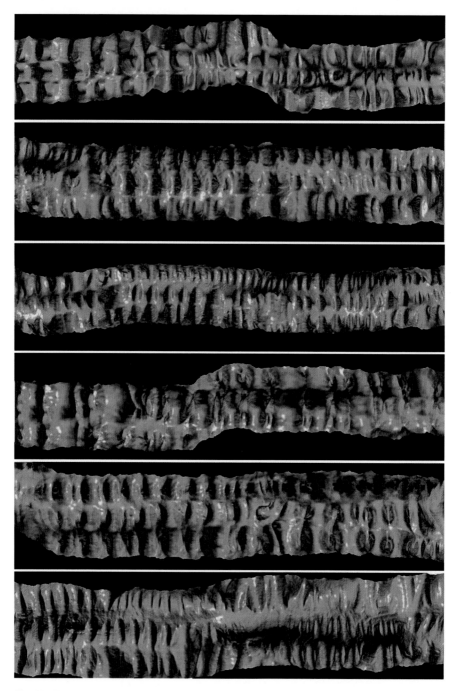

Fig. 13 Flattened results for more datasets processed by our denoise algorithm

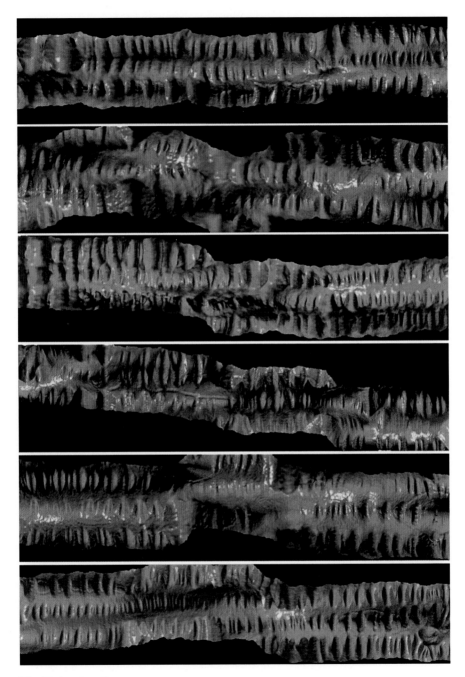

Fig. 13 (continued)

Discussion

The key parts of our method is the new efficient topological denoise algorithm. Our new topological denoise algorithm guarantees the output to be exactly genus 0. As a result, the whole mapping process becomes much faster and more stable.

Acknowledgements The authors would like to thank the support of NSF CCF-0448399, NSF DMS-0528363, NSF DMS-0626223, NSF CCF-0830550, NSF IIS-0916286, NSF CCF-1081424, and ONR N000140910228.

References

1. Hong L, Kaufman A, Wei Y, Viswambharan A, Wax M, Liang Z (1995) 3d virtual colonoscopy. In: IEEE symposium on frontier in biomedical visualization, IEEE CS Press, pp 26–32
2. Hong L, Liang Z, Viswambharan A, Kaufman A, Wax M (1997) Reconstruction and visualization of 3d models of the colonic surface. In: IEEE transactions on nuclear science, IEEE CS Press, pp 1297–1302
3. Pickhardt PJ, Choi JR, Hwang I, Butler JA, Puckett ML, Hildebrandt HA, Wong RK, Nugent PA, Mysliwiec PA, Schindler WR (2003) Computed tomographic virtual colonoscopy to screen for colorectal neoplasia in asymptomatic adults. New Eng J Med 349(23):2191–2200
4. Luboldt PBW, Steiner P (1998) Detection of mass lesions with mr colonoscopy: preliminary report. Radiology 207:59–65
5. Haker S, Angenent S, Kikinis R (2000) Nondistorting flattening maps and the 3d visualization of colon ct images. IEEE Trans. Medic Imag 19:665–670
6. Balogh E, Sorantin E, Nyul LG, Palagyi K, Kuba AG, Werkgartner, Spuller E (2002) Colon unraveling based on electronic field: Recent progress and future work. In: Proceedings SPIE, 4681, pp 713–721
7. Bartrol AV, Wegenkittl R, König A, Gröller E, Sorantin E, Medgraph T (2001) In: Virtual colon flattening. In: VisSym '01 Joint Eurographics - IEEE TCVG Symposium on Visualization, Conference Proceedings, pages 127–136
8. Hong W, Gu X, Qiu F, Jin M, Kaufman A (2006) Conformal virtual colon flattening. In: SPM '06: Proceedings of the 2006 ACM symposium on Solid and physical modeling, ACM, pp 85–93
9. Paik D, Beaulieu C, Jeffrey R, Karadi CA, Napel S (2000) Visualization modes for ct colonography using cylindrical and planar map projections. J Comput Assist Tomograp 179–188
10. Hong W, Qiu F, Kaufman A (2006) A pipeline for computer aided polyp detection. IEEE Trans Visualizat Comput Graph 12:861–868
11. Wang Z, Li B, Liang Z (2005) Feature-based texture display for detection of colonic polyps on flattened colon volume. In: International conference of IEEE engineering in medicine and biology, IEEE CS Press, 4:3359–3362
12. Hong W, Qiu F, Kaufman A (2006) A pipeline for computer aided polyp detection. In: IEEE transactions on visualization and computer graphics, IEEE CS Press, 12(5):861–868
13. Wang S, Li L, Cohen H, Mankes S, Chen J, Liang Z (2009) An em approach to map solution of segmenting tissue mixture percentages with application to ct-based virtual colonoscopy. IEEE Trans Med Imag 28:297–310
14. Hamilton RS (1988) The Ricci flow on surfaces. Mathematics and general relativity (Santa Cruz, CA, 1986). Contemp Math Am Math Soc Providence RI 71

15. Erickson J, Whittlesey K (2005) Greedy optimal homotopy and homology generators. In: Proceedings of the sixteenth annual ACM-SIAM symposium on Discrete algorithms, ser. SODA '05, ACM, pp 1038–1046
16. Jin M, Kim J, Gu XD (2007) Discrete surface ricci flow: Theory and applications. In: IMA conference on the mathematics of surfaces, Springer, pp 209–232
17. Zeng W, Samaras D, Gu XD (2010) Ricci flow for 3D shape analysis. PAMI 32(4):662–677
18. Zeng W, Marino J, Chaitanya GK, Gu X, Kaufman A (2010) Supine and prone colon registration using quasi-conformal mapping. IEEE Trans Visualiz Comput Graph 16 (6):1348–1357

Biography

Wei Zeng is an assistant professor of the School of Computing and Information Sciences at Florida International University. Dr. Zeng received her Ph.D. from Chinese Academy of Sciences in 2008 and her thesis was titled as "Computational Conformal Geometry Based Shape Analysis." Her research interests include computational conformal geometry, Teichmüller quasiconformal geometry, discrete differential geometry, discrete Ricci flow, geometric analysis, and their applications to surface matching, registration, tracking, recognition, and shape analysis. Her research areas span over medical imaging, computer vision, computer graphics and visualization, wireless sensor network, geometric modeling, and computational topology.

Rui Shi is a Ph.D. candidate in the Department of Computer Science at Stony Brook University. He received his BS degree in Automation at University of Science and Technology of China. His research direction towards surface registration and applications of geometric algorithm in Wireless Sensor Network. He has published papers in CVPR, IPMI, InfoCom, IJCV, and so on.

Zhengyu Su is a Ph.D. candidate in the Department of Computer Science at Stony Brook University. He received his B.S. degree in Electrical Engineering at University of Science and Technology of China. His research direction towards area preserving mapping and its applications in Graphics and Medical Imaging. He has published papers in CVPR, IPMI, and so on.

David Xianfeng Gu received his Ph.D. degree in Computer Science from Harvard University in 2003. He is an associate professor of computer science and the director of the 3D Scanning Laboratory in the Department of Computer Science at Stony Brook University. His research interests include computer vision, graphics, geometric modeling, and medical imaging. His major works include global conformal surface parameterization in graphics, tracking and analysis of facial expression in vision, manifold splines in modeling, brain mapping and virtual colonoscopy in medical imaging and computational conformal geometry. He won the US National Science Foundation CAREER award in 2004.

Towards Self-Parameterized Active Contours for Medical Image Segmentation with Emphasis on Abdomen

Eleftheria A. Mylona, Michalis A. Savelonas, and Dimitris Maroulis

Abstract Medical doctors are typically required to segment medical images by means of computational tools, which suffer from parameters that are empirically selected through a cumbersome and time-consuming process. This chapter presents a framework for automated parameterization of region-based active contour regularization and data fidelity terms, which aims to relieve medical doctors from this process, as well as to enhance objectivity and reproducibility. Leaned on an observed isomorphism between the eigenvalues of structure tensors and active contour parameters, the presented framework automatically adjusts active contour parameters so as to reflect the orientation coherence in edge regions by means of the "orientation entropy." To this end, the active contour is repelled from randomly oriented edge regions and is navigated towards structured ones, accelerating contour convergence. Experiments are conducted on abdominal imaging domains, which include colon and lung images. The experimental evaluation demonstrates that the presented framework is capable of speeding up contour convergence, whereas it achieves high-quality segmentation results, albeit in an unsupervised fashion.

Introduction

Medical image segmentation is an essential instrument in computer-aided diagnosis, being potentially crucial for localization of pathologies, study of anatomical structures, computer-integrated surgery, and treatment planning. In particular, abdominal image segmentation allows medical doctors (MDs) to investigate abdominal organs, as visualized by noninvasive imaging modalities. As part of their clinical diagnosis, MDs are typically required to examine and

E.A. Mylona • M.A. Savelonas • D. Maroulis (✉)
Department of Informatics and Telecommunications, University of Athens,
Panepistimiopolis, Ilissia 15703, Athens, Greece
e-mail: emylona@di.uoa.gr; msavel@di.uoa.gr; dmaroulis@di.uoa.gr

A.S. El-Baz et al. (eds.), *Abdomen and Thoracic Imaging: An Engineering & Clinical Perspective*, DOI 10.1007/978-1-4614-8498-1_17,
© Springer Science+Business Media New York 2014

interpret abdominal images obtained by CT scans, in order to extract vital information on abdominal organs, which is associated with their anatomy and pathology. Although such images may contain detailed information, they are often plagued by noise, artifacts, as well as heterogeneity, which yield to inhomogeneous background.

Medical image segmentation has to be a robust and reproducible process without human intervention, so as to substantially support diagnosis and clinical evaluation. However, most segmentation methods are highly parametric, and human intervention is often inevitable. In this regard, automatic medical image segmentation techniques are in demand, so as to ease MDs' workload and bolster the objectivity of the segmentation results.

Region-based active contour models are widely applied for medical image segmentation due to their inherent noise-filtering mechanism and their topological adaptability. Moreover, they are robust to weak edges and intensity inhomogeneity [1–4]. Researchers have developed various region-based active contour variations for abdominal image segmentation. Dhalila et al. [5] propose a semiautomatic active contour variation for the segmentation of the abdominal region of the human body. In the first phase, user intervention is a prerequisite for manual segmentation of a certain number of slices, whereas in the second phase, segmentation is automatic. Jiang et al. [6] propose an approach based on active contour for segmentation of the liver region in abdominal CT images. The active contour model is combined with threshold and morphology-based techniques in order to extract the initial contour and segment the liver slice by slice. Plajer et al. [7] present an active contour algorithm for lung tumor segmentation in 3D-CT image data. The algorithm is based on a mixed internal–external force as well as on a cluster function.

The development of such powerful computational tools contributes to the early diagnosis of the pathology in abdominal organs. However, the vast majority of these tools are dominated by parameters, and although these parameters have a major impact on the segmentation quality, they are empirically determined through the tedious and time-consuming process of trial and error. Parameters are often selected on the basis of a limited amount of experimental results and the visual impression of the domain user, whereas they may be valid for a specific dataset. To this end, the objectivity and reproducibility of the segmentation results are highly questioned. Furthermore, empirical parameterization presumes certain technical knowledge by the end user with respect to the algorithm's intrinsic mechanisms. Nevertheless, this is not the case in the context of medical imaging where the end user is usually a MD.

Previous Work

Several region-based active contour variations have been developed in order to tackle with empirical parameterization. Ma and Yu [8] attempt to balance region-based forces by means of mathematical morphology without separately adjusting each individual parameter. McIntosh and Hamarneh [9] adapt regularization weights across a set of images. Although one weight value may be optimal for some regions in an image, it may not be optimal for all regions. Erdem and Tari [10] and Kokkinos et al. [11] focus on edge consistency and texture cues by utilizing data-driven local cues. However, certain technical knowledge by the domain user is still required. Pluemptiwiriyaweg et al. [12] and Tsai et al. [13] dynamically update active contour parameters during contour evolution. Nonetheless, possible erroneous behavior of the contour in the early stages of evolution, with effects on convergence, has not been considered. Furthermore, parameters are not spatially adaptive, failing to capture local image content. Keuper et al. [14] and Liu et al. [15] propose a method for dynamic adjustment of active contour parameters, applicable on the detection of cell nuclei and lip boundaries, respectively. Both methods require a priori knowledge considering the shape of the target region. Iakovidis et al. [16] and Hsu et al. [17] introduce a framework for optimization of active contour parameters based on genetic algorithms. However, these heuristic approaches converge slowly in locally optimal solutions. Allili et al. [18] present an approach for estimating hyper-parameters capable of balancing the contribution of boundary and region-based terms. In their approach, empirical parameter tuning is still involved. Yushkevich et al. [19] develop an application for level-set segmentation of anatomical structures. Although their GUI is friendly to non-expert users, parameter settings are still empirically determined. Dong et al. [20] present an algorithm to capture brain aneurysms from the vascular tree, by varying the regularization term based on the surface curvature of a pre-segmented vessel. However, the regularization weight does not rely on image content. On the contrary, it depends on the shape of the target region, thus limiting the applicability of the method on different target shapes.

This chapter presents a framework for automated parameterization of region-based active contours, which is applicable on medical image segmentation. The presented framework is inspired by the observation of an isomorphism between the eigenvalues of structure tensors and the active contour regularization and data fidelity parameters. The latter are capable of describing the orientation coherence of edge regions similarly to the former by means of the measure called orientation entropy (OE). This measure obtains low values in structured regions, which contain edges with low orientation variability, and high values in unstructured regions, which contain edges of multiple orientations. Accordingly, OE is capable to adjust forces driving the contour away from unstructured edge regions and guide it towards more structured ones, which are naturally associated with the boundaries of medical objects. Hence, iterations dedicated to false local minima are bypassed, speeding up contour convergence.

The presented framework aims to:

(a) Relieve MDs from the cumbersome and time-consuming process of empirical parameterization
(b) Cope well with the large variability of the shape of target regions in abdominal images

(c) Remain insensitive to noise, artifacts, and heterogeneity
(d) Provide objectivity and reproducibility

Parameter-Adjustment Framework

The presented parameter-adjustment framework exploits the attractive properties
of structure tensor eigenvalues.

Structure Tensors

Structure tensors [21] have been extensively utilized in image analysis for various
tasks such as anisotropic filtering [22] and motion detection [23].

In Weickert's diffusion model [24], the structure tensor D is a symmetric,
semi-positive 2×2 matrix (also called "second-moment matrix"), capable of
describing the orientation coherence of an edge region and is defined as

$$D = (v_1 \ v_2) \begin{pmatrix} \lambda_1 & 0 \\ 0 & \lambda_2 \end{pmatrix} (v_1 \ v_2)^{\mathrm{T}} = (dx \ dy) \begin{pmatrix} I_{xx} & I_{xy} \\ I_{yx} & I_{yy} \end{pmatrix} (dx \ dy)^{\mathrm{T}} \quad (1)$$

where I is the input image, v_1, v_2 are orthonormal eigenvectors, and λ_1, λ_2 are the
corresponding eigenvalues given by

$$\lambda_{1,2} = \frac{1}{2} \left(I_{xx} + I_{yy} \pm \sqrt{(I_{xx} - I_{yy})^2 + 4I_{xy}^2} \right) \quad (2)$$

where the + sign belongs to λ_1. The eigenvectors and eigenvalues of the structure
tensor reflect the local orientation of edge regions. The eigenvectors form the
orthogonal basis so that the variance of the projection on one of the tensor's
axes is maximal and the projection on one of the remaining axes is minimal [25].
The eigenvalues describe the orientation coherence along the corresponding
eigenvectors. It is worth to be noted that λ_1 is the principal eigenvalue and is
longitudinal with respect to the principal axis of the tensor ellipsoid, whereas
λ_2 is the minor eigenvalue and is vertical with respect to the same principal axis.
Figure 1 depicts an elliptical representation of a 2D structure tensor.

Providing that an image region contains either edges of approximately the same
orientation, or edges of multiple orientations, it can be identified by means of a
structure tensor as a structured or unstructured edge region, respectively. The
boundaries of medical objects are naturally associated with structured edge regions,
whereas unstructured edge regions are associated with noise, artifacts, and/or
background clutter. In this light, structure tensors are capable of providing maps
of target and nontarget edge regions in the context of a medical imaging application.

Fig. 1 Elliptical representation of a 2D structure tensor

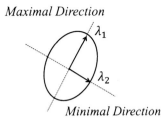

Fig. 2 Elliptical representation of active contour

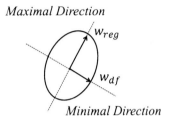

Region-Based Active Contours

The energy functional of the region-based active contours that is minimized can be written as follows:

$$E_{\text{total}} = w_{\text{reg}} \cdot E_{\text{reg}} + w_{\text{df}} \cdot E_{\text{df}} \tag{3}$$

where E_{reg} and E_{df} are the regularization and data fidelity energy terms, respectively, whereas w_{reg} and w_{df} are the corresponding weighting parameters. Energy terms are scalar functions, which most often discard any information associated with the orientation coherence of edge regions. However, forces guiding contour evolution are vectors which are affected by the orientation coherence of edges.

Regularization forces are tangent with respect to the principal axis of the contour, whereas data fidelity forces are vertical, attracting the contour towards target edges. Providing that the contour is initialized as an ellipsoid, the regularization weight w_{reg} is longitudinal with respect to the principal axis of the contour, whereas the data fidelity weight w_{df} is vertical with respect to the same principal axis. Figure 2 depicts an elliptical representation of an active contour.

It can be noted that the regularization weight w_{reg} corresponds to the same direction as the principal eigenvalue λ_1, whereas the data fidelity weight w_{df} corresponds to the same direction as the minor eigenvalue λ_2. This isomorphism associates the regularization and data fidelity parameters with the eigenvalues of the structure tensor.

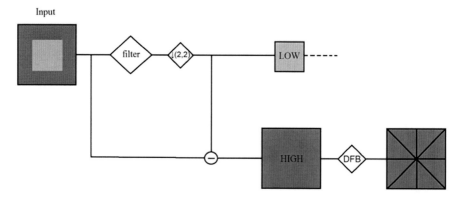

Fig. 3 CTr iterated filter bank. LP provides a downsampled low-pass version and a band-pass version of the image. Consequently, a DFB is applied to each band-pass image

Orientation Estimation

Inspired by the aforementioned observation, regularization and data fidelity parameters of region-based active contours are automated in order to reflect the orientation coherence of edge regions, in a similar fashion to Weickert's diffusion model [24]. The orientation coherence is estimated by means of the orientation entropy (OE). The latter is calculated on directional subbands in each scale of the contourlet transform (CTr) [26], which, apart from intensity, also represents textural information. This approach provides an inherent filtering mechanism, capable of filtering out randomly oriented edges associated with noise, artifacts, and/or background clutter. Moreover, CTr is directly implemented in the discrete domain, as opposed to similar transforms, such as curvelets [27].

The Contourlet Transform

CTr is an anisotropic directional image representation scheme, which effectively quantifies diffusion over contour segments with varying elongated shapes and directions. Aiming at a sparse image representation, it employs a double iterated filter bank, which captures point discontinuities by means of the Laplacian pyramid (LP) and obtains linear structures by linking these discontinuities with a directional filter bank (DFB). The final result is an image expansion that uses basic contour segments. Figure 3 illustrates a CTr iterated filter bank.

The downsampled low-pass and band-pass versions of the image contain lower and higher frequencies, respectively. It is evident that the band-pass image contains detailed information of point discontinuities which are associated with target edges. Furthermore, DFB is implemented by an l-level binary tree which leads to 2^l

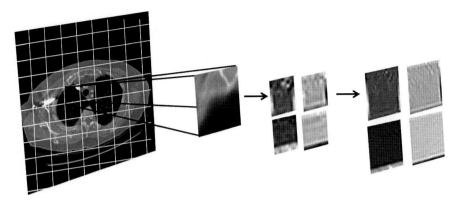

Fig. 4 CTr filter bank on a sample grid of a lung CT scan decomposed to two levels of LP and four band-pass directional subbands

subbands. In the first stage, a two-channel quincunx filter bank [28] with fan filters divides the 2D spectrum into vertical and horizontal directions.

In the second stage, a shearing operator reorders the samples. As a result, different directional frequencies are captured at each decomposition level. The number of iterations depends mainly on the size of the input image. The total number of directional subbands K_{total} is calculated as

$$K_{total} = \sum_{j=1}^{J} K_j \qquad (4)$$

where K_j is a subband DFB applied at the jth level ($j = 1, 2, \ldots, J$).

Figure 4 depicts the CTr filter bank applied on a sample grid of a lung CT scan, decomposed to the finest and second finest scales which are partitioned into four directional subbands. Each $q \times q$ image grid is fed into the CTr filter bank through an iterative procedure. This grid must be appropriately selected in order to preserve the orientation of the main structures of the target region. The band-pass directional subbands represent the local image structure. It should be mentioned that the presented framework is not confined in using CTr and could also embed alternative multi-scale or multi-directional approaches for image representation.

In the context of the presented framework, OE is calculated for each subband image I_{jk} as follows:

$$OE_{jk} = -\sum_{n=1}^{N_{jk}} \sum_{m=1}^{M_{jk}} p_{jk}(m, n) \cdot \log p_{jk}(m, n) \qquad (5)$$

$$p_{jk}(m, n) = \frac{\left|I_{jk}(m, n)\right|^2}{\sqrt{\sum_{n=1}^{N_{jk}} \sum_{m=1}^{M_{jk}} \left[I_{jk}(m, n)\right]^2}} \qquad (6)$$

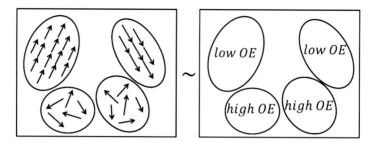

Fig. 5 Schematic representation of (**a**) elliptical structure tensors and (**b**) OE behavior on each structure tensor

where OE_{jk} is the OE of the subband image I_{jk} in the kth direction and the jth level of decomposition, M_{jk} is the row size, and N_{jk} is the column size of the subband image. OE obtains high and low values in cases of unstructured, nontarget and structured, target edge regions, respectively. Figure 5a depicts a schematic representation of several elliptical structure tensors consisting of single and multiple orientations, whereas Fig. 5b depicts the OE behavior on each structure tensor of Fig. 5a.

Automated Parameter Adjustment

Regularization and data fidelity parameters are automatically adjusted according to the following equations:

$$w_{reg}^{auto} \propto (1/w_{df}) \times N \times M, \quad w_{df}^{auto} = arg_{I_{jk}} max\left(OE_{jk}\left(I_{jk}\right)\right) \tag{7}$$

The core idea is to guide the active contour towards structured, target edge regions in the early stages of evolution by appropriately amplifying data fidelity forces in randomly oriented, high-entropy regions. As a result the contour will be repelled and iterations dedicated to erroneous local minima will be bypassed, speeding up contour convergence towards target edges. Equation (7) is an interpretation of orientation entropy values adaptive to the orientation of data fidelity forces. Apart from separately adjusting each parameter, the presented framework also achieves a balanced trade-off between regularization and data fidelity parameters. It should also be noticed that the automated parameterization is spatially adaptive, so as to reflect local variations over the image.

Figure 6 illustrates the improvement in contour evolution achieved by the presented framework as compared to the typical contour evolution obtained by empirical parameterization. Figure 6a depicts a synthetic image containing a target

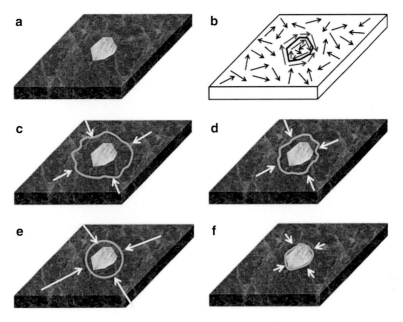

Fig. 6 Contour evolution of the presented framework vs. empirical parameterization, (**a**) synthetic image, (**b**) sketch of orientation variability, (**c, d**) evolution of empirical parameterization, and (**e, f**) evolution of the presented framework

region over an inhomogeneous background, resembling a typical medical image case, whereas Fig. 6b depicts a sketch of orientation variability of the synthetic image. Red arrows correspond to structured, target edge regions, whereas black ones indicate unstructured, nontarget ones.

In the case of empirical parameterization, the contour will be trapped in false local minima associated with background clutter in the early stages of evolution (Fig. 6c). Since region-based forces (short white arrows) are uniformly weighted irrespectively of OE, the contour will be kept away from target edge regions for more iterations (Fig. 6d).

In the case of automated parameterization, OE is considered. For as long as the contour lies in unstructured edge regions associated with background clutter, OE obtains high values and the data fidelity parameter is increased. Thus, region-based forces (long white arrows) are appropriately amplified, repelling the contour away from such regions and navigating it towards more structured ones (Fig. 6e). Once the contour approximates the vicinity of structured edge regions, OE obtains low values and the data fidelity parameter is decreased. Hence, region-based forces (short white arrows) are appropriately reduced in order to facilitate convergence (Fig. 6f). To this end, contour convergence is achieved in less iterations.

Results

The presented framework is embedded into the Chan–Vese model [29] by replacing the optimal fixed parameters with the automatically adjusted parameters, in order to evaluate the segmentation performance of the automated vs. the empirically fine-tuned version. The Chan–Vese model determines the level set evolution by solving the following equation:

$$\frac{\partial \phi}{\partial t} = w_{reg}^{fixed} \cdot \delta(\phi(x, y)) \cdot \mathrm{div}\left(\frac{\nabla \phi}{|\nabla \phi|}\right) - w_{df}^{fixed}(I(x, y) - c_1)^2$$
$$+ w_{df}^{fixed}(I(x, y) - c_2)^2 \tag{8}$$

where ϕ is the level set function, I the observed image, c_1, c_2 the average intensities inside and outside of the contour, respectively, w_{reg}^{fixed} the fixed regularization parameter, and w_{df}^{fixed} the fixed data fidelity parameter. For the empirical case, the optimal parameters are set according to the original paper [29]. For the presented framework, the regularization and data fidelity parameters are automatically calculated according to (7).

Experiments are conducted on three datasets consisting of abdominal imaging modalities such as colon and lung images. Additional experiments are conducted on one dataset containing mammographic images in order to evaluate the presented framework on a different imaging modality comprising abnormalities of various sizes and shapes. All imaging modalities were investigated by MD experts who provided ground truth images.

The first dataset consists of 32 endoscopy frame images containing polyps provided by the Gastroenterology Section, Department of Pathophysiology, Medical School, University of Athens, Greece, and partially by the Section for Minimal Invasive Surgery, University of Tübingen, Germany. The endoscopic data was acquired from sixty-six different patients with an Olympus CF-100 HL endoscope. All frame images consist of small-size adenomatous polyps which are not easily detectable and are more likely to become malignant.

The second dataset consists of 30 axial CT scans of the lung parenchyma obtained by the lung image dataset consortium image collection (LIDC-IDRI) [30]. The aim of segmentation is to separate the lung parenchyma from the surrounding anatomy, which is typically impeded by airways or other "airway-like" structures in the right and left lung. The segmentation result is used for the computation of emphysema measures.

The third dataset consists of 26 CT scans of the thorax obtained by the NSCLC Radiogenomics collection [30]. The segmentation result is used for the evaluation of the condition of the lungs and for further physiological measurements.

The fourth dataset consists of 50 mammographic images containing abnormalities randomly obtained by the Mini-MIAS dataset [31]. The background tissue is characterized as (a) fatty, (b) fatty glandular, and (c) dense glandular,

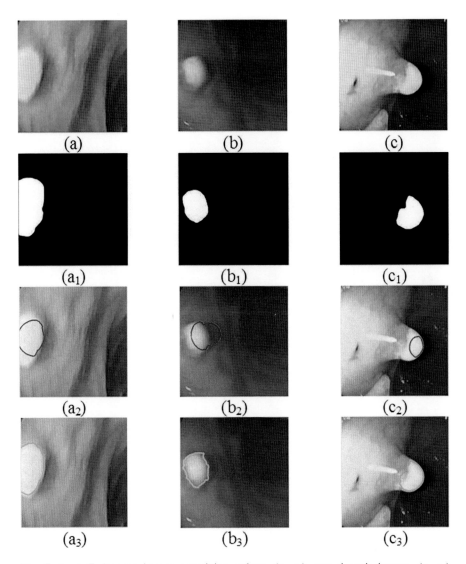

Fig. 7 (**a–c**) Endoscopy images containing polyps, (**a₁–c₁**) ground truth images, (**a₂–c₂**) segmentations obtained by the empirically fine-tuned version, in the same iteration that the automated version has converged, and (**a₃–c₃**) segmentation results of the automated version

whereas the abnormality is classified as (a) well defined/circumscribed and (b) ill defined. In terms of its severity, the abnormality is defined as either benign or malignant. Figures 7, 8, 9, and 10 depict segmentation results obtained by the automated version using the presented framework as well as by the empirical version in the same iteration that the automated version has converged.

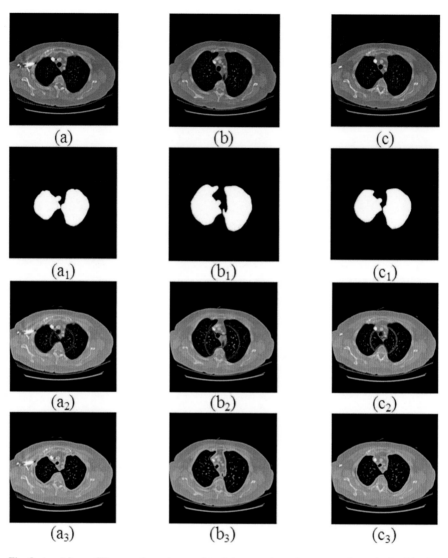

Fig. 8 (**a–c**) Lung CT scans, (**a$_1$–c$_1$**) ground truth images, (**a$_2$–c$_2$**) segmentations obtained by the empirically fine-tuned version, in the same iteration that the automated version has converged, and (**a$_3$–c$_3$**) segmentation results of the automated version

Considering Figs. 7, 8, 9, and 10 and by comparing sub-images (a$_2$)–(c$_2$) to (a$_3$)–(c$_3$), it is evident that contour convergence is delayed in the empirically fine-tuned version. However, in the automated version, contour convergence is accelerated since the former is capable of distinguishing randomly oriented,

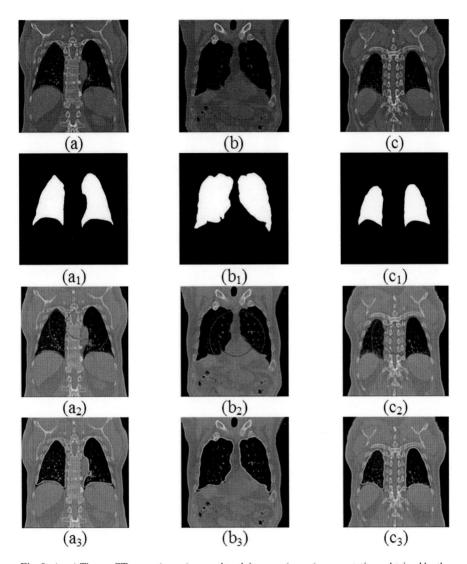

Fig. 9 (**a–c**) Thorax CT scans, (**a$_1$–c$_1$**) ground truth images, (**a$_2$–c$_2$**) segmentations obtained by the empirically fine-tuned version, in the same iteration that the automated version has converged, and (**a$_3$–c$_3$**) segmentation results of the automated version

high-entropy edges from target ones, as explained in Fig. 6. Region-based forces which guide contour evolution are appropriately amplified in unstructured, nontarget edge regions driving the contour away. Hence, iterations dedicated to false local minima, associated with such regions, are avoided.

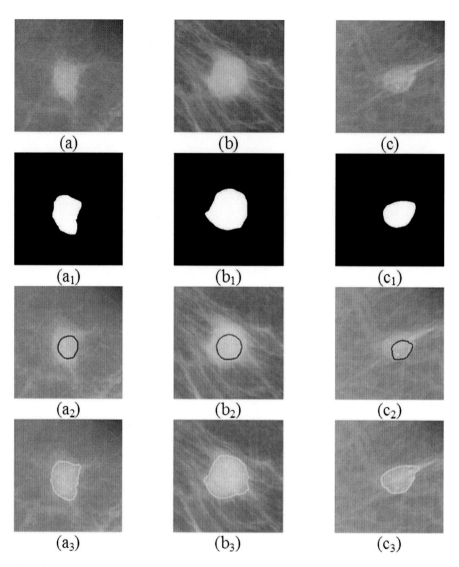

Fig. 10 (**a**–**c**) Mammographic images containing abnormalities, (**a₁**–**c₁**) ground truth images, (**a₂**–**c₂**) segmentations obtained by the empirically fine-tuned version, in the same iteration that the automated version has converged, and (**a₃**–**c₃**) segmentation results of the automated version

Quantitative Evaluation

The experimental results are quantitatively evaluated by means of the region overlap measure, known as the tanimoto coefficient (TC) [32], which is defined by:

$$TC = \frac{N(A \cap B)}{N(A \cup B)} \tag{9}$$

Table 1 TC values obtained by the empirical and automated version, in the iteration that the latter has converged

Dataset	Iterations	TC (%) Empirical	Automated
Endoscopy	6	51.4 ± 3.8	82.3 ± 1.4
Lung	33	49.1 ± 2.2	81.8 ± 0.3
Thorax	23	52.5 ± 4.2	82.7 ± 0.5
Mammogram	19	48.3 ± 6.5	83.2 ± 1.2

Fig. 11 TC for the segmentations of automated vs. empirical parameterization presented in Table 1

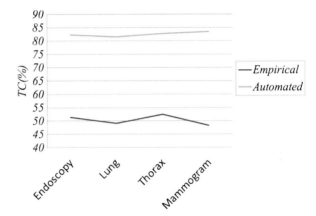

where A is the region identified by the segmentation method under evaluation, B is the ground truth region, and $N()$ indicates the number of pixels of the enclosed region. The automated version achieves an average TC value of 82.9 ± 1.6 %, which is comparable to the TC value of 80.7 ± 1.8 % obtained by the empirically fine-tuned version, with regards to all images tested. Nevertheless, the automated version converges in 10–20 times less iterations. The empirically fine-tuned version achieves a TC value of 52.4 ± 11.3 %, *in the same iteration that the automated version has converged.*

Table 1 shows, for each utilized dataset, the iterations that the automated version has converged as well as TC values obtained by the empirical and automated version, for these same iterations. Figure 11 compares the segmentation performance of the automated vs. empirical parameterization for each utilized dataset presented in Table 1.

The experimental results are also evaluated on the convergence rate of both versions by means of the difference mean intensity value (DMI). DMI is calculated between the inside and outside region terms of the contour according to the following algorithm:

∀ Iteration i

1. Calculate inside $|I(x,y) - c_1|^2$ and outside $|I(x,y) - c_2|^2$ region terms.
2. Normalize and quantize both terms in the range [0, 255].
3. Calculate mean values.
4. Calculate DMI.

Table 2 DMI values obtained by the empirical and automated version, in the early stages of contour evolution

	DMI	
Dataset	Empirical	Automated
Endoscopy	8.2	14.0
Lung	3.4	7.1
Thorax	5.8	8.3
Mammogram	28.2	30.8

During contour evolution, DMI is increased, and once contour converges to the actual target boundaries, DMI obtains its highest value.

Table 2 shows for a sample of each utilized dataset DMI values obtained by the empirical and automated version in the early stages of contour evolution.

It can be observed that DMI reaches higher values in the automated version in the early stages of contour evolution, regardless of the medical imaging modality. This convergence acceleration has been theoretically justified in Section "Parameter-Adjustment Framework."

Conclusion

Medical image segmentation plays a fundamental role in medical research since it aids MDs' clinical evaluation by providing vital information on abdominal organs. Empirical parameterization in segmentation techniques is not accurate since the segmentation results are dependent on the visual impression of a MD. Thus, it is crucial to develop automated algorithms which are accurate and do not require any user intervention.

In this chapter, a framework for automated adjustment of active contour regularization and data fidelity parameters is presented and applied for medical image segmentation. The presented framework is inspired from the properties of structure tensors. The latter are appropriate descriptors of the orientation coherence of edge regions. This information is accordingly incorporated into the active contour parameters by means of OE. In this light, region-based forces are boosted on nontarget, unstructured regions, driving the contour away and guiding it towards the target, structured ones. Thus, iterations dedicated to false local minima are avoided and contour convergence is accelerated. More importantly, MDs are set free from the laborious process of empirical parameterization, and objectivity is bolstered.

The presented framework is evaluated on abdominal imaging modalities, including colon and lung images as well as on mammographic images, by comparing its segmentation performance with the empirically fine-tuned version. The experimental results demonstrate that the automated version is capable of meliorating contour evolution as well as maintaining a high segmentation quality, comparable to the one obtained empirically. Furthermore, it copes well with the variability of target regions and remains insensitive to noise, artifacts, and heterogeneity.

References

1. Shang Y, Yang X, Zhu L, Deklerck R, Nyssen E (2008) Region competition based active contour for medical object extraction. Comput Med Imag Graph 32(2):109–117
2. Wang L, Li C, Sun Q, Xia D, Kao C-Y (2009) Active contours driven by local and global intensity fitting energy with application to brain mr image segmentation. Comput Med Imag Graph 33(7):520–531
3. Xu J, Monaco JP, Madabhushi A (2010) Markov random field driven region-based active contour model (maracel): application to medical image segmentation. In: Proceedings of the 13th international conference on medical image computing and computer-assisted intervention (MICCAI), vol 13, pp 197–204
4. Ramudu K, Reddy GR, Srinivas A, Krishna TR (2012) Global region based segmentation of satellite and medical imagery with active contours and level set evolution on noisy images. Int J Appl Phys Math 2(6):449–453
5. Loncaric S, Kovacevic D, Sorantin E (2000) Semi-automatic active contour approach to segmentation of computed tomography volumes. SPIE Proc 3979:917–924
6. Jiang H, Cheng Q (2009) Automatic 3D segmentation of ct images based on active contour models. In: Proceedings of the 11th IEEE international conference on computer-aided design and computer graphics, Aug 2009, pp 540–543
7. Plajer IC, Richter D (2010) A new approach to model based active contours in lung tumor segmentation in 3D CT image data. In: Proceedings of the 10th IEEE international conference on information technology and applications in biomedicine (ITAB), Nov 2010, pp 1–4
8. Ma L, Yu J (2010) An unconstrained hybrid active contour model for image segmentation. In: Proceedings of the 10th IEEE international conference on signal processing (ICSP), Oct 2010, pp 1098–1101
9. McIntosh C, Hamarneh G (2007) Is a single energy functional sufficient? Adaptive energy functionals and automatic initialization. In: Proceedings of the 10th international conference on medical image computing and computer-assisted intervention (MICCAI), vol 10, pp 503–510
10. Erdem E, Tari S (2009) Mumford-Shah regularizer with contextual feedback. J Math Imag Vis 33(1):67–84
11. Kokkinos I, Evangelopoulos G, Maragos P (2009) Texture analysis and segmentation using modulation features, generative models and weighted curve evolution. IEEE Trans Pattern Anal Mach Intell 31(1):142–157
12. Pluempitiwiriyawej C, Moura JMF, Wu YJL, Ho C (2005) STACS: new active contour scheme for cardiac MR image segmentation. IEEE Trans Med Imaging 24(5):593–603
13. Tsai A, Yezzi A, Wells W, Tempany C, Tucker D, Fan A, Grimson WE, Willsky A (2003) A shape-based approach to the segmentation of medical imagery using level sets. IEEE Trans Med Imaging 22(2):137–154
14. Keuper M, Schmidt T, Padeken J, Heun P, Palme K, Burkhardt H, Ronneberger O (2010) 3D deformable surfaces with locally self-adjusting parameters—a Robust method to determine cell nucleus shapes. In: Proceedings of the 20th IEEE international conference on pattern recognition (ICPR), Aug 2010, pp 2254–2257
15. Liu X, Cheung YM, Li M, Liu H (2010) A lip extraction method using localized active contour model with automatic parameter selection. In: Proceedings of the 20th IEEE international conference on pattern recognition (ICPR), Aug 2010, pp 4332–4335
16. Iakovidis D, Savelonas M, Karkanis S, Maroulis D (2007) A genetically optimized level set approach to segmentation of thyroid ultrasound images. Appl Intell 27(3):193–203
17. Hsu CY, Liu CY, Chen CM (2008) Automatic segmentation of liver PET images. Comput Med Imag Graph 32(7):601–610
18. Allili M, Ziou D (2008) An approach for dynamic combination of region and boundary information in segmentation. In: Proceedings of the 19th IEEE international conference on pattern recognition (ICPR), pp 1–4

19. Yushkevich PA, Piven J, Cody H, Ho S, Gee JC, Gerig G (2005) User-guided level set segmentation of anatomical structures with ITK—SNAP. Insight journal special issue on ISC/NA-MIC/MICCAI workshop on open-source software
20. Dong B, Chien A, Mao Y, Ye J, Osher S (2008) Level set based surface capturing in 3D medical images. In: Proceedings of the 11th international conference on medical image computing and computer-assisted intervention (MICCAI), vol 11, pp 162–169
21. Bigun J, Granlund G, Wiklund J (1991) Multidimensional orientation estimation with applications to texture analysis and optical flow. IEEE Trans Pattern Anal Mach Intell 13 (8):775–790
22. Tschumperlé D, Deriche R (2005) Vector-valued image regularization with PDEs: a common framework for different applications. IEEE Trans Pattern Anal Mach Intell 27(4):506–517
23. Khne G, Weickert J, Schuster O, Richter S (2001) A tensor-driven active contour model for moving object segmentation. In: IEEE international conference on image processing (ICIP), Oct 2001, vol 2, pp 73–76
24. Weickert J, Scharr H (2002) A scheme for coherence-enhancing diffusion filtering with optimized rotation invariance. J Vis Comm Image Represent 13(1–2):103–118
25. Larrey-Ruiz J, Verdú-Monedero R, Morales-Sánchez J, Angulo J (2011) Frequency domain regularization of d-dimensional structure tensor-based directional fields. J Image Vis Comput 29(9):620–630
26. Do MN, Vetterli M (2005) The contourlet transform: an efficient directional multiresolution image representation. IEEE Trans Image Process 14(12):2091–2106
27. Katsigiannis S, Keramidas E, Maroulis D (2010) A contourlet transform feature extraction scheme for ultrasound thyroid texture classification. Engineering Intelligent Systems, Special issue: Artificial Intelligence Applications and Innovations, vol 18(3/4)
28. Vetterli M (1984) Multidimensional subband coding: some theory and algorithms. IEEE Trans Signal Process 6(2):97–112
29. Chan TF, Vese LA (2001) Active contours without edges. IEEE Trans Image Process 10 (2):266–277
30. http://www.cancerimagingarchive.net
31. Suckling J, Parker J, Dance D, Astley S, Hutt I, Boggis C, Ricketts I, Stamatakis E, Cerneaz N, Kok S, Taylor P, Betal D, Savage J (1994) The mammographic images analysis society digital mammogram database. Experta Medica International Congress Series 1069:375–378
32. Crum WR, Camara O, Hill DLG (2006) Generalized overlap measures for evaluation and validation in medical image analysis. IEEE Trans Med Imaging 25(11):1451–1461

Biography

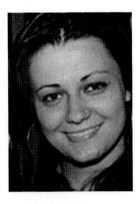

Eleftheria A. Mylona received the B.Sc. degree in Applied Mathematical and Physical Sciences in 2006 from the National Technical University of Athens, Greece, and the M.Sc. degree in Physics in 2007 from the University of Edinburgh, UK. She is currently working towards the Ph.D. degree in Image Analysis at the University of Athens, Greece. For her Ph.D. research, she received a scholarship co-financed by the European Union and Greek National Funds. She has coauthored 11 research articles on biomedical image analysis. Her research interests include image analysis, segmentation, and biomedical applications.

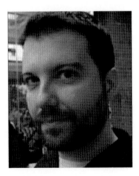

Michalis A. Savelonas received the B.Sc. degree in Physics in 1998, the M.Sc. degree in Cybernetics in 2001 with honors, and the Ph.D. degree in the area of Image Analysis in 2008 with honors, all from the University of Athens, Greece. For his Ph.D. research, he received a scholarship by the Greek General Secretariat for Research and Technology (25 %) and the European Social Fund (75 %). He is currently a research fellow in the Dept. of Electrical and Computer Engineering in the Democritus University of Thrace, as well as in ATHENA Research and Innovation Center, branch of Xanthi. In addition, he is a regular research associate of the Dept. of Informatics and Telecommunications of the University of Athens, Greece, as well as of the Center for Technological Research of Central Greece. In the past, he has served in various academic positions in the University of Athens, University of Houston, TX, USA, Hellenic Air Force Academy and Technological Educational Institute of Lamia. In 2002–2004 he had been working in software industry as responsible for defining, designing, coding, debugging, testing, integrating, and documenting software modules for real-time systems within the context of various projects. Dr. Savelonas has coauthored more than 40 research articles in peer-reviewed international journals, conferences, and book chapters, whereas he has been actively involved in several EU, US, and Greek R&D projects. He is a reviewer in prestigious international journals including Pattern Recognition and IEEE Transactions on Image Processing. His research interests include image analysis, segmentation, pattern recognition, 3D retrieval, and biomedical applications.

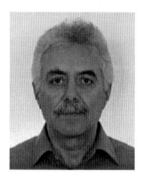

Dimitris Maroulis received the B.Sc. degree in Physics, the M.Sc. degree in Radioelectricity and in Cybernetics with honors, and the Ph.D. degree in Computer Science with honors, all from the University of Athens, Greece. He served as a Research Fellow for three years at the Space Research Department (DESPA) of Meudon Observatory, Paris, France, and afterward he collaborated for more than ten years with the same department. He has also served in various academic positions in the departments of Physics and Informatics of the University of Athens. Currently, he is a Professor in the Department of Informatics and Telecommunications of the same university and leader of the Real-Time Systems and Image Analysis Lab. He has more than 20 years of experience in the areas of data acquisition and real-time systems and more than 15 years of experience in the area of image/signal analysis and processing. He has also been collaborating with many Greek and European hospitals and health centers for more than 15 years in the field of biomedical informatics. He has been actively involved in more than 15 European and National R&D projects and has been the project leader of 5 of them, all in the areas of image/signal analysis and real-time systems. He has published more than 150 research papers and book chapters, and there are currently more than 1,000 citations that refer to his published work. His research interests include data acquisition and real-time systems, pattern recognition, and image/signal processing and analysis, with applications on biomedical systems and bioinformatics.

Bridging the Gap Between Modeling of Tumor Growth and Clinical Imaging

Behnaz Abdollahi, Neal Dunlap, and Hermann B. Frieboes

Abstract This chapter gives a brief overview of the biological processes involved in vascularized tumor growth, followed by a summary of recent mathematical modeling to simulate the biology of tumor growth and angiogenesis. It provides an overview of medical image analysis and describes recent efforts in the area of coupling such tumor models with imaging data. We do not discuss the research of obtaining tumor-specific information from medical imaging data, for which extensive work has been done in image processing and signal analysis. The chapter concludes with a sample simulation of vascularized tumor growth showing the critical role of vascularization in tumor invasiveness and highlighting the potential of gaining further insight into tumor behavior from a more expansive future integration of 3D tumor models with clinical imaging data.

Introduction

Modeling of tumor growth at the centimeter tissue-scale is typically represented using diffusion reaction equations describing the space and time dynamics of mass and diffusible substances (see recent reviews [1–8]). Parameters in these models can be coupled with biological and clinical data in order to more faithfully represent tumor growth and treatment response, including measurements from in vitro cell culture, intravital microscopy, and histopathology [9–16]. Data from medical

B. Abdollahi, Ph.D.
Department of Electrical Engineering, University of Louisville, Louisville, KY 40208, USA

N. Dunlap, M.D., Ph.D.
Department of Radiation Oncology, University of Louisville, Louisville, KY 40202, USA

H.B. Frieboes, Ph.D. (✉)
Department of Bioengineering, Lutz Hall 419, University of Louisville,
Louisville, KY 40208, USA
e-mail: hbfrie01@louisville.edu

A.S. El-Baz et al. (eds.), *Abdomen and Thoracic Imaging: An Engineering & Clinical Perspective*, DOI 10.1007/978-1-4614-8498-1_18,
© Springer Science+Business Media New York 2014

images has also been employed to define values for tumor model parameter values [17–21]. Image series taken from patients contain visual information about anatomical and diffusion properties of tumor tissue. It is challenging, however, to incorporate biological and imaging information into mathematical models of tumor growth. A first step in this process is to synthesize the biological information so that it can be properly represented by mathematical models.

Onset of Cancer

Healthy cells exist with an established pattern of cellular behavior and life expectancy. Each cell in an organism carries a full copy of the organism's DNA, containing the instructions that determine the cell's behavior. Numerous endogenous as well as exogenous mechanisms exist to ensure that cells maintain homeostasis and preserve the integrity of their nuclear DNA in order to maximize the success of an organism's life. For cancer to occur, several of these mechanisms have to jointly fail in order for a cell to start rapid and sustained proliferation with a degenerate DNA or avoid senescence [22]. These mechanisms include cell-induced apoptosis, destruction by macrophages, and DNA repair mechanisms. Once abnormal cell survival persists, a group of cells forms that may grow to around 1–2 mm in size. These cells in the early stages of tumor growth are supported by the preexisting vasculature sustaining the surrounding normal tissue. Nearby capillaries act as a source of oxygen and nutrients (e.g., glucose, glutamine) via diffusion. The size of the growing tumor is thus restrained by its ability to obtain sufficient oxygen and nutrients, and some of the tumor cells may undergo necrosis as a result of an inadequate supply of these substances. It is believed that some tumors may remain for a long time in this state of dormant "equilibrium." However, due to processes that are not fully understood, some of these micro-sized tumors may be driven to grow further; as a result, they will start generating growth factors to stimulate the surrounding vasculature to dramatically increase access to the organism's nutrients. Once a tumor is vascularized, its malignancy is considerably increased.

Onset of Angiogenesis

The angiogenic phenotype is the result of a net balance of endogenous growth factor stimulators and inhibitors of angiogenesis [23]. Both hypoxia and hypoglycemia may stimulate pro-angiogenic expression. Tumor cells prefer glucose as a nutrient, even under aerobic conditions. An increased rate of glycolysis in a system with poor blood and lymphatic vasculature will lead to insufficient removal of lactic acid, thereby increasing the acidity (lowering the pH) of the tumor extracellular matrix with respect to the surrounding tissue. At low pH and O_2, cells (normal or tumorigenic) will increase the net expression of angiogenic stimulators. The expression of angiogenic growth factors (such as fibroblast growth factors [FGF] and vascular endothelial growth factors [VEGFs]) is increased in tumor regions under oxygen and nutrient stress. Possible sources include the cancerous cells and macrophage cells that typically permeate tumors, as well as normal cells in the vicinity.

The angiogenic factors stimulate the surrounding vascular endothelial cells to remodel the existing vessel network to expand without necessarily creating new vessels [24–27]. The secretion of growth factors can also lead to new vessel formation as the vasculature becomes unable to support the metabolic needs of the tumor and normal cells. This process of angiogenesis generates new blood vessels from the preexisting vascular network [28, 29] through endothelial cell sprouting, proliferation, anastomosis, and remodeling. Vessel remodeling and angiogenesis thus cause oxygen and cell nutrients circulating in the vasculature to be transported and released closer to the tumor.

Capillary Development

Angiogenic cytokines act by stimulating vascular endothelial cells in the tumor vicinity to increase in vascular permeability, dilation, and tortuosity. The cells express proteolytic enzymes to degrade the vessel basement membrane, and then they penetrate it via pseudopodia. In this fashion the endothelial cells start migrating through the extracellular matrix separating them from the source of angiogenic stimulation (i.e., along a chemotactic gradient). The cells also prefer to move along a haptotactic gradient of lower fibronectin density. As they migrate, the cells align themselves into small tubular structures, undergoing continuous remodeling and regression. The integrity of these proto-capillaries remains weak until the resynthesis of the basal lamina is complete and the vessel lumen structure is established. The tubules become hollow as the network matures. After reaching a certain distance from the parent vessel, the new capillary sprouts may change direction to meet with each other and fuse together, generating anastomoses. The edge of this network may exhibit a higher rate of branching at the leading edge ("brush-border effect" [30]) as it expands towards the tumor and eventually penetrates it.

The interaction between the surrounding vasculature and tumor cells is abnormal due to incoherent signaling from the tumor cells. The vessels thus produced are inefficient, tortuous, and leaky [31–34]. Compared with vascular networks formed during normal biological processes (e.g., during development and wound healing), tumor-induced vascular networks may be leaky and perform inadequately, producing immature and tortuous vessels [33]. This phenomenon generates increased flow resistance through the network and ultimately leads to a heterogeneous supply of cell substrates within the tumor microenvironment [35].

Fragility of Tumor Vasculature

Most likely due to highly active angiogenesis and microvascular remodeling, most tumor vessels have an irregular diameter and abnormal branching pattern [33]. The vessels leak blood into the tumor tissue, and this leakiness correlates with histological grade and tumor malignancy. At least three sources are implicated in leakage of plasma: openings between cells lining the vessels, holes through the lining cells themselves, and endothelial fenestrae [33]. The bulk of the leakiness is most likely due to the intercellular openings. In some tumors, blood vessels have discontinuous endothelial cell lining, so that blood flows directly past exposed tumor cells. Also, tumor cells may be incorporated as structural elements of the vessel wall. Hemorrhaging may also be caused by sprouting angiogenesis driven by growth factors that predispose to bleeding. Extravasated blood pools, bordered by tumor cells, can exist for several minutes after hemorrhage [33].

Tumor Vascularization and Metastasis

Having obtained access to the organism's vasculature, cancer cells can then proceed to proliferate further beyond the original tumor size. In addition to being porous, tumor vessels are also thin-walled compared to the normal vasculature. The rapid proliferation of tumor cells may cause blood vessels to collapse inside the tumor due to mechanical pressure, thus provoking tumor cell necrosis. For reasons that are not fully clear, some tumor cells may also degrade the vasculature basal lamina and then migrate away from the tumor site to other sites in the organism, where they establish themselves and originate secondary tumors. This process is called metastasis. Intriguingly, it has been observed that metastatic growth can suppress the growth of a primary tumor. Also, a primary tumor may suppress metastasis from a different type of tumor.

Normal Wound Dermal Repair

Angiogenesis and tissue vascularization are not only a property of growing tumors. In cutaneous wounds that are undergoing healing, for example, angiogenesis involves non-leaky vessels with smooth-muscle cells contained in the vessel wall. Normally, the process has three overlapping phases: inflammation, proliferation, and remodeling [36]. The inflammation phase includes blood clot formation and the immune system response, as well as the beginning of epidermis regeneration. The proliferation phase encompasses the migration as a structural unit of macrophages (in the lead), fibroblasts (in the middle), and blood capillaries (in the rear) across the wound bed. The macrophages release chemotactic agents into the wound bed, thus attracting fibroblasts and capillaries into the wound. The fibroblasts build the extracellular matrix that facilitates further cell migration and provides mechanical support for the new blood capillaries. The blood capillaries supply nutrients to the structural unit as it continues to migrate across the wound. The remodeling phase involves wound contraction, maturation of wound bed tissue as it evolves from a highly cellular and vascularized state to form scar tissue (with few cells and blood vessels), and the maturation of the extracellular matrix [36]. Tumor angiogenesis may be viewed as a crude wound healing process gone awry. The normal healing process, dramatically thwarted in cancer, has led some to call tumors as "wounds that never heal."

Modeling of Tumor Growth

Mathematical modeling of vascularized tumor growth has sought to elucidate these complex processes from a biophysical perspective, with the ultimate goal to provide insight to improve patient treatment. Tumor models are typically either discrete or continuum, depending on how the tumor tissue is simulated. Discrete models simulate individual cells according to a specific set of biochemical and biophysical rules. This type of modeling is useful for studying cell-cell and cell-microenvironment interactions, natural selection, carcinogenesis, and genetic instability [1]. Analyses of cell population dynamics have also been used to study biological characteristics that apply to cells in particular populations, such as therapy response.

Continuum models simulate tumors as a collection of tissue, employing principles from continuum mechanics to describe cancer-related variables as continuous fields using partial differential and integro-differential equations [1]. Variables may include cell volume fractions as well as cell substrate concentrations such as oxygen and nutrients. In particular, multiphase (mixture-theory) models are capable of describing interactions between multiple solid cell species, and intra-cellular and extracellular liquids [1].

In contrast to discrete and continuum models, hybrid approaches utilize both continuum and discrete representations of tumor cells and microenvironment components. The goal is to directly fit the discrete scale to molecular and cell-scale data, and then upscale this scale to inform the phenomenological parameters of models at the continuum tissue-scale [1].

Recent reviews on mathematical tumor modeling include [1, 3–8, 37, 38]. In addition to avascular growth, models have focused on tumor-induced angiogenesis and vascular growth [39–41], invasion and metastasis [42], intra-cellular pathways [43], stem cells [44], and treatment [10, 45]. As reviewed in Lowengrub et al. [1], the development of more quantitative and sophisticated models coupled with enhanced computational power has enabled more realistic multiscale tumor models, where temporal and multiple spatial scales are coupled within a single framework [37, 40, 41]. Hybrid models simulating tumor tissue at both single-cell and tissue levels have also been recently developed [46].

Modeling of Tumor Angiogenesis

The process of tumor angiogenesis has been modeled using continuum, fully discrete, composite continuum–discrete, and hybrid continuum–discrete mathematical models (see recent reviews [1–8, 38]). Most models do not couple the tumor and angiogenesis processes dynamically; typically, one of these processes is held static. Models focusing on the angiogenic response have taken two approaches. One of the approaches implements vessels as continuous curves, interconnected lattice patterns, line segments, or collections of individual endothelial cells. Vessel sprout branching and anastomosis have been modeled in this way as well as vascular endothelial cell activation, proliferation and migration via haptotaxis up gradients of ECM-bound chemokines (e.g. fibronectin), chemotaxis up gradients of tumor angiogenic factors (TAFs) (e.g., VEGF), and proteolysis of the extracellular matrix [47–57]. Vascular network remodeling and blood flow have also been simulated (e.g., [58–66]). Additionally, models of tumor growth in static network topologies (e.g., [67, 68]) as well as multiscale models of fluid transport in tumors have also been implemented in this way [69].

Focusing on the angiogenic response, the other approach describes blood vessel densities rather than vessel morphology, using continuum partial differential equations (e.g., [70–81]). In this approach, the dynamics of the vessel densities and angiogenic factors are described by applying continuum conservation laws, and hence these models do not provide blood flow or morphological information about the vasculature. Biochemical and biomechanical models capable of describing the morphology of the vasculature have been developed in the context of vasculogenesis in vitro, accounting for chemotactic response and cell–ECM interactions. Refer, for example, to [82–84] for discrete models and to [85–94] for continuum models.

Coupling of Tumor Modeling and Angiogenesis

Angiogenesis and tumor growth are coupled in that tumor cells in hypoxic regions release a net balance of pro-angiogenic growth factors that attract endothelial cells and stimulate the neovascular network to develop towards the tumor. This process expands the source of oxygen and cell nutrients in the microenvironment. The tumor reacts by increasing cell proliferation in regions where cell nutrients are more abundant. The oxygen changes the distribution of hypoxic tumor regions, which affects the net release of pro-angiogenic factors. A neovascular network also responds to pressure variation introduced by increased tumor cell proliferation and migration in addition to heterogeneous blood flow.

Tumor growth was first fully coupled with tumor-induced angiogenesis for an arbitrary network topology in the model by Zheng et al. [40]. This 2D model coupled a version of the continuum–discrete model of Anderson and Chaplain [48] with the tumor growth model of Cristini et al. [95]. Models of angiogenesis and vascular tumor growth have also been implemented in the context of discrete cell-based systems (e.g., [55, 96–98]). The effects of blood flow through the neovascular network on tumor growth have been considered using cellular automaton models for tumor growth combined with dynamic network models for the vasculature [39, 97, 99–101]. The effects of an arterio-venous network were modeled in Welter et al. [102]. Macklin et al. [41] recently extended the model of [40] by incorporating a version of the dynamic model of tumor-induced angiogenesis developed by McDougall et al. [62] to explicitly analyze the effects of vessel remodeling and blood flow. Lloyd et al. [103] recently simulated the vascular growth of a 2D tumor by coupling an elastic tumor growth model developed earlier with models for angiogenesis, flow through the developing neovascular network and network remodeling. Vascular tumor growth has also been studied in 3D using a tumor mixture model and lattice-free description of tumor-induced angiogenesis [13, 104].

Important aspects in solid tumor growth and vascularization include the flow of interstitial fluid and the associated interstitial fluid pressure (IFP). Theoretical and experimental work has shown that tumors may present elevated IFP, which becomes a physical barrier for small molecules and cell nutrients to be delivered into the tumor. Elevated tumor IFP may also exacerbate biochemical signal gradients (e.g., angiogenic factors) released into the surrounding tissues. This work has helped to understand both biochemical signaling and treatment prognosis.

Mathematical models have been developed to investigate the role of IFP and IFF on tumor-induced angiogenesis and on the transport of TAFs [105–107]. Building upon previous work [48, 58–60, 62, 108, 109], the vascular model of Macklin et al. [41] incorporates vessel sprouting, branching and anastomosis, endothelial cell (EC) migration and proliferation, vascular network remodeling, and blood flow. In the model, the tumor and angiogenesis components are coupled via angiogenic growth factors secreted by tumor cells as well as oxygen released from the blood vessels. The total effects of growth-promoting factors affect the tumor cell phenotype and growth factor secretion, which initiates branching and sprouting in the vasculature. Blood is simulated to flow through the neovascular network once newly formed vessels anastomose. Stresses induced by the blood flow (e.g., shear stresses) as well as the proliferating tumor cells induce continuous remodeling of the vascular network.

This detailed framework was very recently extended in Wu et al. [110] to include fluid/oxygen extravasation as well as a continuous lymphatic field in order to study the micro-environmental fluid dynamics and their effect on tumor growth by accounting for blood flow, transcapillary fluid flux, interstitial fluid flow, and lymphatic drainage. This model further elucidates the nontrivial relationship between key elements contributing to the effects of interstitial pressure in solid tumors. For example, it was found that small blood/lymphatic vessel resistance and collapse may contribute to lower transcapillary fluid/oxygen flux, thus retarding the tumor growth. The results further reveal that poor lymphatic function coupled with elevated interstitial hydraulic conductivity may be a key reason of the development of IFP plateau profiles within tumors (observed experimentally) and leads to solid tumor pressure, a broad-based collapse of the tumor lymphatics, and a more uniform distribution of oxygen. A more elevated vascular hydraulic conductivity within tumors may control the rate that IFF fluxes into the lymphatics and host tissues. The results suggest the intriguing possibility of developing strategies for targeting tumor cells based on examination of the interstitial fluid emanating out of tumors.

Tumor Clinical Image Analysis

The goal of image analysis is to extract particular information from medical images that may be of clinical significance. Medical imaging techniques create images from inside the human body using technologies such as X-ray, CT (computed tomography), MR (magnetic resonance), SPECT (single-photon emission computed tomography), and PET (positron emission tomography); choosing an appropriate imaging technique is based on clinical evaluation of the patient and the disease type. Segmentation, registration, motion detection, and reconstruction can be used to extract particular information from these images. Image segmentation and 3D reconstruction, in which lesions are visualized in three dimensions, are commonly used to screen cancer patients [111], especially those suspected to suffer from lung cancer. Figure 1 shows sample CT image evaluations of patients with lung cancer tumors before and after treatment. The location and shape of the lesions may influence the choice of method to segment the images [112].

Imaging as a Tool for Patient Screening

The importance of cancer screening has been highlighted in the recently published National Lung Cancer Screening Trial (NLST) by demonstrating a 20 % reduction in mortality with the use of low-dose helical CT as opposed to chest X-ray [114]. Screening has the potential to allow for early detection of lung cancer resulting in a phenomenon termed "stage migration." Patients will potentially be diagnosed at an earlier stage and thus more likely cured with treatment. Unfortunately, current diagnostic tools have limitations. In a study by Ko et al. [115], a small nodule size of ≤ 5 mm in diameter (nodule detection sensitivity: ≤ 5 vs. >5 mm, 74 % vs. 82 %), ground-glass opacity nodules (nodule detection sensitivity: ground-glass

Before Therapy   **After Therapy**

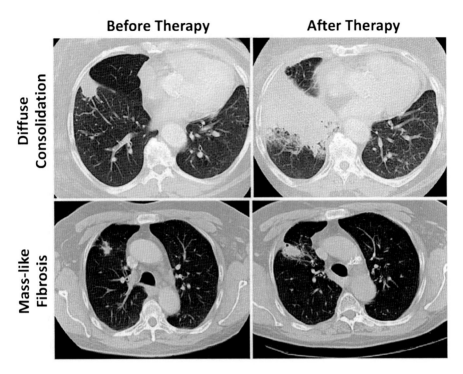

Fig. 1 Representative CT images of patient samples with both diffuse consolidation and mass-like fibrosis before and after stereotactic body radiotherapy [113]. Reprinted with permission from Int J Radiat Oncol Biol Phys, Vol. 84, Dunlap et al., Computed tomography-based anatomic assessment overestimates local tumor recurrence in patients with mass-like consolidation after stereotactic body radiotherapy for early-stage non-small cell lung cancer, p. 1074, Copyright (2012), with permission from Elsevier

opacity vs. solid, 65 % vs. 83 %), and lesion location (nodule detection sensitivity: central vs. peripheral, 61 % vs. 80 %) were shown to be major factors that contribute to the difficulty in detecting nodules. Nodule detection can be improved by advances in computer-aided detection (CAD) systems that are being developed and evaluated to provide a second perspective for nodule detection on CT. The use of CAD can help improve radiologist performance for the detection of unidentified lung cancers during lung cancer screening with CT [116, 117].

When interpreting findings from CT, radiologists must take multiple factors into account when determining whether or not a lesion is malignant or benign. Specific features that must be considered include nodule morphology, growth rate assessment, clinical features incorporated into a Bayesian analysis, hemodynamic characteristics on CT, and metabolic characteristics on ^{18}F-FDG PET. Morphologic criteria allow for predicting the odds ratio of malignancy based on specific radiographic criteria: lobulated margin, a spiculated margin, and the absence of a satellite nodule [118]. Determination of growth rate over a 2-year period has also been shown to be a cost-effective and reliable method. Unfortunately, this method relies heavily on volumetric analysis of a nodule where current segmentation methods are unreliable [119]. Bayesian analysis combines individual probabilities of malignancy in order to estimate the overall odds favoring malignancy. These features include cavities of 16 mm in thickness, irregular or spiculated margin on CT scans, patient complaints of hemoptysis, a patient history of malignancy, patient age >70 years, nodule size of 21–30 mm in diameter, nodule growth rate of 7–465 days, an ill-defined nodule on chest radiographs, patient a current smoker, and nodules with indeterminate calcification on CT scans [120]. Evaluation of tumor vascular with dynamic helical CT has also been proven to be beneficial. Threshold attenuation value can be used to predict the likelihood of malignancy based on changes in Hounsfield units (HU) after contrast administration. Current established standard for differentiating benign from malignant nodules is 15 HU [121]. Finally, incorporating metabolic imaging can improve diagnostic accuracy in a noninvasive way. Studies indicate sensitivity of 88–96 % and a specificity of 70–90 % for malignant nodules [122].

Despite the number of methods clinically available for predicting the likelihood of malignancy, the workup and management relies heavily on clinical interpretation with no one superior model or algorithm. Improvements are required in order to expand diagnostic accuracy while remaining cost-effective from a screening standpoint. By establishing more robust models for predicting malignancy, a larger number of patients can be offered potentially curable treatment with early stage disease.

Extraction of Tumor Model Parameters from Imaging

The spatial reconstruction of a specific lesion depends on many factors, including image resolution, which is scanner-dependent; the contrast level of the tumor tissue; the appearance of very small cells in images; the number and thickness of available slices; and the techniques used for segmentation [111]. Variability in these factors prevents the definition of a uniform set of techniques for extracting tumor model parameter information using medical image analysis. Due to low resolution, imaging techniques cannot accurately localize tumor cells; underestimation or overestimation can be a problem even if the segmentation technique is chosen on technical grounds. If the tumor tissue is not properly isolated, most of the segmentation methods will image through to adjacent tissues with similar intensities. Another issue is that some of the tissues could be mistakenly considered cancerous in CT or MR images. Also, the lesion could be too close to normal tissue in such a way that it is challenging for current segmentation techniques to accurately extract it. These issues suggest that a universal approach for analysis cannot be defined based on currently available imaging methods, and they imply that the power of medical image analysis may be maximized by combining with techniques that take into account other biological aspects. For example, histological information could be indirectly extracted from medical images, as we discuss below.

Table 1 Mean tumor density for different lung cancer types (adapted from [124])

Tumor type	Mean HU before contrast	Mean HU after contrast
Adenocarcinoma	51.5	68.7
Epidermoid carcinoma	60	86
Small cell	50.3	60.2
Large cell	53.4	62.1
Undifferentiated malignant cell	32.3	55.8

The tissue density in CT scans is measured in Hounsfield units (HU). Each organ has a different density, so the CT images show them with a different gray scale. The Hounsfield unit is a normalized value of the calculated X-ray absorption coefficient of a pixel in CT. The tissue appears brighter when the Hounsfield Unit number is higher. Tumors in CT can be detected if the tumor cell density is greater than a certain threshold, which depends on the scanner resolution. Correlation between histology and CT has shown that over half of tumors identified by histology may be missed in CT images [123]. Typically, a tumor with 50 μm in diameter contains ~1,000 cells and a tumor with 200 μm diameter contains ~5,000–8,000 cells [123]. Table 1 shows the mean tumor cell density for different lung cancer types based on experimental results [124].

It is challenging to find a direct relation between a vessel's geometry detected in imaging and histological features like endothelial cell density. Lower density tissues are not shown in MR and CT images. Vessels feeding into tumors are usually newer with low density, so that only the biggest vessels are detected. Yet the relation between tumor vascularization and tumor stage is critical. Histological features of angiogenesis—microvessel density (MVD), identification of receptor for VEGF, and number of circulating endothelia cell (CEC)—fail to provide a complete picture of tumor angiogenesis [125].

Perfusion imaging measures blood volume in tissues; a relation between volume and histological features may be assumed. Perfusion imaging is typically used as a method for determining prognosis in the clinic [126]. In research, imaging of perfusion through a tissue has been used to measure vascular geometry and histological features of tumor angiogenesis and also to estimate microvascular flow through capillaries and venules [127]. Measurements of perfusion flow can provide intravascular blood volume (reflecting the MVD) and mean transit time of blood through the tissue. Some studies show a potential correlation between perfusion imaging and MVD [123, 125, 126, 128], but others did not observe such a correlation [124]. In a clinical study of lung carcinoma angiogenesis using contrast-enhanced dynamic CT images, VEGF and MVD were correlated with maximum values of time attenuation curves instead of perfusion images [125].

Ideally, information obtained about tumor perfusion could be used to model tumor response to blood-borne agents. Recently, a framework for the automated evaluation of vascular perfusion curves measured at the single vessel level through intravital microscopy has been proposed [129]. Primary tumor fragments, collected from triple-negative breast cancer patients and grown as xenografts in mice, were injected with fluorescence contrast and monitored using intravital microscopy. The time to arterial peak and venous delay, two features whose probability distributions were measured directly from time-series curves, were analyzed using a Fuzzy C-mean (FCM) supervised classifier in order to rank individual tumors according to their perfusion characteristics. The resulting tumor rankings correlated inversely with experimental nanoparticle accumulation measurements, enabling prediction of nanotherapeutics delivery into the tumor tissue.

Coupling Tumor Modeling with Image Analysis

The complexity of mathematical tumor models depends in part on the number of biological and physical factors under consideration. It is difficult to extract values for the tumor model parameters from the sparse data available for any particular patient. Medical image analysis can measure the shape, size, volume, and place-ment of tumors from MR and CT images for individual patients, yet these techniques are limited. For instance, the threshold for cell detection is a density of 8,000 cells/mm^3 in MRI, which may miss a significant number of active tumor cells and thus potentially lead to inaccurate prognoses [130, 131]. We review a set of methods by Konukoglu et al. [131] which integrate mathematical modeling of tumor growth with data from patient-specific medical images, with the goal to offer disease development modeling.

Typically, reaction-diffusion equations model tumor growth at the tissue-scale contain terms that describe the change in cells in space and time, and their collective proliferation rate. The local diffusion of the cells is defined as a tensor in the calculations. A typical differential equation may take the form [131]:

$$\frac{\partial u}{\partial t} = \nabla \cdot (D(x)\nabla u) + \rho u(1 - u) \quad \text{where} \quad D\nabla u \cdot \overrightarrow{n_{\partial\Omega}} = 0 \qquad (1)$$

where u is the tumor cell density, D is the local diffusion tensor, ρ is the prolifera-tion rate, and Ω is the boundary of the domain tissue, which in most models that have incorporated imaging data has been the brain. The diffusion term of the tumor cells is $\nabla \cdot (D(x) \nabla u)$ and the reaction term is $\rho u(1 - u)$ [131]. The tumor cell density observed clinically is linked to the reaction-diffusion model by defining a density function based on the image intensity of the lesion [132]. Although the parameter estimation has focused mainly at brain tissue because of image avail-ability and easier tumor identification, the modeling concepts apply generally to solid tumors.

The main challenge of integrating this type of reaction-diffusion model with imaging data is that the model describes the evolution of tumor cell densities in time, while in the image sequences only the shape of the tumor in space is observed [131, 132]. Medical images are usually not available longitudinally in time because most patients are not regularly scanned during the illness progression. As a result, the tumor cell density needs to be estimated from what is observed in the images. Velocity growth of the tumor can be estimated from images (as described below for the example of brain tumors). Parameters such as the real geometry of an organ, estimated speed in different tissues (e.g., white and gray matter in brain), geometry of the tumor margin, tumor cell density and its relation to tumor size would need to be extracted from the images to help formulate the simulated evolution of the tumor in time and space.

The diffusion tensor and the reaction parameters are estimated from the medical images, meaning that the evolution of the tumor equation can be specified for each individual patient. To illustrate this process, we consider in more detail the case of tumors in the brain, for which extensive modeling work has been done (e.g., Hogea et al. [133] and Swanson et al. [134, 135]). These methods usually assume that the velocity of tumor growth differs in different types of tissue (e.g., white and gray matter), so different diffusion tensors are defined based on the location of the tumor. The diffusion tensor for brain tissue is defined as:

$$D(x) = d_g I, \qquad x \in \text{gray matter}$$
$$D(x) = d_w D_{\text{water}}, \qquad x \in \text{whitematter}$$

whereas tumor cells are modeled to diffuse isotropically in the gray matter, the diffusion in the white matter is proportional to the diffusion tensor of water. Tumor cells diffuse isotropically in gray matter with rate d_g, d_w is the diffusion rate in white matter, and D_{water} is the diffusion tensor of water molecules [136]. Medical images provide data to estimate the tumor growth parameters for individual patients: the velocity of the tumor growth (v), the diffusion of the tumor (D), and proliferation rate (ρ). Here, we summarize different mathematical relation between these three parameters. The calculated parameters are based on an assumption that the tumor margin evolves linearly in time [137]. One possible linear relation is defined as: $v^2/4\rho$, which uses Fisher's approximation. The diffusion coefficients in white and gray matters are, respectively, $D_g = v_g^2/4\rho$ and $D_w = v_w^2/4\rho$ [138]. The tumor margin in image sequences approximates the velocity rate [134].

Another mathematical estimation is stated as $v = 2\sqrt{\rho D}$ [135]. The tumor margin advances as a traveling wave, which expands radially and linearly, and the diffusion coefficient D changes centrifugally. If T1 and T2 weighted images are available, then the gradient between these two can be defined as the ratio of diffusion over proliferation [135], where the tumor margin is detected from T1 weighted mages and the edema is detected from T2 weighted images [135]. The gradient has also been defined as $v = 4\sqrt{D\rho}$ [139]. $D\rho$ delineates the kinetics of the tumor growth; simulations have shown that D/ρ can indicate the spatial extent of nonvisible tumor tissue [139]. The results show that utilizing $\sqrt{D/\rho}$ instead of $D\rho$ may reflect the tumor growth rate more accurately [139].

Another method defines a biophysical reaction-diffusion function while adding a mechanical advection term [140]. For individual patients the parameters of the tumor growth are estimated from available image sequences. The mechanical advection term translates the elasticity of the tissue through which the tumor cells diffuse. This model employs different velocities depending on the tumor location; however, the unavailability of serial scans of the lesion precludes the measurement of precise parameter values. The model constraints can be defined in such a way that the problem becomes an optimization exercise with new parameters. The very first scan where the tumor is observed is defined at $t = 0$, and the diffusivity and elastic material coefficients are the new model parameters.

Parameters (e.g., diffusion, velocity, and tumor proliferation) extracted from images through these techniques have been used in modeling the tumor evolution in time and space (spatial-time models). Jbadi et al. [138] modeled the diffusion of tumor cells in anisotropic tissue. They proposed a new definition rate for the diffusion tensor in water, based on calculating the highest eigenvalue of the tensor of water molecules at each point. Another method considers a probabilistic approach [132]. The tumor growth evolution ($\rho(u(t)|\theta_x, \theta_t, \theta_p)$) is a conditional probability where tumor growth parameters describing time, location, diffusion, and proliferation rate are approximated. θ_x is the tumor location parameter, θ_t is the parameter change in time, and θ_p is the personalized parameter: diffusivity and proliferation rate. These parameters are defined based on image sequences.

Some of the modeling work focuses on matching the spatial-time evolution predicted by the model with the known tumor cell density from series of scans that have been prepared independently. The object is to minimize the difference between the estimated tumor cell density calculated from the model with the given tumor cell density from a particular subject [133]. A recent method proposes a modified anisotropic model which models the tumor delineation considering the curved front and the effect of time in its speed [131].

Spatial-time tumor growth models have mainly considered avascularized tumors, whereas it is vascularized tumors that are the most dangerous. Further, the extent of tumor vascularization may affect the chosen treatment. Yet informing the model parameters from vascular imaging information is challenging due to the problem of vessel segmentation. Vessels can be visible in MR and CT images; they usually appear brighter in CTA (computed tomography angiography) and MRA (magnetic resonance angiography) images taken with contrast agents. In general, automatic segmentation vessel trees entail two main steps: extracting features from image slices, and then reconstructing the 3D model of the vessels. Even if the appearance of vessel features is accurately extracted from the images, the 3D reconstruction of curvature is complex: number of vessel branches, curvature shape of the vessel, and numerous other factors affect the accuracy of the segmentation in 3D [141]. Vessels connect to tumors with infinite possibilities: the appearance of vessel branches is different for each individual patient, so one cannot define a predefined model to be able to quantify this information.

Example of Vascularized Tumor Modeling in 3D[1]

Once a model is adequately calibrated, the cell density information in time and space in 3D simulations can be compared to what is observed in imaging in space at a particular time. Further, a prediction of tumor invasiveness may be possible based on vasculature function. Development of this work depends on technology that enables more detailed imaging analysis of tumor vasculature, in particular, involving the extraction of model parameters regarding vascular densities and vessel morphologies. The following simulations highlight the promise of elucidating further insight into tumor behavior by coupling modeling with tumor and vascular parameters that could be obtained from medical imaging. Frieboes et al. [15] simulated the growth of a tumor assuming that the solid (internal tumor) pressure does not shut down any of the vessels. In Fig. 2 ($t = 3$), the tumor is shown starting as a small, round avascular nodule. Angiogenic regulators diffuse from the interior to the outside as necrosis forms in the core (darker color), stimulating the formation of new capillaries in the vicinity of the tumor (small lines) from a preexisting vasculature (not shown). Endothelial cells in these vessels proliferate up a gradient of angiogenic regulators, first forming branches and then looping to conduct blood (darker lines). The nodule is able to grow larger as it becomes surrounded by conducting vessels ($t = 8$). The tumor shape assumes a slightly more asymmetric form ($t = 15$), determined by the heterogeneity in cell proliferation and death, which is in turn based on the availability of cell substrates in the microenvironment as a function of the vasculature. The amount of necrosis remains stable as hypoxic cells gain access to substrates. The simulation shows that viable tumor tissue cuffs around the locations of vessels as observed clinically [13, 104] as well as experimentally [142], with tissue distal from the conducting vessels being necrotic. At later stages ($t = 54$) the tumor continues growing uniformly and fairly compactly in time, consistent with the prediction of Cristini et al. [95], in which nonuniformity in the environment is required for asymmetric growth of vascularized tumors. The vasculature is uniformly distributed around and inside the lesion.

The model predicts that tumor invasiveness depends critically on its coupling with the vasculature. Observations of tumor vasculature function from imaging, when integrated with this type of modeling, could provide further insight into tumor behavior within living patients. Frieboes et al. [15] further simulated the growth of a tumor with one single viable cell species in 3D and included the effects of vessel regression (shutdown) due to the solid (internal tumor) pressure. Figure 3 shows a tumor starting as a small, round avascular nodule at $t = 1$, which becomes surrounded by new capillaries through the process of angiogenesis (e.g., $t = 8$ and $t = 20$). At $t \approx 23$ the cell proliferation exerts enough pressure that the

---

[1] This section contains excerpts reprinted with permission from J Theor Biol, Vol. 264, Frieboes et al., Three-dimensional multispecies nonlinear tumor growth-II: Tumor invasion and angiogenesis, pp. 1254–1278, Copyright (2010), with permission from Elsevier.

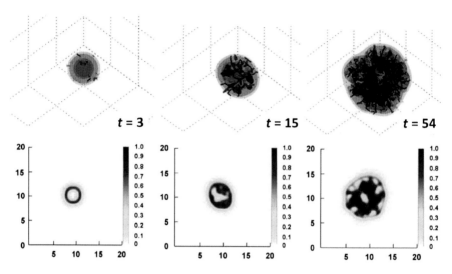

Fig. 2 Simulation of tumor growth in 3D and quantification of tissue density based on vasculari-zation [15]. *Upper three panels*: A tumor grows uniformly and compactly over time as the surrounding capillary vasculature is stimulated through angiogenesis to supply it with increasing oxygen and nutrient. Tumor invasiveness is lessened compared to the case in Fig. 1, since hypoxic cells are better able to gain access to oxygen and nutrients. Viable tumor tissue (*orange/red* color) is shown in 3D contours representing density values of 0.1, 0.2, and 0.6 (min.: 0.0; max.: 1.0). Conducting vessels are shown in *blue* and nonconducting in *gray*. Time unit = 1 day. *Lower three panels*: Slices of tumor (plane $x = 10$) at various times of growth show that viable tumor tissue cuffs around the vessel locations (*darker areas*), as is typically observed clinically for solid tumors, with areas more distal from the vessels being dead. Color coding: density of viable tissue; highest = 1.0 (unit length = 100 μm). Reprinted with permission from J Theor Biol, Vol. 264, Frieboes et al., Three-dimensional multispecies nonlinear tumor growth-II: Tumor invasion and angiogenesis, pp. 1265–1266, Copyright (2010), with permission from Elsevier

blood flow in some of the capillaries becomes impeded, shuts down, and the vascular network regresses. Hypoxia is then locally increased, triggering a higher release of angiogenic factors. The viable cells downgrade their proliferation. Eventually cell homeostasis is disrupted to such an extent that several regions of the tumor undergo necrosis, causing the tumor to regress, thus exacerbating the morphological instabil-ity through uneven shrinking of the tumor mass ($t = 25$). A similar effect has been observed through the model when simulating anti-angiogenic therapy [143], which may shut down the tumor vasculature in an uneven manner and exacerbate tumor break-up and invasion [142, 144–146].

A new round of vessel generation is triggered at $t = 25$ induced by the produc-tion of angiogenic regulators as a result of increased hypoxia in response to continued cell proliferation and tumor necrosis. This second wave of angiogenesis leads to a larger tumor with a more complex morphology than at earlier times, until the pressure from cell proliferation disrupts the blood flow ($t = 49$) once again. By this time, however, the tumor has gained enough mass so that the disruption predominantly affects the right hemisphere, which leads to tissue break-up in this

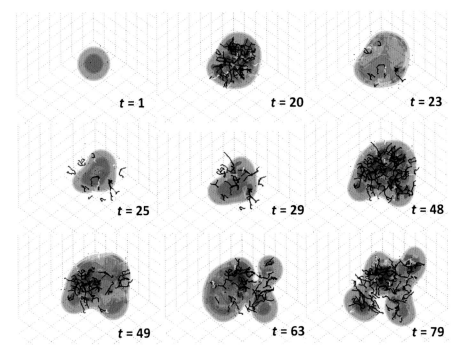

Fig. 3 Simulation of vascularized tumor growth in 3D [15]. Morphological stability of the tumor and its invasiveness are directly linked to the availability of cell substrates regulated by the dynamically evolving vasculature. At time $t = 23$, the supply of cell substrates is shut off by the collapse of vessels due to increasing pressure from the surrounding proliferating cells. The tumor mass then undergoes temporary regression ($t = 25$). By $t = 29$, neovascularization is apparent in response to the increased hypoxia in the interior of the tumor. By $t = 48$ the tumor has re-grown and is once again highly vascularized. At $t = 49$ the vessels in the right hemisphere are crushed by the tumor cells. The tumor morphology becomes more unstable, breaking up into two pieces ($t = 63$). Renewed vascularization eventually helps to restabilize the mass ($t = 79$). Viable tumor tissue (*blue color*) is shown in 3D contours representing density values of 0.1, 0.2, and 0.6 (min.: 0.0; max.: 1.0); complete absence of viable tissue is shown in *gray*. Conducting vessels: *brown*; nonconducting: *white*. Time unit = 1 day (grid length = 200 μm). Reprinted with permission from J Theor Biol, Vol. 264, Frieboes et al., Three-dimensional multispecies nonlinear tumor growth-II: Tumor invasion and angiogenesis, pp. 1267–1268, Copyright (2010), with permission from Elsevier

region. The resulting hypoxia upregulates angiogenesis towards the right side of the tumor, as seen at $t = 54$. The new vascular network is concentrated more towards the center of the tumor and not at the leading clusters, since these have better access to the surrounding (existing) host vasculature (not shown). By $t = 63$ vessels become disrupted on the left lobe, which initially shrinks and furthers the splitting of the tumor into two pieces. As cell proliferation once again increases due to enhanced vascularization, the two parts grow larger and begin to reconnect ($t = 79$). The stability of the tumor morphology and its invasiveness is directly linked to the availability of cell substrates regulated by the evolving vasculature in response to cell proliferation and death.

This simulation shows strong nonlinear coupling between the tumor-induced angiogenesis and the progression of the tumor. The pressure-induced vascular response of constricting the radii of the neovasculature and inhibiting blood-tissue oxygen transfer not only dramatically affects the tumor growth, but also significantly affects the growth of the neovascular network. The modeling thus provides not only a means to quantitatively evaluate the growth of tumors in space and time, but also serves as a means to generate hypotheses from clinical observations.

In conclusion, much work remains to be done to fully integrate mathematical models of tumor growth with data obtained from clinical imaging. As technology is further developed to improve the analysis of this imaging, and as tumor models undergo further refinement to more faithfully represent cancer biology, the gap between modeling and imaging is expected to narrow, thus enabling a more seamless integration to the benefit of cancer patients.

References

1. Lowengrub JS, Frieboes HB, Jin F, Chuang YL, Li X, Macklin P, Wise SM, Cristini V (2010) Nonlinear modelling of cancer: bridging the gap between cells and tumours. Nonlinearity 23: R1–R9
2. Frieboes HB, Chaplain MA, Thompson AM, Bearer EL, Lowengrub JS, Cristini V (2011) Physical oncology: a bench-to-bedside quantitative and predictive approach. Cancer Res 71:298–302
3. Byrne HM (2010) Dissecting cancer through mathematics: from the cell to the animal model. Nat Rev Cancer 10:221–230
4. Astanin S, Preziosi L (2007) Multiphase models of tumour growth. In: Bellomo N, Chaplain M, DeAngelis E (eds) Selected topics on cancer modelling: genesis—evolution—immune competition—therapy. Birkhäuser, Boston, pp 1–31
5. Harpold HL, Alvord EC Jr, Swanson KR (2007) The evolution of mathematical modeling of glioma proliferation and invasion. J Neuropathol Exp Neurol 66:1–9
6. Anderson ARA, Quaranta V (2008) Integrative mathematical oncology. Nat Rev Cancer 8:227–244
7. Deisboeck TS, Zhang L, Yoon J, Costa J (2009) In silico cancer modeling: is it ready for prime time? Nat Clin Pract Oncol 6:34–42
8. Ventura AC, Jackson TL, Merajver SD (2009) On the role of cell signaling models in cancer research. Cancer Res 69:400–402
9. Massey SC, Assanah MC, Lopez KA, Canoll P, Swanson KR (2012) Glial progenitor cell recruitment drives aggressive glioma growth: mathematical and experimental modeling. J R Soc Interface 9:1757–1766
10. Sinek JP, Sanga S, Zheng X, Frieboes HB, Ferrari M, Cristini V (2009) Predicting drug pharmacokinetics and effect in vascularized tumors using computer simulation. J Math Biol 58:485–510
11. van de Ven AL, Wu M, Lowengrub J, McDougall SR, Chaplain MA, Cristini V, Ferrari M, Frieboes HB (2012) Integrated intravital microscopy and mathematical modeling to optimize nanotherapeutics delivery to tumors. AIP Adv 2:11208
12. Frieboes HB, Zheng X, Sun CH, Tromberg B, Gatenby R, Cristini V (2006) An integrated computational/experimental model of tumor invasion. Cancer Res 66:1597–1604

13. Frieboes HB, Lowengrub JS, Wise SM, Zheng X, Macklin P, Bearer EL, Cristini V (2007) Computer simulation of glioma growth and morphology. Neuroimage 37:S59–S70

14. Frieboes HB, Edgerton ME, Fruehauf JP, Rose FR, Worrall LK, Gatenby RA, Ferrari M, Cristini V (2009) Prediction of drug response in breast cancer using integrative experimental/computational modeling. Cancer Res 69:4484–4492

15. Frieboes HB, Jin F, Chuang YL, Wise SM, Lowengrub JS, Cristini V (2010) Three-dimensional multispecies nonlinear tumor growth-II: tumor invasion and angiogenesis. J Theor Biol 264:254–278

16. Frieboes HB, Smith BR, Chuang YL, Ito K, Roettgers AM, Gambhir SS, Cristini V (2013) An integrated computational/experimental model of lymphoma growth. PLoS Comput Biol 9(3): e1003008

17. Gu S, Chakraborty G, Champley K, Alessio AM, Claridge J, Rockne R, Muzi M, Krohn KA, Spence AM, Alvord EC Jr, Anderson AR, Kinahan PE, Swanson KR (2012) Applying a patient-specific bio-mathematical model of glioma growth to develop virtual [18F]-FMISO-PET images. Math Med Biol 29:31–48

18. Swanson KR, Rockne RC, Claridge J, Chaplain MA, Alvord EC Jr, Anderson AR (2011) Quantifying the role of angiogenesis in malignant progression of gliomas: in silico modeling integrates imaging and histology. Cancer Res 71:7366–7375

19. Enderling H, Chaplain MA, Hahnfeldt P (2010) Quantitative modeling of tumor dynamics and radiotherapy. Acta Biotheor 58:341–353

20. Rockne R, Alvord EC Jr, Rockhill JK, Swanson KR (2009) A mathematical model for brain tumor response to radiation therapy. J Math Biol 58:561–578

21. Rockne R, Rockhill JK, Mrugala M, Spence AM, Kalet I, Hendrickson K, Lai A, Cloughesy T, Alvord EC Jr, Swanson KR (2010) Predicting the efficacy of radiotherapy in individual glioblastoma patients in vivo: a mathematical modeling approach. Phys Med Biol 55:3271–3285

22. Hanahan D, Weinberg RA (2000) The hallmarks of cancer. Cell 100:57–70

23. Hanahan D, Folkman J (1996) Patterns and emerging mechanisms of the angiogenic switch during tumorigenesis. Cell 86:353–364

24. Zwick S, Strecker R, Kiselev V, Gall P, Huppert J, Palmowski M, Lederle W, Woenne E, Hengerer A, Taupitz M, Semmler W, Kiessling F (2009) Assessment of vascular remodeling under antiangiogenic therapy using DCE-MRI and vessel size imaging. J Magn Reson Imaging 29:1125–1133

25. Huang J, Soffer S, Kim E, McCrudden K, Huang J, New T, Manley C, Middlesworth W, O'Toole K, Yamashiro D, Kandel J (2004) Vascular remodeling marks tumors that recur during chronic suppression of angiogenesis. Mol Cancer Res 2:36–42

26. Holash J, Maisonpierre PC, Compton D, Boland P, Alexander CR, Zagzag D, Yancopoulos GD, Wiegand SJ (1999) Vessel cooption, regression, and growth in tumors mediated by angiopoietins and VEGF. Science 284:1994–1998

27. Holash J, Wiegand SJ, Yancopoulos GD (1999) New model of tumor angiogenesis: dynamic balance between vessel regression and growth mediated by angiopoietins and VEGF. Oncogene 18:5356–5362

28. Raza A, Franklin M, Dudek A (2010) Pericytes and vessel maturation during tumor angiogenesis and metastasis. Am J Hematol 85:593–598

29. Folkman J (1971) Tumor angiogenesis: therapeutic implications. N Engl J Med 285:1182–1186

30. Gimbrone MA, Cotran RS, Leapman SB, Folkman J (1974) Tumor growth and neovascularization: an experimental model using the rabbit cornea. J Natl Cancer Inst 52:413–427

31. De Bock K, Cauwenberghs S, Carmeliet P (2011) Vessel abnormalization: another hallmark of cancer? Molecular mechanisms and therapeutic implications. Curr Opin Genet Dev 21:73–79

32. Greene J, Cheresh D (2009) VEGF as an inhibitor of tumor vessel maturation: implications for cancer therapy. Expert Opin Biol Ther 9:1347–1356

33. Hashizume H, Baluk P, Morikawa S, McLean JW, Thurston G, Roberge S, Jain RK, McDonald DM (2000) Openings between defective endothelial cells explain tumor vessel leakiness. Am J Pathol 156:1363–1380

34. Jain R (2001) Delivery of molecular medicine to solid tumors: lessons from in vivo imaging of gene expression and function. J Control Release 74:7–25

35. Fukumura D, Jain RK (2007) Tumor microenvironment abnormalities: causes, consequences, and strategies to normalize. J Cell Biochem 101:937–949

36. Gaffney EA, Pugh K, Maini PK, Arnold F (2002) Investigating a simple model of cutaneous wound healing angiogenesis. J Math Biol 45:337–374

37. van Leeuwen IMM, Edwards CM, Ilyas M, Byrne HM (2007) Towards a multiscale model of colorectal cancer. World J Gastroenterol 13:1399–1407

38. Roose T, Chapman SJ, Maini PK (2007) Mathematical models of avascular tumor growth. SIAM Review 49:179–208

39. Owen MR, Alarcón T, Maini PK, Byrne HM (2009) Angiogenesis and vascular remodeling in normal and cancerous tissues. J Math Biol 58:689–721

40. Zheng X, Wise SM, Cristini V (2005) Nonlinear simulation of tumor necrosis, neo-vascularization and tissue invasion via an adaptive finite-element/level-set method. Bull Math Biol 67:211–259

41. Macklin P, McDougall S, Anderson ARA, Chaplain MAJ, Cristini V, Lowengrub JS (2009) Multiscale modeling and simulation of vascular tumour growth. J Math Biol 58:765–798

42. Ramis-Conde I, Chaplain MAJ, Anderson ARA, Drasdo D (2009) Multi-scale modelling of cancer cell intravasation: the role of cadherins in metastasis. Phys Biol 6:016008

43. Novák B, Tyson JJ (2008) Design principles of biochemical oscillators. Nat Rev Mol Cell Biol 9:981–991

44. Michor F (2008) Mathematical models of cancer stem cells. J Clin Oncol 26:2854–2861

45. Enderling H, Chaplain MAJ, Anderson ARA, Vaidya JS (2007) A mathematical model of breast cancer development, local treatment and recurrence. J Theor Biol 246:245–259

46. Kim Y, Stolarska MA, Othmer HG (2007) A hybrid model for tumor spheroid growth in vitro I: theoretical development and early results. Math Meth Appl Sci 17:1773–1798

47. Stokes CL, Lauffenburger DA (1991) Analysis of the roles of microvessel endothelial cell random motility and chemotaxis in angiogenesis. J Theor Biol 152:377–403

48. Anderson A, Chaplain MAJ (1998) Continuous and discrete mathematical model of tumour-induced angiogenesis. Bull Math Biol 60:857–899

49. Tong S, Yuan F (2001) Numerical simulations of angiogenesis in the cornea. Microvasc Res 61:14–27

50. Plank MJ, Sleeman BD (2003) A reinforced random walk model of tumour angiogenesis and anti-angiogenic strategies. Math Med Biol 20:135–181

51. Plank MJ, Sleeman BD (2004) Lattice and non-lattice models of tumour angiogenesis. Bull Math Biol 66:1785–1819

52. Sun S, Wheeler MF, Obeyesekere M, Patrick C Jr (2005) Multiscale angiogenesis modeling using mixed finite element methods. Multiscale Model Simul 4:1137–1167

53. Sun S, Wheeler MF, Obeyesekere M, Patrick CW Jr (2005) A deterministic model of growth factor-induced angiogenesis. Bull Math Biol 67:313–337

54. Kevrekidis PG, Whitaker N, Good DJ, Herring GJ (2006) Minimal model for tumor angiogenesis. Phys Rev E 73:061926

55. Bauer AL, Jackson TL, Jiang Y (2007) A cell-based model exhibiting branching and anastomosis during tumor-induced angiogenesis. Biophys J 92:3105–3121

56. Milde F, Bergdorf M, Koumoutsakos P (2008) A hybrid model for three-dimensional simulations of sprouting angiogenesis. Biophys J 95:3146–3160

57. Capasso V, Morale D (2009) Stochastic modelling of tumour-induced angiogenesis. J Math Biol 58:219–233

58. Pries AR, Secomb TW, Gaehtgens P (1998) Structural adaptation and stability of microvascular networks: theory and simulations. Am J Physiol Heart Circ Physiol 275:H349–H360

59. McDougall SR, Anderson ARA, Chaplain MAJ, Sherratt J (2002) Mathematical modelling of flow through vascular networks: implications for tumour-induced angiogenesis and chemotherapy strategies. Bull Math Biol 64:673–702

60. Stephanou A, McDougall SR, Anderson ARA, Chaplain MAJ (2005) Mathematical modelling of flow in 2D and 3D vascular networks: applications to anti-angiogenic and chemotherapeutic drug strategies. Math Comput Model 41:1137–1156

61. Stephanou A, McDougall SR, Anderson ARA, Chaplain MAJ (2006) Mathematical modeling of the influence of blood rheological properties upon adaptive tumour-induced angiogenesis. Math Comput Model 44:96–123

62. McDougall SR, Anderson ARA, Chaplain MAJ (2006) Mathematical modeling of dynamic adaptive tumour-induced angiogenesis: clinical applications and therapeutic targeting strategies. J Theor Biol 241:564–589

63. Wu J, Zhou F, Cui S (2007) Simulation of microcirculation in solid tumors. IEEE/ICME international conference on complex medical engineering (CME), Beijing, China, pp 1555–1563

64. Zhao G, Wu J, Xu S, Collins MW, Long Q, Koenig CS, Jiang Y, Wang J, Padhani AR (2007) Numerical simulation of blood flow and interstitial fluid pressure in solid tumor microcirculation based on tumor induced angiogenesis. Mech Sin 23:477–483

65. Sun CH, Munn LL (2008) Lattice-Boltzmann simulation of blood flow in digitized vessel networks. Comput Math Appl 55:1594–1600

66. Pries AR, Secomb TW (2008) Modeling structural adaptation of microcirculation. Microcirculation 15:753–764

67. Alarcón T, Byrne HM, Maini PK (2003) A cellular automaton model for tumour growth in inhomogeneous environment. J Theor Biol 225:257–274

68. Betteridge R, Owen MR, Byrne HM, Alarcón T, Maini PK (2006) The impact of cell crowding and active cell movement on vascular tumour growth. Netw Heterogen Media 1:515–535

69. Chapman SJ, Shipley R, Jawad R (2008) Multiscale modeling of fluid transport in tumors. Bull Math Biol 70:2334–2357

70. Byrne HM, Chaplain MAJ (1995) Mathematical models for tumour angiogenesis: numerical simulations and nonlinear wave solutions. Bull Math Biol 57:461–486

71. Orme ME, Chaplain MAJ (1997) Two-dimensional models of tumour angiogenesis and anti-angiogenesis strategies. Math Med Biol 14:189–205

72. de Angelis E, Preziosi L (2000) Advection-diffusion models for solid tumour evolution in vivo and related free boundary problem. Math Models Meth Appl Sci 10:379–407

73. Sansone BC, Scalerandi M, Condat CA (2001) Emergence of taxis and synergy in angiogenesis. Phys Rev Lett 87:128102

74. Levine HA, Pamuk S, Sleeman BD, Nilsen-Hamilton M (2001) Mathematical modeling of capillary formation and development in tumor angiogenesis: penetration into the stroma. Bull Math Biol 63:801–863

75. Levine HA, Sleeman BD, Nilsen-Hamilton M (2001) Mathematical modeling of the onset of capillary formation initiating angiogenesis. J Math Biol 42:195–238

76. Levine HA, Tucker AL, Nilsen-Hamilton MA (2002) Mathematical model for the role of cell signal transduction in the initiation and inhibition of angiogenesis. Growth Factors 20:155–175

77. Hogea CS, Murray BT, Sethian JA (2006) Simulating complex tumor dynamics from avascular to vascular growth using a general level-set method. J Math Biol 53:86–134

78. Peterson JW, Carey GF, Knezevic DJ, Murray BT (2007) Adaptive finite element methodology for tumour angiogenesis modeling. Int J Numer Methods Eng 69:1212–1238

79. Stamper IJ, Byrne HM, Owen MR, Maini PK (2007) Modelling the role of angiogenesis and vasculogenesis in solid tumour growth. Bull Math Biol 69:2737–2772

80. Jain HV, Nor JE, Jackson TL (2008) Modeling the VEGF-Bcl-2-CXCL8 pathway in intratumoral angiogenesis. Bull Math Biol 70:89–117

81. Addison-Smith B, McElwain DLS, Maini PK (2008) A simple mechanistic model of sprout spacing in tumour-associated angiogenesis. J Theor Biol 250:1–15

82. Merks RMH, Brodsky SV, Goligorksy MS, Newman SA, Glazier JA (2006) Cell elongation is key to in silico replication of in vitro vasculogenesis and subsequent remodeling. Dev Biol 289:44–54

83. Merks RMH, Glazier JA (2006) Dynamic mechanisms of blood vessel growth. Nonlinearity 19:C1–C10

84. Merks RMH, Perrynand ED, Shirinifard A, Glazier JA (2008) Contact-inhibited chemotaxis in de novo and sprouting blood-vessel growth. PLoS Comput Biol 4:e1000163

85. Ambrosi D, Gamba A, Serini G (2004) Cell directional and chemotaxis in vascular morphogenesis. Bull Math Biol 66:1851–1873

86. Coniglio A, deCandia A, DiTalia S, Gamba A (2004) Percolation and Burgers' dynamics in a model of capillary formation. Phys Rev E 69:051910

87. Gamba A, Ambrosi D, Coniglio A, deCandia A, DiTalia S, Giraudo E, Serini G, Preziosi L, Bussolino F (2003) Percolation, morphogenesis and burgers dynamics in blood vessels formation. Phys Rev Lett 90:118101

88. Holmes M, Sleeman B (2000) A mathematical model of tumor angiogenesis incorporating cellular traction and viscoelastic effects. J Theor Biol 202:95–112

89. Lanza V, Ambrosi D, Preziosi L (2006) Exogenous control of vascular network formation in vitro: a mathematical model. Netw Heterogen Media 1:621–637

90. Manoussaki D, Lubkin SR, Vernon RB, Murray JD (1996) A mechanical model for the formation of vascular networks in vitro. Acta Biotheor 44:271–282

91. Murray J, Oster G (1984) Cell traction models for generation of pattern and form in morphogenesis. J Math Biol 33:489–520

92. Ngwa G, Maini P (1995) Spatio-temporal patterns in a mechanical model for mesenchymal morphogenesis. J Math Biol 33:489–520

93. Serini G, Ambrosi D, Giraudo E, Gamba A, Preziosi L, Bussolino F (2003) Modeling the early stages of vascular network assembly. EMBO J 22:1771–1779

94. Tosin A, Ambrosi D, Preziosi L (2006) Mechanics and chemotaxis in the morphogenesis of vascular networks. Bull Math Biol 68:1819–1836

95. Cristini V, Lowengrub JS, Nie Q (2003) Nonlinear simulation of tumor growth. J Math Biol 46:191–224

96. Gevertz JL, Torquato S (2006) Modeling the effects of vasculature evolution on early brain tumor growth. J Theor Biol 243:517–531

97. Bartha K, Rieger H (2006) Vascular network remodeling via vessel cooption, regression and growth in tumors. J Theor Biol 241:903–918

98. Wcislo R, Dzwinel W (2008) Particle based model of tumor progression stimulated by the process of angiogenesis. In: Adam J, Bellomo N (eds) Computer science—ICCS. Springer, Heidelberg, pp 177–186

99. Alarcón T, Byrne HM, Maini PK (2005) A multiple scale model for tumor growth. Multiscale Model Simul 3:440–475

100. Lee DS, Rieger H, Bartha K (2006) Flow correlated percolation during vascular remodeling in growing tumors. Phys Rev Lett 96:058104

101. Welter M, Bartha K, Rieger H (2008) Emergent vascular network inhomogenities and resulting blood flow patterns in a growing tumor. J Theor Biol 250:257–280

102. Welter M, Bartha K, Rieger H (2008) Hot spot formation in tumor vasculature during tumor growth in an arterio-venous-network environment. arXiv:0801.0654v2[q-bio.To]

103. Lloyd BA, Szczerba D, Rudin M, Szekely G (2008) A computational framework for modeling solid tumour growth. Philos Trans A Math Phys Eng Sci 366:3301–3318

104. Bearer EL, Lowengrub JS, Chuang YL, Frieboes HB, Jin F, Wise SM, Ferrari M, Agus DB, Cristini V (2009) Multiparameter computational modeling of tumor invasion. Cancer Res 69:4493–4501

105. Phipps C, Kohandel M (2011) Mathematical model of the effect of interstitial fluid pressure on angiogenic behavior in solid tumors. Comput Math Meth Med 2011:843765
106. Stoll BR, Migliorini C, Kadambi A, Munn LL, Jain RK (2003) A mathematical model of the contribution of endothelial progenitor cells to angiogenesis in tumors: implications for antiangiogenic therapy. Blood 102:2555–2561
107. Shields JD, Fleury ME, Yong C, Tomei AA, Randolph GJ, Swartz MA (2007) Autologous chemotaxis as a mechanism of tumor cell homing to lymphatics via interstitial flow and autocrine CCR7 signaling. Cancer Cell 11:526–538
108. Pries AR, Neuhaus D, Gaehtgens P (1992) Blood viscosity in tube flow: dependence on diameter and hematocrit. Am J Physiol Heart Circ Physiol 263:H1770–H1778
109. Pries AR, Cornelissen AJ, Sloot AA, Hinkeldey M, Dreher MR, Höpfner M, Dewhirst MW, Secomb TW (2009) Structural adaptation and heterogeneity of normal and tumor microvascular networks. PLoS Comput Biol 5:e1000394
110. Wu M, Frieboes HB, McDougall SR, Chaplain MAJ, Cristini V, Lowengrub V (2013) The effect of interstitial pressure on tumor growth: coupling with the blood and lymphatic vascular systems. J Theor Biol 320:131–151
111. Pham DL, Xu C, Prince JL (2000) Current methods in medical image segmentation. Annu Rev Biomed Eng 2:315–337
112. Plajer IC, Richter D (2010) A new approach to model based active contours in lung tumor segmentation in 3D CT image data. In: IEEE international conference on Information Technology and Applications in Biomedicine (ITAB), 3–5 Nov 2010, pp 1–4
113. Dunlap NE, Yang W, McIntosh A, Sheng K, Benedict SH, Read PW, Larner JM (2012) Computed tomography-based anatomic assessment overestimates local tumor recurrence in patients with mass-like consolidation after stereotactic body radiotherapy for early-stage non-small cell lung cancer. Int J Radiat Oncol Biol Phys 84:1071–1077
114. National Lung Screening Trial Research Team, Aberle DR, Adams AM, Berg CD, Black WC, Clapp JD, Fagerstrom RM, Gareen IF, Gatsonis C, Marcus PM, Sicks JD et al (2011) Reduced lung-cancer mortality with low-dose computed tomographic screening. N Engl J Med 365:395–409
115. Ko JP, Rusinek H, Naidich DP, McGuinness G, Rubinowitz AN, Leitman BS, Martino JM (2003) Wavelet compression of low-dose chest CT data: effect on lung nodule detection. Radiology 228:70–75
116. Li F, Arimura H, Suzuki K, Shiraishi J, Li Q, Abe H, Engelmann R, Sone S, MacMahon H, Doi K (2005) Computer-aided detection of peripheral lung cancers missed at CT: ROC analyses without and with localization. Radiology 237:684–690
117. Armato SG, Li F, Giger ML, MacMahon H, Sone S, Doi K (2002) Lung cancer: performance of automated lung nodule detection applied to cancers missed in a CT screening program. Radiology 225:685–692
118. Henschke CI, Yankelevitz DF, Mirtcheva R, McGuinness G, McCauley D, Miettinen OS, ELCAP Group (2002) CT screening for lung cancer: frequency and significance of part-solid and nonsolid nodules. AJR Am J Roentgenol 178:1053–1057
119. Ko JP, Rusinek H, Jacobs EL, Babb JS, Betke M, McGuinness G, Naidich DP (2003) Small pulmonary nodules: volume measurement at chest CT—phantom study. Radiology 228:864–870
120. Gurney JW (1993) Determining the likelihood of malignancy in solitary pulmonary nodules with Bayesian analysis. Part I. Theory. Radiology 186:405–413
121. Yamashita K, Matsunobe S, Tsuda T, Nemoto T, Matsumoto K, Miki H, Konishi J (1995) Solitary pulmonary nodule: preliminary study of evaluation with incremental dynamic CT. Radiology 194:399–405
122. Lee J, Aronchick JM, Alavi A (2001) Accuracy of F-18 fluorodeoxyglucose positron emission tomography for the evaluation of malignancy in patients presenting with new lung abnormalities: a retrospective review. Chest 120:1791–1797

123. Kennel SJ, Davis IA, Branning J, Pan H, Kabalka GW, Paulus MJ (2000) High resolution commuted tomography and MRI for monitoring lung tumor growth in mice undergoing radioimmunotherapy: correlation with histology. Med Phys 27:1101–1107

124. Suryanto A, Herlambang K, Rachmatullah P (2005) Comparison of tumor density by CT scan based on histologic type in lung cancer patients. Acta Med Indones 37:195–198

125. Petralia G, Bonello L, Viotti S, Preda L, d'Andrea G, Bellomi M (2010) CT perfusion in oncology: how to do it. Cancer Imaging 10:8–19

126. Ma SH, Le HB, Jia BH, Wang ZX, Xiao ZW, Cheng XL, Mei W, Wu M, Hu ZG, Li YG (2008) Peripheral pulmonary nodules: relationship between multi-slice spiral CT perfusion imaging and tumor angiogenesis and VEGF expression. BMC Cancer 8:186

127. Tateishi U, Kusumoto M, Nishihara H, Nagashima K, Morikawa T, Moriyama N (2002) Contrast-enhanced dynamic computed tomography for the evaluation of tumor angiogenesis in patients with lung carcinoma. Cancer 95:835–842

128. Li Y, Yang ZG, Chen TW, Chen HJ, Sun JY, Lu YR (2008) Peripheral lung carcinoma: correlation of angiogenesis and first-pass perfusion parameters of 64-detector row CT. Lung Cancer 61:44–53

129. van de Ven A, Abdollahi B, Martinez C, Paskett LA, Landis MD, Chang JC, Ferrari M, Frieboes HB (2013) Predictive modeling of nanotherapeutics delivery based on tumor perfusion. New J Phys, in press

130. Swanson KR, Alvord EC Jr, Murray JD (2002) Virtual brain tumors (gliomas) enhance the reality of medical imaging and highlight inadequacies of current therapy. Br J Cancer 86:14–18

131. Konukoglu E, Clatz O, Menze BH, Weber MA, Stieltjes B, Mandonnet E, Delingette H, Ayache N (2010) Image guided personalization of reaction-diffusion type tumor growth models using modified anisotropic eikonal equation. IEEE Trans Med Imaging 29:77–95

132. Menze BH, Leempu KV, Honkela A, Konukoglu E, Weber M-A, Ayache N, Golland P (2011) A generative approach for image-based modeling of tumor growth. Inf Process Med Imaging 22:735–747

133. Hogea C, Davatzikos C, Biros G (2008) An image-driven parameter estimation problem for a reaction-diffusion glioma growth model with mass effect. J Math Biol 56:793–825

134. Swanson KR, Alvord EC Jr, Murray JD (2000) A quantitative model for differential motility of gliomas in grey and white matter. Cell Prolif 33:317–329

135. Swanson KR, Rostomily RC, Alvord EC Jr (2008) A mathematical modeling tool for predicting survival of individual patients following resection of glioblastoma: a proof of principle. Br J Cancer 98:113–119

136. Clatz O, Semesant M, Bondiau P-Y, Delingette H, Wasfield SK, Malandain G, Ayache N (2005) Realistic simulation of the 3D growth of brain tumors in MR images coupling diffusion with biomechanical deformation. IEEE Trans Med Imaging 24:1334–1346

137. Swanson KR, Alvord EC Jr, Murray JD (2004) Dynamics of a model for brain tumors reveals a small window for therapeutic intervention. Discrete Cont Dyn Syst 4:289–295

138. Jbadi S, Mandonnet E, Duffau H, Capelle L, Swanson KR, Pelegrini-Issac M, Guillevin R, Benali H (2005) Simulation of anisotropic growth of low-grade gliomas using diffusion tensor imaging. Magn Reson Med 54:616–624

139. Mandonnet E, Pallud J, Clatz O, Taillandier L, Konukoglu E, Duffau H, Capelle L (2008) Computational modeling of the WHO grade II glioma dynamics: principles and applications to management paradigm. Neurosurg Rev 31:263–269

140. Hogea C, Davatzikos C, Biros G (2007) Modeling glioma growth and mass effect in 3D MR images of the brain. Med Image Comput Comput Assist Interv 10:642–650

141. Lesage D, Angelini ED, Bloch I, Funka-Lea G (2009) A review of 3D vessel lumen segmentation techniques. Models, features and extraction schemes. Med Image Anal 13:819–845

142. Kunkel P, Ulbricht U, Bohlen P, Brockmann MA, Fillbrandt R, Stavrou D, Westphal M, Lamszus K (2001) Inhibition of glioma angiogenesis and growth in vivo by systemic

treatment with a monoclonal antibody against vascular endothelial growth factor receptor-2. Cancer Res 61:6624–6628

143. Cristini V, Frieboes HB, Gatenby R, Caserta S, Ferrari M, Sinek J (2005) Morphologic instability and cancer invasion. Clin Cancer Res 11:6772–6779

144. Rubenstein JL, Kim J, Ozawa T, Zhang M, Westphal M, Deen DF, Shuman MA (2000) Anti-VEGF antibody treatment of glioblastoma prolongs survival but results in increased vascular cooption. Neoplasia 2:306–314

145. Lamszus K, Kunkel P, Westphal M (2003) Invasion as limitation to anti-angiogenic glioma therapy. Acta Neurochir Suppl 88:169–177

146. Bello L, Lucini V, Costa F, Pluderi M, Giussani C, Acerbi F, Carrabba G, Pannacci M, Caronzolo D, Grosso S, Shinkaruk S, Colleoni F, Canron X, Tomei G, Deleris G, Bikfalvi A (2004) Combinatorial administration of molecules that simultaneously inhibit angiogenesis and invasion leads to increased therapeutic efficacy in mouse models of malignant glioma. Clin Cancer Res 10:4527–4537

Biography

Behnaz Abdollahi, Ph.D., recently obtained a Ph.D. in Electrical Engineering from the University of Louisville. She specializes in medical image analysis and machine learning, with emphasis on data evaluation to predict and enhance decision-making with healthcare data. Her areas of interest include developing methods to predict healthcare outcomes using image and healthcare datasets.

Neal Dunlap, M.D., Ph.D., is currently an Assistant Professor and Assistant Residency Director in the Department of Radiation Oncology at the James Graham Brown Cancer Center at the University of Louisville. He received his medical degree at the University of Cincinnati and completed a residency in Radiation Oncology at the University of Virginia. Dr. Dunlap specializes in lung cancer and head and neck cancer treatment. His primary research interests focus on lung cancer imaging, stereotactic body radiation therapy (SBRT), and the mitigation of radiation-related toxicity.

Hermann Frieboes, Ph.D., in Biomedical Engineering from the University of California, Irvine, is an Assistant Professor at the Department of Bioengineering at the University of Louisville, with affiliations at the James Graham Brown Cancer Center and the Departments of Pharmacology/Toxicology and Electrical Engineering. He specializes in applying and integrating mathematical modeling, computational simulation, and experimental techniques to the study of cancer. His interests include the development of quantitative and predictive approaches to the study of tumor growth and treatment, furthering the interaction of basic research with clinical and translational programs, and exploring the use of nanotechnology in disease diagnosis and treatment.

Evaluation of Medical Image Registration by Using High-Accuracy Image Matching Techniques

Zisheng Li and Tsuneya Kurihara

Abstract An effective method for quantitatively evaluating deformable image registration without any manual assessment is developed in the work of this chapter. Fiducial landmarks for spatial evaluation are firstly detected using a feature-point detector in a fixed image, and corresponding points in the registered moving images are localized with a high-resolution image matching algorithm. Distance between the reference points and the correspondences can be used to estimate image registration errors. With the developed method, users can evaluate different registration algorithms using their own image data automatically.

Introduction

Image registration aims to find a spatial transformation that maps points from one image, a moving image, to corresponding points in another image, a fixed image. Medical image registration is fundamentally used in many applications, such as diagnosis, planning treatment, guiding treatment, and monitoring disease progression. Thus, it is necessary to validate whether a rigid/deformable registration algorithm satisfies the needs of an image processing application with high accuracy, robustness, and other performance criteria.

The most straightforward method for estimating image registration error is to compare a given registration transformation with a "gold standard" transformation [1], whose accuracy is high. However, the lack of a gold standard prevents any automatic assessment of registration accuracy. An attempt that stands out in this regard is the "Retrospective Image Registration and Evaluation (RIRE) project" [2] for evaluation of brain-image rigid registration. The RIRE project used bone-implanted fiducial markers to obtain a marker-based rigid transformation as the

Z. Li (✉) • T. Kurihara
Intelligent Media Systems Research Department, Central Research Laboratory,
Hitachi, Ltd., 1-280 Higashi-Koigakubo, Kokubunji-shi, Tokyo 185-8601, Japan
e-mail: zisheng.li.fj@hitachi.com

A.S. El-Baz et al. (eds.), *Abdomen and Thoracic Imaging: An Engineering
& Clinical Perspective*, DOI 10.1007/978-1-4614-8498-1_19,
© Springer Science+Business Media New York 2014

gold standard transformation. Registration error was measured by calculating the error relative to the gold standard over a set of specified regions. For deformable image registration, synthetic images and phantoms were utilized as reference standards to provide qualitative evaluation of registration performance [3–6]. However, such standards lack sufficient realism, compared with that derived from actual patient image data. "Non-rigid Image Registration Evaluation Project (NIREP)" in [7] and recent work in [8, 9] provided intensity-based metrics for evaluating the registration performance of brain images, using manually segmented anatomical regions from actual clinical data. These projects required manual annotation and segmentation to create evaluation databases, and the evaluation data only included brain images. On the other hand, a number of studies utilized expert-determined landmark features to evaluate spatial accuracy of deformable registration for lung images [10–12]. Moreover, the work in [13] utilized both manually labeled regions and expert-determined landmark pairs for evaluation of registration methods on lung images. However, such manual annotation and segmentation require that individuals trained to interpret medical images be involved in the validation of registration algorithm. In addition, the manual assessment tasks are very time-consuming.

The work of this chapter aims to quantitatively evaluate the spatial accuracy of deformable image registration by using automatic feature point matching on lung images. Candidates of fiducial landmarks for spatial evaluation are detected in a fixed image, by using a 3D SIFT (scale-invariant feature transform) keypoint detector [14, 21]. Then, correspondences of such SIFT keypoints in the registered moving image are matched and localized with a 3D phase-based image matching algorithm [15, 29]. By calculating distance between the feature point pairs, it is possible to obtain a quantitative registration error without any manual assessment of the registration algorithm [30].

Framework of Automatic Spatial Accuracy Evaluation

Since it is very difficult and time-consuming to manually annotate actual clinical data to create a ground truth for accuracy evaluation, the development of an automatic method is necessary. In order to obtain a quantitative measurement of image registration error, distance between landmarks or regions in a fixed image and their corresponding ones in a registered moving image should be accurately estimated. It is therefore necessary to develop an accuracy-evaluation framework that mainly consists of two stages: fiducial point detection and corresponding point matching. The framework of the method is illustrated in Fig. 1.

In the procedure of landmark detection, firstly, 3D SIFT keypoint detection [14, 20], which detects local extrema from image pyramids consisting of differences in Gaussian-blurred images at multiple scales, is applied to the fixed image.

After the SIFT feature points detection in the fixed image, a 3D phase-based image matching algorithm is developed to match the corresponding landmarks in the registered moving image. A discrete Fourier transform (DFT) of image blocks around

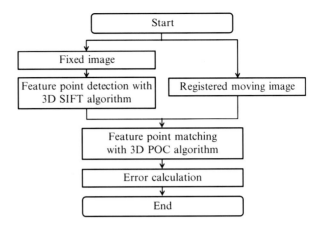

Fig. 1 Framework of registration evaluation

SIFT feature points and that of their candidate correspondences is computed, respectively. Phase components of the image-block pairs in the frequency domain are used to estimate locations of the correspondences. The image-block matching method can achieve high accuracy at the sub-voxel level [15, 29]. Even under rotation, the matching method can give good performance by coarse-to-fine and iterative procedures. As a result, it is possible to measure a registration error by using the distance between the SIFT keypoints and their correspondences. Note that although this work focuses on registration validation on thoracic CT images, the proposed method can be extended to different types and modalities of images, since both the feature detection and image matching algorithms can be applied to general image data.

Feature Point Detection

In this work, a 3D landmark detector is required to extract fiducial landmarks as reference points for spatial accuracy evaluation of image registration. Harkens et al. [16] investigated nine 3D differential operators for the detection of anatomical landmarks in medical images. Recently, the SIFT detector and descriptor introduced by Lowe [17] has become very popular and been widely adopted in research work of medical imaging [14, 18–21, 30]. In this work, SIFT detector, which was extended to 3D in [14, 20], is also adopted to extract candidates of fiducial landmarks for registration evaluation.

Candidate Feature Point Detection

Original SIFT feature points are detected by using difference-of-Gaussian (DoG) images [17]. For a medical image, which is usually a 3D volume, the DoG images can be computed as follows [14]:

Fig. 2 Framework of registration evaluation

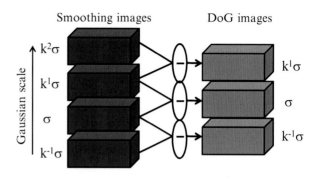

Fig. 3 Local extrema detection. This figure is a modified version of Fig. 2 in [14]

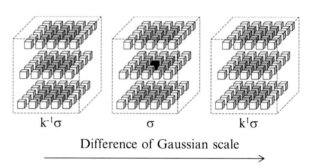

$$D(x, y, z, \sigma) = L(x, y, z, k\sigma) - L(x, y, z, \sigma), \tag{1}$$

where k is a constant multiplicative factor. $L(x,y,z,\sigma)$ is obtained by smoothing the original image $I(x,y,z)$ with a variable-scale Gaussian filter $G(x,y,z,\sigma)$:

$$L(x, y, z, \sigma) = G(x, y, z, \sigma) \times I(x, y, z) = \frac{1}{\left(\sqrt{2\pi}\sigma\right)^3} e^{-\left(x^2+y^2+z^2\right)/2\sigma^2} \times I(x, y, z). \tag{2}$$

Figure 2 illustrates the computation of a group of DoG images. Using such DoG images, local extrema can be detected at the pyramid level of σ. For a voxel v in a DoG image with scale σ, the intensity of v is compared with those of its 80 neighbor voxels (26 neighbor points at the same scale σ, and 27 counterparts at the scale of $k^1\sigma$ and $k^{-1}\sigma$, respectively). The voxel with the most or least extreme value of intensity is considered as a candidate of feature point. Figure 3 illustrates the procedures of local extrema detection. In this work, multi-scale searching parameters are set as that $k = 2.0^{1/3}$ and $\sigma = \{1.00, 1.26, 1.58, 2.00, 2.52, 3.17, 4.00\}$.

Feature Point Refinement and Filtering

For 3D medical images, a large number of candidate feature points, i.e., the scale-space extrema, are usually detected. It is necessary to eliminate candidates that have low contrast or are poorly localized along edges. Moreover, locations of the feature points are needed to be refined to provide better accuracy. In 2D SIFT algorithm [17], an approach was developed to estimate the feature point locations, combined with a thresholding on the local contrast. In addition, edge-like features were removed by testing the relative ratios of 2D Hessian eigenvalues. In this work, following the work in [20], the feature point refinement and filtering procedures are extended to 3D.

Feature Point Localization Refinement

The initial implementation of 2D SIFT [24] simply located keypoints at the coordinate of the detected maxima or minima. Brown and Lowe [25] developed a method for fitting a 3D quadratic function to the local sample points to determine the interpolated locations and scales of the extrema. For 3D medical images, this approach was extended to a fitting problem for a 4D scale-space function, $D(x,y,z,\sigma)$ [20]. The Taylor expansion (up to the quadratic terms) of $D(x,y,z,\sigma)$, at a certain point $\mathbf{x} = (x,y,z,\sigma)^T$, is formulated:

$$D(\mathbf{x}) = D + \frac{\partial D^T}{\partial \mathbf{x}} \mathbf{x} + \frac{1}{2}\mathbf{x}^T \frac{\partial^2 D}{\partial \mathbf{x}^2}\mathbf{x},\tag{3}$$

The location of the extremum, $\hat{\mathbf{x}}$, is determined by taking the derivative of this function with respect to $\mathbf{x}$ and setting it to 0:

$$\frac{\partial D}{\partial \mathbf{x}} + \frac{\partial^2 D}{\partial \mathbf{x}^2}\hat{\mathbf{x}} = 0.\tag{4}$$

Therefore, the sub-voxel location of the extreme is obtained:

$$\hat{\mathbf{x}} = -\frac{\partial^2 D}{\partial \mathbf{x}^2}^{-1} \cdot \frac{\partial D}{\partial \mathbf{x}}.\tag{5}$$

As suggested by Brown and Lowe [25], the Hessian and the derivative of D are approximated by using finite differences of neighboring points.

Removal of Low-Contrast Feature Points

The function value at the extremum, $D(\hat{\mathbf{x}})$, is useful for rejecting unstable extrema with low contrast. $D(\hat{\mathbf{x}})$ can be obtained by substituting (5) into (3):

$$D(\hat{\mathbf{x}}) = D + \frac{1}{2}\frac{\partial D^T}{\partial \mathbf{x}}\hat{\mathbf{x}}.\tag{6}$$

In 2D SIFT method [17], all extrema with a value of $D(\hat{\mathbf{x}})$ less than 0.03 were discarded experimentally. In [20], the threshold of 0.03 was suggested for CT images, whereas a less selective value of 0.01 was suggested for the less contrasted appearance of MR and CBCT images.

Rejecting Poorly Localized Points Along Edges

For stability of image matching, it is not sufficient to reject keypoints with low contrast. The DoG function will have a strong response along edges, even if the location along the edge is poorly determined and unstable to small amount of noise. Such edge responses were eliminated by using the ratio of eigenvalues of 2D Hessian matrix [17].

In this work, adopting an approach developed in [20], the elimination of poorly localized feature points is extended to 3D. Feature points localized along edges and along ridges, other than blob-like structures, are rejected. Such blob-like structures can be characterized by the following properties:

(a) All principal curvatures are of the same sign.
(b) They all have a magnitude of the same order.

Feature points that satisfy the above two conditions are considered as fiducial landmarks for registration evaluation in this work.

Similar to the 2D case, edge responses in 3D space can be measured by a 3×3 Hessian matrix:

$$H = \begin{bmatrix} D_{xx} & D_{xy} & D_{xz} \\ D_{xy} & D_{yy} & D_{yz} \\ D_{xz} & D_{yz} & D_{zz} \end{bmatrix}. \tag{7}$$

The matrix is computed from finite differences at the location and scale of the feature point. And the principal curvatures are proportional to the eigenvalues of $\mathbf{H}$ [26]. Let $\alpha \geq \beta \geq \gamma$ be the three largest eigenvalues in decreasing order of signed magnitude. The trace and the determinant of $\mathbf{H}$ can be computed as:

$$\mathrm{tr}(\mathbf{H}) = \alpha + \beta + \gamma = D_{xx} + D_{yy} + D_{zz}; \tag{8}$$

$$\det(\mathbf{H}) = \alpha\beta\gamma$$

$$= D_{xx}D_{yy}D_{zz} + 2D_{xy}D_{yz}D_{zz} - D_{xx}\left(D_{yz}\right)^2 - D_{yy}\left(D_{xz}\right)^2 - D_{zz}\left(D_{xy}\right)^2. \tag{9}$$

In addition, the sum of principal second-order minors $\sum \det \frac{P}{2}(\mathbf{H})$ is computed as:

$$\left| \sum \det_2^P(\mathbf{H}) \right| = \beta\gamma + \gamma\alpha + \alpha\beta$$

$$= D_{yy}D_{zz} - \left(D_{yz}\right)^2 + D_{zz}D_{xx} - \left(D_{xz}\right)^2 + D_{xx}D_{yy} - \left(D_{xy}\right)^2, \tag{10}$$

When the eigenvalues are either all positive or all negative, condition (a) is satisfied, which corresponds to a dark blob or a bright blob, respectively [27]. This is equivalent to the condition:

$$\sum \det_2^P(\mathbf{H}) > 0, \quad \text{and} \quad \text{tr}(\mathbf{H}) \ \det(\mathbf{H}) > 0. \tag{11}$$

In order to satisfy condition (b) to reject plate-like or tubular structures, let r and s be the ratios such that $\alpha = r\beta$ and $\beta = s\gamma$. Then,

$$\frac{\text{tr}(\mathbf{H})^3}{\det(\mathbf{H})} = \frac{(rs + s + 1)^3}{rs^2}, \tag{12}$$

which depends only on the ratio of the eigenvalues rather than their individual values, and increases with both rs and s. In order to check that the ratio $t = rs$ of principal curvatures is below some threshold, t_{max}, we only need to check:

$$\frac{\text{tr}(\mathbf{H})^3}{\det(\mathbf{H})} < \frac{(2t_{max} + 1)^3}{t_{max}^2}. \tag{13}$$

Otherwise, features look more like edges or ridges than blobs, and are discarded. In [20], an upper threshold $t_{max} = 5$ was experimentally determined for CT images, whereas $t_{max} = 20$ was found to be suited to MR and CBCT images.

Feature Point Matching

To measure distance between the reference points and their correspondences, an image matching method based on a 3D phase-only correlation (POC) function is applied. The original POC function [22, 31, 32] was calculated with a 2D DFT to estimate displacement between image blocks, and it was extended to a 3D implementation while maintaining good performance [15, 29].

3D Phase-Only Correlation Function

POC function [22] is a correlation function used in the phase-based image matching to evaluate similarity between two images. According to [22], image matching with POC can achieve sub-pixel accuracy, and it can be extended to 3D while maintaining the excellent performance [15, 29]. This section will introduce the 3D POC function which is applied in image matching of the accuracy evaluation.

Consider two $N_1 \times N_2 \times N_3$ volumes $r(n_1,n_2,n_3)$ and $f(n_1,n_2,n_3)$, where $n_1 = -M_1, \ldots, M_1, n_2 = -M_2, \ldots, M_2, n_3 = -M_3, \ldots, M_3$ and $N_1 = 2M_1 + 1$, $N_2 = 2M_2 + 1$, $N_3 = 2M_3 + 1$. The 3D DFT of the two volumes is given by

$$R(k_1, k_2, k_3) = \sum_{n_1,n_2,n_3} r(n_1, n_2, n_3) W_{N_1}^{k_1 n_1} W_{N_2}^{k_2 n_2} W_{N_3}^{k_3 n_3}$$

$$= A_R(k_1, k_2, k_3) e^{j\theta_R(k_1,k_2,k_3)}, \tag{14}$$

$$F(k_1, k_2, k_3) = \sum_{n_1,n_2,n_3} f(n_1, n_2, n_3) W_{N_1}^{k_1 n_1} W_{N_2}^{k_2 n_2} W_{N_3}^{k_3 n_3}$$

$$= A_F(k_1, k_2, k_3) e^{j\theta_F(k_1,k_2,k_3)}, \tag{15}$$

where $k_1 = -M_1, \ldots, M_1, k_2 = -M_2, \ldots, M_2, k_3 = -M_3, \ldots, M_3$ and $W_{N_1} = e^{-j\frac{2\pi}{N_1}}, W_{N_2} = e^{-j\frac{2\pi}{N_2}}, W_{N_3} = e^{-j\frac{2\pi}{N_3}}$. $A_R(k_1,k_2,k_3)$ and $A_F(k_1,k_2,k_3)$ are amplitude components, and $e^{j\theta_R(k_1,k_2,k_3)}$ and $e^{j\theta_F(k_1,k_2,k_3)}$ are phase components. The normalized cross spectrum $\hat{P}(k_1, k_2, k_3)$ is defined as

$$\hat{P}(k_1, k_2, k_3) = \frac{R(k_1, k_2, k_3)\overline{F(k_1, k_2, k_3)}}{\left| R(k_1, k_2, k_3)\overline{F(k_1, k_2, k_3)} \right|} = e^{j\{\theta_R(k_1,k_2,k_3) - \theta_F(k_1,k_2,k_3)\}}, \tag{16}$$

where $\overline{F(k_1,k_2,k_3)}$ denotes the complex conjugate of $F(k_1,k_2,k_3)$. The POC function $\hat{p}(n_1, n_2, n_3)$ between $r(n_1,n_2,n_3)$ and $f(n_1,n_2,n_3)$ is the 3D inverse DFT (3D IDFT) of $\hat{P}(k_1, k_2, k_3)$, and is given by

$$\hat{p}(n_1, n_2, n_3) = \frac{1}{N_1 N_2 N_3} \sum_{k_1,k_2,k_3} \hat{P}(k_1, k_2, k_3) W_{N_1}^{-k_1 n_1} W_{N_2}^{-k_2 n_2} W_{N_3}^{-k_3 n_3}. \tag{17}$$

If two image volumes are similar, their POC function gives a distinct sharp peak. If not, the peak drops significantly. The height of the peak can be used as a good similarity measure for image matching, and the location of the peak shows the displacement between the two image volumes.

In order to illustrate how to estimate the sub-voxel displacement between two volumes, let $(\delta_1,\delta_2,\delta_3)$ represent a sub-voxel displacement, and $f(n_1,n_2,n_3)$ be the displaced volume of $r(n_1,n_2,n_3)$ with $(\delta_1,\delta_2,\delta_3)$, i.e., $f(n_1,n_2,n_3) = r(n_1 - \delta_1, n_2 - \delta_2, n_3 - \delta_3)$. In this case, the normalized cross spectrum and the POC function of $r(n_1,n_2,n_3)$ and $f(n_1,n_2,n_3)$ become

$$\hat{P}(k_1, k_2, k_3) \cong W_{N_1}^{-k_1 \delta_1} \cdot W_{N_2}^{-k_2 \delta_2} \cdot W_{N_3}^{-k_3 \delta_3}, \tag{18}$$

$$\hat{p}(n_1, n_2, n_3) \cong \frac{\alpha}{N_1 N_2 N_3} \cdot \frac{\sin\left(\pi(n_1 + \delta_1)\right)}{\sin\left(\frac{\pi}{N_1}(n_1 + \delta_1)\right)} \cdot \frac{\sin\left(\pi(n_2 + \delta_2)\right)}{\sin\left(\frac{\pi}{N_2}(n_2 + \delta_2)\right)}$$

$$\cdot \frac{\sin\left(\pi(n_3 + \delta_3)\right)}{\sin\left(\frac{\pi}{N_3}(n_3 + \delta_3)\right)}. \tag{19}$$

For image matching, the similarity between two images can be estimated by the peak value α, and the image displacement can be estimated by the peak position $(\delta_1, \delta_2, \delta_3)$.

Techniques for High-Accuracy Image Matching Using 3D POC

This section will introduce some techniques for high-accuracy sub-voxel image matching in 3D POC matching algorithm [15, 29].

Windowing to Reduce Boundary Effects

Due to the DFT's periodicity, an image can be considered to "wrap around" at a border, as a result, discontinuities which are not supposed to exist in real world, occur at every border in 3D DFT computation. In order to reduce such discontinuity, 3D window function can be applied to the input volumes. Referring to [29], a 3D Hanning window is used:

$$\omega(n_1, n_2, n_3) = \frac{1 + \cos\left(\frac{\pi n_1}{M_1}\right)}{2} \cdot \frac{1 + \cos\left(\frac{\pi n_2}{M_2}\right)}{2} \cdot \frac{1 + \cos\left(\frac{\pi n_3}{M_3}\right)}{2}. \tag{20}$$

Spectral Weighting Function

For natural images, typically the high frequency components may have less reliability (low S/N ratio) compared with the low frequency components. A low-pass-type weighting function $H(k_1, k_2, k_3)$ can be applied to $\hat{P}(k_1, k_2, k_3)$ in frequency domain and eliminate the high frequency components. The useful weighting function is the DFT of 3D Gaussian function defined as [29]

$$H(k_1, k_2, k_3) = e^{-2\pi^2\sigma^2\left\{\left(\frac{k_1}{n_1}\right)^2 + \left(\frac{k_2}{n_2}\right)^2 + \left(\frac{k_3}{n_3}\right)^2\right\}}, \tag{21}$$

where σ is a parameter that controls the pass-band width. When calculating the POC function, $\hat{P}(k_1, k_2, k_3)$ is multiplied by $H(k_1, k_2, k_3)$ in frequency domain. Therefore, (19) becomes

$$\hat{p}(n_1, n_2, n_3) = \frac{1}{N_1 N_2 N_3} \sum_{k_1, k_2, k_3} H(k_1, k_2, k_3)\hat{P}(k_1, k_2, k_3) W_{N_1}^{-k_1 n_1} W_{N_2}^{-k_2 n_2} W_{N_3}^{-k_3 n_3}$$

$$\cong \frac{\alpha}{2\pi\sigma^2} e^{-\left((n_1+\delta_1)^2 + (n_2+\delta_2)^2 + (n_3+\delta_3)^2\right)/2\sigma^2}. \tag{22}$$

Peak Estimation of POC Function

By calculating the POC function, one can obtain a data array of $\hat{p}(n_1, n_2, n_3)$ for each discrete index (n_1, n_2, n_3). It is possible to find the location of the peak that may exist between image voxels by fitting the function in (22) to the data array around the correlation peak [31], where α, δ_1, δ_2, and δ_3 are fitting parameters. When the POC function obtains the maximum value at $n_1 = a_1$, $n_2 = a_2$, and $n_3 = a_3$, where a_1, a_2, a_3 are integers, δ_1 can be estimated by

$$\delta_1 = \frac{\log\{\hat{p}(a_1 + 1)\} - \log\{\hat{p}(a_1 - 1)\}}{2\log\{\hat{p}(a_1 - 1)\} - 4\log\{\hat{p}(a_1)\} + 2\log\{\hat{p}(a_1 + 1)\}} - a_1, \tag{23}$$

where $\hat{p}(n_1) = p(n_1, n_2, n_3)\big|_{n_2=a_2, n_3=a_3}$. The estimation of δ_2 and δ_3 is in the same way. Using the estimated δ_1, δ_2, δ_3, and (22), peak value of the POC function can be obtained:

$$\alpha = \sqrt{2\pi}\sigma \cdot \hat{p}(a_1, a_2, a_3) \cdot e^{\frac{(a_1+\delta_1)^2 + (a_2+\delta_2)^2 + (a_3+\delta_3)^2}{2\sigma^2}}. \tag{24}$$

Procedures of 3D POC Image Matching

The procedures of image matching using the 3D POC function are described in this section. The algorithm consists of two stages [29, 31, 32]: coarse-to-fine voxel-level correspondence estimation and sub-voxel-level estimation. Figure 4 illustrates the overview of the coarse-to-fine correspondence search procedures.

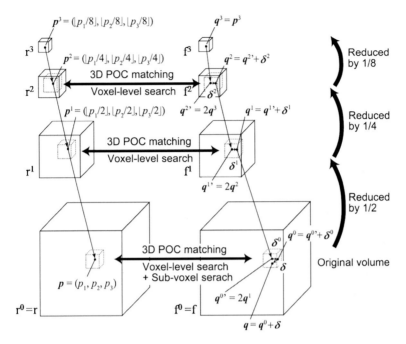

Fig. 4 Coarse-to-fine search procedures. This figure is a modified version of Fig. 1 in [29]

Voxel-Level Estimation

The correspondence search performs POC-based volume block matching, which starts at the coarsest volume layer, and moves the operation to finer layers gradually. Let $p = (p_1, p_2, p_3)$ be one of the reference points in image r, and $q = (q_1, q_2, q_3)$ be the corresponding point in image f, which is the target of the volume block matching.

Step 1
For $l = 1, 2, \cdots, l_{max}$, create volumes r^l and f^l in the l-th layer, i.e., coarser versions of r and f, recursively as follows:

$$r^{l+1}(n_1, n_2, n_3) = \frac{1}{8} \sum_{b_1, b_2, b_3} r^l(2n_1 + b_1, 2n_2 + b_2, 2n_3 + b_3), \qquad (25)$$

$$f^{l+1}(n_1, n_2, n_3) = \frac{1}{8} \sum_{b_1, b_2, b_3} f^l(2n_1 + b_1, 2n_2 + b_2, 2n_3 + b_3), \qquad (26)$$

where $b_1, b_2, b_3 \in \{0,1\}$, and $r^0 = r, f^0 = f$.

Step 2
Assume that at the coarsest layer l_{max}, the coordinates of reference point and their correspondence are the same, which are as follows:

$$p^{l_{max}} = \left(\left|2^{-l_{max}}p_1\right|, \left|2^{-l_{max}}p_2\right|, \left|2^{-l_{max}}p_3\right|\right), \tag{27}$$

$$q^{l_{max}} = \left(\left|2^{-l_{max}}p_1\right|, \left|2^{-l_{max}}p_2\right|, \left|2^{-l_{max}}p_3\right|\right). \tag{28}$$

Next, let $l = l_{max} - 1$, and move to Step 3.

Step 3
At the l-th layer, the coordinate of the reference point p^l is as follows:

$$p^l = \left(\left|2^{-l}p_1\right|, \left|2^{-l}p_2\right|, \left|2^{-l}p_3\right|\right), \tag{29}$$

and the initial value q^l of the correspondence q^l is given by:

$$q^l = 2q^{l+1}. \tag{30}$$

Step 4
For the volume r^l, a searching window (a 3D volume block) centered at p^l is set. Similarly, for the volume f^l, a searching window centered at q^l is also set. According to Sect. 4.1, the displacement δ^l in voxel level can be estimated with the peak position of the POC function of the above two searching blocks. As a result, the coordinate of the correspondence at the l-th layer can be obtained:

$$q^l = q^l + \delta^l. \tag{31}$$

Step 5
Let $l = l - 1$, and iteratively repeat Steps 3–5 until $l = 0$.

Sub-voxel-Level Estimation

At the sub-voxel-level estimation stage, the correspondence search is performed at the basic image layer, i.e., $l = 0$. For the volume $r = r^0$, a searching window centered at $p = (p_1, p_2, p_3)$ is set. Similarly, for the volume $f = f^0$, a searching window centered at q^0 is also set, where q^0 is obtained at the voxel-level estimation stage with (31). The sub-voxel displacement δ can be obtained with the 3D POC function of the searching blocks in the sub-voxel-level estimation stage, using (23). As a result, coordinate of the correspondence in sub-voxel level can be obtained by:

$$q = q^0 + \delta. \tag{32}$$

Iterative Processing

When transformation such as rotation is occurred on the image blocks, it is difficult to obtain accurate matching results by a single run of POC matching. In this case, iterative processing is necessary. Firstly, a rigid transformation is obtained by an initial matching. The transformation is applied to the moving image to reduce the rotation between the image-pairs. Then, block matching is performed again, followed by a resulted transformation. Experimentally, three to five runs of such iterative processing are able to give good matching results for registration evaluation in this work.

Combination of 3D SIFT Detection and 3D POC Matching

Since 3D POC can provide accurate image matching results, it is supposed that distance between corresponding landmark pairs can be used to validate accuracy of an image registration. However, one of the main problems in 3D POC matching is the selection of reference points. In [29], the reference points for image matching are determined by CT value empirically, but this determination is not appropriate for registration evaluation. In this work, 3D SIFT keypoint detector is applied to detect fiducial points in fixed images. Corresponding points in registered moving images are then searched for and localized using the 3D POC image matching. In Sect. 5 of this chapter, it will be proved that the distance between the SIFT feature points and their correspondences (localized by 3D POC image matching) is an appropriate measure of image registration error.

Outlier Removal

Since the accuracy of landmark matching affects the reliability of registration evaluation, outliers in the image matching need to be removed. In this work, a RANSAC algorithm [23] is applied as follows:

Step 1
Randomly select three landmark pairs from the obtained corresponding landmarks p_i and q_i, and estimate a rigid transformation $T_R(x)$, from the selected landmark pairs, where x represents a certain landmark.

Step 2
Apply the rigid transformation to all of the landmarks p_i, and compute the distance between the transformed landmarks and their corresponding ones:
$d_i^2 = q_i - T_R(p_i)^2$.

Step 3

When landmark-pair-distance is smaller than a threshold f_{th}, such landmarks are considered as inliers. Threshold f_{th} is computed by $f_{th} = F_{m_r}^{-1}(\alpha_r)\sigma_r^2$, where $F_{m_r}^{-1}(\alpha_r)$ represents the threshold value of Chi-square distribution with the degrees of freedom m_r; α_r is the proportion of inliers that are determined by the threshold; σ_r is the standard deviation of d_i. In this work, $\alpha_r = 0.9$ is experimentally determined, and the degrees of freedom is $m_r = 3$. As a result, the threshold value is $F_3^{-1}(0.9) = 6.251$.

Step 4

Estimate the iteration number by

$$N_r = \frac{\log(1 - \xi)}{\log\left(1 - (1 - \epsilon)^2\right)}, \tag{33}$$

where ϵ is the current proportion of outliers. Equation (33) ensures that within N_r trials, the probability to obtain a sample set with no outliers is ξ. ξ is set as 0.99 in this work.

Step 5

Repeat Steps 1–4 until the iteration number exceeds N_r.

Step 6

Select the obtained inliers with the largest number within N_r trials.

Experimental Results

In this section, experimental results will be given. Firstly, the accuracy of the image matching based on 3D POC function is measured to prove the effectiveness of the algorithm for image registration evaluation. In the rest experiments, clinical data are used to evaluate the performance of deformable image registration algorithms.

3D Feature Point Matching Error

Five sets of lung CT images of five patients from DIR-Lab dataset [11] were used to validate the accuracy of feature point matching in this work. Fixed and moving images were set as the maximum inhalation and exhalation component phase images, respectively. Each image was cropped to include the entire rib cage and subsampled to 256×256 voxels in the axial plane. The image resolution is 0.97–1.16 mm in the axial plane and 2.5 mm in the z-direction.

　　Pulmonary landmark feature points, typically vessel bifurcations, were manually annotated on the five image-pairs by experts in thoracic imaging. The number of

Table 1 Parameters of POC matching algorithm

Number of coarse-to-fine levels	$l_{max} = 3$
Iteration times	$t_{iter} = 5$
Block size in voxel-level search	$16 \times 16 \times 16$ [voxel]
Block size in sub-voxel-level search	$16 \times 16 \times 16$ [voxel]

Table 2 Inter-observer error and point matching error [mm]

	Case 1	Case 2	Case 3	Case 4	Case 5	Mean
Inter-observer error	0.83	0.74	1.14	0.79	0.95	0.89
Point matching error	0.97	0.93	1.12	1.32	1.40	1.15

registered feature pairs per image-pair ranged from 1,166 to 1,561. For each image-pair, a random set of 300 landmark pairs are publicly available [11].

In this work, such landmark pairs were used to validate the accuracy of the POC matching algorithm. Landmarks on fixed images of the dataset were used as reference points of the POC method, and 3D Euclidean distance of the matched corresponding points and the annotated points on moving images was computed as point matching error. The parameters of the POC matching algorithm are listed in Table 1. Mean computation time of 300 points for the POC matching algorithm was about 6 s.

Such matching error was compared to the repeated registration error measured by Castillo et al. [11]. In [11], random samples of 200 annotated landmarks on each fixed image were selected, and the corresponding landmarks on moving images were re-annotated by a secondary reader. The inter-observer registration error was quantified as the 3D Euclidean distance between the original landmarks on the moving images and the corresponding points re-annotated by the secondary reader. In this work, the matching error of the POC method was compared with the inter-observer error measured in [11]. Table 2 shows the error measurement results.

Mean inter-observer registration error of the five image-pairs in [11] was 0.89 mm, while the point matching error measured in this work was 1.15 mm. One should note that the random point-sets selected in the two experiments are not the same, and the point matching error is larger than the inter-observer registration error only in a small extent. It can be concluded that the POC matching algorithm can provide high accuracy for 3D landmark matching and that it is effective for measuring spatial error of registration quantitatively.

Evaluation of Deformable Registration Results

In the rest parts of the experiments, a deformable registration algorithm based on free-form deformation (FFD) with B-spine functions [28] was developed and evaluated by using the SIFT feature point detection and POC matching techniques in this work.

Clinical data used in the registration experiments are the same data used in Sect. 5.1. The FFD-based deformable registration was applied to the lung CT image-pairs, and registered moving images were created according to the registration results.

In the evaluation experiments, firstly, to improve the point matching accuracy and computational efficiency, lung regions of fixed images were roughly segmented. A CT value threshold (250–800) was experimentally set, and voxels that have a CT value within the threshold range were considered as being inside of the lung regions. SIFT feature points were detected in such regions of each fixed image. Then, the POC matching algorithm was performed to estimate locations of the corresponding points in the registered moving images. The number of SIFT feature points detected from each fixed image was from 1,702 to 3,140. Mean 3D Euclidean distances between SIFT feature points in the fixed images and the matched correspondences in the moving images were computed as the automatically measured spatial errors.

The running time of SIFT feature point detection was about 4 s, and that of POC matching was about 27–48 s. All the evaluation tasks were run on a system with Intel$^{\circledR}$ Core™ i7 3.07-GHz CPU and 12-GB memory. Example results of landmark matching for evaluating a deformable registration are given in Fig. 5 ((a): fixed image; (b): moving image after registration). It is clear that every fiducial point in the fixed image has a corresponding point that is accurately located in the registered moving image.

As ground-truth data for accuracy evaluation, manually annotated landmarks of the DIR-Lab dataset mentioned in Sect. 5.1 were used. Manually evaluated spatial errors were measured by using distances between the annotated landmarks and the transformed corresponding points in the moving images. These manually measured errors were compared with the automatically measured errors, and the results are plotted in Fig. 6. It is clear from the figure that the spatial errors obtained in this work are similar with those obtained by using manually annotated landmarks. In other words, the registration evaluation method in this work is effective and is possible to measure spatial errors of deformable registration quantitatively without any manual assessment.

Conclusion

In the work of this chapter, a method for quantitatively evaluating deformable image registration in an automatic way is developed. With this method, fiducial points of fixed images for the evaluation are detected by 3D SIFT keypoint detector, and corresponding points in the registered moving images are localized with 3D POC image matching algorithm. Experimental results show that the developed

Fig. 5 Example results of landmark matching. (**a**) Fixed image. (**b**) Moving image after registration

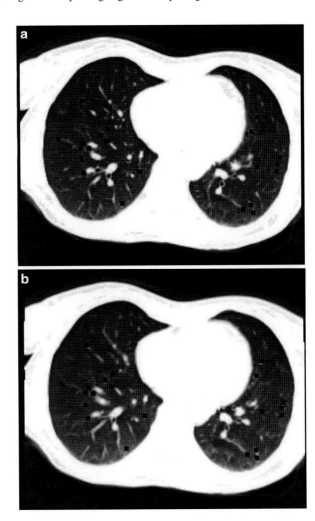

Fig. 6 Comparisons of registration evaluation results

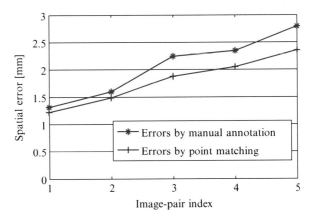

method can provide high enough accuracy that the distance between the fiducial/ corresponding point pairs can be used to measure image registration error. With the proposed method, users can assess their own image data with different registration algorithms quantitatively and automatically.

Acknowledgements The clinical data and the annotated landmarks used in the experiments of this work were provided by Richard Castillo et al., the Deformable Image Registration Laboratory (DIR-Lab), the University of Texas, M.D. Anderson Cancer Center. We would like to thank DIR-Lab for hosting and providing free access to the dataset.

References

1. Hajnal JV (2001) Medical image registration. CRC, Boca Raton
2. West J, Fitzpatrick JM, Wang MY, Dawant BM, Maurer CR Jr, Kessler RM, Maciunas RJ, Barillot C, Lemoine D, Collignon A (1997) Comparison and evaluation of retrospective intermodality brain image registration techniques. J Comput Assist Tomogr 21(4):554–568
3. Lu W, Chen M-L, Olivera GH, Ruchala KJ, Mackie TR (2004) Fast free-form deformable registration via calculus of variations. Phys Med Biol 49(14):3067–3087
4. Guerrero T, Zhang G, Huang TC, Lin KP (2004) Intrathoracic tumor motion estimation from CT imaging using the 3D optical flow method. Phys Med Biol 49(17):41–47
5. Wang H, Dong L, O'Daniel J, Mohan R, Garden AS, Ang KK, Kuban DA, Bonnen M, Chang JY, Cheung R (2005) Validation of an accelerated 'demons' algorithm for deformable image registration in radiation therapy. Phys Med Biol 50(12):2887–2906
6. Kashani R, Hub M, Balter JM, Kessler ML, Dong L, Zhang L, Xing L, Xie Y, Hawkes D, Schnabel JA (2008) Objective assessment of deformable image registration in radiotherapy: a multi-institution study. Medical physics 35:5944–5953
7. Christensen GE, Geng X, Kuhl JG, Bruss J, Grabowski TJ, Pirwani IA, Vannier MW, Allen JS, Damasio H (2006) Introduction to the non-rigid image registration evaluation project (NIREP). In: Biomedical image registration. Springer. Berlin Heidelberg pp 128–135
8. Klein A, Andersson J, Ardekani BA, Ashburner J, Avants B, Chiang M-C, Christensen GE, Collins DL, Gee J, Hellier P (2009) Evaluation of 14 nonlinear deformation algorithms applied to human brain MRI registration. Neuroimage 46(3):786–802
9. Yassa MA, Stark CE (2009) A quantitative evaluation of cross-participant registration techniques for MRI studies of the medial temporal lobe. Neuroimage 44(2):319–327
10. Brock KK (2010) Results of a multi-institution deformable registration accuracy study (MIDRAS). Int J Radiat Oncol Biol Phys 76(2):583–596
11. Castillo R, Castillo E, Guerra R, Johnson VE, McPhail T, Garg AK, Guerrero T (2009) A framework for evaluation of deformable image registration spatial accuracy using large landmark point sets. Phys Med Biol 54(7):1849–1870
12. Wu Z, Rietzel E, Boldea V, Sarrut D, Sharp GC (2008) Evaluation of deformable registration of patient lung 4DCT with subanatomical region segmentations. Med Phys 35:775–781
13. Murphy K et al (2011) Evaluation of registration methods on thoracic CT: the EMPIRE10 challenge. IEEE Trans Med Imaging 30(11):1901–1920
14. Cheung W, Hamarneh G (2009) N-SIFT: n-dimensional scale invariant feature transform. IEEE Trans Image Process 18(9):2012–2021
15. Miyazawa K, Tajima Y, Ito K, Aoki T, Katsumata A, Kobayashi K (2009) A novel approach for volume registration using 3D phase-only correlation. Radiological Society of North America (RSNA), Chicago, USA p 1070.

16. Hartkens T, Rohr K, Stiehl HS (2002) Evaluation of 3D operators for the detection of anatomical point landmarks in MR and CT images. Comput Vis Image Understanding 86(2):118–136
17. Lowe DG (2004) Distinctive image features from scale-invariant keypoints. Int J Comput Vis 60(2):91–110
18. Urschler M, Zach C, Ditt H, Bischof H (2006) Automatic point landmark matching for regularizing nonlinear intensity registration: application to thoracic CT images. In: Medical image computing and computer-assisted intervention–MICCAI 2006, Copenhagen, Denmark pp 710–717
19. Kwon D, Yun ID, Lee KH, Lee S. U (2008) Efficient feature-based nonrigid registration of multiphase liver CT volumes. In: BMVC08, Leeds, UK pp 36.1–36.10
20. Allaire S, Kim JJ, Breen SL, Jaffray DA, Pekar V (2008) Full orientation invariance and improved feature selectivity of 3D SIFT with application to medical image analysis. In: Computer vision and pattern recognition workshops, 2008. CVPRW'08. Anchorage, Alaska, USA pp 1–8
21. Ni D, Qu Y, Yang X, Chui YP, Wong T-T, Ho SS, Heng PA (2008) Volumetric ultrasound panorama based on 3D SIFT. In: Medical image computing and computer-assisted intervention–MICCAI 2008, New York, USA pp 52–60.
22. Takita K, Sasaki Y, Higuchi T, Kobayashi K (2003) High-accuracy subpixel image registration based on phase-only correlation. IEICE Trans Fundam Electron Commun Comput Sci 86(8):1925–1934
23. Fischler MA, Bolles RC (1981) Random sample consensus: a paradigm for model fitting with applications to image analysis and automated cartography. Commun ACM 24(6):381–395
24. Lowe DG (1999) Object recognition from local scale-invariant features. In: The proceedings of the seventh IEEE international conference on computer vision, 1999, vol 2, Kerkyra, Greece pp 1150–1157.
25. Brown M, Lowe DG (2002) Invariant features from interest point groups. In: British machine vision conference, Cardiff, Wales, vol 21, pp 656–665
26. Harris C, Stephens M (1988) A combined corner and edge detector. In: Alvey vision conference, vol 15, Manchester, UK pp 147–152
27. Frangi AF, Niessen WJ, Vincken KL, Viergever MA (1998) Multiscale vessel enhancement filtering. In: Medical image computing and computer-assisted intervention-MICCAI'98, Cambridge, MA, USA pp 130–137
28. Rueckert D, Sonoda LI, Hayes C, Hill DLG, Leach MO, Hawkes DJ (1999) Nonrigid registration using free-form deformations: application to breast MR images. IEEE Trans Med Imaging 18(8):712–721
29. Tajima Y, Miyazawa K, Aoki T, Katsumata A, Kobayashi K (2011) High-accuracy volume registration based on 3D phase-only correlation (in Japanese). IEICE Trans Inform Syst J94-D (8):1398–1409
30. Li Z, Kurihara T, Matsuzaki K, Irie T (2012) Evaluation of medical image registration by using 3D SIFT and phase-only correlation. In: Proceedings of the 4th International conference on abdominal imaging: computational and clinical applications, Nice, France pp 255–264
31. Nagashima S, Aoki T, Higuchi T, Kobayashi K (2006) A subpixel image matching technique using phase-only correlation. In: International symposium on intelligent signal processing and communications, 2006. ISPACS'06, Yonago, Japan pp 701–704
32. Muquit MA, Shibahara T (2006) A high-accuracy passive 3D measurement system using phase-based image matching. IEICE Trans Fundam Electron Commun Comput Sci 89(3):686–697

Biography

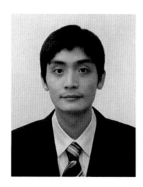

Zisheng Li received B.E. and M.E. degrees from Harbin Engineering University, China, in 2004 and 2007, respectively. He received Ph.D. degree from the University of Electro-Communications, Japan, in 2010. Presently, he is a researcher at Intelligent Media Systems Research Department, Hitachi Central Research Laboratory. His research interests include medical image processing, computer vision, and pattern recognition. He is a member of the Institute of Electronics, Information and Communication Engineers of Japan, and the International Association for Pattern Recognition.

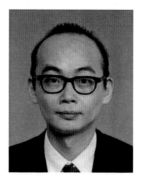

Tsuneya Kurihara is a senior researcher at Hitachi Central Research Laboratory. He received B.E. and M.E. degrees from the University of Tokyo in 1981 and 1983, respectively. He received a Ph.D. in Science from the University of Tokyo in 2009. He was a visiting researcher at Swiss Federal Institute of Technology of Lausanne from 1992 to 1993. His research interests include computer graphics, medical image processing, and augmented reality. He received the Nishita Award from the Institute of Image Electronics Engineers of Japan in 2006. He is a member of the Information Processing Society of Japan, the Institute of Image Electronics Engineers of Japan, and ACM SIGGRAPH.

Preclinical Visualization of Hypoxia, Proliferation and Glucose Metabolism in Non-small Cell Lung Cancer and Its Metastasis

Xiao-Feng Li and Yuanyuan Ma

Abstract Lung cancer is responsible for more deaths than any other cancers; most cancer-related deaths are due to the development of metastatic diseases rather than the progression of the primary tumors. Tumor hypoxia has been commonly observed in a broad spectrum of primary solid malignancies, which is associated with tumor progression, increased aggressiveness, enhanced metastatic potential, and poor prognosis. Hypoxic cancer cells are resistant to radiotherapy and some forms of chemotherapy. In this chapter, nuclear molecular imaging microenvironment including hypoxia, proliferation, and glucose metabolism in lung cancer metastases was discussed.

Introduction

Lung cancer is responsible for more deaths than any other cancer, approximately 85 % human lung cancers are non-small cell lung cancer (NSCLC). Most cancer-related deaths are due to the development of metastatic diseases rather than the progression of the primary tumors [1]. Hypoxic cancer cells are generally more resistant to ionizing radiation and chemotherapy than oxic cells, and hypoxia is an important determinant of relapse-free survival and overall clinical outcome [2–4]. Regions of local hypoxia are common features of most human primary solid

X.-F. Li, M.D., Ph.D. (✉)
Department of Diagnostic Radiology, University of Louisville School of Medicine,
530 S. Jackson Street, CCB-C07, Louisville, KY 40202, USA
e-mail: Linucmed@gmail.com

Y. Ma, M.D., Ph.D.
Department of Pathology, Memorial Sloan-Kettering Cancer Center,
1275 York Avenue, New York, NY 10065, USA
e-mail: yyma121@yahoo.com

A.S. El-Baz et al. (eds.), *Abdomen and Thoracic Imaging: An Engineering & Clinical Perspective*, DOI 10.1007/978-1-4614-8498-1_20,
© Springer Science+Business Media New York 2014

cancers [2, 5–7]. It has been recently demonstrated, in animal models of colorectal cancer and NSCLC, peritoneal cavity microscopic metastases of less than 1 mm diameter are extremely hypoxic [8–12].

In studies of macroscopic tumors, pO_2 probe measurements and noninvasive hypoxic tracers imaging are able to assess hypoxia status. However, assessing of hypoxia in micrometastases may require invasive methods [9], relying on detection of either an exogenous substance such as 2-nitroimidazole compounds pimoni-dazole, EF5, and CCI-103F, which are selectively reduced in hypoxic regions of the tumors (generally when pO_2 <10 mmHg) [13] or the expression of endogenous markers of hypoxia such as hypoxia-inducible factor 1α (HIF1α), carbonic anhydrase 9 (CA9), and glucose transporters 1 [13–16]. Microscopically spatial pattern of these markers can be visualized by immunohistochemical methods. Spatial pattern of binding of radiolabeled hypoxia tracers in tumor sections may be visualized by autoradiography. Radiolabeled tracers including ^{18}F-misonidazole (^{18}F-FMISO) [17–19], copper (II)-diacetyl-bis(N(4)-methylthiosemicarbazone) [20–22], and [124]I-labeled iodo-azomycin galactopyranoside [23, 24] among others have developed for imaging tumor hypoxia. Since the presence and the degree of tumor hypoxia affects disease outcome in patients, from the disease management point of view, noninvasive detection hypoxia and also other microenvironmental components in cancers and/or metastases are critically important for cancer managements and outcome prediction.

Hypoxia, Proliferation and Angiogenesis in Micrometastases

We have recently observed the hypoxic status of microscopic tumors established intraperitoneally and intradermally using the HT29 and HCT-8 colorectal cancer lines [8, 9, 25] and NSCLC A549 and HTB177 cells [11, 12] using pimonidazole immunohistochemical staining technique. In general, submillimeter peritoneal tumor deposits showed intense hypoxia (hypoxic fraction as high as 90 %) with little or no blood perfusion; tumors that ranged from 1 mm to 4–5 mm in diameter seemed relatively well vascularized, well perfused, and generally displayed little hypoxia. In tumors larger than 4–5 mm diameter, hypoxia reappeared in the characteristically perinecrotic distribution pattern seen in macroscopic tumors [8, 26] (Fig. 1). Accordingly, severe hypoxia may be a general feature in peritoneal micrometastases. Future studies need to confirm whether this pattern of micro-metastatic diseases found in mouse models also apply to cancer patients.

Micrometastases may have already existed in many patients when primary cancers were initially diagnosed although lack of imaging evidence of distant metastases. Submillimeter metastases in patients may be avascular and in a state of dormancy [27, 28]. Cell proliferation in dormant tumors had been observed, but results were mixed: cells were either found dividing very slowly or in G0 phase [27–30], others have found proliferation in dormant tumors to be as high as in

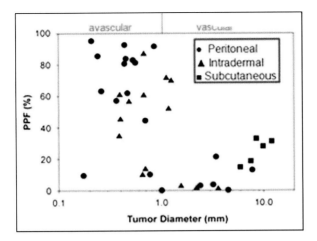

Fig. 1 Scatterplot showing the relationship between tumor size and pimonidazole-positive fraction (PPF) for HT29 tumors. The *x*-axis represents effective tumor diameter (*D*) derived from the cross-sectional area (*A*) of H&E images, $D = 2\sqrt{A/\pi}$ (Li et al. Cancer Res 2007;67:7646)

macroscopic vascularized tumors but that the dormant tumors did not grow beyond a threshold size due to a kinetic balance between proliferation and apoptosis [28, 31], and hypoxia status had not been observed in dormant micrometastases in these studies. In animal model of metastases, we have noted that cellular proliferation was in the nonhypoxic rim, not the interior hypoxic core of submillimeter avascular tumors, whereas proliferating cells were found throughout larger tumors 1–4 mm in diameter which were less hypoxic [8, 9, 25]. This is in good agreement with several studies that cellular proliferation and hypoxia are mutually exclusive in macroscopic tumors [32–34]. Future studies would confirm whether cancer cells in dormant metastases are proliferative; this issue is critically important for systemic chemotherapy, as chemotherapeutic drugs generally target proliferating cancer cells.

Hypoxia has been recognized as a primary physiological regulator of angiogenesis [35, 36]. The existence of severe hypoxia in microscopic tumors may be common irrespective of cell lines and reflects the pre-angiogenic stage of tumor development. As peritoneal and intradermal tumors increased in size to the diameter range ~1–4 mm, there was a drastic reduction in tumor hypoxia coupled with the appearance of functional tumor vascularization [8, 9, 25]. This suggests the sequence of events may be that cells become hypoxic when tumors reach several hundred micrometers, hypoxia drives angiogenesis, previously hypoxic cells become oxygenated, and the neovascularized tumors grow beyond certain size threshold. Apparently, the timing for hypoxia driving angiogenesis switch is critically important for anti-angiogenesis therapy. This is largely unknown in metastases involving other organs and tissues rather than peritoneal cavity.

Animal Models of Metastases

To conduct preclinical study of tumor microenvironment, animal models of cancer and metastases are required. Models of disseminated microscopic malignant disease may be generated in the lung, bone, liver, and peritoneum by intravenous [37–39], left ventricular [37, 40], intrasplenic [41], and intraperitoneal [8, 9, 11, 12, 25] injection of tumor cells, respectively (Fig. 2). We have shown that a model of disseminated microscopic peritoneal and ascites tumors was suitable for studying hypoxia [8, 9, 11, 12, 25]. In the model, disseminated peritoneal microscopic tumors were induced by injecting suspensions of colorectal HT29 and HCT-8 cancer cells or NSCLC A549 and HTB177 cells into the peritoneal cavity of nude mice. Mice sacrificed 4–7 weeks after tumor initiation displayed a distribution of tumors of sizes ranging from a few hundred micrometers up to several millimeters in diameter on or in the intestinal serosa. Ascites fluid containing a distribution of free-floating tumor cell aggregates of up to 1 mm in diameter was frequently presented in mice inoculated with HT29, A549 cells, but was rarely observed in HCT-8 and HTB177 cell lines. Intradermal injection of similar tumor cell suspensions could give rise to unitary microscopic tumors useful for studying hypoxia [8, 25]. An intradermal tumor model has the potential advantage that growth curves for microscopic tumors could be more easily generated via ultrasound or optical imaging. Subcutaneous xenografts generated by subcutaneously injection of cancer cells are widely used for PET study.

Imaging Hypoxia in Metastases

We have recently reviewed that a model system is valid for assessing the microenvironmental features of individual microscopic tumors with targeted PET tracers, including hypoxic status, proliferation, and blood perfusion [10]. Such model system provides a diversity of tumors of differing size and hypoxic status growing in the same animal, thereby reducing or eliminating issues associated with inter-animal variability. To complement the high spatial resolution associated with immunohistochemical detection of hypoxia markers, the intratumoral distribution

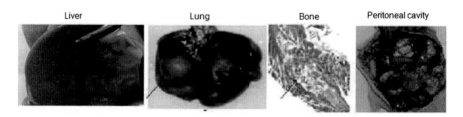

Liver   Lung   Bone   Peritoneal cavity

Fig. 2 Nude mice metastatic models

of radiolabeled hypoxia tracers can be determined by digital autoradiography. Studies comparing the spatial distributions of radiolabeled tracers and hypoxia markers have been reported in macroscopic tumors [22, 33] and microscopic diseases [8].

[18]F-misonidazole [17–19] and [124]I-IAZGP [23, 24, 42] among others are used for in vivo PET imaging of tumor hypoxia. We have recently reported the use of correlative imaging methodologies to examine the uptake of IAZGP and ^{18}F-misonidazole in microscopic [10, 12] and macroscopic [11, 12] tumors and related this to microenviromental factors. Pimonidazole binding and CA9 expression in a small (~1 mm dimension) and relatively large tumor obtained from an animal with disseminated colorectal cancer HT29 peritoneal disease, the smaller tumor shows elevated uptake of ^{131}I-IAZGP and near-ubiquitous staining of pimonidazole and CA9, implying severely hypoxia. The larger tumor shows reduced ^{131}I-IAZGP uptake and low levels of pimonidazole binding and CA9 expression with significant Hoechst 33342 uptake indicating that the tumor was well perfused. Microscopic ascites tumors had high ^{131}I-IAZGP uptake coupled with intense staining of pimonidazole and CA9 [10].

Intratumoral distribution of ^{18}F-misonidazole was observed in subcutaneous xenografts and peritoneal tumors of NSCLC; subcutaneous xenografts and perito-neal metastases were generated utilizing human NSCLC A549 and HTB177 cell types in nude mice. High levels of ^{18}F-FMISO uptake detected by digital autoradiography and pimonidazole binding by immunohistochemical staining were colocalized [11]. Such regions tended to correspond to low levels of cellular proliferation and blood perfusion. Well-oxygenated cancer cells with a high prolif-eration rate had low ^{18}F-misonidazole uptake. Stroma and necrotic zones had lower ^{18}F-misonidazole accumulation [11, 12].

In a PET study [12], we compared the intraperitoneal accumulation of ^{18}F-misonidazole between peritoneal disease-free mice and mice with A549 or HTB177 peritoneal metastases. All image sets for each animal were visually examined using a rotating (cine) three-dimensional display. Figure 3 shows representative PET coronal slices: In metastases-bearing mice, high radioactivity accumulation was found on the left side of abdominal wall, and the overall background in the peritoneal cavity (excluding the intestines) was apparently higher than in the normal mouse. Necropsy revealed that the left peritoneal wall was the site of multiple individual tiny lesions. In both the disease-free and metastases-bearing mice, there was significant uptake of ^{18}F-misonidazole in the gut and bladder and to a lesser extent in the liver. Tumors from the left peritoneal wall were removed for sectioning, H&E staining demonstrated multiple individual micrometastases (generally less 1 mm in diameter), and some of them fused together. The micrometastases had little Hoechst 33342 uptake, indicating a lack of blood perfusion, and a high fraction of pimonidazole binding and high ^{18}F-misonidazole accumulation, indicating severely hypoxic tissue. There was little ^{18}F-misonidazole accumulation in the stroma. Ascites was collected from the peritoneal cavity, and single cells or ascites tumors were harvested by centrifu-gation, and these stained positive for pimonidazole. Therefore, ^{18}F-misonidazole PET is able to detect micrometastases in the peritoneal cavity [12].

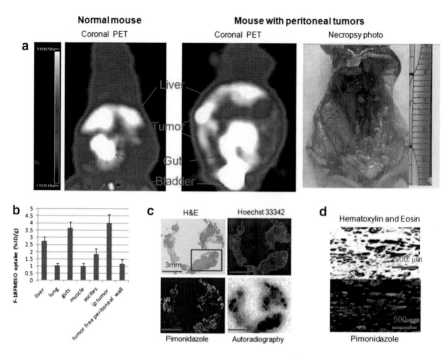

Fig. 3 (a) PET coronal slices of intraperitoneal distribution of ¹⁸F-misonidazole in a peritoneal disease-free mouse (*left*) and a mouse with peritoneal metastases after A549 cell inoculation (*middle*) with necropsy- confirmed peritoneal wall carcinomas (*right*). High radioactivity accumulation was found on the abdominal wall as indicated, and the overall background in the peritoneal cavity (excluding guts) was apparently higher than control. (b) ¹⁸F-misonidazole (¹⁸F-FMISO) distribution in A549 i.p. tumors in mice (*n* = 5). (c) Multiple individual lesions attaching to the peritoneal wall where PET imaging had revealed a high level of ¹⁸F-misonidazole: Hematoxylin and Eosin stain showing multiple individual micrometastases (generally less 1 mm in diameter) which had little Hoechst 33342 uptake, associated with a high fraction of pimonidazole binding and high ¹⁸F-misonidazole accumulation by autoradiography. (d) Single cells or ascites tumors harvested from ascites of the mouse were stained positive for pimonidazole, Hematoxylin and Eosin stain provides as a reference. All scale bars are as indicated. Adapted from [12]

Figure 4 shows a representative ¹⁸F-misonidazole PET mid-coronal slice of a macroscopic A549 subcutaneous tumor, showing considerable heterogeneity in the spatial distribution of the tracer. Autoradiography, pimonidazole, glucose transporter-1 expression, and Hoechst 33342 images were obtained on the same section, and H&E staining was performed on an adjacent section. ¹⁸F-misonidazole colocalized with pimonidazole, which was roughly similar to glucose transporter 1, and these regions mutually excluded Hoechst 33342. Regions of low pimonidazole binding also had low ¹⁸F-misonidazole uptake. Necrosis and stroma were also associated with low ¹⁸F-misonidazole activity. Therefore, ¹⁸F-misonidazole accumulated in hypoxic cancer cells, and low radioactivity regions were either nonhypoxic cancer tissue or stroma and necrosis [12].

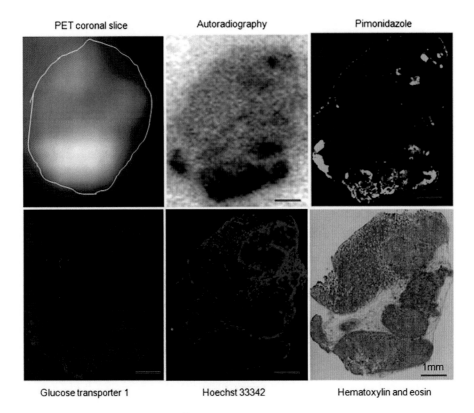

PET coronal slice	Autoradiography	Pimonidazole
Glucose transporter 1	Hoechst 33342	Hematoxylin and eosin

Fig. 4 Intratumoral distribution of ^{18}F-misonidazole in a macroscopic A549 subcutaneous xenograft by PET and autoradiography and its relationship to tumor microenvironment. Autoradiography, pimonidazole, glucose transporter-1 expression, Hoechst 33342, and Hematoxylin and Eosin stains were obtained from the same frozen tissue section. Stroma and pimonidazole-negative cancer cells associated with low ^{18}F-misonidazole accumulation. Glucose transporter-1-expressing regions are much wider than those positive for pimonidazole. All scale bars are 1 mm. Adapted from [12]

In summary, ^{131}I-IAZGP and ^{18}F-misonidazole have been validated as hypoxia imaging tracers in microscopic and macroscopic tumor models colorectal cancer and NSCLC.

Imaging Glucose Metabolism with ^{18}F-FDG

^{18}F-FDG PET has emerged as an important clinical tool for cancer detection, staging, and monitoring of response and is routinely used in the clinical management of several cancer types. The uptake of ^{18}F-FDG, an analog of glucose, is largely proportional to the rate of glucose metabolism enabling this parameter to be quantified [43]. In hypoxic conditions, cancer cells may undergo a switch from aerobic to anaerobic glucose metabolism. This adaptive response involves the coordinated expression of many HIF-regulated proteins, such as glucose transporters 1, and various glycolytic enzymes [44].

In vitro experiments show that incubation in hypoxic conditions induces an increase in cellular ^{18}F-FDG uptake [45–47]. It was recently shown that the intratumoral distribution of ^{18}F-FDG in R3327-AT rat prostatic carcinoma xenografts positively correlated with that of the hypoxic marker pimonidazole [33]. We have recently observed glucose uptake in microscopic tumors grown intraperitoneally in nude mice using ^{18}F-FDG digital autoradiography and to relate this to physiological hypoxia and glucose transporter-1 expression [25]. Human colon cancer HT29 and HCT-8 cells were injected intraperitoneally into nude mice to generate disseminated tumors of varying sizes. Following overnight fasting, animals, either breathing air or carbogen (a gas mixture of 95 % O_2 and 5 % CO_2), were intravenously administered ^{18}F-FDG together with the hypoxia marker pimonidazole and the cellular proliferation marker bromodeoxyuridine 1 h before sacrifice. Hoechst 33342, a perfusion marker, was administered 1 min before sacrifice. The intratumoral distribution of ^{18}F-FDG was assessed by digital autoradiography of frozen tissue sections. This was compared with the distributions of pimonidazole, glucose transporter-1 expression, bromodeoxyuridine, and Hoechst 33342 as visualized by immunofluorescent microscopy. In air-breathing condition, small tumors (generally less than 1 mm in diameter) had high ^{18}F-FDG accumulation and were severely hypoxic with high glucose transporter-1 expression and low proliferation. Larger tumors (1–4 mm diameter) generally had low ^{18}F-FDG accumulation and were not significantly hypoxic with low glucose transporter-1 expression but high proliferation. Carbogen breathing significantly decreased ^{18}F-FDG accumulation and tumor hypoxia in microscopic tumors but had little effect on glucose transporter-1 expression. We concluded that micrometastases have high ^{18}F-FDG uptake, therefore, high glucose demand which is spatially associated with physiological hypoxia and high glucose transporter-1 expression. This enhanced uptake was abrogated by carbogen breathing, indicating that in the absence of physiological hypoxia, high glucose transporter-1 expression, by itself, was insufficient to ensure high ^{18}F-FDG (glucose) uptake [10, 25].

Therefore, ^{18}F-FDG uptake was significantly increased in microscopic peritoneal tumors and only hypoxic regions of macroscopic tumors [11]. This enhanced uptake could be abrogated by carbogen breathing; physiological hypoxia was a necessary condition for increased ^{18}F-FDG uptake.

Intratumoral distribution of ^{18}F-FDG and ^{18}F-misonidazole detected by autoradiography was similar and that both tracers accumulated in hypoxic zones [11]. We extended our observation of ^{18}F-FDG and ^{18}F-misonidazole using PET on the same tumor-bearing animals. ^{18}F-FDG and ^{18}F-misonidazole PET scans were performed separated by a 24 h interval in the same animals. The intratumoral distribution of ^{18}F-FDG and ^{18}F-misonidazole was roughly similar, although areas of mismatch were apparent [12].

Imaging Proliferation with ^{18}F-Fluorothymidine

[18]F-fluorothymidine PET has been used to assess proliferation in cancer. ^{18}F-fluorothymidine preferentially accumulated in areas of tumor that showed high uptake of bromodeoxyuridine and low staining of pimonidazole. This was demonstrated for NSCLC cell lines A549 and HTB177, grown as either subcutaneous xenografts or disseminated peritoneal disease; high ^{18}F-fluorothymidine uptake was found in the regions with high levels of bromodeoxyuridine binding (proliferative) cancer cells where pimonidazole stained negatively indicating well oxygenated. Low ^{18}F-fluorothymidine accumulation was found in cancer cells which were stained positive for pimonidazole (hypoxia) but low for bromodeoxyuridine (low proliferation). Stroma and necrotic zones also associated with low ^{18}F-fluorothymidine accumulation. ^{18}F-fluorothymidine uptake significantly correlated with proliferation index [10, 11].

Discussion

Microscopic tumors derived from colorectal cancer cells and NSCLC cell lines grown intraperitoneally in nude mice are severely hypoxic [8, 9, 11, 12, 25]. PET tracer ^{18}F-misonidazole is able to detect hypoxic cancer cells in microscopic peritoneal metastases and macroscopic xenografts; the hypoxia-specific binding feature of ^{18}F-misonidazole was subsequently verified by autoradiography and immunohistochemical examinations of exogenous and endogenous hypoxia markers of frozen sections obtained after PET scans of the same animals.

Severe hypoxia of peritoneal micrometastases may result in anticancer therapy resistance; hypoxic cells are more resistant than aerobic cells to ionizing radiation and chemotherapy. However, the presence of severe hypoxia may have its advantage as a specific target for molecular imaging of micrometastatic disease, which is still difficult to detect with current anatomic imaging modalities such as CT and MRI. We have examined the capacity of ^{18}F-misonidazole PET and found that the collection of multiple micrometastases was able to be detected noninvasively by ^{18}F-misonidazole PET. Furthermore, there was an apparent increase in ^{18}F-misonidazole activity in ascites in which single cancer cells and clusters of cancer cells were harvested and all were stained positive for pimonidazole. Abnormal accumulation of ^{18}F-misonidazole in the peritoneal cavity would be a sign of the presence of micrometastases, and increased radioactivity in ascites may be a sign of presence of cancer cells which are hypoxic. Current PET technique may be impractical for directly assessing hypoxia in individual microscopic tumors which are too small to be seen [9], but a collection of multiple micrometastases is able to be detected [12].

[18]F-misonidazole in PET may noninvasively detect hypoxic status in NSCLC either on the microscopic or macroscopic level. As the presence of hypoxia is a

general feature of solid malignancies [2, 5–7], to some extent, ^{18}F-misonidazole PET would be useful to distinguish cancers from benign diseases, such as lung nodules in patients; this issue may need further investigation.

In NSCLC mouse models, ^{18}F-FDG also mostly accumulates in hypoxic and nonproliferative cancer cells, and so behaves similarly to ^{18}F-misonidazole in terms of its intratumoral distribution [11]. Tumor microenvironment is fluctuating, and changes in hypoxia have been reported in experimental xenografts growing in animals [48] and solid cancers in patients [49], on a time scale of 1–3 days. ^{18}F-misonidazole and ^{18}F-FDG was compared in the same tumors by PET scans performed 24 h apart, the intratumoral distribution of ^{18}F-FDG and ^{18}F-misonidazole were roughly similar, and some mismatch was present, possibly due to changes in hypoxia occurring over 24 h. Interestingly, serial PET studies indicated that, neither ^{18}F-FDG nor ^{18}F-misonidazole, intratumoral distribution could be fully replicated by subsequent day PET scan (unpublished data).

[18]F-misonidazole accumulated in hypoxic regions of xenografts and therefore can be used to assess the hypoxic volume. We found that low ^{18}F-misonidazole radioactivity regions were either nonhypoxic cancer cells or noncancerous stroma and necrosis. Although hypoxia plays an important role in cancer biology, the presence of oxic cancer cells cannot be ignored. Oxic cancer cells are highly proliferative and, therefore, are of importance for cancer management. ^{18}F-fluorothymidine generally accumulates in proliferating cancer cells [11]; therefore, if ^{18}F-fluorothymidine is injected immediately after ^{18}F-misonidazole PET, the combined scans should visualize both hypoxic and oxic (proliferative) cancer cells. ^{18}F-FDG shares a similar intratumoral distribution pattern with ^{18}F-misonidazole [12], so that a combination of ^{18}F-FDG and ^{18}F-misonidazole for a single PET scan may not provide additional information.

The microenvironment of NSCLC is complex and highly heterogeneous, being composed of viable, minimally proliferative, and hypoxic cancer cells; nonhypoxic and highly proliferative cancer cells; and noncancerous stroma and necrotic zones [5, 11, 50]. In general, cellular proliferation and hypoxia are mutually exclusive [8, 11, 32–34]. We have successfully compared ^{18}F-FDG, ^{18}F-fluorothymidine, and ^{18}F-misonidazole uptake by relating them to specific components of the intratumoral microenvironment. Each of the PET tracers with pimonidazole and bromodeoxyuridine was injected simultaneously; digital autoradiography was compared with histological visualization of tumor hypoxia, proliferation in same or closely adjacent section [25]. Another way to compare PET tracers would be to conduct serial PET scans on the same tumor, and this has been done to compare tumor uptake of ^{18}F-FDG, ^{18}F-fluorothymidine, and ^{18}F-misonidazole, both clinically and preclinically (reviewed in [11]). However, the results have been mixed and controversial. One possibility is that intratumoral microenvironment is fluctuating during the intervals between scans. Rapid change in hypoxia in experimental xenografts growing in animals and solid cancers in patients has been reported. Ljungkvist and coworkers have demonstrated that hypoxic human head–neck cancer cells had a rapid turnover rate; debris from pimonidazole-labeled hypoxic cancer cells was found in the necrotic zone 1–3 days later, and new hypoxia formed during the period [48]. Nehmeh and colleagues found a significant difference in intratumoral ^{18}F-misonidazole distribution between two ^{18}F-misonidazole PET/CT scans in the same head–neck cancer patients over a 3-day interval, which was possibly due to a change in tumor hypoxia during the period [49]. Future investigations would need to address the timing for stability of tumor microenvironment components.

High ^{18}F-fluorothymidine uptake was found in regions where there was greater binding of bromodeoxyuridine. Therefore, ^{18}F-fluorothymidine PET/CT maps the amount of proliferative cells in cancers, and ^{18}F-fluorothymidine may be able to use to observe the change in proliferation following anticancer therapies. Maximal intratumoral uptake of ^{18}F-fluorothymidine is around 30 % of maximal ^{18}F-FDG and ^{18}F-misonidazole uptake. This may be due to the fact that only approximately less than 30 % of the cells in the nonhypoxic zones accumulated ^{18}F-fluorothymidine, whereas all cancer cells in hypoxic zones were presumably able to accumulate both ^{18}F-FDG and ^{18}F-misonidazole [11].

Conclusion

Tumor microenvironment is complex and highly heterogeneous, and the presence of hypoxia is a general feature of most primary solid cancer and in peritoneal microscopic carcinomatosis. ^{18}F-fluorothymidine generally accumulates in proliferating cancer cells, whereas ^{18}F-misonidazole and ^{18}F-FDG mostly accumulate in hypoxic and nonproliferative cancer cells. Accordingly, PET imaging with ^{18}F-misonidazole, ^{18}F-fluorothymidine, and ^{18}F-FDG enables to noninvasively detect the hypoxia status, proliferation, and glucose metabolism in macroscopic tumors and micrometastases.

Acknowledgment The studies presented in this article were partially supported by Kentucky Lung Cancer Research Program Award.

References

1. Soon YY et al (2009) Duration of chemotherapy for advanced non-small-cell lung cancer: a systematic review and meta-analysis of randomized trials. J Clin Oncol 27(20):3277–3283
2. Hockel M et al (1994) Intratumoral pO2 histography as predictive assay in advanced cancer of the uterine cervix. Adv Exp Med Biol 345:445–450
3. Brizel DM et al (1996) Tumor oxygenation predicts for the likelihood of distant metastases in human soft tissue sarcoma. Cancer Res 56(5):941–943
4. Brizel DM et al (1997) Tumor hypoxia adversely affects the prognosis of carcinoma of the head and neck. Int J Radiat Oncol Biol Phys 38(2):285–289
5. Thomlinson RH, Gray LH (1955) The histological structure of some human lung cancers and the possible implications for radiotherapy. Br J Cancer 9(4):539–549

6. Hockel M et al (1991) Oxygenation of carcinomas of the uterine cervix: evaluation by computerized O2 tension measurements. Cancer Res 51(22):6098–6102

7. Koch CJ, Evans SM (2003) Non-invasive PET and SPECT imaging of tissue hypoxia using isotopically labeled 2-nitroimidazoles. Adv Exp Med Biol 510:285–292

8. Li XF et al (2007) Visualization of hypoxia in microscopic tumors by immunofluorescent microscopy. Cancer Res 67(16):7646–7653

9. Li XF, O'Donoghue JA (2008) Hypoxia in microscopic tumors. Cancer Lett 264(2):172–180

10. Li XF et al (2013) A model system for PET radiopharmaceuticals validation: focusing on tumor microenvironment. Int J Med Phys Clin Eng Radiat Oncol 2:19–29

11. Huang T et al (2012) Tumor microenvironment-dependent 18F-FDG, 18F-fluorothymidine, and 18F-misonidazole uptake: a pilot study in mouse models of human non-small cell lung cancer. J Nucl Med 53(8):1262–1268

12. Huang T et al (2013) (18)F-misonidazole PET imaging of hypoxia in micrometastases and macroscopic xenografts of human non-small cell lung cancer: a correlation with autoradiography and histological findings. Am J Nucl Med Mol Imaging 3(2):142–153

13. Airley RE et al (2003) GLUT-1 and CAIX as intrinsic markers of hypoxia in carcinoma of the cervix: relationship to pimonidazole binding. Int J Cancer 104(1):85–91

14. Airley RE, Mobasheri A (2007) Hypoxic regulation of glucose transport, anaerobic metabolism and angiogenesis in cancer: novel pathways and targets for anticancer therapeutics. Chemotherapy 53(4):233–256

15. Oliver RJ et al (2004) Prognostic value of facilitative glucose transporter Glut-1 in oral squamous cell carcinomas treated by surgical resection; results of EORTC Translational Research Fund studies. Eur J Cancer 40(4):503–507

16. Ljungkvist AS et al (2007) Dynamics of tumor hypoxia measured with bioreductive hypoxic cell markers. Radiat Res 167(2):127–145

17. Bentzen L et al (2000) Feasibility of detecting hypoxia in experimental mouse tumours with 18F-fluorinated tracers and positron emission tomography—a study evaluating [18F]Fluoro-2-deoxy-D-glucose. Acta Oncol 39(5):629–637

18. Dubois L et al (2004) Evaluation of hypoxia in an experimental rat tumour model by [(18)F] fluoromisonidazole PET and immunohistochemistry. Br J Cancer 91(11):1947–1954

19. He F et al (2008) Noninvasive molecular imaging of hypoxia in human xenografts: comparing hypoxia-induced gene expression with endogenous and exogenous hypoxia markers. Cancer Res 68(20):8597–8606

20. Vavere AL, Lewis JS (2007) Cu-ATSM: a radiopharmaceutical for the PET imaging of hypoxia. Dalton Trans 43:4893–4902

21. Tatum JL et al (2006) Hypoxia: importance in tumor biology, noninvasive measurement by imaging, and value of its measurement in the management of cancer therapy. Int J Radiat Biol 82(10):699–757

22. O'Donoghue JA et al (2005) Assessment of regional tumor hypoxia using 18F-fluoromisonidazole and 64Cu(II)-diacetyl-bis(N4-methylthiosemicarbazone) positron emission tomography: comparative study featuring microPET imaging, Po2 probe measurement, autoradiography, and fluorescent microscopy in the R3327-AT and FaDu rat tumor models. Int J Radiat Oncol Biol Phys 61(5):1493–1502

23. Iyer RV et al (1998) Preclinical assessment of hypoxic marker specificity and sensitivity. Int J Radiat Oncol Biol Phys 42(4):741–745

24. Zanzonico P et al (2004) Iodine-124-labeled iodo-azomycin-galactoside imaging of tumor hypoxia in mice with serial microPET scanning. Eur J Nucl Med Mol Imaging 31(1):117–128

25. Li XF et al (2010) High 18F-FDG uptake in microscopic peritoneal tumors requires physiologic hypoxia. J Nucl Med 51(4):632–638

26. Bennewith KL, Dedhar S (2011) Targeting hypoxic tumour cells to overcome metastasis. BMC Cancer 11:504

27. Aguirre-Ghiso JA (2007) Models, mechanisms and clinical evidence for cancer dormancy. Nat Rev Cancer 7(11):834–846

28. Naumov GN et al (2006) A model of human tumor dormancy: an angiogenic switch from the nonangiogenic phenotype. J Natl Cancer Inst 98(5):316–325
29. Barnhill RL et al (1998) Tumor vascularity, proliferation, and apoptosis in human melanoma micrometastases and macrometastases. Arch Dermatol 134(8):991–994
30. Aguirre Ghiso JA, Kovalski K, Ossowski L (1999) Tumor dormancy induced by downregulation of urokinase receptor in human carcinoma involves integrin and MAPK signaling. J Cell Biol 147(1):89–104
31. Udagawa T et al (2002) Persistence of microscopic human cancers in mice: alterations in the angiogenic balance accompanies loss of tumor dormancy. FASEB J 16(11):1361–1370
32. Durand RE, Raleigh JA (1998) Identification of nonproliferating but viable hypoxic tumor cells in vivo. Cancer Res 58(16):3547–3550
33. Pugachev A et al (2005) Dependence of FDG uptake on tumor microenvironment. Int J Radiat Oncol Biol Phys 62(2):545–553
34. Kennedy AS et al (1997) Proliferation and hypoxia in human squamous cell carcinoma of the cervix: first report of combined immunohistochemical assays. Int J Radiat Oncol Biol Phys 37 (4):897–905
35. Pugh CW, Ratcliffe PJ (2003) Regulation of angiogenesis by hypoxia: role of the HIF system. Nat Med 9(6):677–684
36. Jain RK (2005) Normalization of tumor vasculature: an emerging concept in antiangiogenic therapy. Science 307(5706):58–62
37. Li XF et al (2006) Visualization of experimental lung and bone metastases in live nude mice by X-ray micro-computed tomography. Technol Cancer Res Treat 5(2):147–155
38. Cameron MD et al (2000) Temporal progression of metastasis in lung: cell survival, dormancy, and location dependence of metastatic inefficiency. Cancer Res 60(9):2541–2546
39. Maniwa Y et al (1998) Vascular endothelial growth factor increased by pulmonary surgery accelerates the growth of micrometastases in metastatic lung cancer. Chest 114(6):1668–1675
40. Hiraga T et al (2007) Hypoxia and hypoxia-inducible factor-1 expression enhance osteolytic bone metastases of breast cancer. Cancer Res 67(9):4157–4163
41. Li XF et al (2002) Benefits of combined radioimmunotherapy and anti-angiogenic therapy in a liver metastasis model of human colon cancer cells. Eur J Nucl Med Mol Imaging 29 (12):1669–1674
42. Riedl CC et al (2008) Imaging hypoxia in orthotopic rat liver tumors with iodine 124-labeled iodoazomycin galactopyranoside PET. Radiology 248(2):561–570
43. Dierckx RA, Van de Wiele C (2008) FDG uptake, a surrogate of tumour hypoxia? Eur J Nucl Med Mol Imaging 35(8):1544–1549
44. Semenza GL (2003) Targeting HIF-1 for cancer therapy. Nat Rev Cancer 3(10):721–732
45. Clavo AC, Brown RS, Wahl RL (1995) Fluorodeoxyglucose uptake in human cancer cell lines is increased by hypoxia. J Nucl Med 36(9):1625–1632
46. Clavo AC, Wahl RL (1996) Effects of hypoxia on the uptake of tritiated thymidine, L-leucine, L-methionine and FDG in cultured cancer cells. J Nucl Med 37(3):502–506
47. Burgman P et al (2001) Hypoxia-Induced increase in FDG uptake in MCF7 cells. J Nucl Med 42(1):170–175
48. Ljungkvist AS et al (2005) Hypoxic cell turnover in different solid tumor lines. Int J Radiat Oncol Biol Phys 62(4):1157–1168
49. Nehmeh SA et al (2008) Reproducibility of intratumor distribution of (18)F-fluoromisonidazole in head and neck cancer. Int J Radiat Oncol Biol Phys 70(1):235–242
50. Graves EE, Maity A, Le QT (2010) The tumor microenvironment in non-small-cell lung cancer. Semin Radiat Oncol 20(3):156–163

Biography

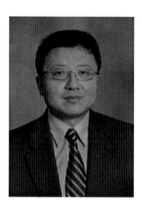

Xiao-Feng Li, M.D., Ph.D., is an assistant professor of radiology in University of Louisville; he earned his medical degree from the Norman Bethune University of Medical Sciences and Ph.D. degree in medical sciences from Kanazawa University. He had his nuclear medicine residency training at Harbin Medical University, clinical nuclear medicine fellowship at Kanazawa University Hospital, and molecular imaging fellowship at Memorial Sloan-Kettering Cancer Center. He conducts researches on tumor hypoxia, angiogenesis, and glucose metabolism; molecular imaging cancer and metastases; and imaging tumor hypoxic microenvironment. He has coauthored numerous peer-reviewed research articles, reviews, and book chapters.

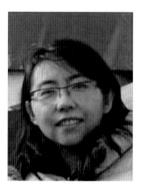

Yuanyuan Ma, M.D., Ph.D., Dr. Ma is a cancer biologist, whose research interests include tumor hypoxia, metastases, cancer metabolism, molecular imaging of cancer, and molecular diagnosis of cancer and metastases.

Thermoacoustic Imaging with VHF Signal Generation: A New Contrast Mechanism for Cancer Imaging Over Large Fields of View

Michael Roggenbuck, Jared Catenacci, Ryan Walker, Eric Hanson, Jiang Hsieh, and S.K. Patch

Abstract Ex vivo thermoacoustic (TA) imaging of large porcine specimens demonstrates the feasibility of performing whole organ TA imaging. A smaller system optimized for ex vivo prostate cancer imaging has been developed and is currently in use to determine whether the TA contrast mechanism can visualize prostate cancer.

Electromagnetic design of the testbeds is detailed. Choice of irradiation frequency is explained and irradiation pulsewidth is matched to transducer bandwidth. Power deposition in specimens is estimated from directional coupler measurements during scanning. These measurements confirm that tissue heating is microdegrees per irradiation pulse.

This work was supported in part by the by National Institutes of Health, #R21 CA137364.

M. Roggenbuck
Epic Software, 1979 Milky Way, Verona, WI 53593, USA

J. Catenacci
Department of Mathematics, NC State University, Raleigh, NC, USA

R. Walker
Department of Mathematics, University of Kentucky, Lexington, KY, USA

E. Hanson
Departments of Mathematics & Physics, McGill University, 805 Sherbrooke St. West, Montreal, QC, Canada

J. Hsieh
GE Healthcare, 3000 N. Grandview Blvd., Waukesha, WI 53188, USA

S.K. Patch (✉)
Department of Physics at UW-Milwaukee, 1900 E. Kenwood Blvd., Milwaukee, WI 53211, USA
e-mail: patchs@uwm.edu

A.S. El-Baz et al. (eds.), *Abdomen and Thoracic Imaging: An Engineering & Clinical Perspective*, DOI 10.1007/978-1-4614-8498-1_21,
© Springer Science+Business Media New York 2014

Introduction

Each diagnostic imaging modality provides different information about tissue properties. Ultrasound (US) reveals mechanical tissue properties whereas X-ray (XR) and X-ray computed tomography (XR CT) reveal projections and reconstructed slices of X-ray attenuation, which is closely related to tissue density. Magnetic resonance imaging (MRI) reveals hydrogen content as well as relaxation properties. Positron emission tomography (PET) reveals metabolic activity. All but PET propagates energy into the imaging region of interest (ROI) and collects the same type of energy. US transmits and receives mechanical pressure waves; XR and XR CT transmit and receive X-rays. MRI propagates very high frequency (VHF) electromagnetic energy to excite magnetic spins and measures fluctuations in the magnetic field caused by those spins. PET provides inverse source images of a radioactive isotope injected into the patient, which is taken up by regions of high metabolic activity. Thermoacoustic computerized tomography (TCT) is a hybrid imaging technique, which provides additional complementary information.

Conversion of electromagnetic (EM) energy into mechanical energy, manifested as ultrasound pulses, is the basis for thermoacoustic (TA) imaging. TCT signals are generated by rapid heating, which causes thermal expansion, exciting mechanical pressure waves. The TCT contrast mechanism therefore is correlated to dielectric, thermal, and mechanical tissue properties. TCT may prove useful for applications that elude current clinical imaging methods, most notably differentiating vulnerable from stable plaque and imaging prostate cancer. Aggressive tumor growth is supported by a large blood supply with high electrical conductivity, which is hypothesized to distinguish cancerous from normal tissue in TA imaging. The patient is irradiated with a short but high-power EM pulse, which rapidly heats the ROI to create outgoing pressure waves. Optimization of both EM and acoustic aspects is required for this technology to gain widespread utilization for the noninvasive detection and pinpoint localization of tumors with dense surrounding vasculature.

Historical Background

Thermoacoustics (TA) is a well-known phenomenon, with a history that dates back more than 100 years to AG Bell's observation of the photoacoustic effect [1]. Ultra-high frequency-induced auditory effects were first observed in the 1960s [2]. The auditory effect was attributed to thermal expansion [3, 4], which was validated experimentally in water [5]. Experimental validation followed in tissue mimicking human head phantoms [6] and in vivo in small animal heads [7].

Application of the thermoacoustic effect to diagnostic imaging was first proposed in the 1980s. Caspers and Conway proposed generating TA signals with submicrosecond microwave pulses with carrier frequency of 9 GHz [8], while

Bowen and colleagues used 2.45 GHz [9, 10]. Experimental thermoacoustic projection images [10, 11] were quickly followed by design of a full-fledged tomographic imaging system [12] and measurements [13]. Kruger pursued photoacoustic (PA) imaging using optical irradiation pulses with 1,064 nm wavelengths, but later moved to lower frequency (433 MHz) excitation. 433 MHz irradiation was used to image the kidney of a small (30 kg) pig [14] and also a human breast [15]. These were relatively easy test cases, compared to in vivo abdominal imaging. The piglet kidney was small, so EM penetration was excellent. The low dielectric constant of fatty breast tissue permits deeper EM penetration than dense organs and muscle. These results provided compelling proof of principle, although the advent of high-field MRI raised doubts about the feasibility of propagating 433 MHz into an adult torso. 300 MHz circularly polarized $\mathbf{B_1}$ fields are routinely propagated into adult heads by 7T MRI scanners, but whole body MRI at 7T remains elusive because it is so difficult to achieve $\mathbf{B_1}$ uniformity throughout an adult abdomen. Two texts [16, 17] and review articles [18, 19] provide excellent overviews.

Governing Equations

Thermoacoustic pressures are governed by the inhomogeneous acoustic wave equation. Following the notation of [17],

$$\left(\frac{\partial^2}{\partial t^2} - v_s^2 \Delta\right) p(\mathbf{x}, t) = \frac{\beta}{\kappa} \frac{\partial^2 T(\mathbf{x}, t)}{\partial t^2} \tag{1}$$

with homogeneous initial and boundary conditions. In soft tissue the speed of sound, $v_s \sim 1.5$ mm/μs, thermal expansion coefficient, $\beta \sim 3.6\mathrm{e}{-4}/°\mathrm{C}$, and compressibility $\kappa \sim 4.6\mathrm{e}{-10}/\mathrm{Pa}$. The heating rate is

$$\frac{\partial T(\mathbf{x}, t)}{\partial t} = \frac{1}{C} \mathrm{SAR} \tag{2}$$

where *SAR* is specific absorption rate of the electromagnetic excitation pulse in W/kg, and $C \sim 4.2$ kJ/kg/°C is the specific heat capacity of soft tissue. In VHF and microwave regimes, SAR is defined as

$$\mathrm{SAR} = \frac{\sigma |\mathbf{E}(\mathbf{x}, t)|^2}{\rho} \tag{3}$$

where σ is electrical conductivity in Siemens/meter and ρ is tissue density. Equation (1) can be written in detail as

$$\left[\frac{\partial^2}{\partial t^2} - v_s^2 \Delta\right] p(\mathbf{x}, t) = \left(\frac{\beta\sigma}{\kappa C\rho}\right)(\mathbf{x})\frac{\partial}{\partial t}|\mathbf{E}(\mathbf{x}, t)|^2 \tag{4}$$

The tissue parameters v_s, κ, β, ρ, and C are often assumed constant but can vary with respect to $\mathbf{x}$. EM loss is proportional to electrical conductivity. Additionally, dispersion cannot be ignored so conductivity is also frequency-dependent, $\sigma = \sigma(\mathbf{x}, f)$ where f denotes frequency. These are all intrinsic tissue properties, but the electromagnetic field, $\mathbf{E}(\mathbf{x}, t)$ is applied by the experimental setup in short, high-power pulses. An idealized system excites with an electric field that is impulsive in time and uniform in space, i.e., $|\mathbf{E}(\mathbf{x}, t)|^2 \sim |\mathbf{E}|^2\delta(t)$.

Most TA systems propagate EM pulses with only 2–3 cm depth penetration. We have developed a benchtop TCT system that provides excellent depth penetration of the EM pulse and yet generates TA pulses of sufficient strength to be detected after travel through 6 cm of soft tissue. The applied electric field is nearly constant in the ROI, but susceptibility effects can cause significant spatial variations. The applied field is not impulsive in time, but it is reasonable to assume that it is separable as $|\mathbf{E}(\mathbf{x}, t)|^2 = |\mathbf{E}(\mathbf{x})|^2 I(t)$ and the governing equation becomes

$$\left[\frac{\partial^2}{\partial t^2} - v_s^2 \Delta\right] p(\mathbf{x}, t) = S(\mathbf{x}) I'(t) \tag{5}$$

where $S(\mathbf{x}) = \left(\frac{\beta\sigma|\mathbf{E}|^2}{\kappa C\rho}\right)(\mathbf{x})$ is the thermoacoustic source term which is recovered from measurements of p at receiver locations, $\mathbf{x}$, located outside of the ROI.

Ideal TCT Pressures

Idealized TCT pressures have straightforward mathematical representation and reconstruction of TCT data bears similarities to reconstruction methods for other imaging techniques. An idealized TCT system propagates impulsively in time so that $I(t) = \delta(t)$ and in this case the pressures generated can be written in terms of spherical means of the source term, S [20].

$$p_\delta(\mathbf{x}, t) = \frac{\partial}{\partial t}\int_{|\mathbf{x}-\mathbf{y}|=v_s t}\frac{S(\mathbf{y})}{4\pi v_s^2|\mathbf{x}-\mathbf{y}|}dy \tag{6}$$

where the subscript, δ, indicates that the pressures were excited impulsively.

Mathematically, idealized TA pressures are equivalent to derivatives of the spherical Radon transform. Physically, TA pressures are nearly equivalent to reflection tomography data. TA pressures generated by impulsive irradiation and reflection tomography data both represent spherical integrals of a source term, S, centered at the transducer focal spot, $\mathbf{x}$. Reflection tomography assumes 2-way travel in which pulses emitted by a transducer are recorded after experiencing only one scattering event. In contrast, TCT measurements represent 1-way travel from object to transducer. TCT sinograms represent internal sources of acoustic pressures, much as PET sinograms represent internal radiation sources. The difference between TCT and PET, however, is that TCT sinograms represent spherical integrals whereas PET sinograms represent line integrals. TCT differs from ultrasound transmission tomography, for which measured pressures are processed to provide line integrals of "slowness" [21, 22], attenuation [23] or both [24–26]. These methods reconstruct line integrals using techniques developed for X-ray CT. Ultrasound tomography accounting for refraction, scattering, and diffraction remains a topic of research. We cite just a few of the numerous results applied to breast cancer imaging [27–29]. Fourier interpolation of diffraction tomography data had long permitted bandlimited recovery of the refractive index of weak scatterers, but backpropagation of the acoustic field improved image quality [30].

Mathematically exact reconstruction of S from measurements of p_δ restricted to a surface surrounding the ROI is a well-studied problem. Explicit inversion formulae for this spherical Radon transform were first derived in series form for circular and spherical measurement apertures [31, 32] while inversion of standard filtered backprojection (FBP) type was derived for a planar measurement geometry [33]. Mathematically exact FBP inversion was derived in [34] and quickly generalized to other measurement geometries [35]. Most of these results assume that the excitation pulse is impulsive in time, but neither ultrasound transducers nor high-power EM amplifiers can transmit true delta functions.

Experimentally Realized TCT Pressures

DuHamel's principle explicitly reveals the extent to which the true pulse, with temporal envelope I, bandlimits TCT pressures

$$p_I(\mathbf{x},t) = [I * p_\delta](\mathbf{x},t) \tag{7}$$

where the convolution is performed with respect to time. This is derived by exploiting linearity of the wave equation and considering the source, S, as a sum of impulsive sources at times $0 < s < t$ [20]. By the convolution theorem,

$$\mathbf{F}p_I(\mathbf{x},f) = \mathbf{F}I(f)\mathbf{F}p_\delta(\mathbf{x},f) \tag{8}$$

where $\mathbf{F}$ denotes the Fourier transform with respect to time. The irradiation pulsewidth therefore directly bandlimits TA pulses, and therefore also bandlimits reconstructed images [36].

Necessary Steps for Translation from Benchtop to Clinical Prototype

Before clinical prototypes can be deployed to validate the TA contrast mechanism in vivo, it is necessary to show that VHF EM pulses can generate useful TA signals without overheating the patient. This requires judicious choice of system parameters, including irradiating EM frequency and pulsewidth as well as choice of ultrasound receivers.

Choice of EM Frequency

TA imaging systems must irradiate with an electric field that penetrates the entire ROI and yet is lossy enough to generate sufficiently strong acoustic pressures to survive the outgoing trip across the ROI. Near infrared radiation (NIR) is extremely lossy in soft tissue, with a typical penetration depth of only 1.7 cm [17]. Microwaves heat tissues with high water content efficiently, but with limited depth penetration [19, 37]. Additionally, diffraction of short wavelength microwaves can cause TA signal dropout [38]. In contrast, VHF frequencies penetrate large tissue volumes well with good uniformity, as witnessed by the success of whole-body 3T MRI, which excites spins using 128 MHz. Precisely because these EM pulses are not lossy in soft tissue, they generate a weaker TA signal than microwave or PA irradiation. Nevertheless, the TA pulses generated are sufficiently strong to survive passage through 5–6 cm of soft tissue [39, 40]. Unlike other systems that irradiate with microwave or optical pulses, 100 MHz EM radiation can penetrate an adult torso, creating the potential for an abdominal TCT system for applications that allow placement of an ultrasound array within just a few centimeters of the ROI.

Both optical and VHF EM energy heat blood, although the contrast mechanisms are dramatically different. NIR energy heats hemoglobin, and by varying optical wavelengths, PA systems discriminate between oxy- and deoxyhemoglobin [41, 42], as do pulse oximeters. Because VHF energy heats ions, blood and physiologic saline each generate a strong TA signal, which is not the case for pure water. The electrical conductivity of physiologic saline ranges from approximately 0.8 S/m at 30 MHz to 1.6 S/m at 100 MHz [43]. Blood is equally lossy near 100 MHz, but the conductivity of pure water is six orders of magnitude lower. Therefore we excite TA signal with a carrier frequency at the top of the frequency modulated (FM) radio band, 108 MHz.

Choice of EM Pulsewidth

Ideal irradiation would be instantaneous, but that is physically unrealizable. TA pulses generated by instantaneous irradiation would be bandlimited only by the content of the tissue. Attenuation limits the clinical utility of high frequency ultrasound for abdominal applications, so an irradiation pulsewidth of 70 ns would essentially bandlimit TA pulses to 14 MHz, approximately the bandwidth of higher frequency clinical ultrasound transducers. The VHF-pulsed amplifier used to generate the results presented here is limited in peak power output and response time. The results presented below were generated by either 900 or 700 ns irradiation pulsewidths, for the large organ and prostate testbeds, respectively.

Optical pulsewidths of order 10 ns are capable of generating PA pulses with essential bandwidth up to 100 MHz. However, such high ultrasound frequencies are quickly attenuated because acoustic attenuation in soft tissue is exponential with respect to both travel distance and frequency:

$$p(\mathbf{x},f) = e^{-a|\mathbf{x}-\mathbf{y}|f^b}p(\mathbf{y},f) \tag{9}$$

In soft tissue b is slightly larger than 1, and a ranges from 0 to 0.2 Np cm^{-1} MHz^{-b} [44].

Small ROI applications are therefore suitable for photoacoustic tomography (PAT). Conversely, microwave and radiofrequency TCT systems struggle to propagate 100 ns pulses; most systems irradiate with 400 ns to 1 μs pulsewidths, generating very low frequency TA (below 1 MHz). Outgoing TA pulses are therefore attenuated very little. Extremely broadband TA signals have been generated [45, 46], but acoustic attenuation quickly decimates the high frequency components of the TA pulse. Because TA bandwidth directly impacts image resolution [36], TCT system design must balance bandwidth, signal strength, and depth penetration. Transmit pulses were optimized for diffraction tomography in [32] and the result applies to EM pulses used to generate TCT signals. Additional care is required for TCT to ensure that the irradiating electric field is sufficiently strong throughout the imaging volume.

Materials and Methods

The testbeds represent slight modifications of the first generation system [47], propagating submicrosecond TE_{10} pulses past the specimen. Testbed design was performed using ANSOFT high frequency structural simulator (HFSS) to minimize reflected power at transitions between air-filled rigid coaxial line and fluid-filled waveguide section. Specifically, S-parameters were optimized to maximize transmission (S_{21}) and minimize reflection (S_{11} and S_{22}). To validate testbed EM performance broadband S-parameters were measured. The basic experimental setup during scanning involves collecting complete 4-channel measurements of incident and reflected pulses at both testbed ports whenever possible. During TCT sinogram acquisition, however, two channels are used to record TCT signal, leaving only two channels for monitoring EM pulses. Ultrasound hardware remains essentially unchanged between systems. The tomographic gantry hardware permits

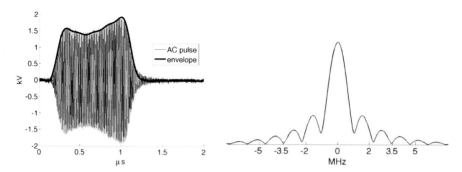

Fig. 1 (*Left*) A single VHF pulse in *grey*. Pulse envelope in *thick black* represents $I^{1/2}$. (*Right*) Spectrum of TA pulse

acquisition of "step-and-shoot" volumetric data. In all systems the axis of rotation and translation runs along the x direction, although the axes are rotated differently in the two systems.

EM Hardware

The testbeds have the dimensions of a TE_{103} cavity, but with different y-dimensions, depending upon the size of the object to be imaged. The testbed designed for imaging large organs was fabricated in the standard orientation of a TE_{10} waveguide, with vertically polarized electric field propagating horizontally along the z-axis. This testbed permits variable height in the y-direction, whereas the testbed optimized for prostate imaging has the y-dimension fixed at 6 cm. Additionally, the orientation of the smaller prostate imaging system is rotated so that the x-axis of translation and rotation is vertical.

Carefully designed coaxial-to-waveguide transitions at each port efficiently propagate TE_{10} pulses through the testbed to a load [47]. Directional coupler line sections and plug-in elements at input and output ports as shown in Fig. 1 allow direct measurement of incident and reflected pulses, from which power loss in the system can be calculated. The SAR in the tissue specimen is estimated by comparing power loss in the loaded vs. the unloaded system. In these benchtop systems SAR during TA signal production is tens of kW/kg, but duty cycle can be extremely low, keeping average SAR is on the order of 1 W/kg.

Active Components

A −10 dBm input pulse from a tunable signal generator (Rohde & Schwarz, SML10) is amplified from a fraction of a milliwatt to a peak power exceeding 40 kW by a custom designed RF amplifier (QEI VHF-50KP). This 3-stage amplifier

Fig. 2 Envelopes of VHF pulses at each stage of the amplifier.

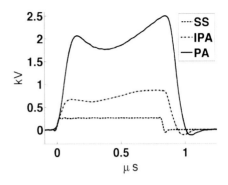

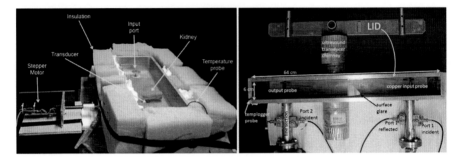

Fig. 3 (*Left*) Large testbed for imaging large organs. (*Right*) Optimized for prostate imaging

propagates pulsewidths no longer than 1 μs. The first stage is solid-state and performs the lion's share of the amplification, sending a 500 W square pulse to the first of two pulsed vacuum tubes. The intermediate pulse amplifier (IPA) is a vacuum tube (CPI #3CPX5000A7). It responds sluggishly, with rise and fall times exceeding 100 ns. This tube generates nearly 6.5 kW near the end of a 880 ns pulse. The final pulse amplifier (PA) tube (#3CPX800A7) further distorts the pulse shape, severely band-passing the irradiation pulse. The first two stages are monitored using directional coupler line sections which provide 27 dB attenuation, and are then further attenuated by an additional 20 dB. The final PA output is attenuated by 62 dB. Envelopes of the pulses generated by a −10 dBm pulse of 880 ns pulsewidth are shown in Fig. 1. High-power pulses propagate along air-filled Electronics Industry Alliance (EIA) 1–5/8″ rigid copper coaxial line to the testbed. A TE_{10} pulse propagates along the fluid-filled testbed. Additional ports added to the testbed permit positioning of the object under test by positioners that extend through a custom designed port outside of the testbed (Fig. 3). The entire setup is housed inside a 100 dB Faraday cage (Lindgren #14-W-5/S-I).

Passive: Common Elements for Both Testbeds

Passive components include testbeds optimized for ex vivo large organ and prostate imaging, as well as the materials that load the testbed. The thermoacoustic testbeds propagate a submicrosecond TE_{10} pulse with carrier frequency 108 MHz and peak power of 40 kW. The dielectric is primarily deionized (DI) water mixed with 15 g/L glycine, which reduces the wavelength by nearly an order of magnitude compared to that in a vacuum. Testbeds have dimensions of a TE_{103} cavity, with $a = 19$ cm and $c = 64$ cm. However, coupling irises were carefully designed to provide a good match between the rigid EIA 1 5/8″ coax attached to each port.

Testbeds exploit reciprocity and efficiently transmit power to a dummy load, so that electromagnetic quality is nearly one. While resonance would increase field strength, it would also diminish our ability to irradiate the object with submicrosecond pulses. Incident and reflected pulses at each port are monitored using line sections (Bird #4715-000) fitted with 50 dB directional coupler slugs (Bird #0274-000). Incident pulses at each port have 2 kV peak amplitude, so they are attenuated by an additional 30 dB (80 dB total) to prevent over-ranging on the oscilloscope (Tektronix DPO 7140). EM pulses are collected using the oscilloscope's full bandwidth of 1 GHz and a sampling rate of 5 GHz. Incident and reflected power at each port are calculated using these measurements (Fig. 3).

US Hardware

The testbeds have dual-channel capability, enabling either faster data acquisition *or* broader bandwidth imaging. Although TA pressures are relatively weak, we choose critically damped transducers over more sensitive lightly damped transducers. This is done because TA pressures tend to be very broadband compared to ultrasound pulse echoes, and the more heavily damped transducers have a broad bandwidth. Focused immersion transducers (Olympus V303, V306) with point target focus of 0. 6″ ~ 1.5 cm and center frequencies 1 and 2.25 MHz were positioned directly below and above the kidney, respectively. This was done to maximize bandwidth of the aggregate measured signal. To minimize scan time when imaging fresh surgical prostate specimens, we use a match pair of 2.25 MHz transducers with 0.8″ point target focus. The 2.25 MHz transducer captures first sidelobe of the power spectrum of a 700 ns irradiation pulse. These lobes lies between 1.4 and 2.9 MHz. TA signal is amplified 54 dB by low noise preamplifiers (Olympus #5662).

EMI Shielding

Great care is taken to electromagnetically shield the transducers and cables. Transducers are recessed 1 cm in an EM cutoff chimney to minimize their exposure to the E-field inside the testbed. Doubly shielded transducer cables (Olympus #BCU-

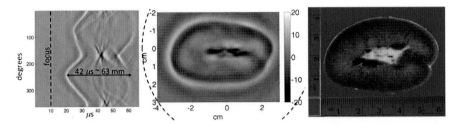

Fig. 4 (*Left*) Filtered sinogram corresponding to slice #31. (*Center*) Slice #31 reconstruction. (*Right*) Photograph from nearby slice

58-10DSW) carry the TA signal to a penetration panel on the Faraday cage. Additionally, standard ductwork is used to further shield the transducer cable from stray electromagnetic interference (EMI) from the amplifier as shown in (Fig. 5). In addition to the cables' mechanical shielding, inline low-pass filters (Mini Circuits) suppress any of the high-power 108 MHz excitation pulse that may still be picked up by the transducer. This is done to protect a 54 dB preamplifier (Olympus, #5662).

Thermal and Mechanical Hardware

Temperature of the glycine solution is monitored by a templogger (TDC D10370003, ThermoWorks, Lindon, UT), whose probe is permanently mounted in one corner of the testbed near port 2. The object under test is rotated and translated by a dual motion actuator and driver (Haydon Kerk #LR35KK4AD-05-940 and #DCM8028, respectively), so that data is collected in "step-and-shoot" mode.

Testbeds: Dimensions and Orientations, E_y for Each

E-field strength along the centerline of the waveguide is estimated using the relative permittivity of water as a function of temperature according to [48]

$$E_y = \sqrt{4\pi f P \mu_o / \beta a b} \tag{10}$$

Here, $\beta = \pi \sqrt{4/\lambda^2 - 1/a^2}$, $\lambda = c/f \sqrt{\in_r(T)}$, c is the speed of light in a vacuum, f is frequency, ε_r is relative permittivity, P is power, μ_o is free-space permeability, and $a = 0.19$ m is the testbed x-dimension. b is the testbed y-dimension, which differs depending upon testbed. $b = 10$ cm for the large testbed and $b = 6$ cm for smaller testbed.

The smaller testbed has $b = 6$ cm and propagates pulses of 700 ns duration and 22.5 kW incident power. Using the empirically estimated relative permittivity for 6 °C glycine of $\varepsilon'_r = 92$ yields a field strength near the input port of $E_y = 15.5$ kV/m. Loss in an unloaded testbed filled with glycine is about 35 %, reducing the field strength to only 10 kV/m near the output port. Prostate specimens are positioned between the ports, and a conservative estimate of electric field strength experienced is 12 kV/m.

Similar calculations for the larger testbed with $b = 10$ cm propagating 900 ns pulses with incident power 25 kW implies a field strength near the input port of 12.6 and 10 kV/m near the kidney. Not only does the smaller testbed concentrate the electric field, but it also permits positioning the ultrasound receivers closer to the specimen. Both effects improve signal to noise ratio (SNR).

Specimen Prep and Scanning

LabVIEW software (2010 version, National Instruments, Austin, TX) controls the tomographic gantry and signal generator (SML-01, Rohde and Schwarz, Columbia, MD), while also controlling data acquisition on a 4-channel digital oscilloscope (DPO 7104, Tektronix, Beaverton, OR). LabVIEW runs directly on the digital oscilloscope, which has an onboard Windows PC. The program communicates to the actuator via a universal serial bus (USB) data acquisition board (#6008, National Instruments), and to the signal generator via a standard general purpose interface bus (GPIB) cable. Both testbeds acquire in step-and-shoot mode over cylindrical measurement apertures.

Great care is taken to prevent tissue damage during scanning. To minimize water absorption 0.2 M glycine (15 g/L glycine powder in deionized (DI) water) serves as acoustic couplant and also as waveguide dielectric. To minimize autolysis the specimen, and therefore couplant, are chilled.

The benchtop systems described below collects complete data in "step-and-shoot" fashion over a cylindrical measurement aperture. The transducer focal point remains outside of the specimen as it rotates, as indicated by the dashed lines in Fig. 4b.

Gantry for Imaging Large Porcine Kidneys

Early work imaging swine kidneys was performed with a horizontal gantry axis and a single 1.8-degree rotation between tomographic views. Because total scan time was not a concern we drove the amplifier at a pulse repetition frequency (PRF) of 20 Hz and translated 2 mm between acquisition slices. "Jerking" of the specimen by rapidly rotating between tomographic views required waiting 3 s after rotation to allow the specimen to come to rest. Hollow-glass positioners were custom designed to maintain the TE_{10} electric field inside the testbed while securely rotating the object. Glass rods had 4 mm OD and 2 mm ID. To preserve the TE_{10} field care was taken to ensure that they were filled with acoustic coupling fluid. One end of each glass rod protruded approximately 1 cm into small cuts in the tissue specimen. The rod which "translated" the specimen was bound securely to the specimen using thread and small hooks in the rods. A custom adapter coupled the stepper motor to positioners. Buoyant forces on an immersed specimen are significant, but nevertheless long kidneys sag somewhat between positioners, degrading positioning accuracy.

Small Testbed for Imaging Fresh Human Prostates

This system has two advantages over the larger system. Firstly, the axis of rotation is vertical, improving positioning accuracy because gravitational forces on the specimen do not change during rotation about a vertical axis. Secondly, EM efficiency is improved because the electric field is concentrated and EM pulsing is optimized.

The third generation testbed gantry also collects volumetric data in "step and shoot" mode, but with gantry axis vertical and perpendicular to the direction of EM propagation. The translation distance between acquisition slices is 3 mm. To avoid suddenly jerking the specimen, each $1.8°$ rotation is executed in 64, $0.028125°$ substeps with a 0.025 s delay between each substep. This smoother specimen rotation approximates the continuous gantry motion of modern-day clinical CT scanners. An additional delay is imposed after the final substep to ensure that the specimen comes to rest before data acquisition commences. An even longer delay is imposed after each translation step. Validation performed using lamb kidneys can be viewed online at http://www4.uwm.edu/letsci/physics/research/patchs/upload/MicrosteppingGantry.mp4.

The system is loaded with fresh prostate specimens that include the whole prostate, as well as varying amounts of surrounding tissue, much of which is adipose tissue situated below the prostate. Samples are suspended below the stepper motor actuator by a monofilament (polydioxanone) surgical suture (PDS*II,0, Ethicon, Somerville, NJ). This study underwent a full committee review and was approved by the Institutional Review Board (IRB) of the Medical College of Wisconsin (MCW). An IRB-approved written informed consent was obtained from each participant prior to the start of any research procedures. Specimens are scanned for no more than 4 h and fixed immediately in formalin. Histology has not been impaired in any of the specimens scanned to date.

Besides concentrating the E-field by mechanically reducing the size of the testbed, software modifications minimize average SAR without degrading TA signal strength, despite a fivefold increase in PRF to 100 Hz. We pulse EM only during data acquisition in order to reduce average SAR. The average acquisition time per tomographic view is approximately 4 s, with more than half this time devoted to specimen positioning. To minimize average SAR the signal generator is switched off during gantry motion, settling time, and data storage. To ensure that recorded data represent a true average of 32 TA pulses, we add 20 % to the signal generator's firing time immediately before recording data to the disk. At a 100 Hz PRF, only 384 ms are required for data averaging. Additionally, the amplifier may fire during the 300 ms switching time. While transmitting 700 ns pulses at a 100 Hz rate, the duty cycle is 0.007 %, but this is reduced conservatively to 0.001 % by switching the amplifier off during specimen positioning and data storage.

We note that our PRF of 100 Hz is limited not by the amplifier, but rather by the mechanical system. Only 50 μs are required for TA data acquisition, but the impulsive EM irradiation causes low frequency vibrations of the testbed, which arrive later and require up to 10 ms to decay. Although our current PRF of 100 Hz is 5 times faster than that of lasers used for photoacoustics, it is still slower than the amplifier's 1 % duty cycle limit. Driving at a PRF of 25 Hz provides extremely stable power output, but 100 Hz makes power output variable, even though pulse shapes are preserved. Incident power upon port 1 of the testbed is variable, but percent loss in the passive testbed is stable.

Reconstruction

For our cylindrical measurement surface, a mathematically exact FBP formula [35] exists for ideal TCT data, which is neither attenuated, nor diffracted.

$$S(\mathbf{x}) = 2 \int_{\mathbf{y} \in \partial \Omega} [p(\mathbf{y}, t) - t p_t(\mathbf{y}, t)]_{t=|\mathbf{x}-\mathbf{y}|/\nu_s} \frac{\mathbf{n} \cdot (\mathbf{x} - \mathbf{y})}{|\mathbf{x} - \mathbf{y}|^3} d\mathbf{y}$$

where $\partial \Omega$ is the cylindrical measurement aperture and $\mathbf{n}$ is the inward unit normal vector.

In practice, however, both attenuation and diffraction degrade data quality so we emphasize small time data by applying an ad hoc weighting scheme only vaguely akin to Parker's half-scan weights [49]

$$w(\mathbf{y}, \mathbf{x}) = \frac{|\mathbf{y}_{conj} - \mathbf{x}|}{|\mathbf{y} - \mathbf{x}| + |\mathbf{y}_{conj} - \mathbf{x}|}$$

where $\mathbf{y}_{conj}$ is the conjugate source location, defined just as the conjugate ray is defined in X-ray CT [50]. Note that $w(\mathbf{y}_{conj}, \mathbf{x}) + w(\mathbf{y}, \mathbf{x}) = 1$.

Backprojecting small time data out of plane implies a strong cone angle. Because our transducers are only mildly directional, we find that backprojecting in plane yields comparable (sometimes better) image quality than volumetric backprojection.

For the prostate specimen data we collect in the small testbed, we exploit the transducers' bandlimited frequency response, and filter by merely applying a Hilbert transform rather than high-pass differentiation. The Hilbert transform plus the transducers' apodized frequency response functions effectively differentiate with respect to time, yielding p_t. To remove noise, TA pulses are bandlimited, typically with lower limit of 100 kHz and upper limit in the range 3–5 MHz. A smooth rolloff was applied to either end of the spectrum. Taking $\nu_s = 1.5$ mm/mus bounds the wavenumber $k = 2\pi f/\nu_s \in (0.42, 15)$ 1/mm. Our transducers are recessed in an EM cutoff chimney. For most points $\mathbf{x}$ inside the reconstruction region, $k|\mathbf{x} - \mathbf{y}| \gg 1$ and the derivative term predominates, $p(\mathbf{y},t) \ll t p_t(\mathbf{y},t)$. Combining this with the fact that we are replacing the surface integral of volumetric backprojection with integrals over the circle for in-plane backprojection yields the approximate reconstruction

$$S(\mathbf{x}) \sim R \int_{\mathbf{y} \in S^1} w(\mathbf{y}, \mathbf{x}) [HBp_{\text{meas}}(\mathbf{y}, t)]_{t=|\mathbf{x}-\mathbf{y}|/\nu_s} \frac{\mathbf{n} \cdot (\mathbf{x} - \mathbf{y})}{|\mathbf{x} - \mathbf{y}|^2} d\mathbf{y}$$

where "H" and "B" denote the Hilbert transform and bandlimiting transforms, R is the radius of the cylindrical measurement surface, and p_{meas} represents the measured data.

Pre-processing

These formulae ignore several strong sources of highly correlated errors in the measured data. In the subsections below we outline methods for removing the most significant sources of error, EMI, and multiple reflections at the tissue-couplant interface.

EMI Correction

EMI is severe in our simple benchtop system because the piezoelectric transducer acts as an antenna and the electronics are too simple to protect the preamps from excessively high voltages. Single element transducers are shielded from the very strong electric field because they are recessed 1 cm in 1″-schedule 40 cutoff chimneys. Nevertheless, they detect the VHF excitation pulse, which is amplified by 54 dB. Additionally, stray RF leakage from the amplifier is detected despite doubly shielded transducer cables (Olympus DSW). Unfortunately, the EMI oscillates with a frequency driven by the EM pulsewidth, which is precisely in the frequency range of the excited thermoacoustic (TA) pressures. Unlike the desired TA pulses, EMI starts immediately and decays (approximately) exponentially, whereas the TA pulses arrive after 10–15 μs and have essential support corresponding to the diameter of the object under test, as shown in Fig. 5. We outline a correction scheme that is effective for removing most EMI, but note that a hardware solution will be required for high-quality and robust clinical imaging.

EMI is an additive error and is typically consistent between views, resulting in ring artifacts in reconstructed images. We utilize a hybrid approach to correction:

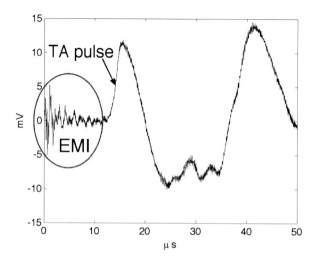

Fig. 5 A raw TCT projection has EMI for $t < 15$ us, and the first arrival of TA pressures occurs at about 12 microseconds

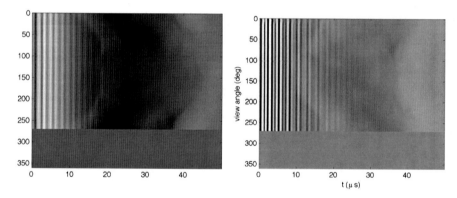

Fig. 6 Raw sinograms suffer significant EMI. (*Left*) Transducer #1. (*Right*) Transducer #2

1. Perform sino-space correction on time- and band-passed data (in that order).
2. Perform Fourier-space correction, nulling as small a number of Fourier components as possible.
3. Time-pass again to remove streaks that were smeared throughout the sinogram and into areas clearly outside the tissue.
4. Combine sinograms from two different transducers before reconstructing. If data quality from one of the two transducers is clearly superior, weight that transducer's data more heavily.

This procedure is detailed on a single slice of a volumetric acquisition in which $270°$ of data were collected by each transducer at each slice. Examples of "raw" sinograms suffering severe EMI are shown below (Fig. 6):

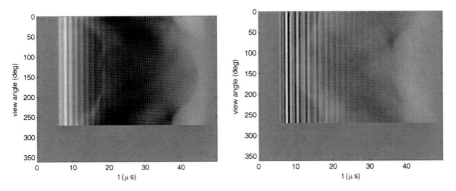

Fig. 7 Time-passed sinograms. (*Left*) Transducer #1. (*Right*) Transducer #2

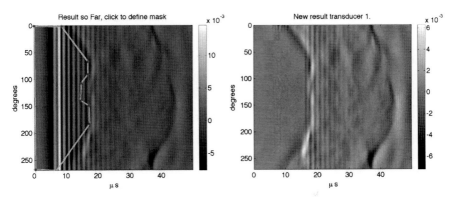

Fig. 8 Bandpassed transducer 1 data. (*Left*) User defined region outlined in blue. (*Right*) After sino-space correction

Note that these sinograms are displayed in the raw view order, and have not yet been adjusted to account for the fact that they are 180° out of phase. Because our transducers are recessed 10 mm inside a cutoff chimney, there cannot be meaningful TA signal during the first 6.5 μs. Similarly, adding the testbed width of 60 to 10 mm offset inside the transducer chimney implies at most a 70 mm acoustic pathlength, so pulses detected after 50 μs clearly are the result of multiple reflections. Therefore we can null all data for $t < 6.5$ mus and 50 mus $< t$. For small specimens these time limits can be tightened. For example, for this specimen we nulled data for $t < 5$ mus and smoothed the temporal window over the next 3 μs, for $5 < t < 8$ mus. Similarly, we smoothed the temporal window from 1 to 0 over the time span of 45–50 mus. The result is shown in Fig. 7.

Next a bandpass filter is applied. The sinograms in Fig. 8 are bandpass filtered with a frequency range between 0.1 and 4 MHz, using a smooth apodization of width 0.05 MHz. An example is shown in Fig. 8 (left). These sinograms are then EMI

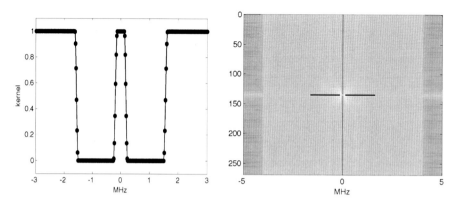

Fig. 9 (*Left*) Kernel. (*Right*) $\log_{10}$ of the absolute value of the 2D FT of the measured views of the sinogram in Fig. 8 (*right*) *after* application of the kernel to the view-angle DC row

corrected manually, using MATLAB subroutines that allow the user to select a region of significant EMI. This region is outside of the specimen, where signal should be zero. The average value of each column inside the selected ROI is subtracted from corresponding columns throughout the image, reducing the remaining EMI for small times. The correction presented in Fig. 8 (right) was performed only for columns that had a minimum of ten rows inside the user-defined ROI.

When EMI persists well into the region of the sinogram containing non-zero pressures, it cannot be corrected by a sinogram space method alone. Additionally, although EMI appears very consistent between rows in Figs. 6 and 7, after sino-space correction slight row-to-row variations become clear. We attempt to minimize the effect of these infrequent and intermittent problems later.

To minimize the EMI remaining in the central part of the sinogram, we resort to a Fourier space correction. Sinogram space is parametrized by view angle, θ, and time, t. Reciprocal space of the 2D Fourier transform of a sinogram is parametrized by k_θ and k_t (temporal frequency). EMI is consistent between tomographic views, and is therefore captured in the $k_\theta = 0$ components of the 2D Fourier transform. Additionally, EMI tends to be driven by the irradiation pulsewidth, and the 700 ns irradiation pulses propagated by our system generate EMI within the frequency range. $k_t \in [0.5, 1.5]$MHz. The remaining EMI is minimized by applying a kernel like that plotted in Fig. 9 (left) to the $k_\theta = 0$ components of the 2D Fourier transform of the sinogram, as depicted in Fig. 9 (right).

The resulting sinograms after inverse Fourier transform are shown in Fig. 10. The vast majority of EMI errors are removed, but not all. EMI is particularly difficult to remove when experimental factors cause slight variations in EMI between views. Transducer #1 suffered only a slight variation in EMI between the first few degrees acquired and the rest of the rotation. Transducer #2, however, suffered significant variation in EMI throughout the 270 acquisition and faint artifacts persist in the sinogram out to nearly 20 μs.

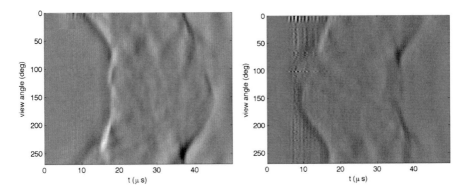

Fig. 10 Sinograms after EMI correction. (*Left*) Transducer #1. (*Right*) Transducer #2

Fourier-space correction can smear streaks throughout the image and into areas outside of the tissue, so time-passing can be performed again at this stage to reduce those. This combined sinogram-space + Fourier-space correction method eliminates most of the EMI in our sinograms.

The ultrasound hardware in our current testbed is sensitive to the electromagnetic irradiation pulse. Therefore, transducers and cables are carefully shielded from the strong electric field to which the object is exposed. In vivo imaging, however, requires that the TRUS probe be located near the ROI—and therefore be exposed to the irradiating E-field. Clinical TCT systems will require far more sophisticated ultrasound hardware to mitigate EMI in the raw signals. Fortunately, such hardware solutions appear feasible. For instance, Verasonics research ultrasound systems have an input signal range of 1.6 V peak-to-peak. At higher voltages, the input diodes conduct and keep the input to the receiver at safe levels. The EMI signal is not likely to damage these diodes and receiver recovery time should be a microsecond or less, before arrival of the TA pulse.

A final correction step to remove artifacts due to acoustic reflections between tissue and acoustic couplant can also be employed to minimize the remaining EMI, inside a user-defined ROI.

Remove Multiple Reflections

Good acoustic couplants are designed to match the acoustic impedance of the tissue being imaged. Our glycine solution is essentially water, which provides a far better match to organ tissue than oils used in microwave-induced TA systems [51]. Nevertheless, the density of most internal organs is greater than that of water and acoustic impedance is not perfectly matched. Acoustic reflections at the tissue/couplant interface are expected. Instantaneous and spatially homogeneous heating of geometrically simple objects is derived in [52]. A theoretical TA pulse generated by a homogeneous sphere that is perfectly matched to the acoustic couplant is a

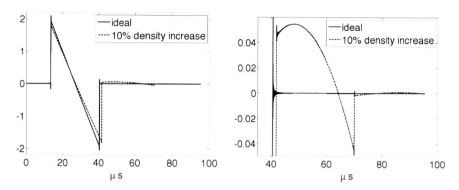

Fig. 11 Idealized TA pulses generated by a homogeneous sphere of radius 20 mm and at distance 40 mm from the receiver. (*Left*) Entire pulse, (*right*) zoomed in on multiple reflections generated by the dense sphere

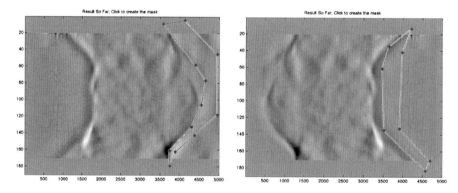

Fig. 12 Temporal mask applied to smooth to zero regions of the sinogram that precede and follow the desired TA signal. (*Left*) User-selected region contains multiple reflections. (*Right*) The sinogram is simply inverted with respect to time and the same method is used to minimize the effect of EMI occurring before arrival of the TA pulse

simple N wave. A sphere that has 10 % greater density generates a train of smaller pulses following the first, as plotted in Fig. 11. These multiple echoes are not accounted for in the analytical inversion formulae discussed in section "Ideal TCT Pressures."

An ad hoc method for removing multiple reflections from sinograms is implemented manually. The user selects a region that should theoretically be zero, as shown in Fig. 12. Data in each row of the masked region is smoothed to zero from left to right, as time increases. This was initially done to minimize the effect of reflections between the tissue and acoustic couplant, which are most detrimental for large times. We have found this technique can be useful to mitigate EMI, which occurs early in the TA pulses Fig. 12 (right).

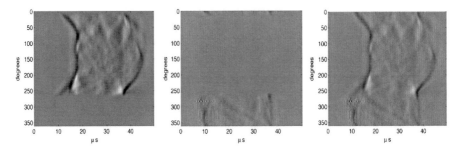

Fig. 13 Corrected and weighted partial-scan sinograms from transducer 1 (*left*) and transducer 2 (*center*). These sinograms are summed to form a complete sinogram ready for reconstruction (*right*)

Combine Partial Scan Datasets to Create a Single Full-Scan Sinogram

Finally, the two sinograms from the different transducers are combined by rotating one of them to account for the difference in view angle, applying partial scan weights and summing the data. When one transducer provides superior data quality compared to the other, the weighting is skewed to use fewer views from the inferior transducer.

In the example shown in Fig. 13, 270° of data were collected by each transducer. Both transducers collected projections over the view-angle ranges [0, 90°) and [180°, 270°). Data collected over these ranges should be identical, but clearly are not. The most significant discrepancy is due to the residual EMI in transducer 2. Time shifts between the sinograms can be caused by mispositioning of a transducer in its chimney. Mispositioning the gantry axis can cause misalignment of the sinograms so they are not precisely 180° out of phase. 2D convolution of overlapping regions in the sinograms is performed via FFT to estimate the shifts in time and view angle, much as motion correction is performed in Propeller MRI [53, 54]. Although they appear to be 180° out of phase, sinogram #2 was shifted by 1.1 mus relative to sinogram #1 in Fig. 13.

Measurements collected by transducer #1 were significantly cleaner than those collected by transducer #2. Therefore, the data from transducer #1 is used preferentially. Data is smoothed over view angle ranges of at least 18°, where data from both transducers is available. In this case the smoothing regions are $\theta \in [0, 18°)$ and $\theta \in [252°, 270°)$. Sinogram #2 is time shifted (if necessary) to properly align the sinograms into a third, complete sinogram, which is used as input to the reconstruction algorithm. Although some errors remain, most of the signal represents physical properties of the specimen.

Parellelizing the Backprojection Step

Reconstruction as outlined above is a classic example of an FBP method. Backprojection is an embarrassingly parallel computation, and by judiciously distributing computational work, nearly linear speed up can be obtained when scaling to multicore clusters. We distributed computational work by view angle.

# Cores	BP time (s)
128	292
64	486
32	825
16	1,501
8	2,879

Table 1 Timing of full volumetric back-projection times vs. number of workers

We used MATLAB Parallel Computing Toolbox's Message Passing Interface functions to run the massively parallel computation on the Milwaukee Institute's MATLAB cluster running the Distributed Computing Toolbox. We observed nearly linear speed up with the number of cores up to 100 cores (2 views per core). Beyond this threshold speed up becomes sublinear as data transfer costs overwhelm the gains from the division of computational labor.

Performance statistics for the reconstruction algorithm on the now defunct MATLAB on the TeraGrid resource are reported below. Timing results are for the reconstruction of simulated spherical phantom data with 200 views, 6,000 time steps, and 21 slices. As this simulated data does not suffer from transducer directionality, full volumetric back-projection includes the contributions from all out of plane slices. Backprojection time is reported in seconds for a $256 \times 256 \times 21$ reconstruction volume (Table 1).

EM Design and Validation

Testbed design was performed using ANSYS HFSS finite element software to optimize power transmitted through the testbed (S_{21}) and minimize reflected power at each port (S_{11} and S_{22}) [47]. Because tissue specimens vary dramatically in size and shape optimization was performed on "unloaded" testbeds, filled only with the desired dielectric. The first generation system was designed assuming room temperature DI water as dielectric, but subsequent systems were designed assuming chilled glycine solution as dielectric.

Broadband Measurements: S-Parameters

Because dielectric properties of pure water are well known, S-parameters were measured and modeled using DI as dielectric. Adding glycine powder to DI was expected to increase permittivity, although we are unaware of publications of dielectric properties of 15 g/L glycine solution. Conductivity and permittivity of glycine solution were therefore empirically estimated by fitting HFSS models to measured S-parameters. Finally, we measured and modeled the S-parameters of the large testbed filled with glycine solution and loaded with an ellipsoidal kidney.

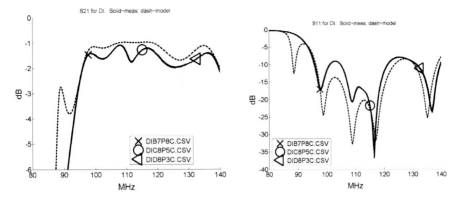

Fig. 14 *S*-Parameters of unloaded testbed, filled with DI water. S21 *left*, S11 *right*

S-Parameters were measured using a network analyzer (E5061A, Agilent, Santa Clara, CA) calibrated using a type *N* calibration standard (#85032E, Agilent). Measurements were taken at 6 °C. Temperatures were recorded using a templogger probe. Modeling was performed using finite element software (ANSYS HFSS, Canonsburg, PA) assuming perfect electric conducting (PEC) testbed walls.

Complex permittivity of DI water at 6 °C is $\varepsilon_\rho = 85.53 - j0.785$, with tan $\delta = 9.179e{-}3$. Electrical conductivity of ultrapure water is $\sigma = 5.5e{-}6$ S/m, so loss is almost entirely due to the complex part of permittivity, rather than conductivity.

$$\tan \delta = \frac{\epsilon''}{\epsilon'} + \frac{\sigma}{\omega \epsilon'} = \frac{0.785}{85.53} + \frac{5.5e-6}{2\pi \cdot 108e6 \cdot 8.85e - 12 \cdot 85.53} \sim 10^{-2} + 10^{-5}$$

HFSS models of the testbeds filled with 6 °C pure water yields good transmission, with $S_{21} > -1$ dB near 108 MHz. *S*-Parameters were measured 3 times, with slightly warmer DI water temperatures near 8 °C.

Measured and modeled *S*-parameters agree well above -10 dBm, although measurements are unable to replicate the dramatic resonances modeled. Measured S_{21} is slightly lower than modeled, indicating slightly greater loss than modeled, as shown in Fig. 14. Assuming PEC boundary conditions underestimates loss slightly. Additionally, the aluminum testbed walls likely create ions in DI water and increase loss. Plots of measured S_{11} (Fig. 14) and S_{21} are both shifted 0.6–0.8 MHz to the left of the model plots, indicating higher relative permittivity in the model than measured. We attribute these shifts to experimental error, or perhaps more accurately, testbed fabrication error.

Adding 15 g/L glycine to DI water dramatically shifts the *s*-parameter plots even further to the left and increases loss slightly. This indicates both relative permittivity and conductivity are higher in glycine solution. We therefore empirically increase both real and imaginary parts of relative permittivity by about 6 % to $\varepsilon_r = 93.32 - j0.9594$. This yields a reasonable approximation but slightly

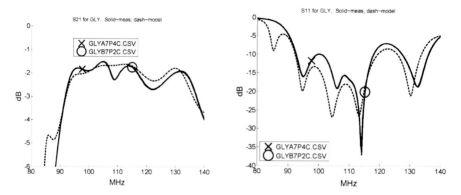

Fig. 15 *S*-Parameters of unloaded testbed, filled with DI water. S21 *left*, S11 *right*

Table 2 Dimensions and masses of physical kidney specimens used to collect TCT data, as well as model *S*-parameters in HFSS

Kidney specimen use	Length (cm)	Width (cm)	Height (cm)	Mass (g)
Cut for scanning	10	6.5	3	147.5
Modeled in HFSS	10	7	3.5	135

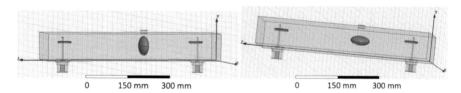

Fig. 16 Ellipsoidal kidney geometry used for simulations. (*Left*) "Vertical" orientation. (*Right*) "Horizontal" orientation

underestimates loss. Increasing conductivity slightly to $\sigma = 4e-3$ S/m yields a good match between measured and modeled S_{21}. For both DI and glycine solution, measured S_{11} fails to demonstrate the dramatic resonances of the models, but agreement is reasonable above -10 dBm and below 120 MHz. Temperature of the glycine solution was closer to 7 °C at time of measurement (Fig. 15).

Finally, to model the large system loaded with a porcine kidney, representative values of kidney permittivity and conductivity were taken from [44]. For both glycine solution and kidney, we used the same loss tangent for DI water. Parameters used in the HFSS simulations are listed in Table 2 (Fig. 16).

A slightly larger kidney specimen was used to collect *S*-parameters, with length 10.5 cm and mass 157 g. *S*-Parameters were collected with the kidney approximately centered along the *x*-axis, and at four different orientations about the *x*-axis. EM loss in the kidney was minimal when it was positioned horizontally, minimizing its surface area exposed to the traveling TE_{10} pulse. Rotating by 90°

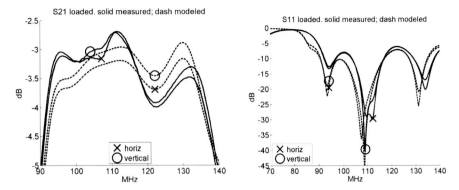

Fig. 17 *S*-Parameters for testbed loaded with chilled glycine and kidney specimen, oriented both horizontally and vertically. *S21* on *left*; *S11* on *right*

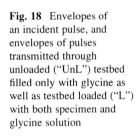

Fig. 18 Envelopes of an incident pulse, and envelopes of pulses transmitted through unloaded ("UnL") testbed filled only with glycine as well as testbed loaded ("L") with both specimen and glycine solution

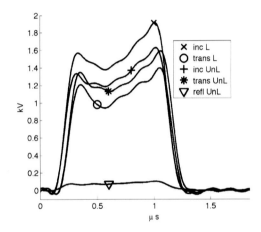

maximized the surface area exposed to the oncoming EM pulse, and loss was maximized. Although the specimen was not symmetric, there was no detectable difference in loss for the two different horizontal or vertical orientations. We note that the kidney specimen was "flatter" in shape than the modeled ellipsoid, which showed almost no difference between orientations (Fig. 17).

Narrowband and Rapid Measurements Immediately Before and After Scanning

High-power, submicrosecond EM pulses and pulse envelopes are shown in Fig. 18. These voltages allow us to compute incident and reflected power at each port. Subtracting port 1 reflected and port 2 incident power from port 1 incident power yields power loss in the system. Power loss in the tissue specimen is estimated by comparing power loss in the loaded vs. the unloaded testbed. We verify that reflected power remains below 2–3 % even when the testbed is loaded with a large specimen.

Peak and average SAR are calculated from voltage envelopes measured at the input and output ports, according to $P = V^2/2\Omega$ where Ω represents impedance of 50 Ω, V represents voltage, and SAR $= P/m$, where m represents specimen mass. Because power output from the amplifier varies from pulse to pulse, we rely upon the fact that power loss in the passive testbed is constant. To estimate power loss in the specimen, we multiply the incident power by the difference in fraction lost between unloaded (containing only glycine solution) and specimen-loaded testbed

$$P_{loss} = P1_{inc}(\%loss_L - \%loss_U) \tag{11}$$

Subscripts L and U denote specimen-loaded and unloaded, respectively. $P1_{inc}$ represents incident power at the input port 1 and P_{loss} represents power lost in the specimen. Normalizing P_{loss} by specimen mass yields peak SAR during EM irradiation; multiplying by the duty cycle yields average SAR.

2-Channel Narrowband Measurements During Scanning

To monitor EM power deposition during TCT scanning, 6 EM pulses are recorded prior to acquiring each single-slice TCT sinogram. During TCT data acquisition, two of the oscilloscope channels are used to collect TCT data, leaving only two channels to capture incident and transmitted EM pulses.

TCT data is acquired by a pair of single element transducers each listening to the TA pulses from opposite sides of the testbed. In principle, when identical transducers are used the specimen needs to be rotated by only 180° before moving on to the next slice. To ensure adequate matching of these limited-angle sinograms, however, we rotate prostate specimens at least 232° per slice, resulting in different specimen orientations about the x-axis when EM pulses are collected.

Because reflected power remains low in the loaded testbed and EM wavelength is large compared to prostates, this gives a reasonable method for monitoring power deposition during data acquisition.

Results

We present reconstructions of large porcine kidney specimens and the tissue heating measurements and reconstructions, SAR, preliminary reconstructions of fresh prostate specimens and system characterization.

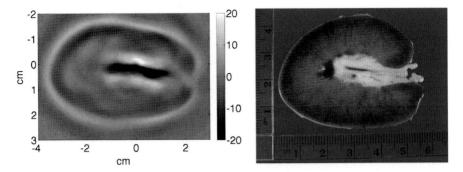

Fig. 19 (*Left*) Slice #26, through the renal pelvis. (*Right*) Photograph from nearby slice

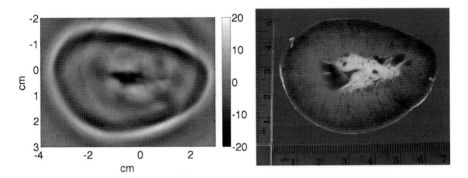

Fig. 20 (*Left*) Slice #12, at other end of kidney. (*Right*) Photograph from nearby slice

Images of Porcine Kidneys

Reconstructions clearly reveal fluid-filled calyces filled with low conductivity glycine solution, which provides strong TA signal contrast with kidney tissue. In Figs. 4, 19, and 20, reconstructions are presented along with photographs of slices cut from approximately the same location. To section the kidney into thin (1.5–2 mm) slices, it was necessary to freeze the kidney. Freezing deformed its shape and made it impossible to slice the kidney at precisely the z-locations corresponding to data acquisition and image reconstruction. However, reconstructions track the progression of multiple small calyces (slice #31) collecting into just a few larger cavities near the renal pelvis (slice #26) and back into small calyces near the other end of the kidney (slice #12). The glycine-filled cavities almost surely changed shape during freezing. Additionally, a slice sensitivity profile (SSP) was generated by scanning a 2.45 mm thick washer with outer diameter of 22.25 mm. Data was collected over a cylindrical aperture of radius 44 mm. The washer was centered at the origin providing the SSP at $r = 11.125$ mm with full width half max of nearly 18 mm, or 6 slice thicknesses, indicating severe

Fig. 21 Slice sensitivity
profile at $r = 11.125$ mm

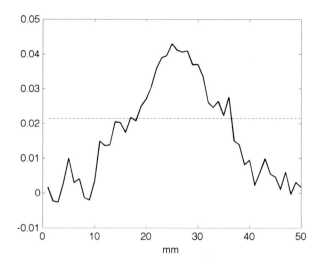

blurring between slices. Therefore, our TCT reconstructions do not faithfully represent the exact size of the cavities during scanning. For instance, calyces in Fig. 3 appear separated in the photographs, but run together in the reconstruction. Nevertheless, the TCT reconstructions consistently detect high-contrast inclusions of only a few mm in size, consistent with in-plane resolution of 5 mm in our single-slice system [39] (Fig. 21).

SAR and Heating of Porcine Kidneys

SAR of the specimen immediately prior to acquisition of each slice is presented in Fig. 22. Note that the peak SAR during EM pulsing is measured in kW/kg—more than four orders of magnitude greater than allowed average SAR. While transmitting 900 ns pulsewidths with 100 Hz repetition frequency, the duty cycle is 0.009 %. For typical porcine kidneys, this typically yields average SAR in excess of 4 W/kg, although for porcine kidneys in this second generation testbed, we have not witnessed SAR greater than 10 W/kg. Because we are working ultimately towards in vivo imaging, we optimized the scanning process to refrain from pulsing during specimen repositioning, keeping average SAR below 4 W/kg. Additionally, this optimized scan process reduces wear and tear on the amplifier tubes. We use the same optimized pulsing approach in our current study imaging surgical prostate specimens.

Several factors contribute to SAR variations between different slices: experimental uncertainty, variation of specimen location and orientation within electric field, temperature variations of glycine solution and specimen, as well as possible leeching of electrolytes from specimen into couplant. During volumetric TCT scanning in our system, the specimen is translated 3 mm between slices and

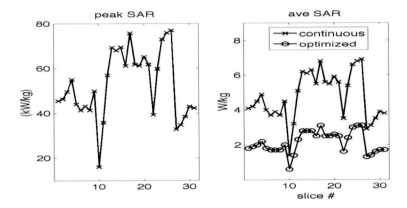

Fig. 22 (*Left*) Peak SAR during EM pulse. (*Right*) Average SAR before optimizing scan procedure denoted by "x", after optimization denoted by "o"

moves along the x-axis of a testbed with dimensions of a TE_{103} cavity of width 19 cm. The ultrasound transducers "listen" along the centerline of the waveguide, where $x = 9.5$ cm and E_y achieves its maximum value. During acquisition of the first slice, the specimen lies entirely in the region $x \leq 9.5$ cm. During subsequent slices, the specimen is progressively more centered with respect to the x-axis, and therefore experiences a stronger E_y field. After the center of the specimen crosses the centerline of the testbed, the field incident upon the specimen decreases. To reduce scan time, we have been acquiring "partial scan" data from many prostate specimens. We sometimes rotate the specimen as few as 234° before translating to acquire the next slice. Therefore, prostate orientation may be rotated about the x-axis for each slice. However, prostate dimensions in the axial directions are less than 6 cm $< \lambda/5$ so rotation about the x-axis should cause minor changes to SAR.

Temperature and pressure jumps induced by a single EM pulse are easily inferred from these measurements. Assuming thermal confinement, homogeneous initial conditions and tissue properties (density, specific heat, and speed of sound), the pressure jump during a single EM pulse is given by integrating (1) [16], so that

$$\delta p = \beta \big/ \kappa \, \delta T \quad \text{where} \quad \delta T \sim 1 \big/ C \, SAR \, \delta t \qquad (12)$$

Multiplying the peak SAR during the EM pulse by pulsewidth and dividing by specific heat yields temperature jumps of approximately 20 microdegrees,

$$\delta T \sim \frac{80 \frac{kW}{kg}}{4 \frac{kJ}{kg°C}} 900e^{-9}s \sim 20e^{-6}°C$$

TA pressures are proportional to temperature jumps, so multiplying by $\beta/\kappa = 0.8$ MPa/° C yields TA pressures on the order of tens of Pascals. These are spatial averages throughout the entire specimen, but TA signal generation varies spatially with electric field strength and tissue properties.

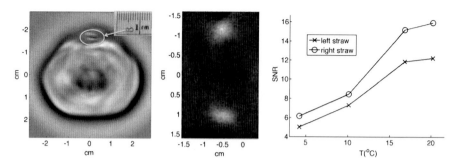

Fig. 23 (*Left*) Reconstruction of a prostate on which surgical staples were affixed. (*Center*) Reconstructions of 3 mm straws filled with PBS. (*Right*) SNR vs. temperature of 4.8 mm straws filled with whole blood product

Preliminary Reconstruction of Sinograms Collected in the Small Testbed

A reconstruction from one of the first prostate specimens we scanned is shown in Fig. 23. 3 mm metallic surgical staples were inadvertently left on the anterior of the specimen, and generated strong artifacts in the reconstruction. We now take care to remove surgical staples prior to positioning the specimen in the testbed. Although the system's ability to localize such small inclusions is encouraging, it also indicates that brachytherapy seeds will wreak havoc with prostate cancer imaging. Straws filled with physiologic saline validate that the system provides at least 3 mm in-plane resolution. Additionally, scanning 4.8 mm straws filled with whole blood product over a range of temperatures verifies the increase in TA signal production with temperature as shown in Fig. 23.

Discussion

These ex vivo results leave little doubt that whole organ TCT imaging is feasible in vivo. Clinical MRI systems routinely propagate VHF excitation pulses into patients with good uniformity. Tissue heating required to generate detectable pulses is low enough that TCT imaging can be performed without causing thermal damage.

Clinical utility of TCT has not yet been demonstrated and will require a clear understanding of the TCT contrast mechanism. Isolating exactly which tissue parameters contribute most to TA signal production is an open question. Pulse echo ultrasound fails to reveal PCa, indicating that mechanical properties of healthy and cancerous prostate tissue are indistinguishable. Additionally, the specific heat capacities of healthy and cancerous prostate tissue appear indistinguishable [55]. TA signal generation is clearly a function of thermal expansion coefficient β, which, in turn, is a function of temperature. β is well understood for pure water: $\beta = 0$ at 4 °C and increases with temperature above 4 °C. Unfortunately, surgical specimens must be kept chilled prior to formalin fixation so we are forced to work at low temperature. We expect that TCT imaging in vivo will generate far stronger signal at body temperature, 37 °C.

Electrical conductivity is clearly an important factor in TA signal production, but few direct measurements of dielectric properties of human prostate tissue have been reported in the VHF regime. Dielectric spectroscopy of fresh prostate tissue at low frequencies (1 kHz to 1 MHz) appears to discriminate between healthy and cancerous tissue [56] and surprisingly, PCa was found to have lower conductivity than glandular and stromal tissue over the frequency ranges of 100 Hz to 100 kHz [56, 58]. Mixed results were reported by Lee et al. [59]: PCa suppressed conductivity from 100 kHz to 2 MHz, but had higher conductivity at 4 MHz. Dielectric properties of rat prostates have also been reported at 915 MHz [60].

There are many limitations of these results, starting with the amplifier used to excite TA pressures, to the transducers that detect those pulses, the simplistic electronics that amplify the measured voltages and finally the need to chill the acoustic couplant. The amplifier was able to generate TA signal using pulsewidths of 700–900 ns, which bandlimited TA pulses produced. EMI will be an issue for any TA imaging system, but this system's electronics passed the submicrosecond EMI signal to the preamplifiers. Single element transducers may be more sensitive than transducer arrays, but they are far more directional and narrowband than clinical transducer array elements. Additionally, they require repositioning the specimen causing lengthy scan times. Because scan times are long, we are forced to keep surgical specimens chilled, which reduced SNR. In vivo TA imaging prototypes can avoid these problems, if sufficient resources are invested into their development.

Many in vivo TA imaging applications will suffer limited angle artifacts, because it will not be possible to position the transducer at all points on a measurement aperture surrounding the ROI. Additionally, it is not clear that in vivo scanning at body temperature will increase TA signal strength enough to offset the sensitivity loss of many clinical transducer array elements compared to the single element transducers.

Exciting with stronger electric fields would increase SAR and induce stronger pressures—and require less signal averaging. Noise in our TA pulses is essentially white, decreasing like $N^{-1/2}$, where N is the number of signal averages required. SAR is proportional to the square of the electric field strength, so a modest increase in field strength allows dramatic reduction in N because the signal-to-noise ratio (SNR) is proportional to $\text{SNR} \propto \sqrt{N}|\mathbf{E}|^2$. Doubling the field strength implies a 16-fold reduction in N. In our small benchtop system, averaging $N = 32$ pulses per view is required to provide adequate SNR for tomographic reconstruction. Increasing electric field strength by a factor of $32^{1/4} = 2.4$ would eliminate the need for signal averaging in our benchtop system. Clinical systems should irradiate with stronger, and probably circularly polarized, electric fields to ensure good field penetration and strong TA signal. Clinical systems could easily maintain low average SAR, either by reducing number of signal averages, shortening EM pulsewidth, or reducing duty cycle. Shortening the EM pulsewidth would increase TA bandwidth and improve resolution of reconstructed images. Reducing duty cycle could be achieved using an ultrasound array rather than single-element transducer. An ultrasound array would capture many TA tomographic views simultaneously and further reduce the number of EM excitations required.

Quantitative information from benchtop studies like this one will be useful for the development of clinical TCT systems. Although it is premature to establish a detailed system design, practical clinical systems will almost surely use ultrasound arrays to provide spatial encoding and propagate the EM pulse from a coil through air, similar to MRI systems. Because TA signal strength is proportional to SAR, in order to generate SAR levels in an adult torso comparable to those we generate in our small benchtop system, we suspect that far stronger VHF pulses must be applied by coils designed to propagate traveling waves [61]. MRI systems require magnetic field homogeneity of parts per million. In contrast, TCT systems could likely tolerate a significant gradient in the electric field, as long as the field strength is known and remains well above zero.

In summary, TA signal generated by high-power, submicrosecond VHF pulses can safely generate detectable TA signal with sufficient depth penetration for whole organ imaging.

Acknowledgment Thanks to J Tropp and J Sidabras, for helpful comments and suggestions. Thanks to J Hass for writing preliminary MATLAB code computing RF power. Thanks to Andrew Eckhart and Jake Maronge for writing preliminary LabView code. Thanks to D Shurilla for providing a power supply and wiring the stepper motors. Thanks to Neal Korfhage for providing glass positioners—usually on short notice.

References

1. Bell A (1881) Production of sound by radiant energy. Manufact Build 13:156–158
2. Frey A (1962) Human auditory system response to modulated electromagnetic energy. J Appl Physiol 17:689–692
3. Guy A, Chou C, Lin J, Christensen D (1975) Microwave-induced acoustic effects in mammalian auditory systems and physical materials. Ann N Y Acad Sci 247:194–218
4. Lin J (1976) Microwave auditory effect—a comparison of some possible transduction mechanisms. J Microw Power 11:77–81
5. Foster K, Finch E (1974) Microwave hearing: evidence for thermoacoustic auditory stimulation by pulsed microwaves. Science 185:256–258
6. Olsen R, Lin J (1981) Microwave pulse-induced acoustic resonances in spherical head models. IEEE Trans Microw Theory Tech 29:1114–1117
7. Olsen R, Lin J (1983) Microwave-induced pressure waves in mammalian brains. IEEE Trans Biomed Eng 30:289–294

8. Caspers F, Conway J (1982) Measurement of Power Density in a Lossy Material by means of Electromagnetically induced acoustic signals for non-invasive determination of spatial thermal absorption in connection with pulsed hyperthermia. Presented at the 12th European Microwave Conference, Helsinki, 1978

9. Nasoni RL, Evanoff GA, Halverson PG, Bowen T (1984) Thermoacoustic emission by deeply penetrating microwave radiation. Presented at the IEEE 1984 ultrasonics symposium, Dallas, TX, 1984

10. Nasoni R, Liew S, Halverson P, Bowen T (1985) Thermoacoustic images generated by a 2450 MHz portable source and applicator. Presented at the IEEE ultrasonics symposium, 1985

11. Olsen R, Lin J (1983) Acoustical imaging of a model of a human hand using pulsed microwave irradiation. Bioelectromagnetics 4:397–400

12. Lin JC, Chan KH (1984) Microwave thermoelastic tissue imaging—system design. IEEE Trans Microw Theory Tech 32:854–860

13. Su J, Lin J (1987) Thermoelastic signatures of tissue phantom absorption and thermal expansion. IEEE Trans Biomed Eng 34:179–182

14. Kruger RA, Kopecky KK, Aisen AM, Reinecke DR, Kruger GA, Kiser WL Jr (1999) Thermoacoustic CT with radio waves: a medical imaging paradigm. Radiology 211:275–278

15. Kruger RA, Miller KD, Reynolds HE, Kiser WL Jr, Reinecke DR, Kruger GA (2000) Contrast enhancement of breast cancer in vivo using thermoacoustic CT at 434 MHz. Radiology 216:279–283

16. Gusev V, Karabutov A (1993) Laser optoacoustics. American Institute of Physics, New York

17. Wang LV, Wu H-I (2007) Biomedical optics: principles and imaging. Wiley-Interscience, Hoboken, NJ

18. Xu M, Wang LV (2006) Photoacoustic imaging in biomedicine. Rev Sci Instrum 77:041101

19. Lin J (2005) Microwave thermoelastic tomography and imaging. In: Lin J (ed.) Advances in electromagnetic fields in living systems, vol 4. Springer, New York, p 41–76

20. John F (1981) Partial differential equations, 4th edn. Springer, New York, NY

21. Glover G, Sharp J (1977) Reconstruction of ultrasound propagation speed distributions in soft tissue: time-of-flight tomography. IEEE Trans Son Ultrason SU-24:229–234

22. Greenleaf J, Johnson S, Samayoa W, Duck F (1975) Algebraic reconstruction of spatial distributions of acoustic velocities in tissue from their time-of-flight profiles. In: Sixth international symposium on acoustical holography, 1975. p 71–90

23. Greenleaf J, Johnson S, Lee S, Herman G, Wood E (1973) Algebraic reconstructions of spatial distributions of acoustic absorption within tissue from their two-dimensional acoustic projections. In: Fifth international symposium on acoustical holography and imaging, Palo Alto, CA, 1973. p 591–604

24. Greenleaf J, Bahn R (1981) Clinical imaging with transmissive ultrasonic computerized tomography. IEEE Trans Biomed Eng BME-28:177–185

25. Carson P, Oughton T, Hendee W, Ahuja A (1977) Imaging soft tissue through bone with ultrasound transmission tomography by reconstruction. Med Phys 4:302–309

26. Greenleaf J, Johnson S, Lent A (1978) Measurement of spatial distribution of refractive index in tissues by ultrasonic computer assisted tomography. Ultrasound Med Biol 3:327–339

27. Wiskin J, Borup D, Johnson S, Berggren M (2012) Non-linear inverse scattering: high resolution quantitative breast tissue tomography. J Acoust Soc Am 131:3802–3813

28. Schmidt S, Duric N, Li C, Roy O, Huang Z-F (2011) Modification of Kirchhoff migration with variable sound speed and attenuation for acoustic imaging of media and application to tomographic imaging of the breast. Med Phys 38:998–1007

29. Huthwaite P, Simonetti F, Duric N (2012) Combining time of flight and diffraction tomography for high resolution breast imaging: initial in vivo results (L). J Acoust Soc Am 132:1249–1252

30. Devaney A (1982) A filtered backpropagation algorithm for diffraction tomography. Ultrason Imaging 4:336–350

31. Norton S (1980) Reconstruction of a two-dimensional reflecting medium over a circular domain: exact solution. J Acoust Soc Am 67:1266–1273
32. Norton S, Linzer M (1979) Ultrasonic reflectivity imaging in three dimensions: reconstruction with spherical transducer arrays. Ultrason Imaging 1:210–239
33. Norton SJ, Linzer M (1981) Ultrasonic reflectivity imaging in three dimensions: exact inverse scattering solutions for plane, cylindrical, and spherical apertures. IEEE Trans Biomed Eng BME-28:202–220
34. Finch D, Patch SK, Rakesh (2003) Determining a function from its mean values over a family of spheres. SIAM J Math Anal 35:1213–1240
35. Xu M, Wang LV (2005) Universal back-projection algorithm for photoacoustic computed tomography. Phys Rev E 71:016706
36. Anastasio M, Zhang J, Modgil D, La Rivière PJ (2007) Application of inverse source concepts to photoacoustic tomography. Inverse Probl 23:S21–S36
37. Tao C, Song T, Yang W, Wu S (2006) Ultra-wideband microwave-induced thermoacoustic tomography of human tissues. Presented at the IEEE nuclear science symposium, 2006
38. Li C, Pramanik M, Ku G, Wang LV (2008) Image distortion in thermoacoustic tomography caused by microwave diffraction. Phys Rev E 77:031923
39. Eckhart A, Balmer R, See W, Patch S (2011) Ex vivo thermoacoustic imaging over large fields of view with 108 MHz irradiation. IEEE Trans Biomed Eng 58:2238–2246
40. Roggenbuck M, Walker R, Catenacci J, Patch S (2013) Volumetric Thermoacoustic Imaging over Large Fields of View. Ultrason Imaging vol. 35, pp. 57–67
41. Esenaliev RO, Larina IV, Larin KV, Deyo DJ, Motamedi M, Prough DS (2002) Optoacoustic technique for noninvasive monitoring of blood oxygenation: a feasibility study. Appl Optics 41:4722–4731
42. Petrov YY, Petrova IV, Patrikeev IA, Esenaliev RO, Prough DS (2006) Multiwavelength optoacoustic system for noninvasive monitoring of cerebral venous oxygenation: a pilot clinical test in the internal jugular vein. Opt Lett 31:1827–1829
43. Stoneman M, Kosempa M, Gregory W, Gregory C, Marx J, Mikkelson W, Tjoe J, Raicu V (2007) Correction of electrode polarization contributions to the dielectric properties of normal and cancerous breast tissues at audio/radiofrequencies. Phys Med Biol 52:6589–6604
44. Duck F (1990) Physical Properties of Tissue. London, San Diego: Academic Press
45. Razansky D, Kellnberger S, Ntziachristos V (2010) Near-field radiofrequency thermoacoustic tomography with impulse excitation. Med Phys 37:4602
46. Telenkov S, Mandelis A (2009) Photothermoacoustic imaging of biological tissues: maximum depth characterization comparison of time and frequency-domain measurements. J Biomed Opt 14:1–12
47. Fallon D, Yan L, Hanson GW, Patch SK (2009) RF testbed for thermoacoustic tomography. Rev Sci Instrum 80:064301
48. Pozar DM (2005) Microwave engineering, 3rd edn. Wiley, Hoboken, NJ
49. Parker D (1982) Optimal short scan convolution reconstruction for fan beam CT. Med Phys 9:254–257
50. Kak A, Slaney M (1988) Principles of computerized tomographic imaging. IEEE Press, New York
51. Wang LV, Zhao X, Sun H, Ku G (1999) Microwave-induced acoustic imaging of biological tissues. Rev Sci Instrum 70:3744–3748
52. Diebold GJ, Khan MI, Park SM (1990) Photoacoustic "signatures" of particulate matter: optical production of acoustic monopole radiation. Science 250:101–104
53. Pipe J (1999) Motion correction with PROPELLER MRI: application to head motion and free-breathing cardiac imaging. Magn Reson Med 42:963–969
54. Patch S (2005) k-space data preprocessing for artifact reduction in MRI. Presented at the radiological society of North America, Chicago, 2005
55. Patch S, Rao N, Kelly H, Jacobsohn K, See W (2011) Specific heat capacity of freshly excised prostate specimens. Physiol Meas 32:N55–N64
56. Halter R, Schned A, Heaney J, Hartov A, Schutz S, Paulsen K (2008) Electrical impedance spectroscopy of benign and malignant prostatic tissues. Urology 179:1580–1586

57. Halter R, Schned A, Heaney J, Hartov A, and Paulsen K (2009) Electrical Properties of Prostatic Tissues: I. Single Frequency Admittivity Properties, J Urol, vol. 182, pp. 1600–1607

58. R. Halter R, Schned A, Heaney J, Hartov A, and Paulsen K (2009), Electrical Properties of Prostatic Tissues: II. Spectral Admittivity Properties, J Urol, vol. 182, pp. 1608–1613

59. Lee B, Roberts W, Smith D, Ko H, Epstein J, Lecksell K, Partin A (1999) Bioimpedance: novel use of a minimally invasive technique for cancer localization in the intact prostate. Prostate 39:213–218

60. Chin L, Sherar M (2004) Changes in the dielectric properties of rat prostate ex vivo at 915MHz during heating. Int J Hyperthermia 20:517–527

61. Kurpad K (2011) Novel orthogonal double solenoid (ODS) volume RF coil for small animal imaging. Presented at the 19th annual meeting—international society of magnetic resonance in medicine, Montreal, 2011

62. Manohar S, Kharine A, van Hespen JCG, Steenbergen W, van Leeuwen TG (2005) The Twente photoacoustic mammoscope: system overview and performance. J Phys Med Biol 50:2543–2557

63. Xia W, Piras D, van Hespen J, van Veldhoven S, Prins C, van Leeuwen T, Steenbergen W, Manohar S (2013) An optimized ultrasound detector for photoacoustic breast tomography. Med Phys 40:1–13

64. Ermilov SA, Khamapirad T, Conjusteau A, Leonard MH, Lacewell R, Mehta K, Miller T, Oraevsky AA (2009) Laser optoacoustic imaging system for detection of breast cancer. J Biomed Opt 14:024007

65. Kunyansky LA (2007) Explicit inversion formulae for the spherical mean Radon transform. Inverse Probl 23:373–383

66. Kunyansky LA (2007) A series solution and a fast algorithm for the inversion of the spherical mean Radon transform. Inverse Probl 23:S11

Biography

Michael Roggenbuck received his B.S. in physics from the University of Wisconsin-Milwaukee in May 2012 and is currently employed by Epic Systems in Verona, Wisconsin.

Jared Catenacci received his B.A. in mathematics from the University of Wisconsin-Milwaukee in May 2012 and is pursuing a Ph.D. in applied mathematics at the University of South Carolina.

Ryan Walker received his B.A. degrees in mathematics and economics from Millersville University and is pursuing his Ph.D. in mathematics at the University of Kentucky.

Eric Hanson is double majoring in mathematics and physics at Mc Gill University.

Jiang Hsieh, Ph.D., earned his doctoral degree in physics at UW-Madison and is a Chief Scientist with GE Healthcare.

S.K. Patch, Ph.D., earned her doctoral degree in applied mathematics at UC Berkeley and is an Associate Professor in physics at UW-Milwaukee.

Automated Prostate Cancer Localization with Multiparametric Magnetic Resonance Imaging

Yusuf Artan, Imam Samil Yetik, and Masoom A. Haider

Abstract Prostate cancer is a leading cause of cancer death for men in the world. Fortunately, the survival rate for early-diagnosed patients is relatively high. Therefore, in vivo imaging plays an important role for the detection and treatment of the disease. Accurate prostate cancer localization with noninvasive imaging can be used to guide biopsy, radiotherapy, and surgery as well as to monitor disease progression. Magnetic resonance imaging (MRI) performed with an endorectal coil provides higher prostate cancer localization accuracy, when compared to transrectal ultrasound (TRUS). However, in general, a single type of MRI is not sufficient for reliable tumor localization. As an alternative, multispectral MRI, i.e., the use of multiple MRI-derived datasets, has emerged as a promising noninvasive imaging technique for the localization of prostate cancer; however, almost all studies are with human readers. There is a significant inter- and intra-observer variability for human readers, and it is substantially difficult for humans to analyze the large dataset of multispectral MRI. To solve these problems, this study presents an automated localization method. We first perform tests to see the best performing combination of multiparametric MRI, then develop localization methods using cost-sensitive support vector machines (SVMs), and show that this method results in improved localization accuracy than classical SVM. Additionally, we develop

Work of Imam Samil Yetik is partially supported by Marie Curie COFUND/TUBITAK Cocirc grant number 112C011.

Y. Artan
Medical Imaging Research Center, Illinois Institute of Technology, Chicago, IL, USA

I.S. Yetik (✉)
Department of Electrical and Electronics Engineering, TOBB Economy and Technological University, Ankara, Turkey
e-mail: yetik@iit.edu

M.A. Haider
Institute of Medical Science, Sunnybrook Research Institute, University of Toronto, Toronto, ON, Canada

A.S. El-Baz et al. (eds.), *Abdomen and Thoracic Imaging: An Engineering & Clinical Perspective*, DOI 10.1007/978-1-4614-8498-1_22, © Springer Science+Business Media New York 2014

a new segmentation method by combining conditional random fields (CRF) with a cost-sensitive framework and show that our method further improves cost-sensitive SVM (C-SVM) results by incorporating spatial information. We test SVM, C-SVM, and the proposed cost-sensitive CRF on multispectral MRI datasets acquired from 21 biopsy-confirmed cancer patients. Our results show that multispectral MRI helps to increase the accuracy of prostate cancer localization when compared to single MR images and that using advanced methods such as C-SVM as well as the proposed cost-sensitive CRF can boost the performance significantly when compared to SVM. We finally discuss potentially effective methods of localization using texture as the next steps of research.

Introduction

Prostate cancer is a major health problem for men, presenting a challenge to urologists, radiologists, and oncologists. Recent cancer studies have determined that 217,730 men were diagnosed and 32,050 died of prostate cancer in the United States in 2010 [1]. Despite the significant mortality rate, prostate cancer treatments have resulted in substantial progress over the past decades [2]. Currently popular methods for the detection of prostate cancer include the digital rectal examination (DRE) and PSA testing and, if needed, transrectal ultrasound (TRUS)-guided biopsy. TRUS-guided biopsy samples are taken from the expert designated regions, and pathologists confirm the presence or absence of cancer in the obtained cores. However, cancer may be invisible on ultrasound or missed due to the limited number of biopsy samples, leading to delayed diagnosis (and thus delayed treatment) of the disease. Accurate image guidance is extremely useful in ensuring that the tissue is collected from suspicious regions for cancer. Therefore, investigation of imaging methods to detect and localize these regions is an active research area.

TRUS is one of the widely used imaging methods for prostate cancer because it is readily available, inexpensive, and repeatable. TRUS enables the accurate determination of prostate size and depicts zonal anatomy, but its ability to detect cancer tissue is limited with sensitivity and specificity varying around 40–50 %. As an alternative to TRUS, MRI has been used to localize prostate cancer with varying degrees of success over the past years [3–5]. MRI provides the best description of the contours of the prostate as well as its internal anatomy. However, both TRUS and MRI lack satisfactory specificity rates for prostate cancer detection as noted in earlier studies [4]. Therefore, researchers investigated methods to boost the performance of prostate cancer localization using MRI. One method is to use additional MR imaging techniques that allow functional assessment such as diffusion-weighted imaging (DWI) and dynamic contrast-enhanced (DCE) MRI. DWI measures the Brownian motion of free water molecules in the tissues, and DCE-MRI depicts the vascularity and vascular permeability of tissue by following the time course of signal over time.

Earlier studies reported that T2-weighted MRI alone has sensitivity and specificity of 22–85 % and 50–99 %, respectively, for tumor detection, depending on the patient population characteristics and technical issues [6]. Similarly, DWI alone has a sensitivity and specificity of 57–93 % and 57–100 %, and DCE-MRI has reported sensitivity and specificity ranges of 52–96 % and 65–95 %. Recently, several studies have demonstrated the potential of combining morphological and metabolic information for localizing cancer [7–10]. Multiparametric MRI, i.e., a combination of DWI and DCE-MRI images, has shown a considerable potential to improve prostate cancer localization accuracy [8–15].

In one study, Haider et al. [10] performed T2-weighted imaging and DWI in 49 patients using an endorectal coil at 1.5 T and showed sensitivity is significantly higher with T2-weighted plus DWI 81 % than with T2-weighted imaging alone 54 %, and T2-weighted plus DWI shows loss in specificity compared with T2-weighted imaging alone 84 % vs. 91 %. In another study, Ocak et al. [8] interpreted DCE-MRI in conjunction with T2-weighted MRI in order to improve the cancer detection. This study reports that 94 % sensitivity and 37 % specificity for T2-weighted image can be improved to 70 % sensitivity and 88 % specificity.

Although various studies have been performed with human observers using multispectral MRI, only a few studies have been done to automatically localize prostate cancer with multispectral MRI [14–16]. There is a significant inter- and intra-observer variability for human readers, and it is difficult for humans to analyze multiple image datasets motivating the need for automated methods. The first part of this chapter is based on support vector machines (SVM) [17], which have demonstrated success in a broad range of applications, including brain tumor detection, microcalcification detection, and cervical cancer segmentation [18, 19]. SVMs are maximum margin classifiers that have strong generalization properties.

However, classical SVM classifiers do not explicitly utilize relative cost of error. To address this, we utilize a cost-sensitive extension of SVM, which is based on prior applications of SVM. This cost-sensitive extension of SVM has been referred to as $2v$-SVM in the literature, and it has found applications in various fields [13]. In this chapter, we apply the cost-sensitive SVM (C-SVM) to prostate cancer localization and compare the results to classical SVM. We also introduce several training methods to obtain the optimal SVM parameters: minimization of the total number of misclassifications, maximization of detection while keeping the false-positive rate below a threshold value, and maximization of the area under the receiver operating characteristic (ROC) curve. During the training stage, each of these training methods will output their optimal SVM parameters to be used in testing. Then, we describe methods that combine spatial information with SVM. Even though SVM is a maximum margin classifier that is superior to many other supervised learning algorithms, it ignores the spatial information for a given segmentation task. Previous studies have noted that most learning tasks involve much richer structure than a simple categorization of the instances into one of the classes [13, 17]. Therefore, it is beneficial to incorporate spatial information in the problem formulation. An earlier study developed a spatial SVM classifier by incorporating neighborhood information in the SVM formulation in an fMRI study [20]. However, this study does not take the cost information into account, and the formulation relies on the extreme sparseness of the data. In this study, we develop a new method that combines the cost-sensitive framework with conditional random fields (CRF) for improved performance of prostate cancer localization.

MRF and CRF are popular probabilistic graphical methods to incorporate contextual information in the segmentation process [21, 22]. MRF is an undirected graphical model proposed for modeling the spatial interaction between neighboring pixels in images, which encourages connected segmentation results by defining pairwise potentials between neighboring labels. However, MRF assumes conditional independence, and interaction among observed data is ignored. Because of the interconnection of the tumor region, tumor pixels are highly dependent on surrounding pixels, and hence, assumption of strong independence is not appropriate.

Unlike generative probabilistic models such as MRF and Hidden Markov Models (HMM), CRF describes the spatial dependencies in a probabilistic framework that directly models the posterior probability distribution over labels, given the observations. In contrast to MRF, CRF allows us to capture dependencies between the observations without resorting to any model approximations and has been shown to be useful in various segmentation applications [21–23]. However, our recent study showed that using CRF in its classical framework does not always yield accurate segmentation results for prostate cancer [16]. This study presents a novel integration of CRF and SVM in a cost-sensitive framework to obtain satisfying localization performance. Although CRF-based methods have not been applied to prostate cancer localization, they have been used in other areas. One study applied CRF in functional MR images, but did not consider combining C-SVM with CRF model [23]. Another study used SVM and CRF together in the area of brain image segmentation [24]; however, that application does not take into account the cost information in the SVM algorithm, and alternative training algorithms for the proper selection of optimal SVM parameters are not considered. Unlike these studies, we propose to combine C-SVM and CRF to achieve accurate prostate cancer localization with various alternatives for training.

The contribution of this chapter is threefold. First we perform a preliminary analysis to determine which combination of multiparametric MRI performs best in terms of localization performance. Secondly, we provide a framework, by using machine learning techniques, to remove the observer variability in tumor identification using multispectral MRI dataset that includes DCE-MRI in addition to DWI and T2-weighted that were used in [15]. We also show that using additional MR image types improves tumor localization significantly compared to a single MR type. The final contribution of this chapter is the introduction of cost-sensitive conditional random fields and its application to prostate cancer localization with multispectral MRI. We present visual, quantitative, and statistical analysis to demonstrate that the proposed cost-sensitive CRF achieves better localization than classical and C-SVM. We also outline methods that utilize texture that will potentially be very effective in prostate cancer localization in the future.

The remainder of the paper is organized as follows. In Section "Methodology," we describe the methodology that is used to select the multiparametric image combination that will be used throughout the study. Then, segmentation methodologies are described. In this section, the basic concepts of SVM, C-SVM, and the proposed cost-sensitive CRF as well as the optimal parameter selection methods are described. Section "Experiments and Results" provides the details of the multispectral MRI dataset used in this study and presents our segmentation results. This section also compares the performances of SVM, C-SVM, and cost-sensitive CRF. In Section "Discussion," we discuss our results and compare our findings with the earlier, mostly human reader, studies. Finally, conclusions are presented in Section "Conclusion."

Methodology

We now briefly describe the basics of support vector machine (SVM) and its cost-sensitive extension. Additionally, we propose a new segmentation method using cost-sensitive CRF and develop training schemes in order to obtain optimal parameters for C-SVM and CRF. Before performing segmentation, multispectral images are needed to be preprocessed as explained next.

Feature Selection to Determine the Optimum Combination of Multiparametric MRI

We have several types of multiparametric MR image types that are available. Therefore, before developing methods for automated cancer localization, we performed a detailed and exhaustive image analysis to determine the most effective MR image types in terms of their ability of cancer localization. For this purpose, all seven quantitative image maps, namely, (1) apparent diffusion coefficient (ADC) maps derived from diffusion-weighted images, (2) T2 maps, (3) k_{ep} derived from DCE MRI, (4) k_{el} derived from DCE MRI, (5) initial area under the curve 30 s (IAUC30), (6) IAUC60, and (7) IAUC90 are usesd. For these seven image types, we have constructed 127 image combinations that include all possible combinations.

Then, for all these combinations, we have calculated the Fisher ratio between two groups of pixels (tumor vs. normal). Then, all these 127 possible combinations were ranked. The highest performing combination was selected as the optimum multi-spectral MRI combination. This combination was T2-ADC-k_{ep} and used throughout the study.

In addition to exhaustive comparison of all possible combinations, we used a feature selection method based on linear programming. Our relevant feature identification is based on the property that minimizing an l_1 norm of linear decision boundary, w, via linear programming yields a sparse hyperplane, in which most

Table 1 Identification of relevant features by minimizing an l_1 norm of linear decision boundary

T2	ADC	k_{ep}	k_{el}	IAUC30	IAUC60	IAUC90
0.6438	0.5210	0.2044	0	0	0	0

components are zero [25]. This linear decision boundary separates the two classes as explained in detail in [25]. The rationale is that zero elements are irrelevant features that would not contribute to the decision process. A tractable convex optimization formulation of this problem has been proposed in earlier studies [25]. Table 1 shows absolute value of the relevancy of each feature with respect to the decision process. Hence, only three features are considered in the rest of our analysis.

Preprocessing and Ground Truth

Multispectral MRI dataset used in this chapter consists of three different types of MR images per the preliminary feature selection study. Each multispectral component represents a particular anatomical and functional response of the prostate gland. Feature vectors used for segmentation are intensity values of multispectral MR images. For each type of multispectral MR images, a single slice of size 256×256 from a 3D MRI is chosen by clinicians to be used in our experiments. The prostate consists of various zones such as transition zone (TZ) and peripheral zone (PZ). However, only the PZ region is considered since 70 % of the prostate cancer occurs in this region [26]. Several other studies presented their sensitivity/ specificity results using only PZ region as well [3, 8]. A manual registration was implemented for each patient to align the PZ region across different image types. All images are median filtered using a 3×3 window to improve signal-to-noise ratio, remove the spikes, and suppress possible registration errors. For each of the multispectral images, applying a simple transformation to the intensity values normalized PZ region intensities. Normalization is applied such that intensities in the PZ region had zero mean and unit standard deviation for all the training and testing subjects for a particular multispectral image. Then,

$$Y_{ij} = \frac{X_{ij} - \mu_j}{\sigma_i} \tag{1}$$

where X_{ij} is the image type i for patient j, Y_{ij} is the normalized image type i for patient j, and μ_j, σ_i refers to the mean and standard deviation of multispectral image type i. This brings intensities of different types of MR images within the same dynamic range, improving the stability of the classifiers. The ground truth is obtained based on pathology. A radiologist transfers the tumor regions on the histological slides to the MR images by viewing the histological slides, ex vivo MR images of these slides, and in vivo MR images. True-positives and true-negatives are defined on a pixel basis, providing a considerable amount of data points for evaluation.

Segmentation Methods

Multispectral MR images show a discernible intensity difference that differentiates between cancerous and normal tissue. Therefore, intensity values of anatomical and functional images are used as our features to construct the classifiers. In the following sections, we present a comparison of the performance of several classification methods, SVM, C-SVM, and the proposed cost-sensitive CRF. A total of 21 patients are used in the training and testing steps. During the experiments, based on the ground truth obtained from pathology, leave-one-out cross validation is implemented using twenty subjects for training and one subject for testing for each of the 21 subjects.

The support vector machine (SVM) is a universal supervised learning algorithm based on statistical learning theory [17]. Learning is the process of selecting the best mapping function $f(x,w)$ from a set of mapping models parameterized by a set of parameters $w \in \Omega$, given a finite training dataset (x_i, y_i) for $i = 1, 2, \ldots, N$, where $x_i \in R^d$ is a d-dimensional input (feature) vector, $y_i \in \{-1, 1\}$ is a class label, and N is the number samples in the training dataset. The objective is to estimate a mapping function $f(x \rightarrow y)$ in order to optimally classify future test samples. Suppose we have a mapping that separates the set of positive samples from negatives. This amounts to finding weights w and the bias b such that

$$y_i < w, x_i > +b > 0 \quad \text{for} \quad i = 1, 2, \ldots, N \tag{2}$$

If there exists a hyperplane satisfying (2), the set is said to be linearly separable. For a linearly separable set, it is always possible to rescale w and b in (2) such that

$$y_i < w, x_i > +b \geq 1 \quad \text{for} \quad i = 1, 2, \ldots, N \tag{3}$$

In this way, closest training point to the dataset has a distance of $1/\|w\|$. Among the alternative hyperplane that satisfy (3), SVM selects the one for which the distance to the closest point in the training data is maximal. Since the distance to the closest point is $1/\|w\|$, SVM finds the hyperplane by minimizing $\|w\|^2$ under constraints given by (3). The quantity $2/\|w\|$ is called the *margin*; hence, SVM is called a maximum margin classifier. When the classes are not linearly separable, constraints are relaxed by adding nonnegative slack variables $(\xi_1, \xi_2, \ldots, \xi_N)$ in the formulation of the optimization problem. The optimum classifier can be found by solving

$$
\begin{aligned}
\min \quad & \frac{1}{2}\|w\|^2 + C\sum_{i=1}^{N}\xi_i \\
\text{st.} \quad & y_i(< w, x_i > +b) \geq 1 - \xi_i \quad \text{for} \quad i = 1, 2, \ldots, N \\
& \xi_i \geq 0 \quad \text{for} \quad i = 1, 2, \ldots, N
\end{aligned}
\tag{4}
$$

where C is the weight for the penalty term for misclassifications. SVM is a frequently used algorithm in image classification applications [19, 27] with several variations. In this study, we use the v-SVM since selection of v is easier than alternatives [28]. The v-SVM has the following primal formulation:

$$\min \quad \frac{1}{2}\|w\|^2 - v + \sum_{i=1}^{N} \xi_i$$
$$\text{st.} \quad y_i(< w, x_i > +b) \geq 1 - \xi_i \quad \text{for} \quad i = 1, 2, \ldots, N$$
$$\xi_i \geq 0 \quad \text{for} \quad i = 1, 2, \ldots, N$$

(5)

In prostate cancer localization, however, there is a disadvantage to v-SVM formulation since it penalizes errors of both classes equally [28]. A reformulation of (5) is called $2v$-SVM, given by

$$\min \quad \frac{1}{2}\|w\|^2 - v + \frac{\gamma}{N}\sum_{i \in I_+} \xi_i + \frac{1-\gamma}{N}\sum_{i \in I_-} \xi_i$$
$$\text{st.} \quad y_i(< w, x_i > +b) \geq 1 - \xi_i \quad \text{for} \quad i = 1, 2, \ldots, N$$
$$\xi_i \geq 0 \quad \text{for} \quad i = 1, 2, \ldots, N$$

(6)

where $\gamma \in [0,1]$ is a parameter controlling the trade-off between false-negatives and false-positives and I_+, I_- are the numbers of training samples that belong to the positive and negative classes, respectively. Solution to above primal formulation is obtained by transforming this convex optimization problem into a corresponding dual formulation resulting in a quadratic cost function. Two parameters in linear $2v$-SVM that determine the classifier performance, γ and v, are selected as explained next.

Optimal parameter selection in SVM [29, 30] is crucial to classifier effectiveness. However, optimal SVM parameters certainly differ depending on the defined error criterion. $2v$-SVM parameter selections require a full grid search over v and γ values to reach the optimum parameters. SVM trained in this way will be referred throughout as C-SVM. One study [13] proposed a variant of coordinate descent algorithm that would speed up the search process. However, due to non-smoothness of the probability of positive and probability of false-negative values, the proposed accelerated algorithm could not be applied in this study. The parameter v was searched in the range [0.01, 0.50] over 50 points, and γ was searched in the range [0.10, 0.90] over 17 points, respectively. These resolutions are chosen in an ad hoc manner based on experience related to the smoothness of the underlying function. Increasing the number of sampling points of v and γ may result in slightly better estimates; however, it would be a computationally intensive task not producing significant differences given typical error functions. Figure 1 shows such a typical error vs. weights values of a single value with 17 samples we use. Notice that minima would not change significantly when the number of samples is increased.

In this study, we utilize and compare three different training methodologies. In our experiments, we implemented $2v$-SVM with the linear kernel based on

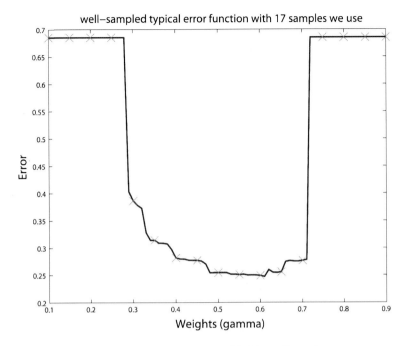

Fig. 1 Error rate vs. γ (weights) of a single υ value with 17 sampling points we use

our preliminary investigation. We trained the 2υ-SVM using cross validation to determine the optimal υ and γ parameters. Now, we describe the proposed training schemes that are used to choose υ and γ parameters.

The objective of the first training method is to minimize the number of pixel misclassifications from both classes. A full grid search is conducted on υ and γ parameters to find the lowest error rate. SVM trained by this method will be referred to as SVM_1 for classical SVM and $C\text{-}SVM_1$ for C-SVM. In the second training method, optimal υ and γ parameters are obtained by performing a full grid search, where υ and γ are selected such that detection probability is maximized while constraining false-positive probability to be below a threshold value referred to as SVM_2 for classical SVM and $C\text{-}SVM_2$ for C-SVM. Third training method utilizes area under the ROC curve (AUC) metric to assess the performance of a classifier. For each υ and γ pair in the grid, Platt's function is used to convert SVM decisions into posterior probabilities [26, 27], and ROC curves are obtained using these posterior probabilities. SVM trained by this method are similarly referred as SVM_3 for classical SVM and $C\text{-}SVM_3$ for C-SVM.

Bias Selection. In the training stage, we determine the optimal υ and γ pair to be used in testing process using one of the training methods mentioned above. However, to make a fair comparison between classical and C-SVM classifiers, the bias of each constructed classifier is adjusted to achieve a false-positive rate of 0.30 for the training dataset. This bias adjustment is performed for all classical SVM and cost-sensitive C-SVM classifiers during the training and not changed for individual test subjects. The false-positive rate used is selected based on a clinically acceptable performance.

Even though SVM benefits from the maximum margin property, it does not utilize spatial information in the classification process. Therefore, we propose a new segmentation method that uses CRF in a cost-sensitive framework as described next. CRF was proposed initially by Lafferty et al. [31] in the context of segmentation and labeling of 1D text sequences. Similar to MRF, it is used to model the spatial interaction in images. For an observed data x and corresponding labels y, MRF models the posterior probability using Bayes' rule:

$$p(y|x) \propto p(x,y) = p(x|y)p(y)$$

where the prior over the labels is assumed to be stationary and Markovian and likelihood is assumed to have a factorized form $p(x|y) = \prod_{i \in S} p(x_i|y_i)$ where S is the set of nodes. Recently, it has been noted [22] that a factorized form of the likelihood model is too restrictive in certain image classification applications because label interactions do not depend on the observed data. Therefore, CRF directly models the posterior probability distribution $p(y|x)$ for a given input image sample x and label y using a Gibbs prior model. Before we present the CRF definition as stated in [31], we first restate the notation. Suppose that the observed features from a given training image are given by $x = \{x_i\}_{i \in S}$ where $x_i \in R^d$ is the feature vector for node i. Corresponding labels at image nodes are given by $y = \{y_i\}_{i \in S}$. CRF constructs a discriminative conditional model $p(y|x)$ from the jointly distributed observations x and y, and the prior, $p(y)$, is not modeled explicitly.

CRF Definition. Let $G = (S, E)$ be a graph such that the vertices of G index y. Then (y, x) is said to be a conditional random field if, when conditioned on x, the random variables y_i obey the Markov property with respect to the graph: $p\left(y_i, x|y_{S-\{i\}}\right)$ $= p\left(y_i, x|y_{S-N_i}\right)$ where S-$\{i\}$ is the set of all nodes in the graph except the node i, N_i is the set of neighbors of the node i in G, and y_Ω represents the set of labels at the nodes in the set Ω [31].

Recently, another study [22] introduced a two-dimensional extension of CRF by using the local discriminative models to capture the class associations at individual nodes as well as the interactions on the neighboring nodes for a 2D graph:

$$p(y|x) = \frac{1}{Z}\exp\left\{\sum_{i \in S} A(y_i, x) + \sum_{i \in S}\sum_{j \in N_i} V\left(y_i, y_j, x\right)\right\} \tag{7}$$

where Z is a normalizing constant known as the partition function, $A(y_i, x)$ is the node potential at node i, and $V(y_i, y_j, x)$ is the edge potential between nodes i and j that encourages spatial smoothness. The terms $A(y_i, x)$ and $V(y_i, y_j, x)$ can be seen as unary data term and smoothness term, respectively. Node potential $A(y_i, x)$ is a measure of how likely the node i will take label y_i given image node x ignoring the effects of other node labels in the image. Generalized linear models are used extensively in statistics to model the class posterior given the observations. In our formulation, $A(y_i,x)$ is modeled using a local discriminative model that outputs the association of the node i with class y_i:

$$A(y_i, x) = \ln\left(\frac{1}{1 + \exp(-y_i w^T x)}\right) \tag{8}$$

where w is the normal to the linear decision boundary that is obtained from C-SVM as explained next in more detail. The edge potential is a function of all observations of x. The aim of the smoothness term is to have similar labels at a pair of nodes for which the node value supports such a hypothesis. For a pair of neighboring nodes (i, j), let μ_{ij} denote a new feature vector obtained by taking the absolute difference of x_i and x_j, $\mu_{ij} = [1, |x_i - x_j|]$, where x_i is simply chosen to be the pixel intensity at node i.

$$V\left(y_i, y_j, x\right) = y_i y_j \kappa^T \mu_{ij} \tag{9}$$

and κ contains the model parameters. The first component of μ_{ij} is fixed to one to accommodate the bias parameter. In summary, the node potential acts as a unary term for individual nodes, while the edge potential is a data-dependent discriminative label interaction (smoothness term). In the classical approach to constructing (7), the parameters of the node potential w and edge potential κ are determined jointly in the training stage, where they are initialized with logistic regression and randomly, respectively [21]. However, in a recent study, we have shown that this approach does not result in accurate prostate cancer segmentation [16].

Therefore, in this chapter, node potential parameter w is obtained from SVM, and edge potential parameter κ is estimated subsequently. Use of a standard maximum-likelihood approach to learn κ parameter involves the evaluation of partition function Z. In general, evaluation of Z is considered as an NP-hard problem [21]. Therefore, we resort to approximation method, pseudo likelihood, to estimate the κ parameter. In this study, we adopted pseudo likelihood [32] to estimate κ due to its simplicity and efficiency. In the pseudo likelihood approach, the factored approximation is

$$\hat{\kappa} = \arg\max_{\kappa} \sum_{m} \sum_{i} \ln p\left(y_i^m \big| y_{N_i}^m, x^m, \kappa\right) \tag{10}$$

where κ refers to the neighbors of the node i and y_i^m is the observed label for node i in the mth training image. Further, (10) can be expressed as shown in (11), where τ is regularization constant. To ensure that the log likelihood is convex and prevent over-fitting due to the pseudo likelihood approximation, we assign a Gaussian prior on κ with zero mean and covariance $\tau^2 I$, where I is the identity matrix. Then we compute the local consistency parameters using its penalized log likelihood:

$$\hat{\kappa} = \arg\max_{\kappa} \sum_{m=1}^{M} \sum_{i \in S} \left\{ \ln\left(\delta\left(y_i w^T x\right)\right) + \sum_{j \in N_i} y_i y_j \kappa^T \mu_{ij}(x) - \ln\left(Z_i^m\right) \right\} - \frac{1}{2\tau^2}\kappa^T \kappa$$

(11)

where

$$Z_i = \sum_{y_i \in \{-1, 1\}} \left\{ \ln\left(\delta\left(y_i w^T x\right)\right) + \sum_{j \in N_i} y_i y_j \kappa^T \mu_{ij}(x) \right\}$$

When τ, chosen by cross validation, is given, the penalized likelihood in (11) is quadratic with respect to κ. Therefore, (11) is convex and can be maximized using a simple gradient descent algorithm. Note that node potentials act as a constant in this optimization process.

Finally, for a given test image x, we perform mean-field inference [33] using the estimated model parameters w and κ to obtain an optimal label configuration y. Next, we describe the multispectral MRI dataset used in this study and present the results obtained using the methods that were described.

Experiments and Results

Description of Multispectral MRI Data

In this chapter, multispectral MR images are obtained from 21 biopsy-confirmed prostate cancer patients. Axial-oblique fast spin-echo (FSE) T2-weighted, echo planar DWI, multi-echo FSE, and DCE-MRI were acquired before surgery using a 1.5-T MRI system (Echospeed or Excite HD; GE Healthcare, Milwaukee, WI) with a 4-channel phased-array surface coil coupled to an endorectal coil (MEDRAD, Warrendale, PA). All data were obtained with the image plane perpendicular to the rectal wall/prostate interface. Median time between imaging and surgery was 33 days (range 1–129 days). Acquisition parameters for T2-weighted MRI were the following: TR/TE = 6,550/101.5 ms; 320 × 256 matrix; echo-train length (ETL) = 16; bandwidth (BW) = 20.83 kHz; number of excitations (NEX) = 3; field of view (FOV) = 14 cm; and no phase wrap. The DWI parameters were the following: TR/TE = 4,000/77 ms; 128 × 256 matrix; ETL = 144; BW = 166.7 kHz; NEX = 10; FOV = 14 cm; and $b = 0, 600$ s/mm^2. Multi-echo FSE images were acquired at ten echo times (9.0–90.0 ms, in 9 ms increments) for T2 mapping (TR = 2,000 ms; 256 × 128 matrix; ETL = 10; BW = 31.25 kHz; NEX = 1; FOV = 20 cm).

Datasets for DCE analyses consisted of T1-mapping from multi-slice, multi-flip fast-spoiled gradient echo images (FSPGR) (flip angles: 2, 5, 10, 20; TR/TE = 8.5/4.2 ms; 256 × 128 matrix; ETL = 8; BW = 31.25 kHz; NEX = 1; FOV = 20 cm), followed by 50 phases of multi-slice FSPGR MRI (flip angle $= 20\infty$; TR/TE $= 4.3/1.9$ ms; 256×128 matrix; BW $= 62.5$ kHz; NEX $= 0.5$; FOV $= 20$ cm; temporal resolution $= 10$s). Two phases were acquired before injection of 20 mL contrast agent (gadopentetate dimeglumine (Magnevist; Bayer Schering Pharma, Berlin, Germany)) at a rate of 4 mL/s, followed by a 20 mL saline flush using a power injector (MEDRAD Spectris MR injection system).

On T2-weighted MRI, cancers exhibit low T2 signal, but common benign processes such as prostatic inflammation, post-biopsy hemorrhage, and fibrosis also exhibit low T2 signal [8], also motivating the need for DWI and DCE-MRI. T2 maps are calculated from a series of echo time measurements and eliminate the fluctuations in signal intensity as a function of proximity to the endorectal coil seen in T2-weighted, as well as providing quantitative values. ADC maps are derived from DWI parametric maps, and several recent studies [10] have shown the usefulness of ADC maps for localizing prostate cancer.

Dynamic contrast-enhanced (DCE) MRI is a well-known method for detecting and quantifying tumor angiogenesis. To obtain DCE-MRI data, contrast agent was injected into the patient, and multiple MR images were acquired at the same spatial location over approximately 10 min. One goal of DCE-MRI is to characterize tissue regions with expectation that certain processes such as blood flow, vascular characteristics, or tissue integrity are different in pathological tissue with respect to normal tissue. The results of dynamic contrast-enhanced MRI are used to calculate time concentration curves, and pharmacokinetic parameters were obtained using Brix model [34] allowing rate constants, such as k_{ep} (wash-in rate), k_{el} (wash-out rate), and A (contrast agent dose and tissue-dependent parameter), to be estimated [35]. Rate constants are known to be elevated in cancerous tissue [5, 7]. Recent studies [8] noted that DCE-MRI improves the specificity of MRI over conventional T2-weighted MRI for the detection and localization of prostate cancer. A full MRI and parametric dataset is shown for an example patient in Fig. 2(a–d).

The available MRI dataset consists of several functional, anatomical, and parametric image types; however, based on preliminary feature selection analysis, we restrict our attention to three types of images (1) T2-maps, (2) ADC, (3) kinetic parameter k_{ep} that have information from three main groups (T2, DWI, and DCE-MRI).

Upon the completion of radical prostatectomy, the extracted prostate was placed in formalin for 24 h and embedded in HistOmer gel prior to ex vivo MRI. T2-weighted (T2w) images were taken at a 5° intervals and the angle corresponding to the plane of in vivo imaging was determined. The gel-embedded prostate was cut into regular 3 mm sections using a rotary blade, along the angle plane determined during the ex vivo imaging sessions. For all sections, standard pathological techniques are used to prepare hematoxylin and eosin (H&E)-stained whole-mount histological slides. A pathologist assesses the whole-mount sections and region of tumor was outlined as ground truth. Then, this tumor location is transferred to the in vivo MRI by an expert radiologist, who views in vivo MRI, histological slide, and the ex vivo MRI of this histological slide. A digitalized

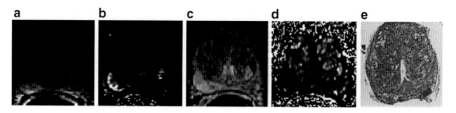

Fig. 2 Prostate MRI and parametric maps. (**a**) T2-weighted MRI, (**b**) T2 maps, (**c**) apparent diffusion coefficient (ADC), (**d**) k_{ep}, (**e**) digitized whole-mount H&E histology slide

histological section of a patient is shown in Fig. 2e from the same patient and location with in vivo MR images shown in Fig. 2(a–d). Histological analysis helps us to determine the malignant and benign prostate tissues with higher accuracy than the analysis of cancer lesion by a radiologist viewing only the in vivo MR images.

Application of Segmentation Methods to Prostate Cancer Localization with Multispectral MRI

In this section, classification methods explained in section "Methodology" are applied and evaluated using multispectral MR images. A comparison of conventional SVM, C-SVM, and the proposed cost-sensitive CRF is presented. Majority (70 %) of cancer nodules are located in the peripheral zone [26]; therefore, we have considered only the peripheral zone of the prostate in this study. Many other studies were conducted using only PZ region of the prostate [3, 8], which would allow us to compare our quantitative results to these previous studies. All experiments are performed using leave-one-out. That is, the test subject is not used in the training stage.

To illustrate the performance improvements through the use of multispectral MR image data visually, we present segmentation results for several subjects in Fig. 3. These example segmentation results from a group of subjects allow us to see the benefit of multispectral MRI visually. Segmentation results using SVM, C-SVM, and cost-sensitive CRF are shown in Fig. 4, where the superiority of the cost-sensitive CRF can also be observed visually.

Statistical and Quantitative Analysis of Results

In addition to visual evaluation, we use several quantitative measures to evaluate the results including specificity, sensitivity, dice measure (DSC) [36], and area under the ROC curve. ROC is a common method used to quantify the classifier performance. To compare performances of different classifiers, we reduce the ROC

Ground Truth   T2   T2ADC   T2ADCk_{ep}

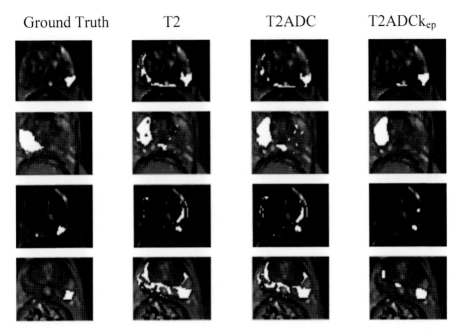

Fig. 3 Segmentation results of cost-sensitive CRF using T2 maps (Column 2), T2 maps and ADC (Column 3), and T2 maps, ADC, and k_{ep} (Column 4). White pixels denote the tumor locations in the image

Ground Truth   SVM   C-SVM   CRF

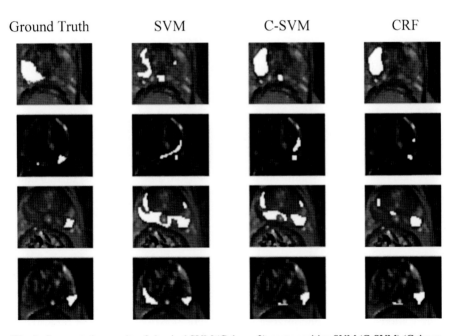

Fig. 4 Segmentation results of classical SVM (Column 2), cost-sensitive SVM (C-SVM) (Column 3), and cost-sensitive CRF (Column 4). White pixels denote the tumor locations in the image

Table 2 Mean ± standard deviation of dice measure using T2, ADC, and k_{ep}

Method	Method1	Method2	Method3
SVM	0.38 ± 0.21	0.36 ± 0.19	0.37 ± 0.20
C-SVM	0.40 ± 0.19	0.37 ± 0.19	0.38 ± 0.21
CRF	0.46 ± 0.26	0.44 ± 0.25	0.43 ± 0.27

Method 1 refers to training scheme using misclassification error minimization, Method 2 to Neyman Pearson, and Method 3 to area under curve

curve to a scalar value, area under curve (AUC), representing the performance of the classifier. In this study, ROC curves are estimated using maximum likelihood and assuming bivariate normal data with ROCKIT software (version 0.9.1-beta, CE Metz, University of Chicago) [37]. We used average AUC values obtained from 21 patients to compare performances of different methods, and also included sensitivity/specificity, and dice measure to assess the performances of the various methods and combinations of MRI types. Sensitivity and specificity are defined as

$$\text{Sensitivity} = \text{TP}/\text{TP} + \text{FN}$$
$$\text{Specificity} = \text{TN}/\text{FP} + \text{TN}$$

where TP and FP denote the numbers of true-positive and false-positive pixels, respectively. Similarly, TN and FN show the numbers of true-negatives and false-negative pixels. DSC (dice measure), a quantity that measures the accuracy of localization for the detected tumor, is

$$\text{DSC}(A, B) = \frac{2|A \cap B|}{(|A| + |B|)}$$

where A is the segmentation result, B is the ground truth, and the operation |.| denotes the number of segmented pixels.

Due to the relatively small number of patients (21 patients), Fisher's exact test [38] is used to measure the statistical significance of our results. It is commonly used in medical image analysis to examine the association of two types of classification. p-value with Fisher's test provides the probability of obtaining a test statistic at least as extreme as the one that was actually observed. Lower p-values indicate a less likely, thus a more significant result. In general, a p-value of less than or equal to 5 % is deemed to be statistically significant.

Table 2 shows the average DSC measures for all three training methods using all three features (T2-ADC-k_{ep}) where we have performed a leave-one-out cross validation and bias adjustment for all 21 patients. Segmentation performances of different training methods are not very different, with Method 1 producing slightly larger DSC values. In the rest of the discussion, we present only results from error minimization (Method 1) resulting in higher DSC. However, we should note that other training schemes proposed might be useful for various other clinical applications. For example, higher specificity or sensitivity might be preferred in the price of decreased DSC.

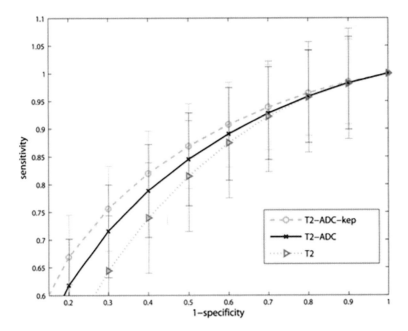

Fig. 5 Average ROC curves and standard deviations of 21 test images for C-SVM using (1) T2 maps (2) T2 maps, ADC (3) T2 maps, ADC, and k_{ep}

Table 3 Mean ± standard deviation for area under curve (AUC) for 21 patients for SVM and C-SVM

Method	T2	T2ADC	T2ADCk_{ep}
SVM$_1$	0.74 ± 0.13	0.76 ± 0.13	0.77 ± 0.11
C-SVM$_1$	0.74 ± 0.13	0.78 ± 0.12	0.79 ± 0.12

Table 4 p-values of area under the curve (AUC) using T2 maps, ADC, and k_{ep} for SVM, C-SVM, and CRF with bias shifting

Method	T2 vs. T2ADC	T2 vs. T2ADC	T2ADC vs. T2ADCk_{ep}
SVM$_1$	0.0133	0.0133	0.0946
C-SVM$_1$	0.0133	0.0133	0.0133

Figure 5 shows the average ROC graph for 21 test patients with leave-one-out applied for all patients. This figure shows that using a richer set of MR images increases the classifier performance considerably. Table 3 shows the average AUC values of 21 patients for several image combinations, and Table 4 shows the p-values for T2, T2-ADC, and T2-ADC-k_{ep} with SVM and cost-sensitive SVM classifiers. We observe that T2-ADC-k_{ep} combination yields the highest AUC values for both methods. This clearly demonstrates the advantage of using multispectral MRI in prostate cancer segmentation. p-values from Table 4 shows that

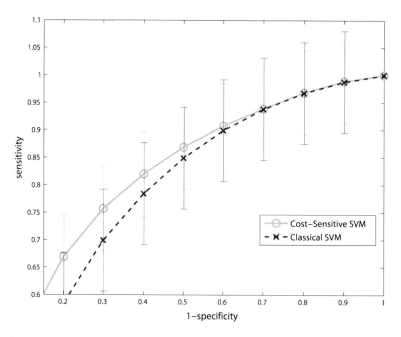

Fig. 6 Average ROC curves and standard deviations of 21 patients using T2, ADC, and k_{ep}

performance improvements are statistically significant as more features are used for both SVM and C-SVM, except for the single case of T2-ADC vs. T2-ADC-k_{ep} with SVM. The performance improvement is statistically significant for the same combinations with C-SVM indicating that C-SVM can better utilize multispectral MRI data.

Further, to show that C-SVM is superior to classical SVM, Fig. 6 shows the average ROC curve of 21 test patients, with leave-one-out for each patient, for classical and C-SVM. We use training Method 1 and all three types of modality images: T2, ADC, and k_{ep} for this figure. In most of the subjects that we have investigated, C-SVM performs better than classical SVM.

On the other hand, Table 5 provides average sensitivity, specificity, and DSC values for performance comparison using different feature vectors with all classification methods. This table shows that combining CRF with C-SVM provides considerably improved performance compared to using only SVM/C-SVM classifiers. There is a noticeable increase in mean values of dice measure (DSC) with the proposed cost-sensitive CRF. However, we can also observe that the sensitivity of the CRF method is inferior to the sensitivity of the other two methods, because CRF is producing much larger specificity values. Therefore, although CRF is preferable when sensitivity and specificity are considered together, a clinical application that particularly needs high sensitivity in the price of decreased specificity can require C-SVM to be used instead of CRF. Also, Tables 6 and 7 present the p-values of dice measures for different classifiers and multispectral images, respectively. Table 6 indicates that the improvements when using three image types

Table 5 Mean $\pm$ standard deviation for sensitivity, specificity, and DSC using T2 maps, ADC, and k_{ep} for SVM, C-SVM, and CRF with bias shifting

Method	Sens/specs	T2	T2ADC	T2ADCk_{ep}
SVM	Sens.	0.68 ± 0.31	0.75 ± 0.24	0.66 ± 0.30
	Spec.	0.63 ± 0.30	0.62 ± 0.22	0.70 ± 0.26
	DSC.	0.35 ± 0.20	0.37 ± 0.19	0.38 ± 0.21
C-SVM	Sens.	0.72 ± 0.27	0.72 ± 0.27	0.73 ± 0.25
	Spec.	0.62 ± 0.27	0.66 ± 0.23	0.67 ± 0.22
	DSC.	0.36 ± 0.19	0.38 ± 0.20	0.40 ± 0.19
CRF	Sens.	0.58 ± 0.39	0.66 ± 0.33	0.64 ± 0.34
	Spec.	0.73 ± 0.14	0.73 ± 0.26	0.78 ± 0.22
	DSC.	0.35 ± 0.28	0.42 ± 0.26	0.46 ± 0.26

Table 6 p-values of dice measure (DSC) using T2 maps, ADC, and k_{ep} for SVM, C-SVM, and CRF with bias shifting

Method	T2 vs. T2ADC	T2 vs. T2ADCk_{ep}	T2ADC vs. T2ADCk_{ep}
SVM	0.0946	0.1917	0.1917
C-SVM	0.0946	0.0392	0.0392
CRF	0.0946	0.0392	0.001

Table 7 p-values of dice measure (DSC) using T2 maps, ADC, and k_{ep} for SVM, C-SVM, and CRF methods

Method	CRF vs. SVM	CRF vs. C-SVM	C-SVM vs. SVM
T2	0.0392	0.0392	0.3318
T2-ADC	0.0946	0.0946	0.0133
T2-ADC-k_{ep}	0.0392	0.0392	0.3318

are statistically significant with CRF. Next, Table 7 shows that the improvements of CRF compared to SVM and C-SVM are statistically significant as evident by p-values when all three-image types are used. These tables show that advanced methods such as CRF and C-SVM can better utilize multispectral MRI data.

Results presented so far were obtained after adjusting the bias of the classifier to achieve 0.70 specificity in the training stage for each patient. Note that specificity values presented in Table 8 are for the test images and they show a specificity value close to 0.70. However, one might wonder how the result would change if we did not perform this shift in classical SVM and used the bias provided by SVM algorithm. Table 8 shows the sensitivity, specificity, and DSC without any bias adjustments with training Method 1. Comparison of Tables 5 and 8 shows that the segmentation performance is considerably improved through the proposed bias adjustment. Note that bias adjustment is done during training, and this bias value does not change for separate test subjects.

Table 8 Mean ± standard deviation for sensitivity, specificity, and DSC using T2 maps, ADC, and k_{ep} for SVM, C-SVM, and CRF without bias shifting

Method	Sens/specs	T2	T2ADC	T2ADCk_{ep}
SVM	Sens.	0.80 ± 0.20	0.83 ± 0.19	0.74 ± 0.25
	Spec.	0.40 ± 0.24	0.47 ± 0.23	0.60 ± 0.24
	DSC.	0.32 ± 0.16	0.34 ± 0.19	0.36 ± 0.19
C-SVM	Sens.	0.85 ± 0.19	0.84 ± 0.19	0.70 ± 0.29
	Spec.	0.50 ± 0.25	0.48 ± 0.22	0.68 ± 0.29
	DSC.	0.34 ± 0.18	0.35 ± 0.18	0.38 ± 0.21
CRF	Sens.	0.73 ± 0.30	0.81 ± 0.24	0.66 ± 0.33
	Spec.	0.60 ± 0.31	0.57 ± 0.28	0.72 ± 0.28
	DSC.	0.34 ± 0.23	0.39 ± 0.20	0.42 ± 0.27

In summary, the visual, quantitative, and statistical results presented here show that proposed cost-sensitive CRF is superior to the classical techniques of SVM and C-SVM, and using multispectral MRI significantly improves localization performance when compared to single type of MRI.

Prostate Cancer Localization with Texture

General image segmentation studies often utilize filter banks in their analysis. Filter banks are known to be the most efficient and accurate way to derive texture features. Recently, Leung et al. [39] introduced a set of filter banks known as Leung-Malik (LM) filters for natural image segmentation study. We plan to combine filter bank-derived features with random walker (RW) algorithm [40] to develop robust, accurate image segmentation technique. We present quantitative and qualitative performance comparison between pixel intensity and filter bank-derived features using toy images. We show that filter bank and RW combination results in better segmentation in general image segmentation tasks.

Filter Banks. Filter banks have been ubiquitously used in image segmentation applications. Recently, Leung-Malik (LM) filter banks received significant attention due to their high performance in segmenting natural scene images [39]. The LM filter set is a multi-scale, multi-orientation filter bank with 48 filters. It consists of first and second derivatives of Gaussians at 6 orientations and 3 scales, making a total of 36; 8 Laplacian of Gaussian (LOG) filters; and 4 Gaussians. The components of LM filter bank are shown in Fig. 7. Given input image is convolved with each of the filters shown in Fig. 7, after each filtering step, we smooth the response image by applying a low-pass filter on the response image. In order to show the effectiveness of the random walker image segmentation with filter banks, we have used toy examples. For quantitative comparison between intensity and filter-based RW algorithms, we use the dice measure. In our experimental setting, we have an image with a set of initialization points referred as seeds that indicates

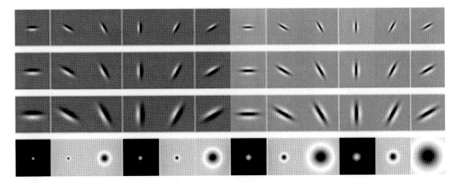

Fig. 7 The Leung-Malik filter bank. The filter bank consists of an edge and bar filter both at scales 3 and 6 orientations and 2 rotationally symmetric filters of 49 × 49 pixels

different classes. Segmentation results using a set of simple images are shown in Fig. 8 using intensity and filter bank-based random walker.

Table 9 shows the quantitative dice measure for both segmentation schemes. Difference between the mean values clearly shows the benefit of using filter banks with random walker algorithm. Notice that from Fig. 8 intensity alone is not able to capture the texture properties, hence results in a worse segmentation.

Since the tumors on the prostate, especially in the transition zone, show considerable difference in texture when compared to the normal tissue, localization methods using texture are potentially very effective and need to be further investigated.

Discussion

There exist several prostate cancer segmentation studies with multispectral MRI in the literature [8, 10, 14]. However, most of these are with human readers; therefore, a direct comparison of our results with those studies is difficult. There is a notable inter- and intra-observer variability for human readers, and it is tedious for humans to analyze multiple image datasets. Therefore, automated methods have an intrinsic advantage over human readers since they remove observer variability and can easily be repeated.

Another difficulty for comparison is that the study population differs from one study to another and sensitivity/specificity critically depends on the sampling variation. Girouin et al. [9] report sensitivity/specificity value of 50–60 % and 13–21 % over 46 patients using only T2-weighted (1.5 T) MRI in cancer detection. Further, Girouin presents sensitivity/specificity value of 78–81 % and 32–56 % for the same dataset using T2-weighted (3.0 T) MRI. Futterer et al. [5] present their results for six patients using T2-weighted (1.5 T) MRI, and their results show a

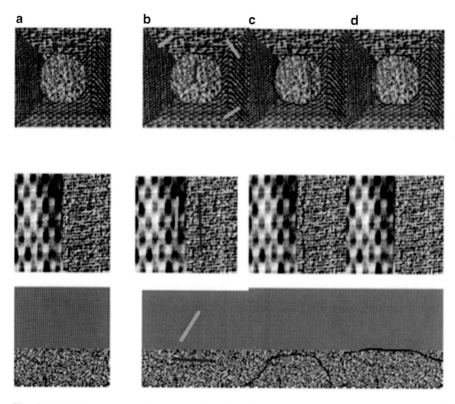

Fig. 8 (**a**) Original image, (**b**) Seed points, *blue* (foreground), *green* (background), and *red* (boundary), using (**c**) intensity RW (**d**) LM-based RW

Table 9 Mean ± standard deviation for DSC using random walker with intensity and filter bank features

Measure	RW	LM filter RW
DSC	0.73 ± 0.15	0.93 ± 0.06

significantly higher values, sensitivity/specificity is 83 % and 83 %, respectively. However, studies that include higher number of patients do not confirm Futterer's results [3, 8, 41]. Clinical results with DCE-MRI at 1.5 T have been inconsistent with sensitivities and specificities varying from 51 % to 89 % and 67 % to 87 %, respectively [42]. A recent study by Ocak et al. [8] interpreted DCE-MRI in conjunction with T2-weighted MRI in order to improve the cancer detection. This study reports that 94 % sensitivity and 37 % specificity for T2-weighted image can be improved to 70 % sensitivity and 88 % specificity. We were able to achieve 64 % sensitivity and 78 % specificity with 21 patients using the automated localization methods presented in this chapter. Note that automated localization avoids any human interference in the decision process, therefore, allows us to remove observer variability. Furthermore, automated methods are more efficient in tumor localization. On the other hand, they may not be able to capture certain aspects of the human experience that clinicians learn over many years.

The limitations of this study are the limited number of patients and possible misalignment between pathology and ground truth. Since the alignment is not 100 % accurate, we anticipate a certain amount of error in the location and size of the tumor.

Conclusion

In this chapter, we presented a framework for selecting the most effective combination of multiparametric MRI for prostate cancer localization and methods for automatically localizing prostate cancer with multispectral MR images using supervised classification algorithms. Currently, the most often used invasive method for prostate cancer detection requires needle biopsy samples that are guided by TRUS images. However, TRUS is used only to locate the prostate and cannot accurately localize the cancer.

Multispectral MR imaging has shown promising results in detecting prostate carcinoma more accurately. However, almost all of these studies are with human readers, causing significant observer variability. The only automated method that was applied to prostate cancer is classical SVM [15] and is a supervised method that does not utilize training data [14]. In this study, we presented automated methods for prostate cancer segmentation with multispectral MRI using supervised classification algorithms: SVM, which was used in earlier studies and included for comparison purposes, C-SVM, and the proposed cost-sensitive CRF. Automated methods are not only more efficient but also remove the inter-observer variability, which is a particularly severe problem with multispectral MRI.

In this study, we used additional parameters to control class-related cost in the SVM formulation, which allowed us to increase overall segmentation accuracy. Next, we noticed that, even though classical SVM and C-SVM allow a simple categorization of instances into one of the classes, they do not use spatial information from the images. Therefore, we incorporated probabilistic graphical models to utilize the structure in the images. A probabilistic graphical model, CRF, allows one to use image structure for segmentation purposes. However, our previous results have shown that using classical CRF with logistic regression initialization of w parameter does not yield accurate segmentation results. Therefore, we integrated the C-SVM algorithm developed for classification of independent instances with graphical models that can exploit the inherent structure in the image result, yielding a novel cost-sensitive CRF technique.

In this chapter, we have also used three training schemes and compared their performances. Each of these training schemes achieves a different objective. In our discussion, we presented results using training Method 1 since it resulted in higher

DSC values for this dataset. However, the other training schemes could be useful for certain other clinical applications. For instance, there could be cases where the sensitivity or specificity is more important than DSC measure for a particular application. After performing experiments using real MRI data, our results concur with the findings of earlier studies with human readers showing that increasing the number of MR types increases the accuracy of detection and localization. From our results, the following can be deduced:

- Most effective combination of multiparametric MRI for prostate cancer localization consists of T2maps-ADC-k_{ep}.
- C-SVM is superior to classical SVM in prostate cancer segmentation using multispectral MRI. For instance, Table 3 shows that average AUC increases from 0.77 for classical SVM to 0.79 for C-SVM. Figure 4 presents an illustration of the performance of classical and C-SVM for several test patients.
- Average specificity/sensitivity and dice measure results considerably improve when proposed cost-sensitive CRF is used. Table 5 shows that dice measure increases from a mean value of 0.38 for classical SVM to 0.46 for CRF if we use T2-ADC-k_{ep} features to construct the classifier.
- Shifting the bias to achieve a constant false-positive rate yields better localization results compared to using the bias provided by SVM. A comparison of the corresponding values between Tables 5 and 8 shows such improvements for the majority of the cases. For example, cost-sensitive CRF dice measure increases from 0.39 to 0.42 for T2-ADC combination when we adjust the bias with the proposed method.

Fisher's exact test is also used to show that almost all of these improvements are statistically significant. Future work will include a more comprehensive comparison of the integrated SVM-CRF model to other discriminative models. Considering the lack of shape of the prostate tumors, and the fact that the tumor and healthy regions may have overlapping intensities, context-based segmentation methods for prostate cancer detection have to be investigated further. We have also discussed a group of methods that use texture for prostate cancer localization that potentially can be very effective in the future.

References

1. American Cancer Society (2010) Surveillance and health policy research. American Cancer Society, Atlanta
2. Villeirs GM, Verstraete L, De Neve WJ, De Meerleer GO (2005) Magnetic resonance imaging anatomy of the prostate and periprostatic area: a guide for radiotherapists. Radiother Oncol 76:99–106
3. Ito H, Kamoi K, Yokoyama K, Yamada K, Nishimura T (2003) Visualization of prostate cancer using dynamic contrast-enhanced MRI. Comparison with transrectal power doppler ultrasound. Br J Radiol 76(909):617–624

4. van Dorsten FA, van der Graaf M, Engelbrecht MR, van Leenders GJ, Verhofstad A, Ripkema M, de la Rosette JJ, Heerschap A (2004) Combined quantitative enhanced MR imaging and (1)H MR spectroscopic imaging of human prostate cancer. J Magn Reson Imaging 20(2):279–287
5. Futterer J, Heijmink S, Scheenen TW, Veltman J, Huisman HJ, Vos P, Hulsbergen-Van de Kaa CA, Witjes JA, Krabbe PF, Heerschap A, Barentsz JO (2006) Prostate cancer localization with dynamic contrast-enhanced MR imaging and proton MR spectroscopic imaging. Radiology 241(2):449–458
6. Turkbey B, Albert PS, Kurdziel K, Choyke PL (2009) Imaging localized prostate cancer. Current approaches and new developments. Am J Roentgenol 192(6):1471–1480
7. Futterer JJ, Barentsz J, Heijmink S (2009) Imaging modalities for prostate cancer. Expert Rev Anticancer Ther 9(7):923–937
8. Ocak I, Bernardo M, Metzger G, Barrett T, Pinto P, Albert PS, Choyke PL (2007) Dynamic contrast-enhanced MRI of prostate cancer at 3 T. A study of pharmacokinetic parameters. Am J Roentgenol 189(4):192–200
9. Girouin N, Mege-Lechevallier F, Senes S, Bissery S, Rabilloud M, Colombel M, Lyonnet D, RouviÔøΩre O (2007) Prostate dynamic contrast-enhanced MRI with simple visual diagnostic criteria. Is it reasonable? Eur J Radiol 17(6):1498–1509
10. Haider M, van der Kwast TH, Tanguay J, Evans AJ, Hashmi AT, Lockwood G, Trachtenberg J (2007) Combined T2-weighted and diffusion weighted MRI for localization of prostate cancer. Am J Roentgenol 189(2):323–328
11. Scheidler J, Hricak H, Vigneron DB et al (1999) Prostate cancer. Localization with three dimensional proton MR spectroscopic imaging-clinicopathologic study. Radiology 213:473–480
12. Yoshikazo T, Wada A, Hayashi T, Uchida K, Sumura M, Uchida N, Kitagaki H, Igawa M (2008) Usefulness of diffusion-weighted imaging and dynamic contrast enhanced magnetic resonance imaging in the diagnosis of prostate transition-zone cancer. Acta Radiol 49 (10):1208–1213
13. Davenport MA, Baraniuk RG, Scott CD (2006) Controlling false alarms with support vector machines. In: Proceedings of IEEE international conference on Acoustics, Speech, and Signal Processing (ICASSP), MIT Press, Cambridge, MA, pp 589–593
14. Liu X, Yetik IS, Wernick M et al (2009) Prostate cancer segmentation with simultaneous estimation of the MRF parameters and the class. IEEE Trans Med Imaging 28:906–915
15. Chan I, Wells W, Mulkern RV, Haker S, Zhang J, Zou KH, Maier SE, Tempany CM (2003) Detection of prostate cancer by integration of line-scan diffusion, T2-mapping and T2-weighted magnetic resonance imaging; a multichannel statistical classifier. Med Phys 30 (9):2390–2398
16. Artan Y, Yetik IS, et al (2009) Prostate cancer segmentation with multispectral MRI using cost sensitive conditional random fields. In: Proceedings of IEEE International Symposium on Biomedical Imaging (ISBI), pp 226–230
17. Vapnik V (1998) Statistical learning theory. Wiley, New York
18. Ricci E, Perfetti R (2007) Retinal blood vessel segmentation using line operators and support vector classification. IEEE Trans Med Imaging 26:1357–1365
19. El-Naqa I, Yang Y, Wernick M, Galatsanos NP, Nishikawa P (2002) A support vector machine approach for detection of microcalcifications. IEEE Trans Med Imaging 21:1552–1563
20. Liang L, Cherkassy V, Rottenberg DA (2006) Spatial SVM for feature selection and fMRI activation detection. In: International Joint Conference on Neural Networks (IJCNN), pp 1463–1469
21. Vishvanathan SV, Schaudarolph NN, Schmidt M, Murphy KP (2006) Accelerated training of conditional random fields with stochastic gradient methods. In: Proceedings of International Conference on Machine Learning (ICML), pp 969–976

22. Kumar S, Hebert M (2004) Discriminative random fields. A discriminative framework for contextual interaction in classification. In: Proceedings of IEEE Conference on Computer Vision and Pattern Recognition (CVPR), pp 1150–1157
23. Wang Y, Rajapakse J (2006) Contextual modelling of functional MR images with conditional random fields. IEEE Trans Med Imaging 25:804–812
24. Lee CH, Greiner R, Schmidt M, (2005) Support vector random fields for spatial classification. Lecture notes in computer science 3721:121–132, Springer
25. Bhattacharyya C, Grate LR, Rizki A et al (2002) Simultaneous relevant feature identification and classification in high-dimensional spaces: an application to molecular profiling data. Signal Process 83:729–743
26. Carrol CL, Somer FG, McNeal JE, Stammey TA (1987) The abnormal prostate. MR imaging at 1.5-T with histopathologic correlation. Radiology 163(2):521–525
27. Chew HG, Bogner RE, Lim CC (2001) Dual-v support vector machines and applications in multi-class image recognition. In: Proceedings of IEEE international conference on Acoustics, Speech, and Signal Processing (ICASSP), pp 1269–1272
28. Scholkopf B, Smola AJ, Williamson RC, Bartlett PL (2000) New support vector algorithms. Neural Comput 12:1207–1245
29. Steinwart I (2003) On the optimal parameter choice for v-support vector machine. IEEE Trans Pattern Anal Mach Intell 25:1274–1284
30. Chalimourda A, Scholkopf B, Smola AJ (2004) Experimentally optimal v-support vector regression for different noise models and parameter settings. Neural Netw 17(1):127–141
31. Lafferty J, McCallum A, Pereira F (1986) Conditional rando fields: a probabilistic model. J R Stat Soc 48(3):259–302
32. Besag J (1986) On the statistical analysis of dirty pictures. J R Stat Soc 48(3):259–302
33. Weiss Y (2001) Comparing mean field method and belief propagation for approximate inference in MRFs. Advanced mean field inference methods. MIT Press, Cambridge, MA
34. Brix G, Semmler W, Port R, Schad LR, Layer G, Lorenz WJ (1991) Pharmacokinetic parameters in CNS Gd-DTPA enhanced MR imaging. J Comput Assist Tomogr 15(4):621–628
35. Tofts PS (1997) Modeling tracer kinetics in dynamic Gd-DTPA MR imaging. J Magn Reson Imaging 7(1):91–101
36. Fisher RA (1954) Statistical methods for research workers. Oliver and Boyd, Edinburgh
37. Metz CE, Herman BA, Shen JH (1998) Maximum likelihood estimation of receiver operating characteristic curves from continuously distributed data. Stat Med 17:1033–1053
38. van Rijsbergen CJ (1979) Information retrieval. Butterworth-Heinemann, Newton, MA
39. Malik J, Belongie S, Leung T, Shi J (2001) Contour and texture analysis for image segmentation. Int J Comput Vis 43:7–27
40. Artan Y, Haider MA, Langer DL, Yetik IS (2010) Semi-supervised prostate cancer segmentation with multiparametric MRI. In: Proceedings of 2010 International Symposium on Biomedical Imaging (ISBI), pp 648–651
41. Schlemmer HP, Merkle J, Grobholz R (2004) Can operative contrast-enhanced dynamic MR imaging for prostate cancer predict microvessel density in prostatectomy specimens? Eur Radiol 14:309–317
42. Yu KK, Hricak H (2000) Imaging prostate cancer. Radiol Clin North Am 38(1):59–85

Biography

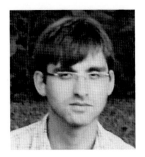

Yusuf Artan received his B.S. degree in Electrical Engineering from Rensselaer Polytechnic Institute in 2006 and his M.S. degree from Lehigh University in 2008. Since 2008, he has been a Ph.D. candidate in Medical Imaging Research Center at Illinois Institute of Technology. His research interest includes medical imaging, machine learning, and semi-supervised image segmentation.

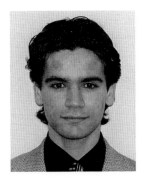

Imam Samil Yetik received his B.S. degree from Bogazici University, Bebek, Istanbul, in 1998, M.S. degree from Bilkent University, Ankara, Turkey, in 2000, and the Ph.D. degree in electrical engineering from University of Illinois, Chicago, in 2004. Between 2005 and 2006, he was a Postdoc at University of Illinois-Chicago and University of California at Davis, and a faculty member at Medical Imaging Research Center, Illinois Institute of Technology, between 2007 and 2013. Currently, he is an Associate Professor in the Department of Electrical and Electronics Engineering, at TOBB Economy and Technological University, Ankara, Turkey. His research interests are in the areas of biomedical signal and image processing with statistical approaches and machine learning techniques. His most recent focus areas are on prostate cancer localization, dynamic PET imaging, and oxygen tension imaging of the retina. Dr. Yetik is a senior member of IEEE.

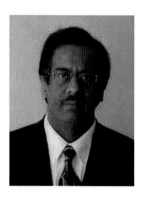

Masoom A. Haider received his B.Sc. degree in computer science from the University of Waterloo, Canada, in 1990 and MD degree from the University of Ottawa, Canada, in 1986. He completed a Radiology Residency at the University of Toronto, Canada, in 1994 and a Fellowship in Abdominal Imaging at the Cleveland Clinic Foundation in Cleveland, OH, in 1995. He is an American Board of Radiology certified radiologist and a Fellow of the Royal College of Physicians and Surgeons of Canada. He has been a Staff Radiologist at the Princess Margaret Hospital since 1995 and has been the Head of Abdominal MRI for the University Health Network and Mount Sinai Hospital since 1998. He has been a member of the Faculty of Medicine, Department of Medical Imaging at the University of Toronto since 1995 and has been an Associate Professor since 2006. Dr. Haider is a Fellow of the International Caner Imaging Society. He is a Clinician Scientist in the appointment in the Ontario Institute of Cancer Research with a research focus on MRI and CT of cancer of the prostate. Dr. Haider has held peer-reviewed grants from the Prostate Cancer Research Foundation of Canada and the National Cancer Institute of Canada for MRI-related prostate cancer research.

Ultrasound-Fluoroscopy Registration for Intraoperative Dynamic Dosimetry in Prostate Brachytherapy

Ehsan Dehghan, Nathanael Kuo, Anton Deguet, Yi Le, Elwood Armour, E. Clif Burdette, Danny Y. Song, Gabor Fichtinger, Jerry L. Prince, and Junghoon Lee

Abstract Low-dose-rate prostate brachytherapy is a treatment option for low- and mid-risk prostate cancer through introduction of radioactive seeds into the prostate. Seed placement deviations are common and associated with postoperative complications. Dynamic dosimetry is a method to accurately localize the true

E. Dehghan, Ph.D.
Clinical Informatics, Interventional, and Translational Solutions (CIITS), Philips Research North America, 345 Scarborough Road, Briarcliff Manor, NY 10510, USA
e-mail: ehsan.dehghan@philips.com

N. Kuo, M.S.
Department of Biomedical Engineering, Johns Hopkins University, 3400 North Charles Street, Clark 204, Baltimore, MD 21218, USA
e-mail: nkuo8@jhmi.edu

A. Deguet, M.S.
Laboratory for Computational Sensing and Robotics, Whiting School of Engineering, Johns Hopkins University, 3400 North Charles Street, Hackerman 137B, Baltimore, MD 21218, USA
e-mail: anton.deguet@jhu.edu

Y. Le, Ph.D. • E. Armour, Ph.D., D.A.B.R. • D.Y. Song, M.D. • J. Lee, Ph.D. (✉)
Department of Radiation Oncology and Molecular Radiation Sciences, Johns Hopkins University, 401 North Broadway, Weinberg 1440, Baltimore, MD 21231, USA
e-mail: yle1@jhmi.edu; earmour1@jhmi.edu; dsong2@jhmi.edu; junghoon@jhu.edu

E.C. Burdette, Ph.D.
Acoustic MedSystems, Inc., 208 Burwash Avenue, Savoy, IL 61874, USA
e-mail: clifb@acousticmed.com

G. Fichtinger, Ph.D.
School of Computing, Queen's University, 25 Union St, 557 Goodwin Hall, Kingston, ON, Canada K7L 3N6,
e-mail: gabor@cs.queensu.ca

J.L. Prince, Ph.D.
Department of Electrical and Computer Engineering, Johns Hopkins University, 3400 North Charles Street, Clark 201B, Baltimore, MD 21218, USA
e-mail: prince@jhu.edu

A.S. El-Baz et al. (eds.), *Abdomen and Thoracic Imaging: An Engineering & Clinical Perspective*, DOI 10.1007/978-1-4614-8498-1_23,
© Springer Science+Business Media New York 2014

position of the seeds inside the tissue, calculate the delivered dose, and adapt the implant plan accordingly to compensate for seed placement deviations in the operating room. A practical method for dynamic dosimetry relies on localization of the implanted seeds in 3D space from several C-arm images and registering them to a 3D ultrasound volume of the prostate region. In this chapter we introduce a system and workflow for intraoperative dosimetry for prostate brachytherapy. In the suggested workflow, C-arm images are acquired from different angles and are used to reconstruct the seeds in 3D space. For this purpose, we rely on a method based on dimensionality reduced linear programming to match the projections of a seed in different images and localize the seed positions after automatic C-arm pose correction. In the next step of the workflow, the reconstructed seeds are registered to an ultrasound volume of the prostate in a point-to-volume registration scheme. We tested our method on data from 16 patients and compared our dosimetry results with results from Day-1 CT. In comparison, we achieved absolute error of 2.2 $\pm$ 1.8 % (mean $\pm$ STD) in estimating the percentage of the prostate volume that receives 100 % of the prescribed dose ($V100$) and absolute error of 10.5 $\pm$ 9.5 % in prediction of the minimum dose delivered to 90 % of the prostate ($D90$).

Introduction

Prostate cancer is the leading cancer and the second cause of cancer death among men in the United States [1]. Radical prostatectomy, external beam radiation therapy, and prostate brachytherapy are treatment options for prostate cancer. Low-dose-rate prostate brachytherapy (hereafter, brachytherapy) is an outpatient treatment option that has shown at least equal or better outcomes with high rate of cancer-free survival and fewer side effects compared to the radical prostatectomy which is considered as the gold standard. Low-dose-rate prostate brachytherapy is a form of radiation therapy in which radioactive seeds are implanted inside the cancerous prostate to irradiate the cancerous tissue. The most common seeds used in practice are I-125, Pd-103, and Cs-131 and are almost as small as a grain of rice. The seed positions are accurately planned before implantation to assure delivery of sufficient dose to the target gland yet sparing the organs at risk such as urethra, rectum, and bladder. The quality of the treatment depends on the accuracy of seed placement.

During the operation, a transrectal ultrasound (TRUS) probe mounted on a stepper that allows translation and rotation of the probe is used for image guidance. A guiding template—a grid with holes—is also mounted on the stepper that allows the needles to move nominally parallel to the long axis of the TRUS probe. C-arm fluoroscopy is frequently used to visualize the distribution of the implanted seeds (see Fig. 1) and oftentimes needle positioning during the procedure.

Seeds can deviate from their planned positions for many reasons, including prostate motion and deformation [2], prostate swelling due to insertion trauma [3], needle deflection [4], and seed migration. Therefore, the real distribution of the

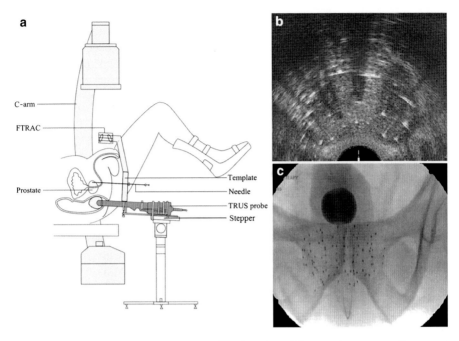

Fig. 1 (**a**) Brachytherapy setup, showing the TRUS probe, guiding template, stepper, C-arm, and radio-opaque fluoroscope tracking fiducial (FTRAC). (**b**) A sample axial TRUS image of the prostate with implanted seeds. (**c**) A sample X-ray image showing the seeds

implanted seeds never perfectly matches the plan. The resultant suboptimal dose distribution can lead to under-dosing of the cancerous gland or overdosing of the organs at risk. Consequences are complications such as sexual and urinary dysfunction, rectal ulceration, and cancer recurrence.

The treatment quality is assessed traditionally using CT one day or up to 4 weeks after the operation, when modifications to the treatment are difficult or impossible. Accurate localization of the implanted seeds in real time during the operation would enable the physician to detect the under-dosed regions and predict the regions with high chance of over-radiation while the patient is still on the operating table. In this case, optimal dose coverage could be achieved before the patient leaves the operating room. Real-time seed localization followed by dose calculation and modification, a process called "Dynamic Dosimetry", has been a topic of extensive research during the past decade [5, 6]. In addition to providing real-time evaluation of the procedure, dynamic dosimetry can simplify the quantitative postoperative dosimetry by replacing the postimplant CT.

Since TRUS is the main imaging modality during prostate brachytherapy, an extensive body of research has been dedicated to seed localization in ultrasound. Methods such as processing the B-mode images [7], singular spectrum analysis [8], analyzing the radio-frequency signal [9], trans-urethral ultrasound [10], Doppler ultrasound imaging of magnetically vibrated seeds [11], and vibroacoustography [12] have been tried. However, ultrasound-only seed localization methods have not shown the necessary robustness for clinical application. Ultrasound (US) images are of relatively low quality when the tissue is implanted with metallic seeds. For example, distal seeds (with respect to the US probe) can be located in the shadow of proximal seeds. Some seeds are oriented at an angle with respect to the incoming ultrasound beam that causes reflection of the beam away from the probe, rendering them invisible. US images are also rife with seed-looking artifacts caused by calcifications and air bubbles (see Fig. 1). In fact, it has been shown that even careful manual identification of the seeds in B-mode images cannot result in reliable dosimetry [13].

A commercially available method for an approximate dynamic dosimetry is to manually identify the seeds on the sagittal ultrasound image as they are ejected from the needle. Although this method has shown successful results [5, 14], it cannot account for seed motion after deposition. Therefore, the final resting place of the seeds remains unknown and the actual dose is not known with great accuracy.

A promising alternative for ultrasound-only seed localization and dosimetry is multimodality integration of ultrasound and fluoroscopy. C-arm fluoroscopy is widely used in brachytherapy practice for projection visualization of the seeds. Several X-ray images taken from different angles can be used to reconstruct the seed positions in 3D. However, C-arm fluoroscopy images have almost no soft-tissue contrast (see Fig. 1). Since for dosimetry the seeds must be localized with respect to prostate boundaries, seeds localized with C-arm fluoroscopy should be registered to ultrasound.

In this chapter, we introduce a fully automatic and practical system and workflow for reconstruction of the seeds in 3D using C-arm fluoroscopy and registering them to ultrasound images.

Dynamic Dosimetry Using Ultrasound-Fluoroscopy Registration

A possible workflow for dynamic dosimetry using ultrasound-fluoroscopy registration consists of the following. (1) During the operation, when needed, a TRUS volume of the prostate region is acquired. The TRUS volume can be reconstructed from axial images taken during the retraction of a tracked TRUS probe from the prostate base to apex (see Fig. 2a, b). Alternatively, the volume can be reconstructed from sagittal images acquired during a rotational sweep. (2) Following US imaging, at least 3 C-arm fluoroscopy images are acquired at different C-arm positions (see Fig. 2c). Conveniently, these images are taken by rotating the C-arm in a cone around the anterior-posterior (AP) axis of the patient. The TRUS probe is retracted before C-arm imaging to avoid occlusion of the seeds. (3) The X-ray images are processed for seeds and fiducials that are used for C-arm

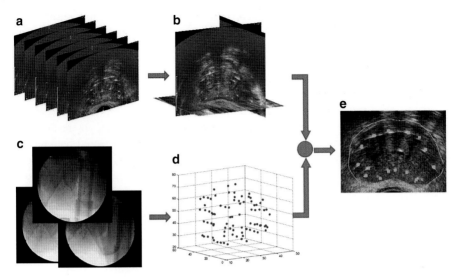

Fig. 2 The workflow for dynamic dosimetry using ultrasound-fluoroscopy registration. (**a**) Several axial slices of TRUS images. (**b**) A reconstructed TRUS volume. (**c**) Three X-rays acquired at different angles. (**d**) Reconstructed seeds in 3D space. (**e**) A sample axial slice of TRUS volume overlaid with the registered seeds (*green squares*), prostate contour (*red*), and 100 % isodose line (*green*)

pose computation. (4) The seeds are reconstructed in 3D by solving a matching problem that finds the correspondence between different seed projections of a particular seed in different images (Fig. 2d). (5) Finally, the reconstructed seeds are registered to the TRUS volume and used for implant evaluation and dosimetry (Fig. 2e). Based on the dosimetry information, the under-dosed and likely-to-be overdosed regions can be identified and the rest of the implant plan can be modified accordingly.

Reconstruction of Seeds in 3D Space

An essential component in our dynamic dosimetry system is the reconstruction of seeds in 3D space from several X-ray images taken from different angles. Two main methods have been devised for seed reconstruction in 3D—digital tomosynthesis and matching-based methods. In the former, the background is removed from the X-ray images and the seed projection regions are back-projected toward the corresponding X-ray sources. The corresponding back-projections for each seed intersect in the seed location. Digital tomosynthesis inherently solves the matching problem and recovers hidden seeds [15–20]. Since tomosynthesis-based reconstruction methods only require separation of the seeds from the background in a binary image; hence, explicit localization of the seed projection centers in the images and declustering are not necessary. However, tomosynthesis-based methods suffer from false positives and are relatively time-consuming. In the matching-based seed reconstruction methods, a seed is localized in 3D space by triangulation. In order to do so, the correspondence between the seed projections in different X-ray images should be known. Since this correspondence is not known, the matching problem and the reconstruction are solved together. For matching-based reconstruction methods, seed projection centroids should be identified in the images. However, in every image there can be several overlapping or hidden seeds, where the seed centroids cannot be reliably identified. Recent studies have engineered seed reconstruction methods that can solve the matching problem and recover the hidden seeds [21–25]. Compared to tomosynthesis-based methods, matching-based seed reconstruction requires fewer X-ray images.

Most reconstruction methods assume accurately known pose of the C-arm during image acquisition obtained through external tracking of the C-arm device or accurate geometry of radiotherapy simulators. External tracking of a C-arm device is not always practical and radiotherapy simulators are not available in every brachytherapy operating room. As a solution, seeds have been used as fiducials to improve an initial estimation of C-arm pose during seed reconstruction [19, 26–29]. In our work, we use reduced dimensionality matching for prostate brachytherapy seed reconstruction with automatic pose correction (APC-REDMAPS) [25, 29]. This is a fast, practical, and robust matching-based method that is able to concurrently estimate the pose of the images as well as solve for the matching problem despite presence of hidden seed projections.

Our seed reconstruction method requires seed projection centroids to be segmented in the X-ray images. In addition, a relatively accurate C-arm pose is required for fast and successful reconstruction. The C-arm pose can be calculated using a fluoroscope tracking fiducial, named FTRAC, introduced by Jain et al. [30] that consists of 2 ellipses, 3 parallel lines, and 9 beads as shown in Fig. 3. The FTRAC can be mounted on the guiding template used for prostate brachytherapy. The C-arm pose can be recovered after segmentation of the projections of the FTRAC in the X-rays with the tracking accuracy of $0.33°$ in rotation and 0.56 mm in translation [30]. In the following, we describe the algorithms for segmentation of the fiducial and seed projections in the X-ray images as well as our method for solving the matching problem and pose correction.

Seed and Fiducial Segmentation in X-Ray Images

Our X-ray processing algorithm is responsible for automatic segmentation of the FTRAC ellipses, lines, beads as well as the center of seed projections in the image without a manually selected region of interest [31]. In addition, if some seed projections are overlapped, the image processing can detect and separate them into their constituent projections. We assume that the X-rays are corrected for image distortions caused by the image intensifier. The correcting function parameters can be calculated preoperatively using a calibration device which is

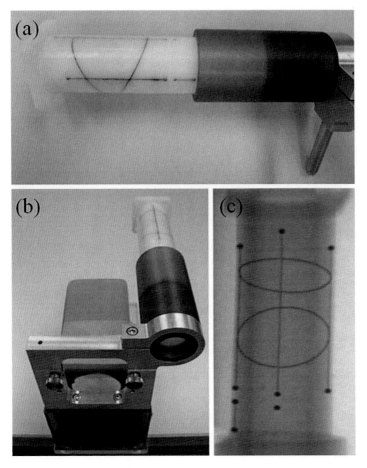

Fig. 3 (**a**) The fluoroscope tracking fiducial (FTRAC). (**b**) FTRAC mounted on the guiding template. (**c**) An X-ray image of FTRAC, showing the projections of the ellipses, lines, and beads

also used to identify the C-arm calibration parameters. We also assume that the seeds and FTRAC are fully visible in the C-arm images and the FTRAC image does not overlap with the seed projections (Fig. 4). This can be achieved by limiting the C-arm rotation to a ±10° cone around the patient's AP axis. The image processing algorithm requires that the FTRAC appears on the right side of seeds and in an almost vertical position in the X-ray image. Mounting the FTRAC on the grid as shown in Fig. 3b satisfies this requirement (see Fig. 4 for an example).

Fiducial Segmentation

The X-ray processing starts with segmenting the FTRAC lines and beads. The FTRAC specific design, in which the beads are positioned on the top of the three parallel lines, is taken into account for simultaneous segmentation. The algorithm

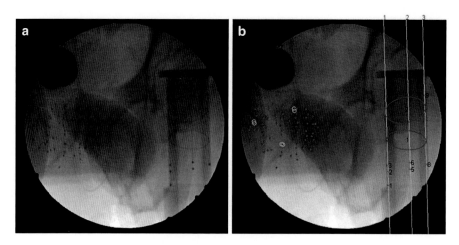

Fig. 4 The result of seeds and FTRAC segmentation on a clinical image. (**a**) The original image. (**b**) Segmented seeds, ellipses, beads, and lines (shown by numbers). *Magenta dots* indicate single seeds are marked by *magenta dots* and separated overlapping seeds by *cyan circles*

starts with generating a binary image by applying a top-hat by reconstruction operation using a disk-shaped structuring element on the complemented X-ray image followed by the Otsu thresholding [32]. The region properties of the connected components including their area, eccentricity, solidity, and location are used to distinguish beads from seeds. As the beads are located on parallel lines, the Hough transform is applied to the image and the strongest three parallel lines in an almost vertical orientation on the right side of the image are selected. The line positions are further refined and then used to localize the beads in the image [31].

Following the detection of the FTRAC beads and lines, a pipeline of morphological image filters including top-hat operation and image opening, thresholds, and edge thinning algorithms are applied to the images to detect the edges of the ellipses. Then, knowing the position of the beads, the candidate edges for the two ellipses are separated. Finally, an ellipse detection algorithm based on random sample consensus (RANSAC) is employed to fit two ellipses to the detected edges. For more details on the ellipse detection we refer the readers to [31].

Seed Segmentation

Once the FTRAC is segmented, the X-ray processing can continue onto seed segmentation without interference from the fiducial. The pipeline continues with generating a binary image by applying a top-hat by reconstruction operation using a disk-shaped structuring element on the complemented X-ray image followed by the Otsu thresholding. To reduce false positives, connected components within the region of the FTRAC or outside the densest seed cloud region of connected components are removed.

Most of the remaining connected components correspond to single seed projections, although some may correspond to multiple overlapping seed projections. A metric based on the rearrangement of Beer's law can serve as an estimate of the number of seed projections within each connected component:

$$I_x(x,y) = I_0 e^{-\mu \int dz}$$

$$-\ln \frac{I_x(x,y)}{I_0} = \mu \int dz \tag{1}$$

$$\iint -\ln \frac{I_x(x,y)}{I_0} dxdy = \mu \iiint dxdydz = \mu V$$

Here, $I_x(x,y)$ is the X-ray image intensity at position (x, y), I_0 is the incident X-ray intensity, z is the axis orthogonal to the image plane along the line of projection, and V is the volume of the object(s) imaged. Therefore, a calculation of $\iint -\ln \frac{I_x(x,y)}{I_0}$ $dxdy$ can serve as a metric for estimating the number of seed projections within each connected component, since the resulting value is a constant μV for single seed projections and n times the constant μV for n seed projections. For more details on the metric, we refer the readers to [31].

The coordinates of the seed projections can finally be calculated through application of the k-means clustering algorithm [33], which partitions data into a user-defined number of clusters. For this case, the input data are the pixel coordinates within a specific connected component weighted by intensity, and the number of clusters is the now computed metric for the connected component. The output partition separates any overlapping seeds and the centroid of each partition results in the desired seed projection position.

Solving the Matching Problem

As mentioned, we need at least three X-ray images taken at different angles to reconstruct the seeds. Without loss of generality and for the sake of simplicity, we assume that we have only three X-rays. Assume that the images are processed so the seed projections are segmented in the images. To start with, let's assume that the C-arm poses (the relative positions and orientations of the X-ray images in 3D space) and the correspondences between the seed projections in different images are known (see Fig. 5 for an example). For each of the corresponding seed projections p_{i1}, p_{i2} and p_{i3} in images 1, 2 and 3, respectively, there is a line $L_{ij}, j \in \{1,2,3\}$ that connects that projection to its corresponding C-arm source

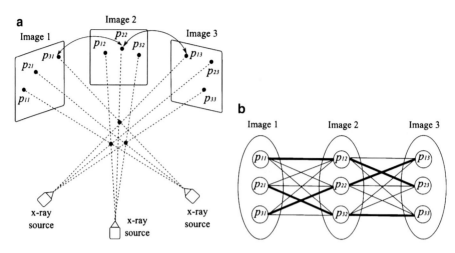

Fig. 5 (**a**) Schematic diagram of reconstruction of three seeds from their projections in 3 X-ray images. The correspondence between the seeds and different projections are shown. (**b**) All possible matching solutions between the seed projections in different images. Each edge in this figure has a weight equal to the reconstruction accuracy. The correct matches for the simple case shown in (**a**) are indicated by thick edges

position r_j, $j \in \{1,2,3\}$. Then, the reconstructed seed position s_i is the point with minimum aggregate distance from these lines and is calculated as:

$$s_i = \left[\sum_{j=1}^{3} \left(I - v_{ij} v'_{ij} \right) \right]^{-1} \sum_{j=1}^{3} \left(I - v_{ij} v'_{ij} \right) r_j, \qquad (2)$$

where, v_{ij} is the unit vector along L_{ij}, I is the identity matrix, and $(.)'$ denotes the transpose of a matrix or a vector. We define the "reconstruction accuracy" as the root mean square distance from the reconstructed seed to L_{ij}'s [25], which is zero in ideal case with known image poses.

In the problem of seed reconstruction for prostate brachytherapy, the correspondence between seed projections is not known. In addition, there are hidden seed projections in the images. Therefore, seed localization and the correspondence problem should be solved jointly. This problem can be formulated as a combinatorial optimization problem:

$$\min_{x_{ijk}} \sum_{i=1}^{N_1} \sum_{j=1}^{N_2} \sum_{k=1}^{N_3} c_{ijk}(\Phi, \mathbf{t}) x_{ijk}, \qquad (3)$$

$$\text{s.t.} \sum_{j=1}^{N_2} \sum_{k=1}^{N_3} x_{ijk} \geq 1, \forall i$$

$$\sum_{i=1}^{N_1} \sum_{k=1}^{N_3} x_{ijk} \geq 1, \forall j$$

$$\sum_{i=1}^{N_1} \sum_{j=1}^{N_2} x_{ijk} \geq 1, \forall k \tag{4}$$

$$\sum_{i=1}^{N_1} \sum_{j=1}^{N_2} \sum_{k=1}^{N_3} x_{ijk} = N$$

$$x_{ijk} \in \{0, 1\}, \forall i, j, k$$

where N is the total number of implanted seeds, N_1, N_2, N_3 are the numbers of segmented seed projection centroids in images 1, 2, 3, respectively. c_{ijk} is the cost of matching the seed projection i from image 1 with seed projection j from image 2 and seed projection k from image 3. The variable x_{ijk} is equal to 1 if seed projections i in image 1, j in image 2, k in image 3 are selected as a match, i.e., originate from the same physical seed, and equal to 0 otherwise. The matching cost c_{ijk} is a function of C-arm pose rotation $\boldsymbol{\Phi} = (\phi_1, \phi_2, \phi_3)$ and translation $\mathbf{t} = (t_1, t_2, t_3)$. We use the reconstruction accuracy as the matching cost [25, 29]. Since x_{ijk} is binary, this combinatorial optimization problem becomes a binary integer programming problem. The inequalities in (4) guarantee that each seed projection is selected at least once. Seed projections are allowed to be selected more than once to recover the hidden seeds. The equality constraint assures that the number of reconstructed seeds is equal to the number of implanted seeds.

Due to the large number (around 100) of implanted seeds during a brachytherapy session, the above mentioned problem is of large dimensionality and cannot be solved fast enough for practical purposes. Therefore, APC-REDMAPDS reduces the dimensionality of this matching problem through a pruning algorithm [25]. Lee et al. has shown that over 99 % of the variables in (3) can be eliminated [25]. Moreover, the dimensionality reduced binary programming in (3) can be solved using linear programming with relaxed fractional constraints in near real time. If the C-arm poses are known relatively accurately, the reduced linear programming renders a binary solution that is global optimum of (3). However, if the C-arm pose is not known very accurately, the solution may not be binary and, if rounded, may not be globally optimal. Therefore, APC-REDMAPS is designed to solve the matching problem and improve the pose estimations, iteratively.

Automatic Pose Correction

In order to solve the matching problem 100 % correctly, the pose of the C-arms should be known precisely, which is not the case in clinical practice. However, the linear programming approach described above has shown to correctly recover most of the seed correspondences for image pose errors up to $5°$ in rotation and 10 mm in translation [25].

   If the C-arm poses are precisely known, the lines that emanate from corresponding seed projections intersect at a single point. Therefore, if the reconstructed seed is projected back on the images, the distance between the projection of the reconstructed seed and the corresponding segmented seed projection on each image should be zero. However, in the presence of C-arm pose errors, there are errors between the projections of the reconstructed seed and its segmented seed projections on the images. We use the term "projection error" for this error. The projection error is employed within APC-REDMAPS to improve the pose estimation accuracy. The matching and pose improvement problems are solved iteratively until convergence.

   Let $s_i^W = [s_{ix}^W, s_{iy}^W, s_{iz}^W, 1]'$ represent the position of the ith seed in the 3D homogeneous world coordinate system. The projection of this seed on the jth image can be calculated in the image homogeneous coordinate system as:

$$p_{ij} = \begin{bmatrix} f/\sigma_x & 0 & o_x & 0 \\ 0 & f/\sigma_y & o_y & 0 \\ 0 & 0 & 1 & 0 \end{bmatrix} \begin{bmatrix} R(\phi_{j1}, \phi_{j2}, \phi_{j3}) & t_j \\ 0 & 1 \end{bmatrix} s_i^W, \qquad (5)$$

where the left matrix is the projection matrix that consists of the C-arm focal length f, the origin of the image (o_x, o_y), and the pixel spacings (σ_x, σ_y), all of which can be preoperatively calibrated. The right matrix is the C-arm pose matrix which is defined by the C-arm rotation and translation parameters. Equation (5) renders the x-y coordinates of the seed projection as $\begin{bmatrix} p_{ij}^x & p_{ij}^y \end{bmatrix}'$. Then, the projection error for seed i in image j can be calculated as:

$$\Delta e_{ij} = \begin{bmatrix} p_{ij}^x(\Phi_i, t_i) \\ p_{ij}^y(\Phi_i, t_i) \end{bmatrix} - \begin{bmatrix} q_{ij}^x \\ q_{ij}^y \end{bmatrix}, \qquad (6)$$

where, $\begin{bmatrix} q_{ij}^x & q_{ij}^y \end{bmatrix}'$ denote the position of the segmented seed centroid in the image. A linear approximation of Δe_{ij} with respect to the pose error can be written as:

$$\Delta e_{ij} = J \begin{bmatrix} \Delta\phi_{j1} \\ \Delta\phi_{j2} \\ \Delta\phi_{j3} \\ \Delta t_{j1} \\ \Delta t_{j2} \\ \Delta t_{j3} \end{bmatrix} = J\Delta E_j \qquad (7)$$

The Jacobian matrix J can be explicitly calculated as detailed in [29]. The pose error ΔE is estimated from (7) using Newton's method [34]. Each C-arm pose is iteratively updated using:

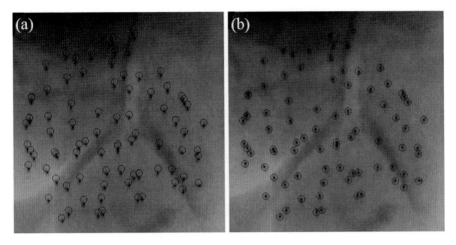

Fig. 6 Reconstruction results without (**a**) and with (**b**) automatic pose correction. The reconstructed seeds are projected back on the clinical image and are shown as *purple circles*. The segmented seed centroids are shown as *red dots*

$$R_j^{k+1} = R_j^k \Delta R_j^k, \quad \mathbf{t}_j^{k+1} = \mathbf{t}_j^k + \Delta \mathbf{t}_j^k, \tag{8}$$

where, ΔR_j^k and $\Delta \mathbf{t}_j^k$ are calculated from ΔE_j^k and k is the iteration number.

APC-REDMAPS has been extensively validated on simulated and clinical data sets. Trial on clinical data sets showed that APC-REDMAPS can significantly improve the seed reconstruction results and achieve matching rates of $\geq$99.4 %, reconstruction error of $\leq$0.5 mm, and the matching solution optimality of $\geq$99.8 % [29]. Figure 6 shows the necessity of automatic pose correction and the efficacy of APC-REDMAPS in pose correction.

Ultrasound-Fluoroscopy Registration

Registration of ultrasound and fluoroscopy (RUF) for image guidance in prostate brachytherapy has been extensively studied before. Todor et al. [35] put radio-opaque markers on the TRUS probe and used it for registration. Jain et al. [36] used mechanical registration of the FTRAC to the TRUS probe for this purpose and French et al. [37] used the images of the probe in the X-rays. For C-arm imaging the TRUS probe should be retracted, at least partially, to avoid occlusion of the seeds. This results in motion and deformation of the prostate in the posterior direction as the physicians usually press the probe against the prostate to achieve a good acoustic coupling. However, the marker- and fiducial-based registration methods rely on a relationship between the seed positions and the fiducials or marker that change by the retraction of the probe.

A seed-based registration method was used by Su et al. [38], Orio et al. [39], and Tutar et al. [40] in which manually selected seeds in ultrasound images were registered to seeds reconstructed from X-rays. Manual seed localization in ultrasound is difficult, time-consuming, subjective, and prone to errors. Moradi et al. [41] proposed a method for automatic yet partial seed segmentation in ultrasound using 3D template matching of radio-frequency signal. However, the detection rate in this method is low.

Fallavollita et al. [42] introduced an image-based ultrasound to fluoroscopy registration employing several filters such as phase congruency, noise reduction, and beam profiling to filter the ultrasound volume. They achieved successful registrations in a phantom study; however, their study on a single-patient data set showed only qualitative good results despite the complexity of the filters used.

We also use an image-based point-to-volume registration method that registers the reconstructed seeds from X-rays to an ultrasound volume of the prostate. Ultrasound and fluoroscopy are not generally compatible for intensity-based registration as fluoroscopy images have almost no soft tissue contrast. However, seed implantation inside prostate changes the ultrasound images, advantageously. Metallic seeds are hyper-echoic and result in bright regions in ultrasound images that correlate with the C-arm reconstructed seeds. We take advantage of this correlation for our registration purpose. However, the ultrasound volume should be processed such as described below in order to enhance the seed footprints and increase the robustness of the registration.

Ultrasound Image Processing

In the first step, a volume of interest (VOI) is selected. The VOI is selected as a cube that encloses the prostate and the seeds within. Image cropping can be done automatically, if the prostate contours are available. However, manual selection of the VOI is also fast and easy. As the seeds are hyper-echoic, they appear as outliers in VOI image intensity distribution (see Fig. 7a). Therefore, a threshold based on the image intensity statistics can be used to remove the background such that:

$$I_T(x, y, z) = \begin{cases} 0 & \text{if } I_u(x, y, z) \leq \mu_u + \alpha\sigma_u \\ 1 & \text{if } I_u(x, y, z) \geq \mu_u + \alpha\sigma_u \end{cases} \tag{9}$$

where μ_u and σ_u are the mean and standard deviation of image intensity in the VOI, respectively, and α is the threshold parameter. If α is too large, many of the true seeds will be removed and there will not be sufficient number of seeds for registration. On the other hand, if α is too small, the thresholded image contains many false positives that can produce local optimums for the registration. We chose $\alpha = 2.5$ throughout this work for all of our phantom and clinical data sets. We have shown in [43] that our registration algorithm is robust to reasonable variations in α. In fact, we have shown that changing $\alpha \in \{2, 2.5, 3\}$ results only in submillimeter

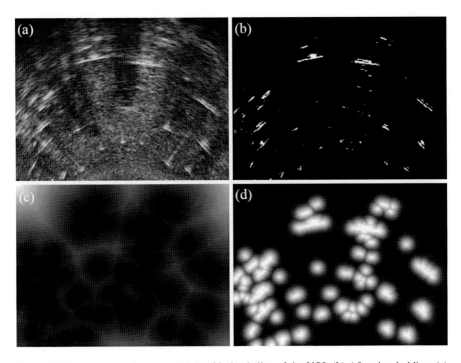

Fig. 7 US image processing steps. (**a**) A mid-gland slice of the VOI. (**b**) After thresholding. (**c**) After distance transform. (**d**) After Gaussian blurring

variations in the position of the registered seeds. The result of the thresholding step can be seen in Fig. 7b. Note that this threshold does not detect all the seeds nor remove all the false positives. However, our registration algorithm is robust to these missing seeds and false positives as it uses mutually present seeds in ultrasound volume and C-arm reconstructed seeds to calculate the registration parameters.

A binary image is not suitable for registration as it does not have an intensity gradient to guide the optimizer. As it can be seen in Fig. 7b, I_T is a sparse binary image. Therefore, variation of the registration parameters in an optimization loop may result in no or very small variation in the objective function—similarity metric in our case—if the initial registration is not very accurate. An image with a smooth intensity variation, on the other hand, increases the basin of convergence and the likelihood of arriving at the global optimum. In order to create such an image, we first apply a Euclidian distance transform to each slice of the binary image to create a distance transform image I_D such that:

$$I_D(x, y, z) = \min_{x_s, y_s} \sqrt{(x - x_s)^2 + (y - y_s)^2}$$
$$\text{s.t.} I_T(x_s, y_s, z) = 1. \tag{10}$$

In other words, the intensity of the distance transform image $I_D(x,y,z)$ is equal to the distance of a pixel to the closest white pixel in the same slice (see Fig. 7c).

Finally, an image with a smooth intensity variation I_G is produced by applying a Gaussian blurring function to the distance transform image I_D, such that:

$$I_G(x, y, z) = \exp\left(-\frac{I_D^2(x, y, z)}{2\sigma^2}\right), \tag{11}$$

where, σ is the standard deviation of the Gaussian blurring function. As shown in Fig. 7d, the Gaussian blurred image has a smooth intensity variation with maximum values around the seed candidates. This can act as an attractive force to, iteratively, drive the C-arm reconstructed seeds toward the seeds in ultrasound volume. The parameter σ plays an important role in the behavior of the registration algorithm. If σ is too small, the seeds are not spread enough and the optimization will not have a sufficiently large capture range. If σ is too large, the optimization algorithm can be trapped in local minima as the effect of false positives is enhanced. In this work, we chose σ such that the Gaussian function decreases to 75 % of its peak value at 1 mm away from the center of a seed.

Affine Transformation

As mentioned, retraction of the probe for C-arm imaging results in deformation of the prostate. As the probe pressure is mainly in the AP direction and fairly uniform, we use a 1D scaling in AP direction to compensate for it. To this end, we assume a TRUS coordinate system such that the x axis is parallel to the horizontal axis of the image from left to right, the y axis is parallel to the vertical axis of the image from bottom to top, and the z axis runs in the superior-inferior direction. We use an affine transformation $T : \mathbb{R}^3 \rightarrow \mathbb{R}^3$ between the C-arm coordinate system and TRUS coordinate system as:

$$T(\mathbf{x}) = \begin{bmatrix} 1 & 0 & 0 \\ 0 & \lambda^{-1} & 0 \\ 0 & 0 & 1 \end{bmatrix} R(\boldsymbol{\theta})\mathbf{x} + \mathbf{t}, \tag{12}$$

where, R is the rotation matrix, $\boldsymbol{\theta} = (\theta_x, \theta_y, \theta_z)$ represents the rotations around different axes, $\mathbf{t} = [t_x, t_y, t_z]'$ is the translation vector, λ is the scaling factor, and x represents the coordinates of a point in the C-arm coordinate system.

Point to Volume Similarity Metric

In order to achieve a computationally fast registration, we assume that the TRUS volume is fixed in space and the C-arm reconstructed seeds can move and rotate as a set of points. We need to define a similarity metric between a set of points and a 3D image volume. To this end, we assume cuboids of the size $\Delta x \times \Delta y \times \Delta z$ around each C-arm reconstructed seed and measure the processed TRUS volume intensity inside all the cuboids. Note that the axes of the cuboids are always parallel to the TRUS coordinate axes (there is no need to rotate the cuboids). The size of a cuboid in this work is $2 \times 2 \times 6$ mm^3 that is slightly bigger than a seed. The cuboids are used to guide the C-arm seeds toward the center of the bright regions in the processed TRUS volume. Therefore, we define our point to volume similarity metric as the summation of image intensity over all the cuboids and formulate it as:

$$
S = \sum_{n=1}^{N} \int_{-\frac{\Delta z}{2}}^{\frac{\Delta z}{2}} \int_{-\frac{\Delta y}{2}}^{\frac{\Delta y}{2}} \int_{-\frac{\Delta x}{2}}^{\frac{\Delta x}{2}} I_G \left(T(s_i) + \begin{bmatrix} x \\ y \\ z \end{bmatrix} \right) dxdydz, \tag{13}
$$

where s_i represents the coordinates of seed i in the C-arm coordinate system.

Optimizer

For our registration, we have three rotation parameters $\boldsymbol{\theta}$, three translation parameters $\mathbf{t}$, and one scale to optimize. We impose realistic constraints on our registration parameters and formulate the registration problem as the following constrained optimization:

$$
(\boldsymbol{\theta}^*, \mathbf{t}^*, \lambda^*) = \text{argmin} \quad S(\boldsymbol{\theta}, \mathbf{t}, \lambda)
$$
$$
\text{s.t.} \begin{cases} \boldsymbol{\theta}_{\min} \leq \boldsymbol{\theta} \leq \boldsymbol{\theta}_{\max} \\ \mathbf{t}_{\min} \leq \mathbf{t} \leq \mathbf{t}_{\max} \\ \lambda_{\min} \leq \lambda \leq \lambda_{\max} \end{cases} \tag{14}
$$

We employ the Covariance Matrix Adaptation-Evolutionary Strategy (CMA-ES) for optimization [44]. This is a robust and efficient stochastic optimization method capable of optimizing nonlinear and nonconvex problems. For each iteration of the optimization, CMA-ES calculates the similarity metric over a set of randomly distributed samples. The samples are drawn from a multivariate normal distribution. The samples with the highest similarity metric in the population and information from the previous iterations are used to update the covariance matrix of the normal distribution as the iterations continue. Given a relatively good initial estimate for the registration parameters, as we discuss later, the constrained optimization in (14) can deliver successful registration.

Experiments and Results

Validation on Phantom

First, we conducted a phantom experiment on a commercial CIRS-053 prostate brachytherapy training phantom (CIRS Inc., VA, USA). The phantom, implanted with 48 dummy seeds, was imaged using ultrasound and CT. In this experiment, we employed CT instead of fluoroscopy because it was easier to obtain a ground truth registration between CT and US. However, the seeds were segmented in CT, turned into a set of points, and treated as C-arm reconstructed seeds. In order to obtain a ground truth registration between the TRUS and CT coordinate systems, the phantom was equipped with some fiducials visible in CT that defined the phantom coordinate system. During TRUS imaging, both the probe and the fiducials were tracked using a Cetrus optical tracker (NDI, ON, Canada) and a calibrated pointer (Traxtal Inc., ON, Canada) to provide the registration between the TRUS and phantom coordinate systems (see Fig. 8). The TRUS calibration was performed following the method described in [45]. After CT imaging, the fiducials were carefully localized in CT images and were used to establish the registration between CT and phantom coordinate systems, and consequently between TRUS and CT coordinate systems. The segmented seeds in CT were transformed to the TRUS coordinate system using this registration and assumed as ground truth seed positions.

In order to test the performance of the registration algorithm, independent perturbations of ±15° around each axis and ±15 mm along each axis were applied to the ground truth seeds. We simulated the effect of the missing seeds by adding some seeds to the ground truth CT seeds. Similarly, the effect of false positive seeds was simulated by removing some seeds from the ground truth CT seeds.

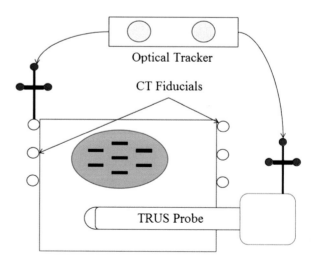

Fig. 8 The phantom experiment setup. The ground truth registration between the TRUS and CT coordinate system is defined by optically tracking fiducials visible in CT

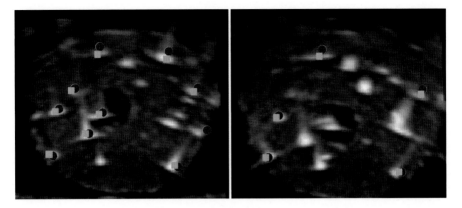

Fig. 9 Two transverse slice images of the phantom overlaid with ground truth seeds (*red circles*) and registered seeds (*green squares*)

	Registration error (mm)
Seed cloud	Mean ± SD (Max)
Complete	0.77 ± 0.40 (1.99)
Missing 5	0.79 ± 0.40 (2.01)
Missing 10	0.84 ± 0.42 (2.18)
Extra 5	0.86 ± 0.46 (3.10)
Extra 10	0.93 ± 0.52 (3.81)
Overall	0.84 ± 0.45

Table 1 Mean and standard deviation (SD) of registration errors for phantom study

For example, to simulate the effect of missing seeds in the TRUS volume, we added 5 or 10 seeds, at random positions, to the CT seeds. As these seeds do not have a counterpart in the TRUS volume, they act as missing seeds in the TRUS volume. The positions of these additional seeds were randomly selected for each value of perturbation. Similarly, in order to simulate false positives in the TRUS volume, we randomly removed 5 or 10 seeds from CT seeds data set. Since the TRUS seeds that corresponded to these seeds in the complete set do not correspond to any seeds in the reduced set, they act as false positives. These seeds were randomly removed from the complete set for each value of perturbation. We limited the search region to $t_{max} = -t_{min} = [20,20,20]'$ mm and $\theta_{max} = -\theta_{min} = [20°, 20°, 20°]$ and $1 \leq \lambda \leq 1.3$.

The registration algorithm successfully converged close to the ground truth seeds with a maximum average registration error of 1.34 mm in all 930 simulations. This shows the large capture range of our algorithm as well as its high accuracy. The registration error was measured as the average seed-to-seed distance between the registered and the ground truth seeds. Figure 9 shows two transverse slices of the phantom with overlaying registered and ground truth seeds. The registration error for different simulation conditions is summarized in Table 1.

Validation on Clinical Data Sets

We also tested our dosimetry system on 16 patient data sets treated at the Johns Hopkins Hospital, Baltimore, MD, USA. The clinical workflow started by anesthetizing the patient. Then the TRUS probe was mounted on the stepper and inserted into the patient's rectum. The TRUS probe position was adjusted until good imaging quality was achieved. Several transverse TRUS images of the patient's prostate with slice spacing of 5 mm were acquired and used for dose planning. The operating physician contoured the prostate and the organs at risk (rectum and urethra) on these images and planned the position of the seeds to achieve sufficient prostate coverage while having a tolerable dose on the organs at risk. After planning, the seeds were delivered using needles and a Mick applicator (Mick Radio-Nuclear Instruments, NY, USA). The patients in our study received 60–105 (median = 77) Pd-103 seeds (Model 200, TheraSeed, Theragenics, GA, USA). A BK Pro Focus (BK Medical, MA, USA) ultrasound machine was used during the implant for image guidance.

Right after all the seeds were implanted, the physician acquired a set of transverse TRUS slices by retracting the probe from a 5–10 mm superior to the prostate base to 5–10 mm inferior to the apex. The margins were chosen to ensure that all the seeds were covered during the imaging. The standard brachytherapy treatment system automatically recorded the images taken at 1 mm intervals, while the physician was continuously retracting the TRUS probe. The axial slices have in-plane pixel spacing of 0.19 mm. The TRUS probe was fully retracted after volume acquisition. Then 9 X-ray images were acquired by rotating a GE OEC 9600 mobile C-arm (GE Healthcare, WI, USA) around the patients' AP axis within a 20° cone. The FTRAC was mounted on the guiding template during C-arm imaging. We made sure that all the seeds and FTRAC are in the image and the FTRAC is located on the right side of the seeds in the image. The C-arm device was postoperatively calibrated using a special calibration phantom to measure its image pixel spacing, image center, focal length, and image distortion correction parameters.

In our study, the X-ray images were corrected for geometric distortion and the seeds and FTRAC were segmented using the method explained in section "Seed and Fiducial Segmentation in X-Ray Images." An initial estimate of the C-arm poses was obtained from the FTRAC and passed to the seed reconstruction algorithm along with the seed projection centroids. APC-REDMAPS solved for the matching problem in the presence of some hidden seeds and corrected for the pose estimation errors. The seeds were reconstructed in 3D from 5 to 6 images and passed to the registration algorithm.

The VOI in x-y plane was chosen in an axial image of the mid-gland as a rectangle that tightly encloses the prostate. All the acquired TRUS slices were included in the VOI, so the VOI covers the whole volume in the z direction. The VOI was processed using the filters described in section "Ultrasound Image Processing." In order to achieve higher registration speed, the Gaussian blurred VOI was subsampled in axial planes by a factor of two to a pixel size of 0.38×0.38 mm^2.

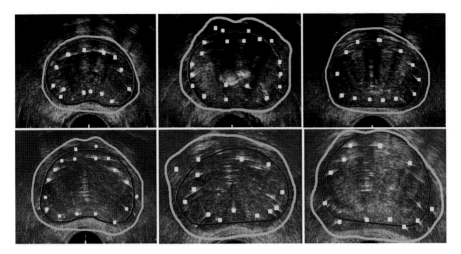

Fig. 10 The results of ultrasound-fluoroscopy registration shown for the mid-gland slice of some of the patients. The seeds are shown as *yellow squares*. The *red* contours show the prostate contours. The *green* contours show the 100 % prescribed isodose line

The registration algorithm was initialized by aligning the center of mass of the C-arm seeds with the center of the VOI. The rotation parameters were initialized by registering the seeds to their planned positions using the iterative closest point (ICP) method. The scale factor was initialized to $\lambda = 1$. For the study on the clinical data, the translation, rotation, and scale parameters were constrained to $\mathbf{t}_{max} = -\mathbf{t}_{min} = [15,15,15]'$ mm, $\boldsymbol{\theta}_{max} = -\boldsymbol{\theta}_{min} = [15°, 15°, 15°]$, and $1 \leq \lambda \leq 1.3$, respectively. These search regions are sufficiently large for our application. A translational search region of ± 15 mm is larger than 50 % of the prostate for a supermajority of cases. Also the seeds as a whole are unlikely to rotate more than $15°$ with respect to their planned position. Since the probe is always pushing against the prostate and compressing it, we assumed $\lambda \geq 1$. We visually inspected the results of registration to ensure a successful registration. Several mid-gland slices of TRUS images overlaid with registered seeds are shown in Fig. 10.

As part of the clinical protocol, CT scanning was done one day after the implant (Day-1) to perform postoperative dosimetry. The seeds were localized in CT images by a board-certified medical physicist, and the prostate, urethra, and rectum were contoured by a radiation oncologist. The localized seeds and organ contours were used to calculate the dose coverage and dosimetry parameters. In order to evaluate the performance of the seed reconstruction algorithm, the reconstructed seeds were compared against the CT seeds. The number of reconstructed seeds from X-rays always matched the number of seeds identified in CT. We measured the seed reconstruction as the seed-to-seed distance between the reconstructed seeds and CT seeds after a rigid registration. In order to do so, after the rigid registration, a one-to-one relation is established between each seed in the CT seeds set and the reconstructed seeds using the Hungarian algorithm. The results for the seed

Table 2 Validation results on clinical data, showing the number of implanted seeds, mean ± SD of reconstruction errors, prostate volume in CT and US, and the dose parameters calculated from CT- and RUF-based dosimetry

Patient ID	Num Seeds	Recon error (mm)	Prostate vol (cc)		V100 (%)		D90 (%)	
			CT	US	CT	RUF	CT	RUF
1	76	2.1 ± 1.8	38.6	34.5	98.2	94.2	124.9	121.5
2	90	2.1 ± 2.5	46.3	40.1	98.1	98.2	132.1	146.1
3	64	1.2 ± 0.7	31.6	29.9	92.4	96.0	102.5	114.2
4	105	2.2 ± 1.5	54.3	47.2	99.0	97.6	117.6	111.1
5	91	1.7 ± 0.9	41.9	41.6	99.0	97.6	128.7	132.3
6	73	1.8 ± 1.8	36.5	37.0	95.3	95.4	109.3	114.7
7	61	2.3 ± 1.9	20.7	30.3	99.9	97.3	165.8	127.6
8	67	2.3 ± 0.9	32.0	31.5	96.4	95.1	113.8	120.5
9	102	1.3 ± 0.8	48.8	51.5	98.7	97.7	126.9	131.8
10	78	2.2 ± 4.2	49.5	40.5	98.9	97.6	124.0	140.3
11	76	2.1 ± 1.1	49.3	32.2	92.2	96.8	104.3	108.7
12	85	1.2 ± 0.7	53.1	33.8	92.7	98.2	106.8	127.4
13	78	2.0 ± 1.0	40.3	31.2	99.7	96.7	140.5	126.1
14	83	2.6 ± 5.0	42.3	29.8	98.8	93.9	121.2	120.9
15	60	4.8 ± 2.0	31.6	25.6	96.1	97.5	108.6	110.9
16	73	1.9 ± 1.8	30.8	24.6	99.9	99.8	152.7	169.0

reconstruction errors are shown in Table 2. All the seeds were included in calculating the reconstruction errors (false reconstructions were not excluded). Therefore, some large reconstruction errors in Table 2 can be influenced by 1–2 falsely reconstructed seeds in the whole batch. It should be noted that the C-arm reconstructed seeds are from X-rays acquired right after the implant (Day-0), while the CT images are acquired on Day-1. Therefore, the position of the seeds in these two modalities can differ due to edema-induced changes in the prostate volume and deformation of the prostate.

Since there is no ground truth available for the position of the seeds in TRUS images, we cannot directly evaluate the performance of the registration algorithm. Therefore, we evaluated our registration algorithm in a dosimetry study. In such a comparison, the delivered dose parameters are calculated using the TRUS-Fluoroscopy registration and compared against the CT-based dosimetry results. Since we need both seed positions and organ contours to calculate the dose parameters, prostate was contoured in the TRUS images as well by the operating radiation oncologist. For nine patients (patients 1–9), the operating radiation oncologist contoured the prostate in the postimplant TRUS images, while only preimplant organ contours were available for the rest of the patients (patients 10–16).

The dose parameters calculated in this work are: the percentage of the prostate volume covered with 100 % of the prescribed dose ($V100$), and the minimum percentage of prescribed dose delivered to 90 % of the prostate volume ($D90$). We followed TG-43 formalism for dose calculation [46]. Table 2 shows these dose parameters using Day-1 CT and ultrasound-fluoroscopy registration.

Table 3 Comparison of dosimetry parameters calculated based on Day-1 CT and registration of ultrasound and fluoroscopy

Parameter	Mean ± SD (%)	Range (%)
$V100_{CT}$	97.2 ± 2.7	92.2–99.9
$V100_{RUF}$	96.8 ± 1.6	93.9–99.8
$D90_{CT}$	123.7 ± 17.7	102.5–165.8
$D90_{RUF}$	126.4 ± 15.5	108.7–169.0
e_{V100}	0.4 ± 2.9	−5.5–4.9
e_{D90}	−2.7 ± 14.2	−20.6–38.2
$|e_{V100}|$	2.2 ± 1.8	0.0–5.5
$|e_{D90}|$	10.5 ± 9.5	0.4–38.2

We also calculated the following prediction errors, compared to Day-1 CT-based dosimetry:

$$e_{D90} = D90_{CT} - D90_{RUF}$$
$$e_{V100} = V100_{CT} - V100_{RUF},$$
(15)

where, $D90_{CT}$ and $V100_{CT}$ are the dose parameters calculated based on Day-1 CT and $D90_{RUF}$ and $V100_{RUF}$ are the same dose parameters calculated based on RUF. Table 3 shows a summary of comparison between the dose parameters calculated based on Day-1 CT and RUF. As it can be seen in this Table, our registration method resulted in errors of less than 5.5 % in prediction of $V100$ with an average absolute error of 2.2 %. A paired t-test failed to show statistically significant difference between the CT-based and RUF-based $V100$ at a 5 % significance level (p-value = 0.624). We achieved an average absolute error of 10.5 % for prediction of $D90$. Once again, a paired t-test failed to show statistically significant difference between the CT-based and RUF-based $D90$ calculation at a 5 % significance level (p-value = 0.459).

Discussion

We compared our dosimetry results against CT which is the standard of care. The comparison results show the potentials of our method as an intraoperative dose assessment method. Several factors can affect the dose parameters prediction accuracy, such as seed localization error, registration error, and errors in delineation of organs in CT and ultrasound.

The prostate swells as a reaction to the trauma of needle insertion. As a result the prostate volume increases during the operation. As the edema subsides after the operation, the prostate volume decreases. Therefore, there is an inherent difference between the prostate volume during CT imaging and TRUS imaging. The prostate swelling results in movement of the seeds inside the prostate as well.

Fig. 11 Preimplant prostate contour overlaid on a mid-gland slice of postimplant prostate. The discrepancy between the contour and the real prostate boundaries is easily detectable at the prostate lateral lobes

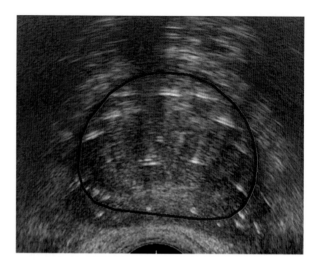

Therefore, the relative position of the seeds at the time of CT imaging is not the same as the relative position of the seeds at the time of C-arm imaging. In addition, there are some errors in segmentation of seed projections and in matching and reconstruction of the seeds that can be seen in Table 2 and result in some errors in prediction of dose parameters.

Another source of error stems from differences in delineation of the prostate in two different modalities—CT and TRUS. As mentioned, CT images do not show sufficient soft tissue contrast and as a result, prostate delineation in CT is different from TRUS. In addition, our prostate delineations in TRUS were performed postimplant for patients 1–9 and preimplant for patients 10–16. Prostate delineation in preimplant prostate is easier. However, it does not show the changes in prostate volume during the operation (see Fig. 11). Moreover, the registration between the preimplant contours and the postimplant prostate volume is established via tracking of the TRUS probe. Therefore, any motion of the prostate with respect to the probe is not taken into account. On the other hand, postimplant prostate delineation is more accurate as it takes into account the prostate swelling and motions of the prostate with respect to the probe. However, prostate contouring in postimplant TRUS images is difficult as the seeds deteriorate the quality of ultrasound images (see Fig. 10). These errors contribute to the discrepancy between the CT and RUF dose parameter calculations. Lindsay et al. [47] showed that the uncertainties in prostate segmentations can affect the dosimetry results as severely as uncertainties in seed localizations. For comparison, we define the prostate volume measurement error e_v as the difference between the prostate volumes segmented in CT and TRUS. As Table 4 shows, there is a statistically significant difference between e_v's computed using preimplant prostate contour and postimplant prostate contour. However, it did not result in a statistically significant difference in the dose parameter prediction errors.

Table 4 Effect of prostate delineation on dosimetry parameters: nine patients havepostimplant contours and seven have preimplant contours

	Prostate segmentation	Mean ± STD	p-value
e^v(cc)	Preimplant	11.3 ± 5.2	0.0012
	Postimplant	0.8 ± 5.1	
$|e_v|$(cc)	Preimplant	11.3 ± 5.2	0.0031
	Postimplant	3.7 ± 3.4	
e^{v100}(%)	Preimplant	−0.3 ± 3.8	0.4437
	Postimplant	0.9 ± 2.1	
$|e_{v100}|$(%)	Preimplant	3.0 ± 2.1	0.1649
	Postimplant	1.7 ± 1.4	
e^{D90}(%)	Preimplant	−6.4 ± 12.2	0.3715
	Postimplant	0.2 ± 15.6	
$|e_{D90}|$(%)	Preimplant	10.7 ± 8.1	0.9683
	Postimplant	10.5 ± 11.0	

The most significant prostate contouring error can be seen for patient 7, for whom the postimplant prostate contouring in TRUS resulted in a prostate volume of almost 50 % larger than that of Day-1 CT. Such a change in prostate volume is unlikely. If we remove this patient from our cohort, the prediction error for $D90$ for patient with postimplant prostate contour decreases to 7.0 ± 3.8 %.

It should be noted that prostate contouring is not necessary for the physician to spot the cold spots or the likely hot spots as he/she can rely on his/her dose distribution visualization within the prostate. In such a scenario, the isodose contours are calculated based on the registered positions of the seeds and overlaid on the TRUS images, without updating or contouring the prostate or other organs at risk.

Our data was collected after all the seeds had been implanted. In such a case, our initialization method resulted in initial registrations sufficiently close to the optimal value for the registration algorithm to converge. We envisage our intraoperative dosimetry method to be used at several occasions during the operation when only a portion of the seeds are implanted. In such a case, aligning the center of the reconstructed seeds with the center of the TRUS volume may not provide a good translational initial condition. Although this matter requires further validation, aligning the center of reconstructed seeds with the center of planned seeds up to that point can provide a good initialization. However, as our registration algorithm is computationally fast, it can be run several times with different initial conditions, if necessary.

All parts of our image processing, seed reconstruction, and registration were implemented in Matlab. The X-ray image processing is done during the image acquisition as soon as an image is acquired, while the operator moves the C-arm to the next image acquisition pose. So, image acquisition and preprocessing add less than a minute to the current workflow. The average time for seed matching, automatic pose correction, and seed reconstruction is 6 s on a PC with 2.5 GHz CPU. The final ultrasound-fluoroscopy registration takes 30 s on average. Including the time for image acquisition, verification of the results after each step, and rarely required manual correction, our intraoperative dosimetry can provide the results in a few minutes. Hence, it has great potential for practical clinical use.

The seed segmentation method described here was optimized for segmentation of Pd-103 seeds. I-125 seeds have a different seed projection that is longer than Pd-103 seeds. Therefore, overlapping seed projections are more common. Alternative solutions for I-125 seed segmentation using region-based active contours and separation of overlapping projections using template-based declustering technique have been proposed and validated [48, 49]. In addition, tomosynthesis-based reconstruction methods can be used to localize the seeds in 3D as shown in [19, 20].

We used the FTRAC to get an initial estimate of the C-arm pose. An alternative to explicit segmentation of the FTRAC in the images is pose recovery using an intensity-based registration of the FTRAC [50]. If the motion of the C-arm in limited to rotation, the C-arm pose can be estimated using accelerometers attached to the C-arm [51, 52]. Likewise, the rotation of the C-arm can be measured using protractors. This approach combined with motion compensation can be used to reconstruct seeds in both matching- and tomosynthesis-based reconstructions as reported in [19, 28].

Conclusions and Future Work

We introduced a fully automatic and complete system for intraoperative prostate brachytherapy dosimetry. Our system is based on registration of ultrasound and fluoroscopic imaging and includes an X-ray image processing module for segmentation of the seed projections and tracking fiducial, a seed reconstruction module with automatic pose correction for 3D localization of the seeds, and an image-based nonrigid ultrasound-fluoroscopy registration module for registering the reconstructed seeds to the ultrasound prostate volume.

We have tested our method on 16 clinical data sets and compared our dosimetry parameters with Day-1 CT as ground truth. We achieved absolute prediction errors of 2.2 ± 1.8 % and 10.5 ± 9.5 % for $V100$ and $D90$, respectively. Considering the accuracy of our results, minimal manual interaction requirement, computation time, and ease of use, our algorithm is a promising tool for enabling intraoperative dynamic dosimetry and improving prostate brachytherapy treatment quality.

Acknowledgments This research was supported in part by the National Institute of Health/ National Cancer Institute (NIH/NCI) under grant 2R44CA099374 and grant 1R01CA151395, and in part by the Department of Defense (DOD) under grant W81XWH-05-1-0407. The first author was with the Queen's University and the Johns Hopkins University while carrying out this research and was supported in part by the Ontario Ministry of Research and Innovation Postdoctoral Fellowship.

References

1. Siegel R, Ward E, Brawley O, Jemal A (2011) Cancer statistics, 2011. CA Cancer J Clin 61 (4):212–236
2. Lagerburg V, Moerland MA, Lagendijk JJ, Battermann JJ (2005) Measurement of prostate rotation during insertion of needles for brachytherapy. Radiother Oncol 77(3):318–323
3. Yamada Y, Potters L, Zaider M, Cohen G, Venkatraman E, Zelefsky MJ (2003) Impact of intraoperative edema during transperineal permanent prostate brachytherapy on computer-optimized and preimplant planning techniques. Am J Clin Oncol 26(5):e130–e135
4. Nath S, Chen Z, Yue N, Trumpore S, Peschel R (2000) Dosimetric effects of needle divergence in prostate seed implant using I125 and Pd103 radioactive seeds. Med Phys 27(5):1058–1066
5. Nag S, Ciezki JP, Cormak R, Doggett S, Dewyngaert K, Edmundson GK, Stock RG, Stone NN, Yan Y, Zelefsky MJ (2001) Intraoperative planning and evaluation of permanent prostate brachytherapy: Report of the American Brachytherapy Society. Int J Radiat Oncol Biol Phys 51(5):1422–1430
6. Polo A, Salembier C, Venselaar J, Hoskin P (2010) Review of intraoperative imaging and planning techniques in permanent seed prostate brachytherapy. Radiother Oncol 94(1):12–23
7. Wei Z, Gardi L, Downey DB, Fenster A (2006) Automated localization of implanted seeds in 3D TRUS images used for prostate brachytherapy. Med Phys 33(7):2404–2417
8. Feleppa EJ, Ramachandran S, Alam SK, Kalisz A, Ketterling JA, Ennis RD, Wuu C-S (2002) Novel methods of analyzing radio-frequency echo signals for the purpose of imaging brachytherapy seeds used to treat prostate cancer. In: Proc. SPIE
9. Wen X, Salcudean SE, Lawrence PD (2010) Detection of brachytherapy seeds using 3D transrectal ultrasound. IEEE Trans Biomed Eng 57(10):2467–2477
10. Holmes DR III, Robb RA (2004) Improved automated brachytherapy seed localization in trans-urethral ultrasound data. In: Proc. SPIE
11. McAleavey S, Rubens D, Parker K (2003) Doppler ultrasound imaging of magnetically vibrated brachytherapy seeds. IEEE Trans Biomed Eng 50(2):252–254
12. Mitri F, Trompette P, Chapelon J-Y (2004) Improving the use of vibro-acoustography for brachytherapy metal seed imaging: a feasibility study. IEEE Trans Med Imaging 23(1):1–6
13. Han BH, Wallner K, Merrick G, Butler W, Sutlief S, Sylvester J (2003) Prostate brachytherapy seed identification on post-implant TRUS images. Med Phys 30(5):898–900
14. Nath R, Bice WS, Butler WM, Chen Z, Meigooni AS, Narayana V, Rivard MJ, Yu Y (2009) AAPM recommendations on dose prescription and reporting methods for permanent interstitial brachytherapy for prostate cancer: report of task group 137. Med Phys 36(11):5310–5322
15. Persons TM, Webber RL, Hemler PF, Bettermann W, Daniel Bourland J (2000) Brachytherapy volume visualization. In: Proc. SPIE
16. Messaris G, Kolitsi Z, Badea C, Pallikarakis N (1999) Three-dimensional localisation based on projectional and tomographic image correlation: an application for digital tomosynthesis. Med Eng Phys 21(2):101–109
17. Tutar IB, Managuli R, Shamdasani V, Cho PS, Pathak SD, Kim Y (2003) Tomosynthesis-based localization of radioactive seeds in prostate brachytherapy. Med Phys 30:3135–3142
18. Brunet-Benkhoucha M, Verhaegen F, Reniers B, Lassalle S, Beliveau-Nadeau D, Donath D, Taussky D, Carrier J-F (2009) Clinical implementation of a digital tomosynthesis-based seed reconstruction algorithm for intraoperative postimplant dose evaluation in low dose rate prostate brachytherapy. Med Phys 36(11):5235–5244
19. Dehghan E, Moradi M, Wen X, French D, Lobo J, James Morris W, Salcudean SE, Fichtinger G (2011) Prostate implant reconstruction from C-arm images with motion-compensated tomosynthesis. Med Phys 38(10):5290–5302
20. Lee J, Liu X, Jain A, Song D, Burdette E, Prince J, Fichtinger G (Dec. 2009) Prostate brachytherapy seed reconstruction with Gaussian blurring and optimal coverage cost. IEEE Trans Med Imaging 28(12):1955–1968

21. Narayanan S, Cho P, Marks R (2002) Fast cross-projection algorithm for reconstruction of seeds in prostate brachytherapy. Med Phys 29:1572–1579

22. Lam ST, Cho PS, Marks RJ II, Narayanan S (2004) Three-dimensional seed reconstruction for prostate brachytherapy using Hough trajectories. Phys Med Biol 49(4):557–569

23. Su Y, Davis BJ, Herman MG, Robb RA (2004) Prostate brachytherapy seed localization by analysis of multiple projections: identifying and addressing the seed overlap problem. Med Phys 31(5):1277–1287

24. Kon R, Jain A, Fichtinger G (2006) Hidden seed reconstruction from C-arm images in brachytherapy. In: IEEE international symposium on biomedical imaging: nano to macro

25. Lee J, Labat C, Jain AK, Song DY, Burdette EC, Fichtinger G, Prince JL (2011) REDMAPS: reduced-dimensionality matching for prostate brachytherapy seed reconstruction. IEEE Trans Med Imaging 30(1):38–51

26. Tubic D, Zaccarin A, Beaulieu L, Pouliot J (2001) Automated seed detection and three-dimensional reconstruction. II. Reconstruction of permanent prostate implants using simulated annealing. Med Phys 28(11):2272–2279

27. Jain A, Fichtinger G (2006) C-arm tracking and reconstruction without an external tracker. In: Proc. medical image computing and computer assisted intervention (MICCAI)

28. Dehghan E, Jain AK, Moradi M, Wen X, Morris WJ, Salcudean SE, Fichtinger G (2011) Brachytherapy seed reconstruction with joint-encoded C-arm single-axis rotation and motion compensation. Med Image Anal 15:760–771

29. Lee J, Kuo N, Deguet A, Dehghan E, Song DY, Burdette EC, Prince JL (2011) Intraoperative 3D reconstruction of prostate brachytherapy implants with automatic pose correction. Phys Med Biol 56(15):5011–5027

30. Jain AK, Mustufa T, Zhou Y, Burdette C, Chirikjian GS, Fichtinger G (2005) FTRAC-A robust fluoroscope tracking fiducial. Med Phys 32(10):3185–3198

31. Kuo N, Deguet A, Song DY, Burdette EC, Prince JL, Lee J (2012) Automatic segmentation of radiographic fiducial and seeds from X-ray images in prostate brachytherapy. Med Eng Phys 34(1):64–77

32. Otsu N (1979) A threshold selection method from gray-level histograms. IEEE Trans Syst Man Cybern 9(1):62–66

33. Seber G (2004) Multivariate observations. Hoboken, NJ, Wiley-Interscience

34. Bertsekas PD (1999) Nonlinear programming, 2nd edn. Athena Scientific, Belmont, MA

35. Todor DA, Zaider M, Cohen GN, Worman MF, Zelefsky MJ (2003) Intraoperative dynamic dosimetry for prostate implants. Phys Med Biol 48(9):1153–1171

36. Jain A, Deguet A, Iordachita I, Chintalapani G, Vikal S, Blevins J, Le Y, Armour E, Burdette C, Song D, Fichtinger G (2012) Intra-operative 3D guidance and edema detection in prostate brachytherapy using a non-isocentric C-arm. Med Image Anal 16(3):731–743

37. French D, Morris J, Keyes M, Goksel O, Salcudian SE (2005) Intraoperative dosimetry for prostate brachytherapy from fused ultrasound and fluoroscopy images. Acad Radiol 12 (10):1262–1272

38. Su Y, Davis BJ, Furutani KM, Herman MG, Robb RA (2007) Seed localization and TRUS-fluoroscopy fusion for intraoperative prostate brachytherapy dosimetry. Comput Aided Surg 12(1):25–34

39. Orio PF III, Tutar IB, Narayanan S, Arthurs S, Cho PS, Kim Y, Merrick G, Wallner KE (2007) Intraoperative ultrasound-fluoroscopy fusion can enhance prostate brachytherapy quality. Int J Radiat Oncol Biol Phys 69(1):302–307

40. Tutar IB, Gong L, Narayanan S, Pathak SD, Cho PS, Wallner K, Kim Y (2008) Seed-based transrectal ultrasound-fluoroscopy registration method for intraoperative dosimetry analysis of prostate brachytherapy. Med Phys 35(3):840–848

41. Moradi M, Sara Mahdavi S, Dehghan E, Lobo JR, Deshmukh S, James W, Fichtinger G, Salcudean SE (2012) Seed localization in ultrasound and registration to C-arm fluoroscopy using matched needle tracks for prostate brachytherapy. IEEE Trans Biomed Eng 59 (9):2558–2567

42. Fallavollita P, Karim-Aghaloo Z, Burdette E, Song D, Abolmaesumi P, Fichtinger G (2010) Registration between ultrasound and fluoroscopy or CT in prostate brachytherapy. Med Phys 37(6):2749–2760
43. Dehghan E, Lee J, Fallavollita P, Kuo N, Deguet A, Le Y, Clif Burdette E, Song DY, Prince JL, Fichtinger G (2012) Ultrasound-fluoroscopy registration for prostate brachytherapy dosimetry. Med Image Anal 16(7):1347–1358
44. Hansen N (2006) The CMA evolution strategy: a comparing review, vol 192. Springer, Berlin, Heidelberg, pp 75–102
45. Chen TK, Thurston AD, Ellis RE, Abolmaesumi P (2009) A real-time freehand ultrasound calibration system with automatic accuracy feedback and control. Ultrasound Med Biol 35 (1):79–93
46. Rivard MJ, Coursey BM, DeWerd LA, Hanson WF, Saiful Huq M, Ibbott GS, Mitch MG, Nath R, Williamson JF (2004) Update of AAPM task group No. 43 report: a revised AAPM protocol for brachytherapy dose calculations. Med Phys 31(3):633–674
47. Lindsay PE, Van Dyk J, Battista JJ (2003) A systematic study of imaging uncertainties and their impact on 125I prostate brachytherapy dose evaluation. Med Phys 30(7):1897–1908
48. Moult E, Fichtinger G, Morris W, Salcudean S, Dehghan E, Fallavollita P (2012) Segmentation of iodine brachytherapy implants in fluoroscopy. Int J Comput Assist Radiol Surg 7 (6):871–879
49. San Filippo C, Fichtinger G, Morris W, Salcudean T, Dehghan E, Fallavollita P (2013) Declustering n-connected components: an example case for the segmentation of iodine implants in C-arm images. In: Int. conf. information processing in computer-assisted interventions (IPCAI), Heidelberg, Germany
50. Fallavollita P, Burdette EC, Song DY, Abolmaesumi P, Fichtinger G (2011) Technical note: unsupervised C-arm pose tracking with radiographic fiducial. Med Phys 38(4):2241–2245
51. Grzeda V, Fichtinger G (2010) C-arm rotation encoding with accelerometers. Int J Comput Assist Radiol Surg 5(4):385–391
52. Wolff T, Lasso A, Ebenkamp M, Wintermantel E, Fichtinger G (2013) C-arm angle measurement with accelerometer for brachytherapy — an accuracy study. Int J Comput Assist Radiol Surg:1–8

Biography

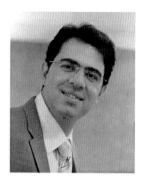

Ehsan Dehghan received the B.Sc. and M.Sc. degrees in electrical engineering from Sharif University of Technology, Tehran, Iran, in 2001 and 2003, respectively, and the Ph.D. degree in electrical and computer engineering from the University of British Columbia, Vancouver, BC, Canada, in 2009. From 2009 to 2012, he was a Postdoctoral Fellow at Queen's University, Kingston, ON, Canada, and Johns Hopkins University, Baltimore, MD, USA. He is currently with Philips Research North America, Briarcliff Manor, NY. His research interests include image-guided and computer-assisted intervention and therapy, medical image analysis, soft tissue modeling and simulation, medical robotics, finite element modeling, and control systems.

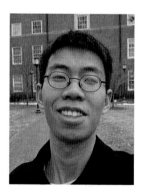

Nathanael Kuo is a Ph.D. candidate in the Department of Biomedical Engineering at Johns Hopkins University, where he works with Dr. Jerry L. Prince in the Image Analysis and Communications Laboratory, and Dr. Emad M. Boctor in the Medical UltraSound Imaging and Intervention Collaboration. Having graduated highest honors from the University of Illinois at Urbana-Champaign with a B.S. in

Electrical Engineering and minors in Computer Science and Mathematics, he currently specializes in image-guided therapy within the broader field of medical imaging. His dissertation research focuses on seed localization in prostate brachytherapy dynamic dosimetry systems and involves several imaging modalities including X-ray, ultrasonic, and photoacoustic imaging.

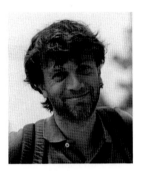

Anton Deguet completed his M.S. degree in Computer Science at Grenoble's Joseph Fourier University in 1994. After several years as a Ph.D. candidate, he started working for the Johns Hopkins University in 2000 as a research engineer. His primary interests are software engineering and robotics for medical applications. More specifically, he has worked on the integration of technologies for prostate brachytherapy, including C-arm calibration and tracking, seed reconstruction, and robotic needle template.

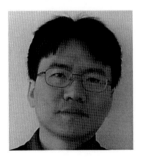

Yi Le received his B.S. and M.S. degree in Physics from University of Science and Technology of China (USTC) in 1996 and 1998, respectively. In 1998 he went to United States to pursue his Ph.D. degree in experimental particle physics and obtained his Ph.D. degree from Johns Hopkins University in 2004. He switched his focus to therapeutic radiation physics and was a postdoctoral research fellow in radiation oncology department at Virginia Commonwealth University from 2004 to 2006. Since 2006, he has been a medical physicist in department of radiation oncology and molecular radiation science at Johns Hopkins University School of

Medicine. His research interest is using multimodality imaging techniques to guide radiation therapy including brachytherapy. He is also interested in using functional imaging techniques to do radiation treatment assessment.

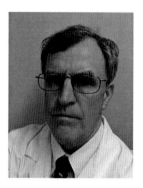

Elwood P. Armour received his Ph.D. degree in Biomedical Sciences from the Univ. of Texas, GSBS at Houston. He completed a postdoctoral fellowship in Radiation Cancer Biology at Stanford University. He subsequently held positions in Radiation Biology and Medical Physics at the University of Texas MD Anderson Cancer Center and William Beaumont Hospital. He is currently the Chief Medical Physicist in the Radiation Oncology and Molecular Radiation Sciences Department at Johns Hopkins University Medical School.

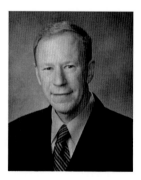

Everette C. Burdette is President/CEO of Acoustic MedSystems, Inc., a company dedicated to image-guided medical interventions and localized therapies for cancer and benign disease. He serves on the corporate boards of Presence Covenant Medical System Central IL Region, Oncology Systems, Inc., Acoustic MedSystems, Inc. and Precision Therapeutics, Inc. He was Vice President of Research and Clinical Design at Computerized Medical Systems (CMS) and President of the Image Guidance Division. He was President of Burdette Medical Systems from its inception in 1997 until its acquisition in 2002. He is an innovator of image-guided cancer management methods and was principal scientist in developing the first intraoperative dosimetry and image guidance system for radiation implants. He holds Ph.D. and M.S. degrees in Electrical Engineering and in Physics, and B.S. in Physics from the Georgia Institute of Technology, and a Ph.D. in Physiology from Emory University. He was Director of Advanced Technology Development for Dornier Medical Systems, Inc. from 1992-97. He was President of Labthermics Technologies, Inc., a medical therapeutic equipment company, from 1986 to 1992. He was a faculty member at the University of Illinois at Urbana-Champaign, Emory University School of Medicine, and Georgia Tech. He has worked in the radiation oncology, hyperthermic oncology, ultrasound imaging, and urological fields for 28 years and prior to that worked in the development of radar systems and micro-wave devices for military applications for 7 years. His product development spans medical imaging, image guidance of therapeutic ablation tools, radiotherapy treat-ment planning systems, and high power needle/catheter-based ultrasound devices for interventional ablative therapy. He has authored over 200 conference proceedings, scientific papers, and book chapters and holds 43 patents.

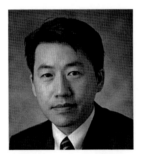

Danny Y. Song serves as the Clinical Director and Director of Brachytherapy in the Department of Radiation Oncology and Molecular Radiation Sciences at the Johns Hopkins University School of Medicine. His research focus is on technological innovations and image guidance for improving the practice of prostate radiother-apy, as well as clinical research in radiotherapy for prostate cancer and other genitourinary malignancies.

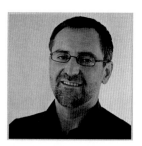

Gabor Fichtinger received the Ph.D. degree in computer science from the Technical University of Budapest, Budapest, Hungary, in 1990. He is currently a Professor in the School of Computing, with cross appointments in the departments of Mechanical and Material Engineering, Electrical and Computer Engineering, and Surgery, Queen's University, Kingston, ON, Canada, where he also directs the Percutaneous Surgery Laboratory. He is also adjunct professor in Radiology and Computer Science at the Johns Hopkins University, Baltimore, USA. His research specializes on medical image computing and computer-assisted interventions, primarily for the diagnosis and therapy of cancer. Dr. Fichtinger is a Senior Member of IEEE, Distinguished Lecturer of IEEE EMBS, and a Fellow of MICCAI. Dr. Fichtinger also holds a Level-1 Cancer Care Ontario Research Chair in Cancer Imaging.

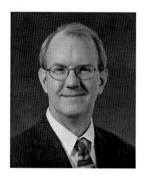

Jerry L. Prince received the B.S. degree from the University of Connecticut in 1979 and the S.M., E.E., and Ph.D. degrees in 1982, 1986, and 1988, respectively, from the Massachusetts Institute of Technology, all in electrical engineering and computer science. He worked at the Brigham and Women's Hospital, MIT Lincoln Laboratories, and The Analytic Sciences Corporation (TASC). He joined the faculty at the Johns Hopkins University in 1989, where he is currently William B. Kouwenhoven Professor in the Department of Electrical and Computer Engineering and holds joint appointments in the Departments of Radiology, Biomedical Engineering, Computer Science, and Applied Mathematics and Statistics. Dr. Prince is a Fellow of the IEEE, Fellow of the MICCAI Society, and a member of Sigma Xi. He also holds memberships in Tau Beta Pi, Eta Kappa Nu, and Phi

Kappa Phi honor societies. He was an Associate Editor of IEEE Transactions on Image Processing from 1992-1995, an Associate Editor of IEEE Transactions on Medical Imaging from 2000-2004, and is currently a member of the Editorial Board of Medical Image Analysis. Dr. Prince received a 1993 National Science Foundation Presidential Faculty Fellows Award and was Maryland's 1997 Outstanding Young Engineer. He is also co-founder of Diagnosoft, Inc., a medical imaging software company. His current research interests are in image processing and computer vision with primary application to medical imaging and has published over 300 articles and abstracts on these subjects.

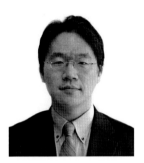

Junghoon Lee is Assistant Professor in the Department of Radiation Oncology and Molecular Radiation Sciences and Assistant Research Professor in the Department of Electrical and Computer Engineering at the Johns Hopkins University, Baltimore, MD. He received B.S. degree in Electrical Engineering and M.S. degree in Biomedical Engineering in 1997 and 1999, respectively, both from Seoul National University, Seoul, Republic of Korea. He received Ph.D. degree from Purdue University, West Lafayette, IN in Electrical and Computer Engineering in 2006. In 2007, he joined the Department of Electrical and Computer Engineering and the NSF Engineering Research Center for Computer-Integrated Surgical Systems and Technology at the Johns Hopkins University as a Postdoctoral Fellow and continued to work as Associate Research Scientist from Jan. 2009 to Oct. 2010. His current research interests are in medical image processing and analysis, specifically in novel reconstruction algorithm and image-guided interventions, surgery, and radiation therapy.

Multi-Atlas-Based Segmentation of Pelvic Structures from CT Scans for Planning in Prostate Cancer Radiotherapy

Oscar Acosta, Jason Dowling, Gael Drean, Antoine Simon, Renaud de Crevoisier, and Pascal Haigron

Abstract In prostate cancer radiotherapy, the accurate identification of the prostate and organs at risk in planning computer tomography (CT) images is an important part of the therapy planning and optimization. Manually contouring these organs can be a time-consuming process and subject to intra- and inter-expert variability. Automatic identification of organ boundaries from these images is challenging due to the poor soft tissue contrast. Atlas-based approaches may provide a priori structural information by propagating manual expert delineations to a new individual space; however, the interindividual variability and registration errors may lead to biased results. Multi-atlas approaches can partly overcome some of these difficulties by selecting the most similar atlases among a large data base, but the definition of similarity measure between the available atlases and the query individual has still to be addressed. The purpose of this chapter is to explain atlas-based segmentation approaches and the evaluation of different atlas-based strategies to simultaneously segment prostate, bladder, and rectum from CT images. A comparison between single and multiple atlases is performed. Experiments on atlas ranking, selection strategies, and fusion-decision rules are carried out to illustrate the presented methodology. Propagation of labels using two registration strategies is applied and the results of the comparison with manual delineations are reported.

O. Acosta (✉) • G. Drean • A. Simon • P. Haigron
INSERM, U1099, Rennes 35000, France

Université de Rennes 1, LTSI, Rennes 35000, France
e-mail: oscar.acosta@univ-rennes1.fr

J. Dowling
The Australian e-Health Research Center-CSIRO, Brisbane, Australia

R. de Crevoisier
INSERM, U1099, Rennes 35000, France

Université de Rennes 1, LTSI, Rennes 35000, France

Département de Radiothérapie, Centre Eugène Marquis, Rennes 35000, France

A.S. El-Baz et al. (eds.), *Abdomen and Thoracic Imaging: An Engineering & Clinical Perspective*, DOI 10.1007/978-1-4614-8498-1_24,
© Springer Science+Business Media New York 2014

Introduction

Prostate cancer is one of the most commonly diagnosed male cancers worldwide [1], with 190,000 new cases diagnosed in USA in 2010 [2] and 71,000 new cases in France in 2011 [3]. In Australia, prostate cancer is the most commonly diagnosed cancer behind skin cancer and is the second highest cause of cancer-related deaths behind lung cancer [4]. External beam radiation therapy (EBRT) is a major clinical treatment for prostate cancer which has proven to be efficient for tumor control [5]. EBRT uses high-energy X-ray beams combined from multiple directions to deposit energy (dose) within the patient tumor region (the prostate) to destroy the cancer cells. Modern treatment techniques offer nowadays improved treatment accuracy through a better planning, delivery, visualization, and the correction of patient setup errors.

The standard clinical protocol for EBRT treatment planning is shown in Fig. 1. During the planning step, CT images from patients are acquired. The treatment targets (prostate and potentially seminal vesicles) along with important normal tissues (rectum, bladder, and femoral heads) are manually delineated using the scans. If MRI is used for the prostate definition then alignment of the MRI and the CT is performed to transfer the MRI structure contours to the CT scan. A defined prostate volume is then expanded to constitute the Planning Target Volume (PTV) for treatment (Fig. 2). These spatial margins between the organs and the PTV allow for uncertainties in delineation, patient setup, motion, and organ deformations [6–8].

The next step is the use of computer planning tools to determine the directions, strengths, and shapes of the treatment beams which will be used to deliver a prescribed dose to the defined target while minimizing the dose to the normal tissues, according to a certain number of recommendations (e.g., [9]). Thus, a treatment plan consists of dose distribution information over a 3D matrix of points overlaid onto the individual's anatomy. Dose volume histograms (DVHs) summarize the information contained in the 3D dose distribution and may serve as tools for quantitative evaluation of treatment plans. The International Commission on Radiation Units and Measurements (ICRU) 50 and 62 reports define and describe several target and critical structure volumes that aid in the treatment planning process and that provide a basis for comparison of treatment outcomes. For example, to comply with ICRU recommendations for prostate, 95 % of the PTV is irradiated with at least 95 % of the prescribed dose. For the rectal wall the maximal dose should be less or equal than 76 Gy and the irradiated volume at 72 Gy must be less than 25 %. Finally, during the dose delivery step, which may last several weeks, the patient is carefully positioned at the accelerator and the treatment is performed according to the planning. A frequent method to align the patient for treatment is to use small implanted fiducial markers in the prostate. These are visible under X-ray imaging and show precise prostate position within the body. Image guidance may also be used to align the treatment target each day for the entire course (Fig. 3).

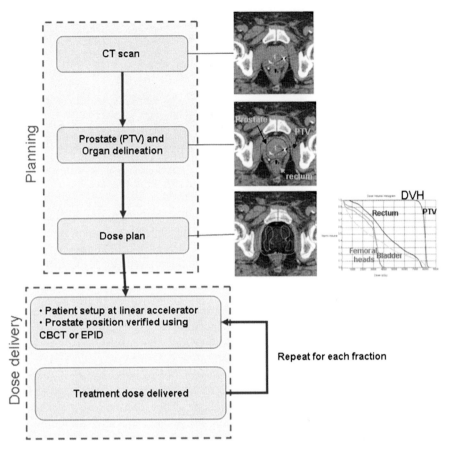

Fig. 1 Workflow for traditional prostate cancer image-guided radiation therapy. The prescribed radiation dose for EBRT is generally delivered over several weeks in small daily amounts (fractions)

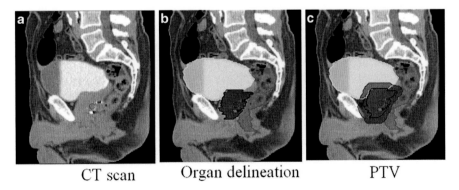

Fig. 2 Sagittal views of a male pelvis showing the original CT scan (**a**) with overlaid delineations of the bladder, rectum and prostate (**b**) and with the planning target volume (PTV) (**c**) defining the area which will receive the prescribed radiation dose

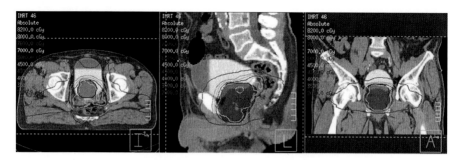

Fig. 3 Typical intensity modulated radiation therapy (IMRT) plan (axial, coronal, and sagittal views) showing iso-dose curves and the (PTV), obtained after organ delineations

One of the main challenges in prostate radiotherapy is to control the tumor, by accurately targeting the prostate, while sparing neighboring organs at risk (OAR) (bladder and rectum). Several strategies have been developed in order to improve local control, particularly by increasing the radiation dose with highly conformal techniques demonstrating a strong dose-effect relationship [10]. The precision of treatment delivery is steadily improving due to the combination of intensity modulated RT (IMRT) and image-guided RT (IGRT) and intraprostatic fiducial markers. New delivery systems are also populating clinical centers (ARC-Therapy, cyberknife). Hence, the possibilities for achieving better control by increasing the dose are within reach. However, dose escalation is limited by rectal and urinary toxicity [11, 12]. Toxicity events (incontinence, rectal bleeding, stool lose) are frequent with standard prescribed doses (70–80 Gy) and may even significantly increase for higher doses [13]. Thus, accurate delineation of both prostate and OARs (i.e., bladder, rectum) from planning images are crucial to exploit the new capabilities of the delivery systems [14]. Identifying the boundaries of pelvic structures are of major importance not only at the planning step, but also in other radiotherapy stages such as patient setup correction, accumulating dose computation when IGRT is used [15, 16], or for toxicity population studies [17] (Fig. 4).

Nowadays, the organ contouring tasks are mainly carried out manually by medical experts. However, the CT offers poor soft tissue contrast and therefore segmenting pelvic organs is highly time-consuming (between 20 and 40 min to delineate each). Manual contouring requires training and is prone to errors, especially in the apical and basis regions [18, 19]. These uncertainties lead to large intra- and inter-observer variation [20] and may impact treatment planning and dosimetry [19, 21]. Previous studies, for instance, have reported a prostate delineation variance of 20:60 % [20]. For the rectum and bladder this difference may be as high as 2.5 to 3 % [19]. Although improved organ contrast may be obtained with Magnetic Resonance Images (MRI), and several studies are in progress to introduce MRI in the radiotherapy planning [22, 23], CT scans are still required to perform this task since dose computation relies on electron density.

Therefore, there is a strong case for more reliable semi- or fully automatic CT segmentation techniques. When dealing with automatic segmentation methods for

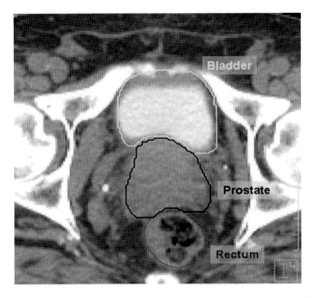

Fig. 4 Axial view of manual segmentation of bladder, prostate, and rectum overlaid on CT scan

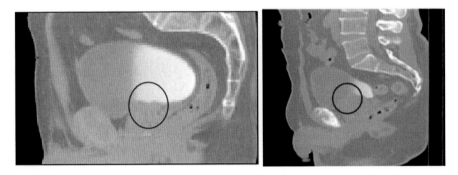

Fig. 5 Two examples of pelvic structures in CT (sagittal views). The poor contrast between structures hampers organ segmentation

prostate cancer treatment, there are several difficulties which may arise. Firstly, there is a poor contrast between prostate, bladder, and rectum and, secondly, there may exist a high variability in the amount of bladder and rectum filling. These challenges restrict the use of classical intensity-based segmentation methods. In addition the high intra- and interindividual variability may cause model-based methods to fail [24] (Fig. 5).

Atlas-based approaches are common methods for organ segmentation, not only for obtaining a final contour, but also to provide initial organ positions for further segmentation algorithms. In atlas-based methods a precomputed segmentation or prior information in a template space is propagated towards the image to be segmented via spatial normalization (registration). These methods have been largely used in brain MRI [25, 26], head and neck CT Scans [27–29], cardiac aortic CT [30], pulmonary lobes from CT [31], and prostate MR [32, 33]. In the atlas-based methods image registration is a key element, as label propagation relies on the registration of one or more templates to a target image.

In this chapter a brief overview of image registration and atlas methods will be provided. Atlas-based methods which can perform the segmentation of the individuals' pelvic structures, prostate, and OAR from CT scans will be discussed and evaluated against clinical datasets.

Image Registration

Introduction

Atlas-based segmentation is heavily dependent on the quality of image registration. Medical image registration involves determining the spatial transform which maps points from a moving image to homologous points on an object in a fixed image. The general idea of the registration may be summarized as in Fig. 6.

The basic input data to the registration process are two images: one is defined as the *fixed image F(X)* and the other as the *moving image M(X)*. The output of the registration is a spatial transformation T allowing the warping or the alignment of the moving image, on the fixed image, according to a similarity metric.

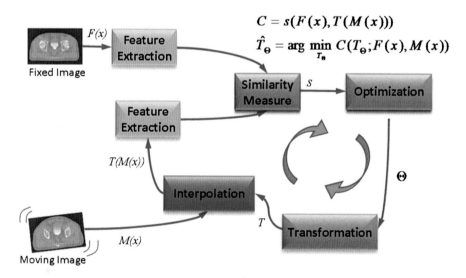

$$C = s(F(x), T(M(x)))$$

$$\hat{T}_\Theta = \arg \min_{T_\Theta} C(T_\Theta; F(x), M(x))$$

Fig. 6 Computerized registration framework

As depicted in Fig. 6, there are four main components involved in image registration: a similarity measure between two images; the transformation model used to map points between images; a method to find the optimal transform parameters; and finally an interpolator to calculate moving image intensities at non-grid positions [20].

In this sense, registration may be seen as an optimization problem

$$\hat{T}_\Theta = \arg \min_{T_\Theta} C(T_\Theta; F(x), M(x)) \tag{1}$$

aimed at estimating the spatial mapping that better align the moving image with the fixed image according to a cost function:

$$C = s(F(x), T(M(x))) \tag{2}$$

where $s(F(x), T(M(x))$ is the similarity which provides a measure of how well the fixed image is matched by the transformed moving image. This measure forms the quantitative criterion to be optimized over the search space defined by the parameters of the transform. The similarity may lie on control points, features, anatomical structures, intensities, etc. Here, we restricted the study to the intensity similarity metrics.

Transform

The transform component $T(X)$ represents the spatial mapping of points from the fixed image space to points in the moving image space. The transformation model can either apply to the entire volume (global) or to each voxel (local).

The two global methods are: rigid registration which allows only rotations and translations; and affine registration which extends rigid registration with the addition of skew and scaling parameters.

Deformable (also known as nonrigid or nonlinear) registration affects individual voxels within the volume. This enables the matching of soft tissues which may deform between scans (e.g., a patient's bladder on two CBCT volumes) or when performing interindividual mapping. Typically a regularization constraint is also implemented to constrain the allowable solution space. Deformable methods can be complex and difficult to validate [34]. Common deformable transforms include BSpline free form deformation (FFD) [35], thin plate splines [36], and optical flow-inspired approaches (Demons algorithm) [37]. The output from deformable registration is generally a volume (the deformation field) which contains displacement vectors for each voxel as illustrated in Fig. 7.

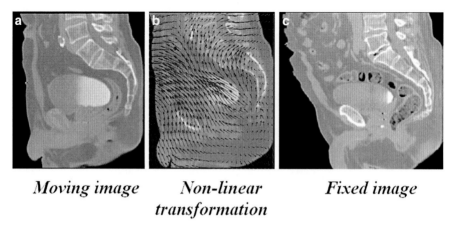

Moving image   Non-linear   Fixed image
transformation

Fig. 7 Example of a nonlinear transformation (**b**) obtained when registering the moving image (**a**) into the space of the fixed image (**c**)

Image Similarity Metrics

When the similarity between two images is based on intensity levels, several metrics can be considered [38]. These can be computed via their voxel-wise differences, for example, with the sum of squared differences (SSD), or via the cross-correlation (CC) or the mutual information (MI). These metrics are computed over the whole image as follows:

$$\text{SSD} = \frac{1}{n}\sqrt{\sum_i \left(F(x_i) - T(M(x_i))\right)^2} \tag{3}$$

where $F(x_i)$ is the fixed image and $T(M(x_i))$ represents the transformed moving image. The CC as

$$\text{CC} = \frac{\sum_i \left(F(x_i) - \overline{F}(x)\right)\left(T(M(x_i)) - T\left(\overline{M}(x)\right)\right)}{\sqrt{\sum_i \left(F(x_i) - \overline{F}(x)\right)^2}\sqrt{\sum_i \left(T(M(x_i)) - T\left(\overline{M}(x)\right)\right)^2}} \tag{4}$$

and the MI, computed as

$$\text{MI}(F, M) = H(F) + H(M) - H(F, M) \tag{5}$$

where $H(x)$ is the individual entropy of an image x, given by

$$H(F) = -\sum_i p(i)\log p(i) \tag{6}$$

and

$$H(F,M) = -\sum_{i,j} p(i,j)\log p(i,j) \tag{7}$$

is the joint entropy and p the joint probability. The idea behind the term $-H(F,M)$ is that maximizing MI is related to minimizing joint entropy. A more robust version of the MI is the normalized mutual information (NMI) proposed by Studholme et al. [39] and computed as

$$\text{NMI}(F,M) = \frac{H(F) + H(M)}{H(F,M)} \tag{8}$$

An important consideration with similarity metrics is the computational cost and the need of a large number of samples for the algorithms to be robust. Novel ways of computing MI have been proposed [40], yielding comparable results with less samples. This approach approximates the entropy computation using the high-order description. For a complete survey of MI, the reader may refer to [41].

Optimization

The images (or image features) are ideally related to each other by some transformation T. As shown in Fig. 6, the iterative process of optimization aims at finding T with a cost function determined by the similarity metric. As the cost function may have multiple local minima, a weighted regularization term may be added to penalize undesirable deformations as

$$C = s(F(x), T(M(x))) + w\Psi \tag{9}$$

Examples of Ψ include the curvature, the elastic energy, or volume preserving constraints. This term ensures smoothness of T in the nonparametric approaches. There are several ways to perform the optimization of T. These include the deterministic gradient-based algorithms such as gradient descent, quasi-Newton, or nonlinear gradient descent; or the stochastic gradient-based algorithms such as the Kiefer-Wolfowitz, simultaneous perturbation, Robins Monro and Evolution Strategy, where they derive search directions with stochastic approximations of the derivative.

A full evaluation of optimization techniques in a nonrigid registration context was presented by Klein et al. [32]. They compared several methods with respect to speed, accuracy, precision, and robustness. By using a set of CT images of heart and MR images of prostate, it was shown that a stochastic gradient descent technique, the Robins-Monro process outperformed the other approaches. Acceleration factors of approximately 500 compared to a basic gradient descent method were achieved.

Interpolation

As depicted in Fig. 6, after a transformation is applied to the moving image, an interpolation is performed which enables evaluation of the moving image intensities at non-grid positions. To resample the moving image in the fixed image grid, the transformation can be applied either in a forward or backward manner. In the forward way, each voxel from the moving image can be directly transformed using the estimated mapping functions. Because of the discretization, this approach can produce holes and/or overlaps in the transformed image.

Hence, the backward approach is more convenient and usually implemented. In this approach, the image interpolation takes place on the regular grid in the space of the fixed image. Thus, the registered image data from the moving image are determined using the coordinates of the target voxel and the inverse of the estimated transformation. In this way, neither holes nor overlaps can occur in the output image. Thus, depending on the required precision different alternatives exist for this resampling, for instance the nearest neighbor (NN), tri-linear, BSpline (BS), Cubic interpolations (CI), etc. However, some artifacts may be introduced as a consequence of the iterative process. These interpolation-related errors in image registration have been studied by Pluim et al. [42]. Thevenaz et al. [43] have proposed a different approach to image resampling. Unlike the other methods, their resampling functions do not necessarily interpolate the image intensity levels but values calculated as certain functions of the intensities. The authors demonstrated how this approach outperforms traditional interpolation techniques. Several survey papers on resampling techniques have been published recently [44–47].

In practical terms, although higher-order methods may yield good result in terms of accuracy, the tri-linear interpolation offers a very good trade-off between accuracy and computational complexity. Cubic or spline interpolation is recommended when the transformation involves significant geometrical differences, as several voxels may be interpolated in between available information. Nearest neighbor interpolation produces several artifacts, but is advised when the image to be transformed contains low number of intensities. For example, when propagating labels in atlas-based segmentation approaches, this is the preferred approach.

General Atlas Construction and Segmentation Strategies

Introduction

The key idea in atlas-based segmentation is to use image registration to map one or more pre-labeled images (or "atlas") onto a new patient image. Once a good correspondence between structurally equivalent regions in the two images is achieved, the labels defined on the atlas can be propagated to the image. Rohlfing et al. [48] have identified four main methods to generate the atlas which is

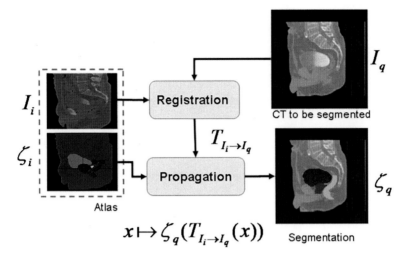

Fig. 8 Atlas-based segmentation strategy

registered to a target volume: i) using a single-labeled image, ii) generating an average shape image, iii) selecting the most similar image from a database of scans; or finally iv) registering all individual scans from a database and using multi-classier fusion to combine the pair-wise registration results.

An atlas A_i is constituted by a template image I_i and, a set of generated labels ζ_i defined in the same coordinate system. In the case of pelvic structures from CT scans, the set of labels $\zeta_i = \{\text{prostate,rectum,bladder}\}$. The general framework of atlas-based segmentation, as depicted in Fig. 8, relies on the registration of the template I_i, to the query image I_q in order to obtain a transformation $T_{I_i \to I_q}$, that maps ζ_i into I_q. If the mapping is anatomically correct, the yielded segmentation is accurate and anatomically meaningful. It is worth nothing that the similarity between the images I_i and I_q, as explained in previous sections, may impact the registration results and therefore the segmentation.

Several issues may arise under this framework in order to produce accurate segmentations. Firstly, the selection and generation of the initial patient scan which may be representative of a population; secondly, the registration strategy to bring I_i into the space of I_q; and finally, the propagation of the labels ζ_i into I_q.and the subsequent generation of the new segmentation ζ_q.

Concerning the first issue, a typical individual from a given population may constitute an atlas, where the segmentation ζ_i may be manually generated on I_i. This is the simplest strategy, but with the problems related to the interindividual variability and inter-observer rating arising. However, in order to attenuate the dependency on a single observer, a group of experts can generate the set of labels, adding robustness to the definition of ζ_i. To cope with the interindividual variability, several individuals from a population can be used to constitute the atlas. In this case, two kinds of strategies may be followed. Either an atlas is built

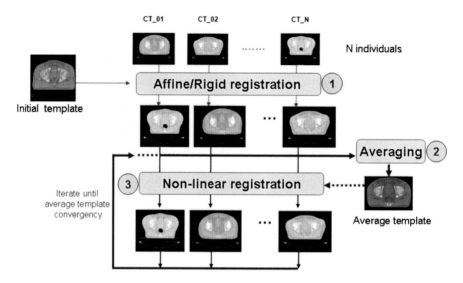

Fig. 9 Iterative averaging for obtaining a template

from the population by averaging the data $(I_i, \zeta_i\ i = 0, \ldots, M)$ or alternatively each individual is considered as a single atlas. In that case, for a given query, there is a previous selection of the best n atlases $A_i, i = 0, \ldots, M$ which better fit to the query I_q. The last strategy allows for a reduction of the bias inherent to using a single template, but new questions arise concerning the best atlas selection strategy and label fusion decisions to constitute the final segmentation ζ_q. These points are detailed in the following sections. Proposed experiments compare the performances of those for segmenting prostate, bladder, and rectum.

Average Atlas Construction

An atlas can be computed in an iterative process as depicted in Fig. 9. This approach was used in a comparative study that we presented in [17], but also is detailed in [49]. In this scheme, an arbitrary but representative individual is selected as the initial template, defining the atlas space alignment. The first iteration involves the registration of every other individual to the selected template using a rigid or affine registration method (i.e., robust block matching approach [50], followed by a nonrigid registration [37] in the subsequent iterations). At the end of each iteration, a new average atlas is generated and used in the subsequent iteration.

After the average template is obtained, a probabilistic set of soft labels ζ_i (probability maps) is eventually generated by propagating the manual segmentations of these organs for each case using the obtained affine transform and deformation field into the atlas space. Figure 10 shows an example of the obtained

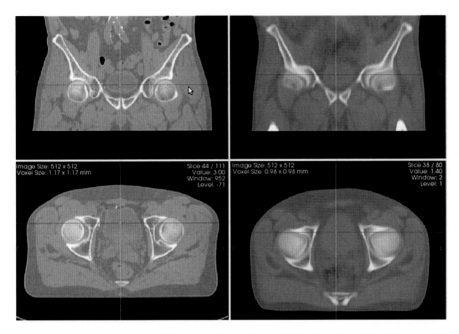

Fig. 10 Coronal (*top*) and axial (*bottom*) views of an individual's male pelvis CT scan (left column) and an averaged template (right column)

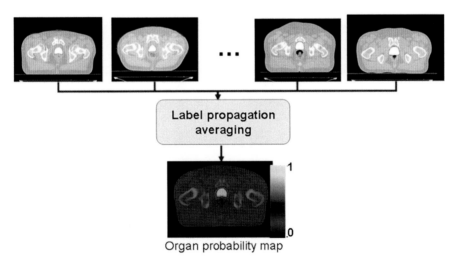

Fig. 11 Generation of organ probability maps by propagating labels into the common template

template after five iterations and Fig. 11 depicts an overlaid of the probabilistic labeling for the prostate in the atlas coordinate system.

The drawbacks of this strategy within the context of CT pelvic segmentation come from the large interindividual variability and the poorly contrasted average

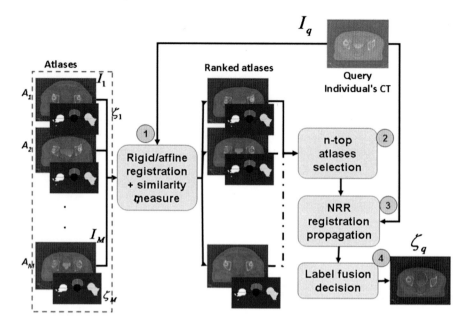

Fig. 12 Multi-atlas-based segmentation process. Atlas are first ranked according to the similarity to the query image, then, labels from the top n-ranked atlases are propagated towards the individual CT and finally, in a fusion-decision step, organ segmentations are obtained

atlas which is produced after several iterations. In order to diminish the bias inherent to using a single template, one potential strategy is to select one patient among typical individuals from a database, who is quite similar to the majority of individuals. Additional benefits may be brought to the segmentation by combining the results from multiple atlases, improving the accuracy as explained in the next section.

Multi-Atlas Strategy: Selecting the N Best Atlas from a Database

Previous works have shown the benefits of combining multiple atlases (multi-atlases-based approaches), improving the segmentation accuracy (e.g., [25, 26, 30, 51]). Thus, given a query individual, different possibilities appear. Either the closest individual from the database is selected as the best atlas or all the atlases are combined together as in the strategy depicted in Fig. 12. In this approach, the atlases are firstly ranked according to the similarity to the query image. This is done after a rigid or affine registration step which allows for the interindividual differences to be assessed. Then, in the steps 2 and 3, labels from the top *n*-ranked atlases are propagated towards the individual CT via nonrigid registration to more accurately match template anatomies. Finally, in a fusion-decision step, organ segmentations are obtained by combining different labels. The particular case $n = 1$ corresponds to the most similar individual atlas strategy.

The questions arising in this scheme concern (i) the method for selecting the atlases to be used and particularly the most convenient similarity metric, (ii) the nonrigid registration technique, and (iii) the fusion-decision rules (discussed in the next subsection).

The similarity measure can be based on the difference of intensity levels, for example, as explained in previous sections: the SSD, the cross-correlation, or the mutual information. The similarity can be also based on information obtained from the deformation [52], such as the Jacobian. The drawback of the Jacobian is the dependency on the registration method used to align the images. Two registration strategies are tested and discussed later in a further section, namely FFD [35] and the demons algorithm [53].

Label Fusion

For both the average and multi-atlas approaches, a method for combining labels is required. This fusion step occurs at the voxel level during each training iteration of average atlas construction, and when combining propagated labels from selected atlases in a multi-atlas scheme.

Majority voting simply counts the number of label overlaps (or votes) on a single voxel from each registered atlas and chooses the voxels receiving the most votes to produce the final label. In a probabilistic voting scheme, the labels mapped to the each voxel are combined to give an estimate of label likelihood (i.e., a value of 0 means that no labels were mapped to that voxel location, and a value of 1 for a voxel means that all labels were mapped to that voxel location). The probabilistic segmentation can then be thresholded at a particular probability (typically 0.5) to give a degree of confidence for the label location. A more elaborate approach assigns a weight to voxels that are located at a particular location (e.g., the center of a structure of interest) or which contain more similar intensities (both within the training image-labeled regions, or globally) [30, 54].

An alternate method to fusing labels which has been applied to prostate segmentation was proposed in the Selective and Iterative Method for Performance Level Estimation (SIMPLE) approach. In this method the labels to fuse are selected according to a similarity metric. The quality of the label segmentation is then improved by discarding the poorly correlated labels from the fused result. This process then iterates until a desired level of label similarity is achieved [55].

The Simultaneous Truth and Performance Level Estimation (STAPLE) is a popular approach which uses Expectation Maximization to iterate between the estimation of the "true" consensus segmentation and the estimation of reliability parameters for each of the propagated segmentations [56]. The sensitivity and specificity of each propagated label are used to weight the contributions when generating the consensus label estimate. The current consensus estimate can, in turn, be used to measure the reliability of the raters and this forms the basis of the EM iterations [25].

Experiments and Results

Average Atlas-Based Segmentation

This section describes the construction and application of an average atlas to perform segmentation using a single template. The work in this section was motivated by the importance of applying spatial specific predictive models for toxicity [17].

Data and Methods

The study consisted of 19 patients who were receiving EBRT for prostate cancer. Each patient underwent a planning CT scan and 8 more weekly CT scans. All CT scans were acquired without contrast enhancement. The size of the images in the axial plane was 512×512 pixels with 1 mm resolution 3-mm thick slices. For each patient, the femur, the bladder, the rectum, the prostate, and the seminal vesicles (SV) were manually contoured by the same observer of these organs for each case using the obtained affine transform and deformation field previously computed.

An arbitrary but representative case in our database was selected as the initial atlas, defining the atlas space alignment. A pipeline as detailed in Fig. 9 was applied to generate an average template. The first iteration involved the registration of every other case to the selected individual case using a robust block matching approach [50], followed by a diffeomorphic demons nonrigid registration [37] in the subsequent iterations. At the end of each iteration, a new average atlas was generated and used in the subsequent iteration. In this study, five iterations were performed.

After generation of the probabilistic labels (Prostate, rectum, bladder) in the common space, the atlas was used in a segmentation step to constrain the organs of interest. Thus, a scheme based on affine, followed by a diffeomorphic Demons nonrigid registration, led us to map the atlas onto each individual's CT scan. The obtained affine transform and deformation fields were then used to map the probabilistic labels onto each individual scan. These registered labels were thresholded at 50 % to provide the organ segmentations for each individual scan.

Results

The generated atlas and an example of probabilistic label are shown in Fig. 13. Figure 14 depicts the overlap between the atlas and a single individual. The nonrigid registration scheme obtains good correspondence between the two images, although the soft tissue contrast is still quite low. Notably the bladder and rectum alignment is better with the template than the prostate, as the intensity contrast in those organs is higher. The automatic hard segmentations were quantitatively compared against the manual segmentations using the Dice Similarity Coefficient (DSC) [57]:

$$DSC = \frac{2|X \cap Y|}{|X| + |Y|} \tag{10}$$

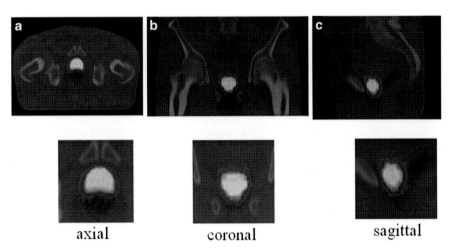

axial   coronal   sagittal

Fig. 13 Prostate probability maps overlaid on the generated average atlas orthogonal axial (**a**), coronal (**b**) and sagittal (**c**) views

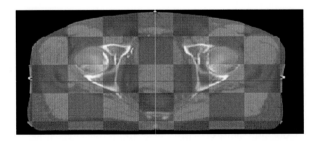

Fig. 14 Axial slice showing registration result between the atlas and a single individual

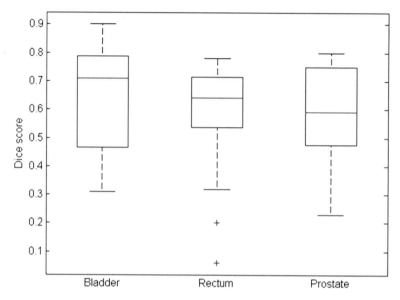

Fig. 15 Results from leave-one-out validation using the average atlas. DSC results are displayed for all labeled organs (bladder, rectum, and prostate)

A leave-one-out cross-validation was performed (at each iteration a single individual was extracted from the training data and used as a test). The DSC results appear summarized in Fig. 15.

In general a good agreement was obtained with this approach. The main cause of error in the automatic segmentation results is related to interindividual organ variation. Obesity appears to be a source of error, as it induces a quite important variability to the training data set. We must also consider the high inter-observer variability which also creates bias in the obtained results. This could be alleviated with the contribution of additional subjects to the atlas or with the computation of a set of atlases to stratify subjects. This will allow to group portions of the populations that can be further mapped together into a single template.

Discussion

The automatic segmentation of the prostate, rectum, bladder from CT images using a probability atlas scheme had reasonable correspondence with the manual segmentation and may provide useful initial constraints for further segmentation methods, such as active contours or statistical models (e.g., [58, 59]). However, these examples point out the main concerns of a single average atlas. The contrast is very low, there is a large interindividual variability, and considered structures are heterogeneous leading in several cases to low DSC scores.

Several problems appear when a single patient scan is used as the initial target for average atlas construction since the atlas is biased towards that patient's anatomy. It is expected that further improvement is brought by the selection and combination of several scans which are more similar to the query image as explained in the next section.

Evaluation of Multi-Atlas-Based Segmentation

In this section, we evaluated several multi-atlas-based strategies, as an extension of [51], taking into account the different stages of the pipeline depicted in Fig. 12. (i) Selection of the atlases based on three different metrics: SSD, cross-correlation, and mutual information; (ii) nonrigid registration using both FFD and the demon's algorithm with multi-atlas label propagation; (iii) multi-label decision fusion using classical voting rule compared to the STAPLE method [56]. Figure 16 summarizes the considered methods.

Data and Methods

The images used in this experiment consisted of 30 patients treated for prostate cancer, who underwent a planning CT scan. All CT scans acquired were 2-mm slice thickness with 512×512 pixels of 1 mm in the axial plane. For each patient, the organs were manually contoured by the same expert observer, following the clinical protocol for the therapy. In this study, only the segmented prostate, bladder, and rectum were considered.

Following a leave-one-out cross-validation scheme we assessed the impact of the atlas selection methods by comparing individual's manual segmentations with the obtained hard segmentations using the DSC. Thus, at each iteration a single individual was extracted from the training data and used as a test. The comparisons were done in two steps: first after affine alignment, aimed at quantifying the reliability of the similarity criteria; then, as depicted in Fig. 16, the set of atlas was ranked according to a given similarity criteria and the ith-ranked atlases were considered. This atlas was used to segment the query image via two nonrigid registration strategies (FFD and Demons) that were compared. In a further experiment, a multiple atlas strategy allowed for two label fusion methods (VOTE and STAPLE) to be compared.

Selecting Only the *i*th-Ranked Atlas

For each template, the registered individuals were ranked according to the similarity criteria computed on the masks of the union of the prostates, the union of the bladders, and the unions of the rectums after a rigid registration. Then we computed the average dice score for only the *i*th-top-ranked individual (with $i = 1 \ldots 30$). Finally, Pearson score (R) was computed between the rank and the average dice score with the aim of assessing the best similarity metric able to predict the best template from a database.

Increasing the Number of Ranked Atlas. Selection of the Best n-Ranked Atlas

In an additional experiment, we assessed the effect of the number of atlases selected after ranking, by progressively including a new atlas to the segmentation step. The two schemes of decision rule were tested, voting and STAPLE, and two nonrigid registration strategies were compared (FFD and Demons) as depicted in Fig. 20.

Results

We first computed the average DSC when using only the *i*th-ranked atlas to segment, where *i* spans 1 to 29. Figure 16 depicts for a single individual an example of overlapping between top-ranked and bottom-ranked atlases and a single individual. A significant difference between propagated structures appears depending on the atlas used to segment. In average, the SSD seems to be a better predictor of overlapping for the prostate and the rectum. The results of correlations between ranking and DSC for three organs and similarity measures are summarized in Table 1. The largest dependency with the rank appears in the bladder when the CC is used. Indeed, this organ is very prone to deformations and exhibits a high interindividual variability that was better detected with the CC ($R = 0.76$) than with the SSD $R = 0.45$. Unlike these measures, the MI offers a poor agreement, therefore it was not considered in the following experiments. We are in a monomodality context, and MI would be supposed to work better for measuring similarities between multimodal images.

A significant improvement in the overlap was brought by the demons nonrigid registration. In average, for the prostate 23.2 % ($p < 0.0001$), for the rectum 24.8 % ($p < 0.0001$), and for the bladder 35.0 % ($p < 0.0001$). Further, with the demons algorithm the dependency on the selected *i*th-ranked atlas tends to become weaker, as shown by the correlation coefficients, which for some cases tends to be lower. This is due to the fact that the nonrigid registration is more accurate, which compensates for large differences between individuals. Consequently, the overlap was significantly improved when the lower-rank atlases were selected. The poor contrast

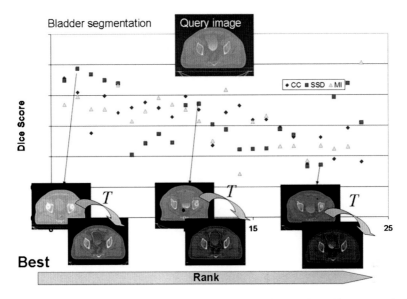

Fig. 16 *Top*: example of bladder segmentation with three different atlases (from top-ranked to bottom-ranked). The query individual is matched to the atlas data set via three similarity metrics: CC, SSD, and MI. The most similar atlas yields a better result

Table 1 Correlation (R) between the average Dice score and the rank of the atlas used to segment, firstly, after affine registration (AFF) and then after nonrigid registration (NRR)

Organ	Registration	MI	CC	SSD
Prostate	AFF	0.10	−0.53	−0.65
Bladder	AFF	0.27	−0.76	−0.45
Rectum	AFF	0.47	−0.56	−0.62
Prostate	NRR	0.38	−0.55	−0.63
Bladder	NRR	0.50	−0.72	−0.42
Rectum	NRR	0.60	−0.54	−0.67

between the prostate and bladder led in some cases to mis-registration problems when the images are quite dissimilar. The rectum, when not empty, was also poorly registered, although the results are still dependant on the rank of the selected atlas.

Increasing the Number of Ranked Atlases Within the Segmentation

Results of progressively increasing the number of atlas within the segmentation are depicted in Figs. 17 to 24. Firstly, a comparison between different registration strategies (rigid, FFD, Demons) are depicted (Figs. 17 to 20). In this case, the majority vote was used for label fusion because it yielded the best result to compare. It can be seen that as the number of atlas increases, there is a clear improvement

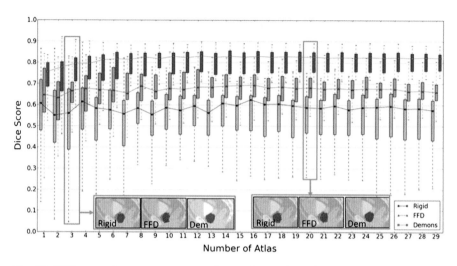

Fig. 17 DSC scores for prostate segmentation as the number atlases increased. Comparison between the different registration strategies

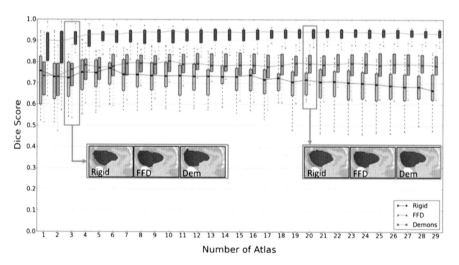

Fig. 18 DSC scores for bladder segmentation as the number atlases increased. Comparison between different registration strategies

when using demons. The same trend exists for the three obtained organ segmentations after the inclusion of 20 atlases shown in Fig. 20.

Figures 21, 22, 23 and 24 compare STAPLE to majority vote. In case of STAPLE, the trust given to each atlas was the same. It is shown that as the number of selected atlases increased, the performance of the segmentations was firstly improved in both cases. Then, after several atlases were included the quality

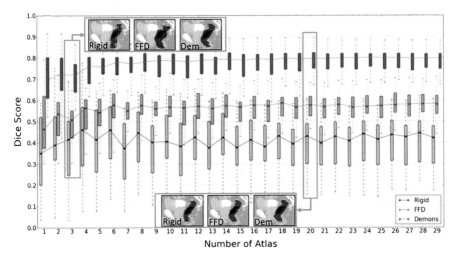

Fig. 19 DSC scores for rectum segmentation as the number of atlases increased. Comparison between different registration strategies

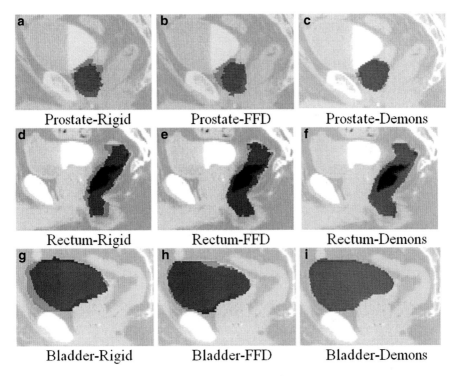

Fig. 20 Example of segmentations for prostate, rectum, and bladder, after including 20 atlases. Comparison between rigid, FFD, and demons registration. Label fusion with majority voting. *Blue* label is the ground truth, *red* is the obtained segmentation

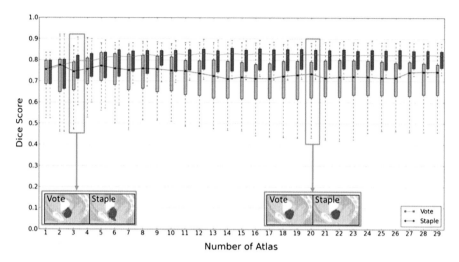

Fig. 21 Dice scores for prostate segmentation as a function of the number of best atlases used. Comparison between vote and STAPLE

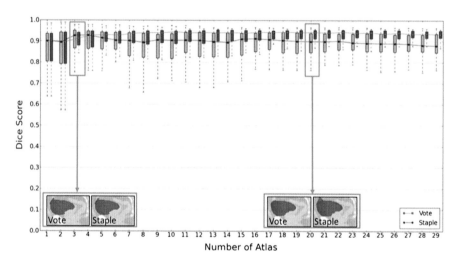

Fig. 22 Dice scores for bladder segmentation as a function of the number of best atlases used. Comparison between vote and STAPLE

tends to a stable value with a lower variance for the vote, unlike STAPLE, which exhibits a different behavior. Indeed for the three organs the quality of the segmentations steadily decreases for STAPLE. Results on these data suggest that the vote-decision rule is more robust to high interindividual variability. In average, for the prostate and the rectum the differences between both methods became statistically significant ($p < 0.0001$) after 12 top-ranked atlases were combined. For the bladder, these differences are significant ($p < 0.01$) after 23 atlases.

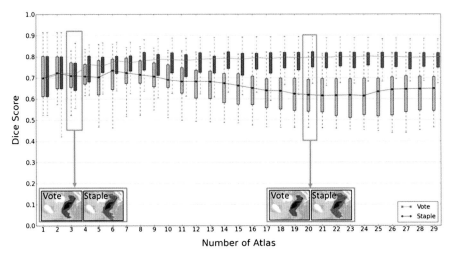

Fig. 23 Dice scores for rectum segmentation as a function of the number of best atlases used. Comparison between vote and STAPLE

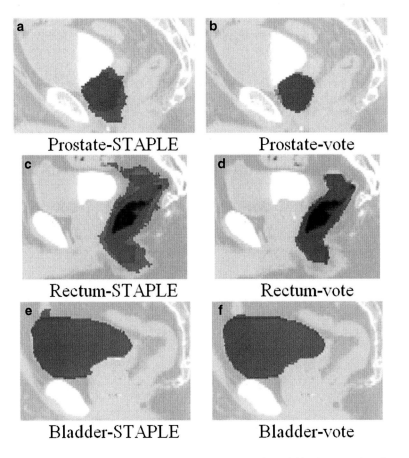

Fig. 24 Comparison between vote and STAPLE after inclusion of 20 atlases (registration was performed with demons)

Conclusion

We have presented a study aimed at evaluating different atlas selection strategies for segmentation of organs in pelvic CT for prostate cancer radiotherapy planning. We quantified the influence of multiple atlas selection based on three similarity measures and computed both the effects of the ranking according to these measures and the dependency on the number of atlases used. Results suggest that SSD is a better predictor for mapping than the MI and is slightly similar to the CC. Considering the fusion-decision rules the majority vote performed better than STAPLE. With the vote, combining more than one similar atlas may be more robust, but as the number of dissimilar atlases increased, the results tend to remain stable, at the expense of computation time. A good compromise would be to use the top 20 % ranked atlases. To increase the specificity of similarity measures as predictors for segmentation, more local similarity measures may be used, computed only in regions close to the considered organs or including other individual's characteristics, such as the patient weight. Another possibility relates to the inclusion of additional individuals within the atlas data base for query. Finally, different nonrigid registration methods can be validated within the same framework.

Summary

Atlas-based methods provide very useful tools for image analysis and generating automatic organ labels. This chapter has provided an overview of atlas-based analysis applied to planning images in EBRT treatment for the prostate.

All atlas-based approaches depend on the quality of image registration used. Careful decisions need to be made about the transformation model, similarity metric, and the optimization method used to deform a moving volume onto a target volume.

Two main types of atlas have been described. The first is an average atlas approach where a single average volume is generated from a training set along with a set of labels. This average atlas is then registered to a target volume, and the same transform or deformation is then applied to the atlas labels to provide automatic label, or segment, the target volume. A constraint with the average atlas approach is that atlas is biased towards the initial target patient selected during atlas construction and the atlas may not generalize to a wider population with different anatomy.

The second, multi-atlas, approach involves pair-wise registration between each volume in an atlas set and the target volume. Following this, the registered volumes and the target volume are compared and the transformed labels from the most similar registration results are combined (or fused) to provide an automatic segmentation. There are a number of methods to fuse labels; however, the most common method involves a simple voting approach.

A number of previous papers have suggested that when adequate patients are included in the atlas set, the multi-atlas approach has been found to lead to improved segmentation results. Experiments involving both types of atlas have been presented in this chapter, and the results have found that for CT monomodal atlas-based analysis the use of a multi-atlas approach with correlation or SSD is better suited to handle large inter-patient anatomical variations.

References

1. GLOBOCAN (2012) Prostate Cancer Incidence and Mortality Worldwide in 2008
2. Jemal A, Bray F, Center MM, Ferlay J, Ward E, Forman D (2011) Global cancer statistics. CA Cancer J Clin 61:69–90
3. INCa (2011) La situation du cancer en France en 2011-Rapport Institut National Du Cancer. INCa, rapport 14 Novembre 2011
4. AIHW (2007) Cancer in Australia: an overview. Australian Institute of Health and Welfare (AIHW) & Australasian Association of Cancer Registries (AACR) Cancer series no. 37
5. Grimsley SJS, Khan MH, Lennox E, Paterson PH (2007) Experience with the spanner prostatic stent in patients unfit for surgery: an observational study. J Endourol 21:1093–1096
6. Mangar SA, Huddart RA, Parker CC, Dearnaley DP, Khoo VS, Horwich A (2005) Technological advances in radiotherapy for the treatment of localised prostate cancer. Eur J Cancer 41:908–921
7. Guckenberger M, Flentje M (2007) Intensity-modulated radiotherapy (IMRT) of localized prostate cancer: a review and future perspectives. Strahlenther Onkol 183:57–62
8. Cheung P, Sixel K, Morton G, Loblaw DA, Tirona R, Pang G, Choo R, Szumacher E, Deboer G, Pignol JP (2005) Individualized planning target volumes for intrafraction motion during hypofractionated intensity-modulated radiotherapy boost for prostate cancer. Int J Radiat Oncol Biol Phys 62:418–425
9. Beckendorf V, Guerif S, Le Prise E, Cosset JM, Bougnoux A, Chauvet B, Salem N, Chapet O, Bourdain S, Bachaud JM, Maingon P, Hannoun-Levi JM, Malissard L, Simon JM, Pommier P, Hay M, Dubray B, Lagrange JL, Luporsi E, Bey P (2011) 70 Gy versus 80 Gy in localized prostate cancer: 5-year results of GETUG 06 randomized trial. Int J Radiat Oncol Biol Phys 80:1056–1063
10. Zietman AL, DeSilvio ML, Slater JD, Rossi CJ Jr, Miller DW, Adams JA, Shipley WU (2005) Comparison of conventional-dose vs high-dose conformal radiation therapy in clinically localized adenocarcinoma of the prostate: a randomized controlled trial. JAMA 294:1233–1239
11. Fonteyne V, Villeirs G, Speleers B, De Neve W, De Wagter C, Lumen N, De Meerleer G (2008) Intensity-modulated radiotherapy as primary therapy for prostate cancer: report on acute toxicity after dose escalation with simultaneous integrated boost to intraprostatic lesion. Int J Radiat Oncol Biol Phys 72:799–807
12. Fiorino C, Rancati T, Valdagni R (2009) Predictive models of toxicity in external radiotherapy: dosimetric issues. Cancer 115:3135–3140
13. de Crevoisier R, Fiorino C, Dubray B (2010) Dosimetric factors predictive of late toxicity in prostate cancer radiotherapy. Cancer Radiother 14:460–468
14. Njeh CF (2008) Tumor delineation: the weakest link in the search for accuracy in radiotherapy. J Med Phys 33:136–140
15. Cazoulat G, Lesaunier M, Simon A, Haigron P, Acosta O, Louvel G, Lafond C, Chajon E, Leseur J, de Crevoisier R (2011) From image-guided radiotherapy to dose-guided radiotherapy. Cancer Radiother 15:691–698

16. Chen T, Kim S, Zhou J, Metaxas D, Rajagopal G, Yue N (2009) 3D meshless prostate segmentation and registration in image guided radiotherapy. Med Image Comput Comput Assist Interv 12:43–50

17. Acosta O, Dowling J, Cazoulat G, Simon A, Salvado O, de Crevoisier R, Haigron P (2010) Atlas based segmentation and mapping of organs at risk from planning CT for the development of voxel-wise predictive models of toxicity in prostate radiotherapy. In: Presented at prostate cancer imaging. Computer-aided diagnosis, prognosis, and intervention, international workshop in MICCAI 2010

18. Collier DC, Burnett SS, Amin M, Bilton S, Brooks C, Ryan A, Roniger D, Tran D, Starkschall G (2003) Assessment of consistency in contouring of normal-tissue anatomic structures. J Appl Clin Med Phys 4:17–24

19. Fiorino C, Reni M, Bolognesi A, Cattaneo GM, Calandrino R (1998) Intra- and inter-observer variability in contouring prostate and seminal vesicles: implications for conformal treatment planning. Radiother Oncol 47:285–292

20. Gual-Arnau X, Ibanez-Gual MV, Lliso F, Roldan S (2005) Organ contouring for prostate cancer: interobserver and internal organ motion variability. Comput Med Imaging Graph 29:639–647

21. Fiorino C, Vavassori V, Sanguineti G, Bianchi C, Cattaneo GM, Piazzolla A, Cozzarini C (2002) Rectum contouring variability in patients treated for prostate cancer: impact on rectum dose-volume histograms and normal tissue complication probability. Radiother Oncol 63:249–255

22. Greer PB, Dowling JA, Lambert JA, Fripp J, Parker J, Denham JW, Wratten C, Capp A, Salvado O (2011) A magnetic resonance imaging-based workflow for planning radiation therapy for prostate cancer. Med J Aust 194:S24–S27

23. Dowling JA, Lambert J, Parker J, Salvado O, Fripp J, Capp A, Wratten C, Denham JW, Greer PB (2012) An atlas-based electron density mapping method for magnetic resonance imaging (MRI)-alone treatment planning and adaptive MRI-based prostate radiation therapy. Int J Radiat Oncol Biol Phys 83:e5–e11

24. Costa MJ, Delingette H, Novellas S, Ayache N (2007) Automatic segmentation of bladder and prostate using coupled 3D deformable models. Med Image Comput Comput Assist Interv 10:252–260

25. Aljabar P, Heckemann RAA, Hammers A, Hajnal JVV, Rueckert D (2009) Multi-atlas based segmentation of brain images: atlas selection and its effect on accuracy. Neuroimage 46:726–738

26. Wu M, Rosano C, Lopez-Garcia P, Carter CS, Aizenstein HJ (2007) Optimum template selection for atlas-based segmentation. Neuroimage 34:1612–1618

27. Han X, Hoogeman MS, Levendag PC, Hibbard LS, Teguh DN, Voet P, Cowen AC, Wolf TK (2008) Atlas-based auto-segmentation of head and neck CT images. Med Image Comput Comput Assist Interv 11:434–441

28. Commowick O, Gregoire V, Malandain G (2008) Atlas-based delineation of lymph node levels in head and neck computed tomography images. Radiother Oncol 87:281–289

29. Ramus L, Thariat J, Marcy PY, Pointreau Y, Bera G, Commowick O, Malandain G (2010) Automatic segmentation using atlases in head and neck cancers: methodology. Cancer Radiother 14:206–212

30. Isgum I, Staring M, Rutten A, Prokop M, Viergever MA, van Ginneken B (2009) Multi-atlas-based segmentation with local decision fusion—application to cardiac and aortic segmentation in CT scans. IEEE Trans Med Imaging 28:1000–1010

31. van Rikxoort EM, Prokop M, de Hoop B, Viergever MA, Pluim JP, van Ginneken B (2010) Automatic segmentation of pulmonary lobes robust against incomplete fissures. IEEE Trans Med Imaging 29:1286–1296

32. Sanda MG, Dunn RL, Michalski J, Sandler HM, Northouse L, Hembroff L, Lin X, Greenfield TK, Litwin MS, Saigal CS, Mahadevan A, Klein E, Kibel A, Pisters LL, Kuban D, Kaplan I,

Wood D, Ciezki J, Shah N, Wei JT (2008) Quality of life and satisfaction with outcome among prostate-cancer survivors. N Engl J Med 358:1250–1261

33. Dowling JA, Fripp J, Chandra S, Pluim JPW, Lambert J, Parker J, Denham J, Greer PB, Salvado O (2011) Fast automatic multi-atlas segmentation of the prostate from 3D MR images. Prost Cancer Imaging Image Anal Image Guid Interv 6963:10–21

34. Yoo TS (2004) Insight into images. A K Peters, Ltd, Wellesley

35. Rueckert D, Frangi AF, Schnabel JA (2003) Automatic construction of 3-D statistical deformation models of the brain using nonrigid registration. Med Imaging IEEE Trans 22:1014–1025

36. Davis BC, Foskey M, Rosenman J, Goyal L, Chang S, Joshi S (2005) Automatic segmentation of intra-treatment CT images for adaptive radiation therapy of the prostate. Med Image Comput Comput Assist Interv 8:442–450

37. Vercauteren T, Pennec X, Perchant A, Ayache N (2009) Diffeomorphic demons: efficient non-parametric image registration. Neuroimage 45:S61–S72

38. Tang CI, Loblaw DA, Cheung P, Holden L, Morton G, Basran PS, Tirona R, Cardoso M, Pang G, Gardner S, Cesta A (2008) Phase I/II study of a five-fraction hypofractionated accelerated radiotherapy treatment for low-risk localised prostate cancer: early results of pHART3. Clin Oncol (R Coll Radiol) 20:729–737

39. Studholme C, Hill DLG, Hawkes DJ (1999) An overlap invariant entropy measure of 3D medical image alignment. Pattern Recognit 32:71–86

40. Rubeaux M, Nunes J-C, Albera L, Garreau M (2010) Edgeworth-based approximation of mutual information for medical image registration. In: Presented at IPTA 10, international conference on image processing theory, tools and applications, Paris

41. Pluim JP, Maintz JB, Viergever MA (2003) Mutual-information-based registration of medical images: a survey. IEEE Trans Med Imaging 22:986–1004

42. Pluim JPW, Maintz JBA, Viergever MA (2000) Interpolation artefacts in mutual information-based image registration. Comput Vis Image Underst 77:211–232

43. Thevenaz P, Blu T, Unser M (2000) Interpolation revisited. IEEE Trans Med Imaging 19:739–758

44. King CR, Lehmann J, Adler JR, Hai J (2003) CyberKnife radiotherapy for localized prostate cancer: rationale and technical feasibility. Technol Cancer Res Treat 2:25–30

45. Parker J, Kenyon RV, Troxel DE (1983) Comparison of interpolating methods for image resampling. IEEE Trans Med Imaging 2:31–39

46. Grevera GJ, Udupa JK (1998) An objective comparison of 3-D image interpolation methods. IEEE Trans Med Imaging 17:642–652

47. Zitova B, Flusser J (2003) Image registration methods: a survey. Image Vis Comput 21:977–1000

48. Rohlfing T, Brandt R, Menzel R, Maurer CR (2004) Evaluation of atlas selection strategies for atlas-based image segmentation with application to confocol microscopy images of bee brains. Neuroimage 21:1428–1442

49. Rohlfing T, Brandt R, Maurer CR, Menzel R (2001) Bee brains, B-splines and computational democracy: Generating an average shape atlas. In: IEEE workshop on mathematical methods in biomedical image analysis, proceedings, pp 187–194

50. Dowling J, Fripp J, Freer P, Ourselin S, Salvado O (2009) Automatic atlas-based segmentation of the prostate: a MICCAI 2009 Prostate Segmentation Challenge entry. In: Worskhop in Med Image Comput Comput Assist Interv, pp 17–24

51. Acosta O, Simon A, Monge F, Commandeur F, Bassirou C, Cazoulat G, de Crevoisier R, Haigron P (2011) Evaluation of multi-atlas-based segmentation of CT scans in prostate cancer radiotherapy. Biomedical Imaging: From Nano to Macro, 2011 IEEE International Symposium on, vol., no., pp.1966,1969, March 30 2011–April 2 2011. doi: 10.1109/ISBI.2011.5872795

52. Commowick O, Malandain G (2007) Efficient selection of the most similar image in a database for critical structures segmentation. In: Ayache N, Ourselin S, Maeder A (eds) Medical image

computing and computer-assisted intervention MICCAI 2007, vol. 4792, lecture notes in computer science. Springer, Berlin, Heidelberg, pp 203–210

53. Roche A, Mériaux S, Keller M, Thirion B (2007) Mixed-effects statistics for group analysis in fMRI: a nonparametric maximum likelihood approach. Neuroimage 38:501–510

54. Artaechevarria X, Munoz-Barrutia A, Ortiz-de-Solorzano C (2009) Combination strategies in multi-atlas image segmentation: application to brain MR data. IEEE Trans Med Imaging 28:1266–1277

55. Langerak TR, van der Heide UA, Kotte ANTJ, Viergever MA, van Vulpen M, Pluim JPW (2010) Label fusion in atlas-based segmentation using a selective and iterative method for performance level estimation (SIMPLE). IEEE Trans Med Imaging 29:2000–2008

56. Warfield SK, Zou KH, Wells WM (2004) Simultaneous truth and performance level estimation (STAPLE): an algorithm for the validation of image segmentation. IEEE Trans Med Imaging 23:903–921

57. Dice LR (1945) Measures of the amount of ecologic association between species. Ecology 26:297–302

58. Chandra S, Dowling J, Shen K, Raniga P, Pluim J, Greer P, Salvado O, Fripp J (2012) Patient specific prostate segmentation in 3D magnetic resonance images. IEEE Trans Med Imaging 31:1955–1964

59. Martin S, Troccaz J, Daanenc V (2010) Automated segmentation of the prostate in 3D MR images using a probabilistic atlas and a spatially constrained deformable model. Med Phys 37:1579–1590

Biography

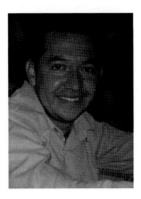

Oscar Acosta, Ph.D., is since 2010 an associate professor at the Signal and Image Processing Laboratory (LTSI—INSERM 1099), University of Rennes 1, France. He was awarded a Bachelors degree in Electrical Engineering in 1995 and subsequently a Master of Sciences degree in 1997 by the University of Andes in Bogotá, Colombia. In 2004 he received a Ph.D. degree in Signal Processing and Telecommunications from the University of Rennes 1, France, in 2004. Between 2005 and 2009 he worked as a research scientist for CSIRO in Australia. Based first at Westmead Hospital in Sydney (where he undertook the segmentation of pediatric CT images) and then at the Australian e-Health Research Centre in Brisbane where the focus of his research was in medical image processing for the study of Alzheimer's Disease as being part of the biomedical imaging team. Today, his main research activities are in image processing and computational methods for Prostate Cancer Radiotherapy in collaboration with the Centre Eugene Marquis for cancer treatment. Further details at http://blogperso.univ-rennes1.fr/oscar.acosta

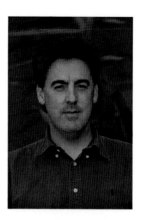

Jason Dowling, B.App.Sc. (Psych.,Comp.), B.Comp. (Hons I), Ph.D., is a research scientist and project leader at the Commonwealth Scientific and Industrial Research Organisation (CSIRO) in Australia. A major focus of his current work is the use of MRI in radiation oncology (focusing on MRI-alone treatment planning), particularly for prostate and cervical cancer radiation therapy treatment. This work involves automatic detection and segmentation of organs of interest and the development of methods to automatically assign electron density information from MRI (generating pseudo-CTs) for dose calculations (currently this is not possible as MRI scans lack the electron density information required to calculate radiation dose). Further details are available at http://www.ict.csiro.au/staff/jason.dowling/

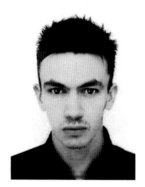

Gaël Dréan received his M.Sc. degree in 2010 in applied mathematics. After work experience in the genetic of algae and in astrophysics for the European GAIA mission, he began in 2010 his Ph.D. at the Laboratory of Signal and Image processing (LTSI, INSERM U1099) from the University of Rennes1. He is currently working on the building of 3D predictive models of toxicity in prostate cancer radiotherapy in the perspectives of treatment adaptation and patient-specific treatment. He also used to be a teaching assistant in financial mathematics.

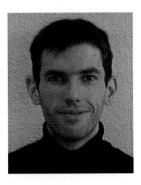

Antoine Simon received the Ph.D. degree in Signal Processing and Telecommunications from the University of Rennes 1, Rennes, France, in 2005. He is currently an Assistant Professor in the Laboratory of Signal and Image Processing, University of Rennes 1 and INSERM U-1099. His research interests include medical image processing and computer-aided medical interventions, with applications to Image-Guided and Adaptive Radiotherapy and to Cardiac Resynchronization Therapy.

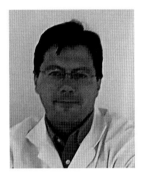

Renaud de Crevoisier (M.D., Ph.D.) is Professor at the University of Rennes 1 and radiation-oncologist at the Regional Cancer Center (CRLCC) Eugène Marquis, Rennes, France. His research and clinical activities are in the field of image-guided radiotherapy. He spent two years (2003–2005) as a researcher at MD Anderson Cancer Center (University of Texas, Houston, USA) and was the coordinator of large clinical randomized studies focused in IGRT/adaptive RT in France. He is currently co-responsible for the IMPACT research team at LTSI-Inserm U1099, Rennes, France.

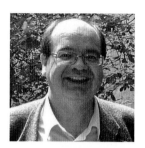

Pascal Haigron is Professor at the University of Rennes 1, Rennes, France. He is co-responsible for the IMPACT team (Images and Models for Planning and Assistan Ce to Therapy and surgery) at the LTSI-Inserm U1099. He received the Ph.D. in Signal Processing and Telecommunications, from the University of Rennes 1, France, in 1993. His experience is related to 3D shape reconstruction, virtual endoscopy, medical image registration, and image-guided therapy.

Propagating Segmentation of a Single Example to Similar Images: Differential Segmentation of the Prostate in 3-D MRI

Emmanouil Moschidis and James Graham

Abstract In this chapter, we address the online and real-time segmentation propagation from one example onto similar images. We consider segmentation as a process consisting of two stages: the localization of the anatomy of interest and its boundary delineation. For each stage, we identify and evaluate different potential candidate methods. All methods are assessed regarding their ability to tackle the differential segmentation of the prostate on a dataset of 22 three-dimensional magnetic resonance images of individuals with benign prostatic hyperplasia (BPH). The estimation of the volume of different anatomical zones of the prostate is important for monitoring the progress of the disease. Differential segmentation of the prostate is challenging due to contrast challenges at different locations from surrounding tissues. Also, the high variation of appearance of the prostate across individuals affects the repeatability of frameworks that leverage prior knowledge from one image example. Our observation is that the repeatability is improved, when a two-stage methodology is employed, based on DROP (deformable registration using discrete optimization) registration followed by graph cuts-based segmentation. Our methodology achieves automatically results close to the ground truth, which can serve as an advanced starting point of an interactive process with reduced human operator workload.

Introduction

The main objective of this study is to offer assistance in the context of an interactive framework for building models of three-dimensional (3-D) medical images. In such a framework, a human operator obtains by interaction the surfaces of the anatomy

E. Moschidis (✉) • J. Graham
Centre for Imaging Sciences, Institute of Population Health, The University of Manchester, Stopford Building, Oxford Road, Manchester M13 9PT, UK
e-mail: emmanouil.moschidis@manchester.ac.uk

A.S. El-Baz et al. (eds.), *Abdomen and Thoracic Imaging: An Engineering & Clinical Perspective*, DOI 10.1007/978-1-4614-8498-1_25,
© Springer Science+Business Media New York 2014

of interest, which will be subsequently modeled. These surfaces are extracted from images, which are similar to each other in the sense that they depict the same anatomy of interest and they are acquired by the same imaging modality using the same protocol.

While the extraction of the organ surfaces can be tackled interactively on each image separately, this approach results in an inefficient pipeline with increased workload. As segmentation advances, the number of processed images and therefore the knowledge about the anatomy of interest increases. If this insight is exploited, there is the potential for the design of a framework, which can reduce the amount of user intervention by predicting the segmentation of unseen images. The accuracy of the prediction with respect to the ground truth is associated with the reduction of the amount of intervention that is further required until the desired segmentation is obtained; an accurate prediction requires fewer interactive maneuvers than an inaccurate one. Consequently, the provision of an accurate segmentation prediction reduces the operator's workload.

In this chapter, we address the problem of minimizing the user interaction when similar images are processed, given a *single* previously segmented image as an example of the desired outcome. We tackle this by propagating the segmentation example onto the subsequently processed images. This way the user is freed from the entire process and may intervene only if necessary at a later refinement stage or in case the framework fails to provide satisfactory outcomes. Our main assumption is that the processed images do not exist as a dataset, but they rather appear one at a time (online), as often happens in real life. Therefore, groupwise approaches are not included in the evaluation. Also, since one single image cannot capture the variation of a population, we exclude model-based methods and we restrict our study to data-driven ones. We illustrate the approach using the example of differential segmentation of the prostate in fat-suppressed T2-weighted magnetic resonance (MR) images. The prostate is anatomically divided into several zones, but in MR images, two regions can be identified: the central gland and the peripheral zone. Figure 1 shows a schematic diagram of the relationship between these regions and examples of their appearance in MR images.

We consider segmentation as a process that consists of two distinct tasks: the localization/recognition of the anatomy of interest and its boundary delineation, as suggested in [2]. Consequently, we suggest a two-staged framework that handles these two tasks separately. For each stage we identify and evaluate potential candidate methods against ground truth. Our evaluation can be regarded as an assessment of the extent of the effectiveness of data-driven methods towards the solution of this particular problem.

The results of the experimental work presented in this chapter demonstrate that the suggested framework can provide results close to the ground truth, without any user interaction, serving as an advanced starting point of an interactive process with a small number of further interactive maneuvers. Moreover, we observe that the framework's repeatability improves when the segmentation task is tackled in two distinct stages. Parts of the work that is discussed in this chapter have also appeared in [3–5].

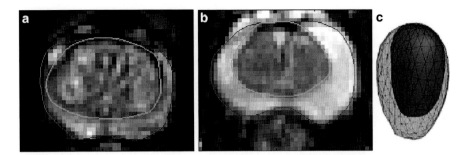

Fig. 1 Two axial midsections of the prostate of fat-suppressed T2 MRI from different individuals (the *red* and *green* contours delineate the peripheral zone and the central gland respectively) (**a, b**) and a three-dimensional schematic depiction of the anatomical zones of the prostate (**c**) [1] © 2006 IEEE

Background

Differential Segmentation of the Prostate

The prostate is a gland of the size and shape of a chestnut [6]. It exists only in men and is located immediately below the urinary bladder, where it surrounds a part of the urethra. Its function is the production of a slightly alkaline fluid (40 % of the volume of the semen), which assists towards the neutralization of the acidity of the vaginal tract, thus prolonging the sperm lifespan. In addition, it assists the motility of the sperm cells [6]. Benign prostatic hyperplasia (BPH) is a noncancerous enlargement of the prostate that affects 50 % of men over 60 years old [7]. Approximately a third of them will develop lower urinary tract symptoms, and a quarter of them will need to be operated. For the remaining BPH patients, drug treatment is increasingly utilized [7, 8].

The prostate is anatomically divided into the peripheral (PZ), central (CZ), transitional (TZ), and fibromuscular (FZ) zones. In BPH, the prostatic enlargement is mainly due to the volumetric increase in the TZ. Therefore, the estimation of the TZ volume and the TZ ratio (TZ volume/total prostate volume) is important for monitoring the progress of the disease and the effectiveness of drug treatments [8]. In MRI, two regions are identified: the PZ and the central gland (CG), which includes the other three anatomical zones (Fig. 1). However, in BPH, the TZ is the predominant zone in the CG, due to its expansion, and therefore TZ and CG can be considered as equivalent [1]. Differential segmentation—identifying the surfaces of both the CG and PZ—is challenging. The appearance of the central and peripheral glands varies significantly among individuals (Fig. 1). Furthermore, surrounding tissue (seminal vesicles, blood vessels, the urethra, and the bladder) present contrast challenges at different locations.

While a number of studies recently have addressed segmentation of the prostate in MR images [9–19], segmentation of separate zones has attracted rather less attention [3, 20–24]. These studies fall into two categories: those that employ algorithms trained on multiple image examples in an attempt to model in detail the morphology and shape of the different zones of the prostate and those that tackle the segmentation task interactively. Of the former group, Allen et al. [1] combine a 3-D point distribution model with a Gaussian mixture model, while others apply trained classifiers, such as an evidential C-means classifier in [20] and a Random Forest classifier used within a contextual Markov random field model in [21], or trainable graph-based models [22]. Litjens et al. [18] report that a trained linear discriminant classifier outperforms a multi-atlas approach. Interactive or semi-interactive methods [3, 24] base the segmentation on graphical representations. Given the difficulties in the segmentation task, we have taken the direction in this study of seeking to reduce the workload of interactive methods by leveraging the prior knowledge arising from a single previously segmented example.

Segmentation Propagation from One Image Example

As differential segmentation of the prostate is a challenging task, we assume that expert interaction will be required and investigate methods for minimizing the workload required to achieve a final segmentation. It can often be the case that images are acquired in a sequential (online) manner, rather than being available in a group. In this study we consider the use of a single example as a guide for further segmentations, reducing the level of intervention in subsequent cases. Forward propagation of the template segmentation results in an approximate segmentation for new cases. If this approximate segmentation is accurate, the interactive work-load required is correspondingly reduced.

One of the few studies of the literature, which addresses the same problem as we formulate it in this chapter, is the study of Cootes and Taylor in [25]. They adopt a shape representation based on finite element methods (FEMs) [26, 27] when prior knowledge is based on a single image example, whereas they employ an active shape model [28] strategy when multiple image examples are available. When only a single example is available, the allowable shape variation is expressed in terms of the vibrational modes of the FEM model. As further examples are added, this artificial representation of variability is replaced by observed statistical variability.

A single image example is also employed by Rother et al. [29] in a method they call *cosegmentation*. This denotes simultaneous segmentation of the common parts of a pair of images. In order to tackle this task, they employ an algorithm, which matches the appearance histograms of the common parts of the images. At the same time, the imposition of MRF-based spatial constrains guarantees the spatial coher-ence of the resulting segmented regions. Results are presented for applications such as video tracking and interactive cosegmentation. Similar ideas have been reported in [30–35]. Most of these methods aim at segmenting 2-D colored natural images.

Photographs generally demonstrate good contrast between foreground and background and, due to the variation in color, simple statistics such as color histograms can offer effective discrimination of segments (e.g., [29]). However, histogram-based classification has little to offer in the context of segmentation of greyscale medical images, especially in cases where foreground and background demonstrate similar intensity variations or in case of images with complex appearance.

Active Graph Cuts (AGC) [36] leverages previous segmentations to achieve convergence in a new image in a different way. AGC, when provided with an initial cut, constructs two disjoint subgraphs from the original graph. The initial cut defines the boundary of the two subgraphs. Subsequently, the max-flow/min-cut problem is solved on each of these two subgraphs separately. The combined solution from these subgraphs provides the overall segmentation outcome in the image. We consider and evaluate AGC in our work. To the best of our knowledge, it is the first time that this algorithm is implemented and evaluated independently with respect to its performance on 3-D medical image segmentation tasks.

Atlas-based segmentation is one additional segmentation approach in which often a single image example, termed the *atlas*, is employed as the prior knowledge about the anatomy of interest [37]. An atlas constitutes a complete description of the geometrical constraints and the neighborhood relationships of the anatomy of interest and is often created by manual segmentation of one image. The segmentation of subsequent images is obtained via registration of the processed image and the atlas. Registration constitutes a procedure, which establishes a point-to-point correspondence between two images [38]. When deformable registration is employed for achieving the dense correspondence of the two images, the atlas is deformed and its labels are mapped onto the processed image, also termed *reference image* or *target image*. This process is often referred to as *warping, fusion,* or *matching* [38].

One issue associated with frameworks leveraging prior knowledge is the effect of the latter on their performance. If the sample that encapsulates the prior knowledge is representative of the processed population, good results are obtained. However, in the case that it consists of one image, as in this study, the results decline drastically if this image is an outlier with respect to the population. This in turn reduces the framework's repeatability. This is an issue which has attracted considerable attention in the context of atlas-based segmentation [37]. Solutions towards this problem typically involve the combination of multiple atlases into a mean atlas or alternatively the selection of a single atlas that demonstrates a high degree of similarity with the processed image from a group of atlases. A more recent approach is the multi-atlas label fusion [37]. In the context of this strategy, the segmentation suggestions from multiple atlases onto the target image are utilized as individual classifiers, which are combined via a voting scheme. These approaches improve the repeatability of atlas-based methods. However, they all employ multiple atlases. In our study, we are restricted to utilize one single example as prior knowledge. Therefore, the repeatability issue remains.

In the work presented in this chapter, we follow an approach that is driven by registration, similarly to atlas-based segmentation. However, in order to improve its repeatability, we employ a two-staged strategy, as outlined above. Each of the stages, localization/recognition of the anatomy of interest and delineation of its boundary, is tackled separately. In the first stage, the localization task is tackled via registration; in the second stage, a semi-automatic refinement of the segmentation boundary is realized via graph cuts [39, 40]. We show that adopting this strategy improves the repeatability of the framework (in comparison to the single-stage processing approach) and the sensitivity to unhelpful templates is reduced. While we address this in the context of interactive segmentation, a similar conclusion applies in "automatic" atlas-based segmentation, especially on occasions where a single atlas is employed. In addition, for each stage of our approach we identify and evaluate potential candidate methods against ground truth. Therefore, our study can also serve as a comparative performance evaluation of registration and segmentation strategies. In the next sections, we will discuss further the different components of the suggested framework.

Methods

Figure 2 summarizes our segmentation strategy, its constituent stages, and the operations performed in each of these stages, illustrated here in two-dimensions for the sake of clarity. The segmented example consists of the raw image and a binary mask.

The registration (warping) stage is followed by boundary delineation using graph cuts. As we shall discuss further in the following sections, we employ graph cuts to operate on a zone, which is created via successive erosions and dilations of the warped binary mask produced by the framework's first stage. This operation aims at the refinement of the boundary of the anatomy of interest, in cases where registration has failed to provide an accurate segmentation boundary.

Dataset

We use a dataset consisting of 22 3-D T2 fat-suppressed MR images of the prostate from individuals with BPH. T2 fat-suppressed MRI provides good contrast not only between the prostate and its surrounding tissue but also between the prostatic anatomical zones. The images were acquired using a 1.5 T Philips Gyroscan ACS MR scanner. After their acquisition, all images were manually cropped close to the prostate (Fig. 3). The ground truth for each image is a binary volumetric mask produced after averaging the manual delineation of two radiologists on the cropped images. Prior to the experiments, the intensities of all images were normalized to lie in the bounded interval [0, 255]. Lastly, all images were resampled to allow for an iso-voxel resolution and volumes of equal sizes to be created.

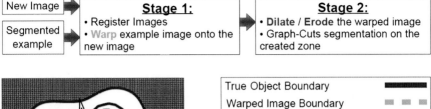

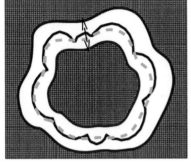
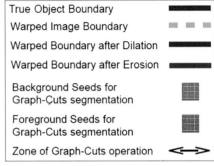

Fig. 2 Overview of the suggested framework

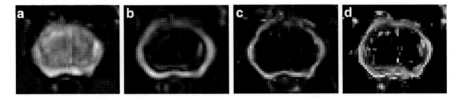

Fig. 3 An axial midsection of a T2 fat-suppressed image of the prostate (**a**), and the raw responses of a Canny (**b**), a Phase Congruency (**c**), and a SUSAN (**d**) feature detector. The settings of the parameters of each detector are outlined in the experiments section of this chapter

Localization of the Anatomy of Interest

The framework's first stage addresses the localization of the anatomy of interest. We evaluate four different registration methods and AGC. In the following paragraphs, we provide the necessary background information with respect to these techniques.

a. *Registration*

Registration is a process that establishes a point-to-point correspondence between two images. The images are considered to be identical, but one of them is treated as being corrupted by spatial distortions; therefore, they cannot be aligned in their current form. The two images are known as *target* and *floating* image. The terms *reference* or *fixed* and *template* or *moving* image respectively are also encountered in the literature [38, 41]. The aim of registration is to compute the exact geometrical transformation that the floating image needs to suffer, in order to match the target image. For a more comprehensive review of registration and its constituent components as a framework, readers can refer to the relevant literature (e.g., [38, 41, 42]).

In the context of our framework, the example image plays the role of the template image (Fig. 2). The registration scheme computes the spatial transformation, which best aligns this image to the image to be segmented, denoted as New Image in Fig. 2. Subsequently, the spatial transformation is applied to the template image's binary mask. The deformed (warped) binary mask constitutes the segmentation suggestion of the framework's first stage. It also represents the prior knowledge with respect to the segmentation outcome, in the new image's coordinate system.

The registration methods that we assess are the B-Spline-based registration method of Rueckert et al. which employs nonrigid free-form deformations [43]; Thirion's demons registration method [44]; the deformable registration method of Glocker et al. [45], which employs MRFs and discrete optimization [46]; and the groupwise registration method of Cootes et al. [47], utilized here in a pair-wise fashion. The implementations of Kroon and Slump [48] were used for the first two registration methods, whereas the authors' implementations were provided for the latter two methods. In the next paragraphs, we highlight briefly the main components of these registration methods.

The B-Spline method of Rueckert et al. [43] employs a hierarchical transformation model, which combines global and local motion of the anatomy of interest. Global motion is described by an affine transformation, whereas local motion is described by a free-form deformation, which is based on cubic B-Splines. The overall transformation is performed within a multi-resolution setting, which reduces the likelihood of occurrence of a deformation field with invalid topology due to folding of the control points (grid points). The similarity metric employed in this method is normalized mutual information, and the optimization component is based on a gradient descent approach [49].

The underlying concept of the original demons method [44] is that every voxel of the template image is displaced by a local force, which is applied by a demon. The demons of all voxels specify a deformation field, which describes fluidlike free-form deformations; when this field is applied to the template image, the latter deforms so that it matches the reference image. The algorithm operates in an iterative multi-resolution fashion for increased robustness and faster convergence. The original demons algorithm, as presented in [44], is data driven and demonstrates analogies with diffusion models and optical flow equations. Since its original conception, several variants have emerged in the literature [50]. In our study, we use and evaluate the implementation of Kroon and Slump [48], which employs a variant suggested by Vercauteren et al. in [51]. In this variant, the authors follow an optimization approach to demons image registration; more specifically, they employ a gradient descent minimization scheme and operate over a given space of diffeomorphic spatial transformations. Diffeomorphic transformations can be inverted, which is often desirable in image registration. Lastly, Kroon and Slump employ the joint histogram peaks as the similarity metric of their implementation, which allows for the computation of local image statistics [48].

The registration method of Glocker et al. [45], denoted as DROP (deformable image registration using discrete optimization), follows a discrete approach to deformable image registration. Similarly to the method of Ruckert et al., local motion of the anatomy of interest is modeled by cubic B-Splines. The difference, however, is that image registration is reformulated as a discrete multi-labeling problem and modeled via discrete MRFs. In addition, their optimization scheme is based on a primal-dual algorithm, which circumvents the computation of the derivatives of the objective function [46, 52]. This is due to its discrete nature. In their approach, they also follow a multi-resolution strategy, which is based on a Gaussian pyramid with several levels. Moreover, diffeomorphic transformations are guaranteed through the restriction of the maximum displacement of the control points. The authors' implementation, which is available online [53], features a range of well-known similarity metrics. In this study, the sum of absolute differences was employed.

The registration method of Cootes et al. [47], denoted as GWR, belongs to the groupwise approaches to image registration. Groupwise registration methods aim to establish dense correspondence among a set of images [47], as opposed to pair-wise approaches. In the context of groupwise registration, every image in the set is registered to the mean image, which evolves as the overall process advances. Groupwise registration is often employed in the context of automatic building of shape and appearance models from a group of images, given few annotated examples (e.g., [54]). Conversely, models of shape and appearance can assist registration, when integrated in the process, by imposing certain topological constraints in the spatial deformations. As a result of this integration, Cootes et al. follow a model-fitting approach in their registration method; for each image that is registered to the reference (mean) image, the parameters of the mean texture model are estimated, so that the texture model fits the target image. The overall aim in the process is to minimize the residual errors of the mean texture model with respect to the images of the set. This is achieved via an information theoretic framework, which is based on the minimization of description length (MDL) principle, described in [55]. Piecewise affine transformations are employed for the spatial transformations, which guarantee invertibility of the deformation field. A simple elastic shape model is employed to impose shape constraints to the transformation. Similarly to the previous methods, the registration technique of Cootes et al. follows a multi-resolution approach [47]. In our work, we utilize this method in a pair-wise fashion. We achieve this by employing the reference image to play the role of the mean image. Consequently, the texture and shape model are derived from this single image.

b. *Active Graph Cuts*

AGC [36] exploits an approximate segmentation as initialization, in order to compute the optimal final segmentation outcome via max-flow/min-cut algorithms. The authors pose no restriction on the nature of images that this algorithm may process and they claim that convergence is achieved even when the approximate segmentation is very different from the desired one. In the context of our study, this approximate solution is provided by the surface of the segmented example image. While it does not perform registration, AGC does provide a method of propagating an initial segmentation and is a likely candidate method for the first stage of our framework. For the needs of our experimental work, we realized our own implementation of the method in MATLAB®. To the best of our knowledge, this is the first independent implementation and evaluation of this technique in the context of 3-D medical image segmentation. In the following paragraphs, we provide further details about the method.

AGC is a graph-based method; therefore, in the context of this technique, an image is represented as a graph. Its initialization, termed "initial cut", is a set of contiguous graph edges, which separates the overall graph into two subgraphs that form two independent flow networks. The vertices adjacent to the initial cut are connected to the source graph terminal. Their t-link weight is equal to the capacity of the adjacent graph edge, which is part of the initial cut. In order to solve the max-flow/min-cut problem, different algorithms may be employed. In [36], the authors suggest a preflow-push [56] approach to tackle this problem on the subgraphs. Preflow-push strategies operate locally and thus flood the network gradually. This in turn generates intermediate cuts as the algorithm progresses. However, in our work, we are rather interested in the final min-cut instead of the intermediate cuts. Therefore, we employ an implementation of a max-flow/min-cut algorithm [57], which follows the augmenting paths approach as described in [58]. The final segmentation outcome is provided by the aggregation of the solutions of the max-flow/min-cut problem on the two subgraphs.

The authors provide no instruction about the positioning of the sink graph terminal on the two subgraphs in [36]. In our work, we observed that different choices may significantly affect the segmentation outcome. For the sake of consistency, with respect to this problem, in all our experiments, the voxels at the image borders were connected to the sink graph terminal of the subgraph that lies outside the initial cut, whereas for the subgraph that is contained by the initial cut, the voxels at a fixed distance, using a distance transform, from the centroid of the initial cut were connected to the sink.

Delineation of the Anatomical Boundary

In the previous sections, we highlighted the candidate methods for the first stage of our framework: localization of the anatomy of interest in the "New Image" of Fig. 2. The second stage of our framework aims for the delineation of an accurate boundary of the anatomy of interest, given the output of the first stage as initialization.

In a previous study [57], we demonstrated that graph cuts segmentation [39, 40] offers significant advantages over several other methods in the context of interactive segmentation. In the work presented in this chapter, we employ graph cuts in a semi-automated fashion to refine the boundary of the anatomy of interest. As shown in Fig. 2, graph cuts (GC) operates in a zone that surrounds the initial boundary defined by successive erosions and dilations of the initial binary segmentation. Erosion and dilation are morphological operations, which result into contraction and expansion of a binary object respectively [59]. The width of the zone is controlled via a user-defined parameter and depends on the number of erosions and dilations performed on the segmented image example. This is the only interaction that takes place during delineation of the anatomy of interest.

For this stage of our framework, we employ GC with a modified objective function and assess its performance as a means of accurate boundary delineation against the original GC. More specifically, we modify the objective function's boundary term, in order to enable GC to couple with feature detectors. The concept of employing feature detectors to enhance the boundary localization ability of GC is recent. A similar approach to our work [4–6] is followed by Krčah et al. [60], who employ the Hessian matrix as means of increasing the contrast at the boundaries of bones in three-dimensional CT scans. However, the GC boundary term that they employ is not the same as the one that we suggest. In our work, we couple GC with three well-known edge detectors, namely, Canny [61], phase congruency [62], and SUSAN [63]. The three GC variants are denoted as GC + C, GC + PC, and GC + S, respectively. Subsequently, we evaluate the performance of these variants with respect to their ability to provide accurate delineation of the anatomy of interest, as part of our framework's second stage. In the following paragraphs, we provide further details about our modified boundary term and the boundary detectors that we apply.

a. *Coupling Graph Cuts with Feature Detectors*

In interactive GC segmentation [39, 40], an image is represented as a graph. The user selects voxels that belong to the interior and the exterior of the object of interest, referred to as foreground and background seeds, respectively. The optimal foreground/background boundary is then obtained via global minimization of a cost function with min-cut/max-flow algorithms (e.g., [58]). Such a function is usually formulated as

$$E(A) = \lambda \cdot R(A) + B(A) \tag{1}$$

where

$$R(A) = \sum_{p \in P} R_p(A_p) \tag{2}$$

$$B(A) = \sum_{\{p,q\} \in N} B_{\{p,q\}} \cdot \delta(A_p, A_q) \tag{3}$$

and

$$\delta\left(A_p, A_q\right) = \begin{cases} 1, & \text{if} \quad A_p \neq A_q \\ 0, & \text{otherwise} \end{cases} \tag{4}$$

$R(A)$ and $B(A)$ are the regional and boundary term of the energy function, respectively. The coefficient λ weighs the relative importance between the two terms. N contains all the unordered pairs of neighboring voxels and A is a binary vector, whose components A_p, A_q assign labels to pixels p and q in P, respectively, on a given 2-D or 3-D grid.

The regional term assesses how well the intensity of a pixel p fits a known model of the foreground or the background. These models are either known a priori or estimated by the user input, when this is sufficient. Otherwise, the regional term is weighted low relative to the boundary term or in practice $\lambda = 0$. This approach is followed in [39] as well as in this study. The boundary term encompasses the boundary properties of the configuration A, represented in the weighted graph. Each edge in this graph is usually assigned a high weight if the pixel intensity difference of its adjacent nodes is low and vice versa. The exact value of these weights is calculated with the following Gaussian function [40]:

$$B_{\{p,q\}} = K \cdot \frac{1}{\text{dist}(p, q)} \cdot \exp\frac{-\left(I_p - I_q\right)^2}{2\sigma^2} \tag{5}$$

where I_p and I_q are the intensities of two pixels p and q and $\text{dist}(p,q)$ the Euclidean distance between them. $\text{dist}(p,q)$ is set to 1 in case of equally spaced grids (iso-voxel volumes) when only the immediate neighbors are taken into account. Setting K to 1 leads to a Gaussian function with its peak equal to 1, which is useful for the normalization of the graph weights. σ therefore is the only free parameter, which controls the full width at half maximum of the Gaussian function.

In (5), the effect of the $\left|I_p - I_q\right|$ term is to position the min-cut at locations where neighboring voxels demonstrate high-intensity difference, which corresponds to peaks and valleys in the gradient image. This works well for images that demonstrate boundaries with good contrast between foreground and background. However, medical images are often noisy and often demonstrate weak contrast or textured boundaries which are further compromised by partial volume effects. In such challenging boundary conditions, the previous approach can face difficulties in localizing the boundary accurately. To address this problem, we suggest a modification in GC's boundary term, which allows the method to couple with feature detectors. The modified boundary term is described below.

Feature detectors typically produce a response (voxels with high grey-level intensity values) at image locations where, based on local image evidences, the likelihood for the presence of a salient feature is high. In order to allow GC to couple with feature detectors, we modify its weighting function as follows. As we wish the min-cut to occur at maxima (ridges) in the feature output, we replace the $\left|I_p - I_q\right|$ term in this function with $(R_p + R_q)/2$, where R_p and R_q is the response of the feature detector on pixel p and q, respectively. Consequently, we have the modified boundary term:

$$B_{\{p,q\}} = \exp - \left(\varepsilon \cdot \left(R_p + R_q \right)^2 \right) \tag{6}$$

where $\varepsilon = 1/8\sigma^2$. Similarly to σ in (5), ε controls the full width at half maximum of the peak of the Gaussian function. Within the following sections, we briefly describe the three well-known feature detectors that we use: Canny [61], phase congruency [62], and SUSAN [63]. Figure 3 also depicts the raw response of these feature detectors on an example T2 fat-suppressed image of the prostate.

b. *Canny Edge Detector*

The Canny edge detector was derived to be an "optimal" edge detector. Its implementation is straightforward in two and three dimensions due to the separability of the Gaussian filter, which is its main computational element [61]. The parameters of the Canny edge detector implementation are the size of the Gaussian filter and its standard deviation. Due to the fact that Canny is a gradient-based edge detector, the strength of its response at a certain image location depends on the magnitude of the gradient at this location.

c. *Feature Detection from Phase Congruency*

In [62], Kovesi employs the Fourier domain of an image to identify image features. His work is based on the local energy model, introduced by Morrone et al. [64] and Morrone and Owens [65], which suggests that humans perceive features at image locations that demonstrate maximal phase congruency in their Fourier components. Phase congruency can be calculated using log Gabor wavelets. A Gabor wavelet is a filter, which is constructed via the modulation of a Gaussian kernel function by a sinusoidal plane wave [66]. The computation of phase congruency is complex as it involves the use of multiple filters at different scales (wavelengths) and orientations. In addition, phase congruency is susceptible to noise. Therefore, a noise reduction strategy is routinely followed prior to its computation [62]. Also, due to the fact that image features are identified in the frequency domain, the strength of the phase congruency response, as a feature detector, does not depend on the gradient of the image. This is a major qualitative difference between feature detection based on phase congruency and gradient-based schemes, such as Canny detection. We computed phase congruency employing the code available from [67].

d. *The SUSAN Feature Detector*

SUSAN is an acronym, which stands for smallest univalue segment assimilating nucleus [63]. The SUSAN edge detection scheme employs a circular mask (sphere in 3-D), which is moved over the processed image. The advantage of circular masks is that they provide isotropic responses. The typical radius of the SUSAN mask is

3.4 voxels, which corresponds to a mask that covers an area of 37 pixels in 2-D and 179 voxels in 3-D. During edge detection, the nucleus of the mask is placed at each voxel of the image. Then, the brightness of each voxel within the mask is compared with the brightness of the nucleus. Those voxels that demonstrate similar brightness to the nucleus (within a user-specified tolerance) belong to the USAN area. The size of the USAN area plays an important role in this feature detection scheme. The USAN area reaches its maximum size when the mask is over image areas that demonstrate relatively uniform voxel intensity, whereas its size gets smaller when the mask approaches an edge or a corner. The SUSAN detector is devised to provide responses, when the USAN area is smaller than a predefined threshold and no response otherwise [63]. The SUSAN edge detection scheme does not need any noise reduction, it does not involve the computation of image derivatives, and it is computationally efficient. In our work, we implemented the SUSAN edge detector in MATLAB®.

Evaluation Framework

We assess the performance of our methodology with a score of classification accuracy (CA), the Tanimoto coefficient (Tc), and the maximum point to surface distance between the segmentation and the ground truth surface (MaxDist).

In order to calculate the CA metric, all the voxels are classified into true- and false-positives (TP, FP) and true- and false-negatives (TN, FN). The CA score is then defined as

$$CA\ (\%) = 100 \times \frac{|TP| + |TN|}{|TP| + |TN| + |FP| + |FN|}\ \% \tag{7}$$

The Tc score is computed as

$$Tc\ (\%) = 100 \times \frac{|TP|}{|TP| + |FP| + |FN|}\ \% \tag{8}$$

Finally, the MaxDist score is calculated via a 3-D distance transform. The distance is given in voxels, but since we use images with isotropic voxels, the results can be report in millimeters as well.

In the case of CA and Tc scores, accurate segmentation outcomes are represented by large values, whereas in case of the MaxDist score, accurate segmentation outcomes are represented by small values.

Experiments and Results

Localization of the Anatomy of Interest

This section concerns the performance evaluation of the four deformable registration methods discussed in the previous sections and AGC. These methods are employed to provide the localization of the anatomy of interest in a new unseen image, given a single image as an example with respect to the desired segmentation outcome. During the experiments, each image in every dataset was selected once as a template image and its ground truth surface was propagated to the remaining images of the same dataset with each of the assessed methods.

When propagation of the segmentation surface was performed via registration, for each pair of images, the spatial transformation was first computed, and then the template image's ground truth surface was warped onto the target image's space to produce the new segmentation outcome. When propagation of the segmentation surface was performed via AGC, a similar strategy was followed: each image's ground truth surface was set as the initial cut for the remaining images of each dataset, providing thus the required initialization for the AGC algorithm.

In these experiments, all registration methods were employed with their default settings. Figure 4 summarizes the results of the performance evaluation of the four registration methods and AGC. GWR provided results that demonstrated (in most cases) the best mean values of the three employed scores that quantify segmentation accuracy, with DROP providing comparable results. More specifically, GWR demonstrated mean values of the three performance scores of CA = 93.5 %, Tc = 69.6 %, and MaxDist = 5.5 mm for the total prostate segmentation task

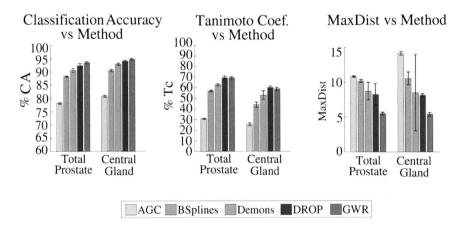

Fig. 4 Summary of the performance of the first stage's candidate methods with respect to the accuracy metrics. The error bars represent the $\pm 1.96 \times$ standard error of the mean

and CA = 94.8 %, Tc = 58.9 %, and MaxDist = 5.4 mm for the central prostatic gland segmentation task. DROP achieved mean values of the three scores of CA = 92.3 %, Tc = 69.6 %, and MaxDist = 8.3 mm for the total prostate segmentation task and CA = 94.1 %, Tc = 60.2 %, and MaxDist = 8.1 mm for the central prostatic gland segmentation task.

In terms of computational efficiency, DROP was by far the most computationally efficient method and GWR the most expensive. For instance, GWR required more than an hour to register two prostate images, whereas DROP performed the same task in few seconds. Computational efficiency is a favorable quality in the context of interactive segmentation systems. Therefore, DROP was adopted as the most appropriate method for our framework's first stage.

In our experiments, AGC consistently failed to produce plausible segmentation outcomes. This is quantitatively depicted in the results presented in Fig. 4. It is conceivable that segmentation of medical images is a challenging task for a max-flow/min-cut segmentation strategy, which is not provided with a good initialization. It is easier to understand this if we recall that AGC employs only the boundary term of a GC objective function. Therefore, in complex images, when wrong initial labeling is provided, the algorithm is susceptible to the detection of undesirable edges, thus providing erroneous segmentation outcomes.

Delineation of the Anatomical Boundary

In this section, we present the results of the evaluation of candidate methods for our framework's second stage, using different GC variants operating in a zone surrounding the boundary defined by the first stage. The voxels that lie within the eroded warped volume are selected as foreground seeds for the GC segmentation, whereas the voxels that lie outside the dilated warped volume are selected as background seeds (see Fig. 2). The zone width is a user-defined parameter that was kept constant for every dataset, to allow for unbiased experimental results. More specifically, this zone was 6 voxels wide (2 voxels outside and 4 voxels inside the boundary suggested by DROP) for segmentation of the prostatic central gland and 9 voxels wide (3 voxels outside and 6 voxels inside the DROP boundary) for the total prostate. We decided to create an asymmetric zone due to the frequent misplacement of the segmentation boundary by the registration stage outside the anatomy of interest. The width of the zone for the central gland is narrower than for the total prostate because this anatomical structure is relatively small. Consequently, a large number of erosions may leave no foreground seeds for GC to operate.

The following parameter settings were used throughout the experiments: when GC was employed with its original boundary term (5), σ was set equal to 1.5; in the case of our modified boundary term (6), ε was set equal to 0.02. The Canny edge detector used a Gaussian kernel of length 7, with standard deviation 0.7. In case of phase congruency, log Gabor filters with 6 different scales and 6 orientations were

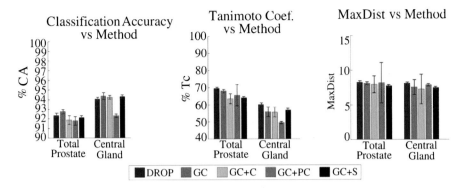

Fig. 5 Summary of the performance of the second stage's candidate methods with respect to the accuracy metrics. The error bars represent the $\pm 1.96 \times$ standard error of the mean

utilized. The minimum wavelength (smallest scale) was set to 5 voxels. Lastly, the SUSAN tolerance threshold was set to 24 (levels of grey). The output of all feature detectors was normalized to lie in the interval [0,255]. All parameters were set to these values via manual experimentation on few images.

The raw response of Canny and SUSAN edge detectors is readily computed in 3-D. However, the code employed for the computation of phase congruency in this study only tackles the task in 2-D. In order to produce an estimate of phase congruency in 3-D, the measure was computed along the three different anatomical planes, and the results were combined by selecting the maximum value from every plane for each voxel. Computation of phase congruency directly in 3-D is obviously preferred; however, such a task is nontrivial. For example, the orientations that need to be considered in 3-D are many more than in 2-D. Rajpoot et al. [68] suggest the use of the monogenic filter to tackle the computation of phase congruency in 3-D. However, when we experimented with their code, their approach produced noisier raw responses than the one we employed.

Figure 5 summarizes the results of the performance evaluation of the candidate methods for the second framework stage. The results of the DROP registration without further segmentation are also included, to allow for direct observation of the effect of the additional processing on the DROP outcome. Overall, the changes in segmentation performance with respect to accuracy due to it are small. The main effect is a slight reduction of the MaxDist error.

In the segmentation of the central gland, GC + S gave less variable results than GC. However, in the total prostate, the use of edge detectors did not seem to provide any advantage over the original GC, possibly due to the already good object/background contrast.

In the case of the central gland segmentation, the paired t-test suggests that there is no significant difference between the performances of GC + S and GC, when the accuracy is assessed with the CA metric. However, this test suggests that GC + S performs significantly better than GC ($p < 0.03$), when the Tc and MaxDist scores

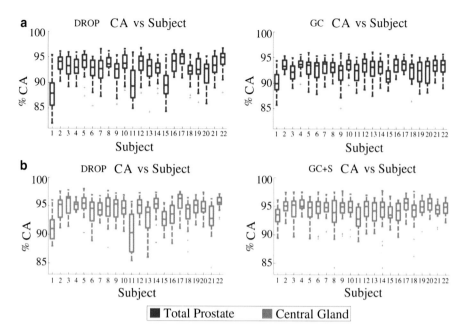

Fig. 6 Pairs of box and whisker plots depicting the repeatability of stage 1 (*left* image) and stage 2 (*right* image) for each segmentation task with respect to the CA score. The whiskers are 1.5 × the interquartile range. Values outside them are considered outliers (*red crosses*) [4] © 2011 IEEE

are used. The Wilcoxon signed-rank test [69] suggests that GC + S performs significantly better than GC ($p < 0.01$), in case of all the employed accuracy scores. The Wilcoxon signed-rank test does not assume that the compared samples are normally distributed. This statistical test may be more appropriate for our assessment, as there is no guarantee that our experimental measurements are normally distributed.

The major advantage of the additional processing step is the increase of the framework's repeatability, compared to the repeatability of the framework when we employ a single-stage processing approach based on DROP registration. Figures 6, 7, and 8 show the variation in segmentation accuracy as different examples are employed as templates, with and without application of the GC stage, using the CA, Tc, and MaxDist metrics, respectively. This improvement is clearest when the framework's performance is measured using the CA and MaxDist metric (Figs. 6 and 8). These figures suggest that in all datasets the second stage offers a reduction of the framework's dependency on the selected template. A qualitative example of the effect of the framework's second stage is also depicted in Fig. 9.

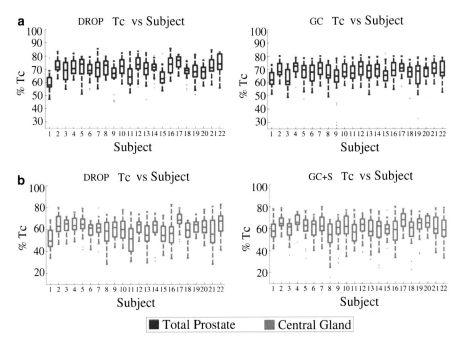

Fig. 7 Pairs of box and whisker plots depicting the repeatability of stage 1 (*left* image) and stage 2 (*right* image) for each segmentation task with respect to the Tc score. The whiskers are 1.5 × the interquartile range. Values outside them are considered outliers (*red crosses*)

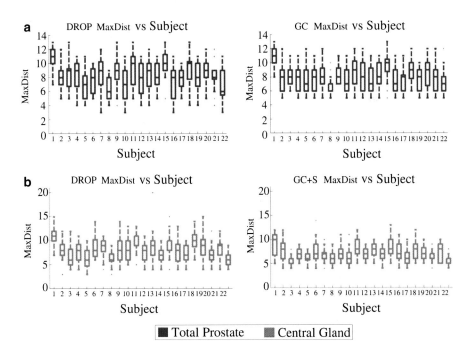

Fig. 8 Pairs of box and whisker plots depicting the repeatability of stage 1 (*left* image) and stage 2 (*right* image) for each segmentation task with respect to the MaxDist score. The whiskers are 1.5 × the interquartile range. Values outside them are considered outliers (*red crosses*)

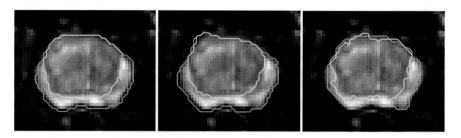

Fig. 9 An example of axial midsection of a prostate, depicting the ground truth (*left*), the segmentation outcome produced by DROP (*middle*), and GC initialized by DROP (*right*). The *yellow* and *cyan* contours delineate the central gland and the total prostate, respectively. The result of the GC+S variant is depicted for the segmentation of the central gland

Summary

In this chapter, we presented the results of a performance evaluation study of candidate methods for an interactive segmentation framework, which leverages prior knowledge from one single image example, in order to minimize the amount of required user intervention when similar images are processed. The suggested framework operates in two stages: localization (registration) followed by delineation (segmentation). The experimental results suggest that this framework can provide results close to the ground truth, without any user interaction, for a challenging segmentation task, when a deformable registration is followed by a graph cuts segmentation. These results can serve as an advanced starting point of an interactive process that can lead to the desired segmentation outcome with a small number of further interactive maneuvers.

Using segmentation of the central gland and total prostate in 3-D MR images as an example application, we show that one of the effects of the additional processing step is the decrease of the MaxDist error. While the CA and Tc scores give overall indications of agreement between the segmentation outcome and the ground truth, they are rather insensitive to local segmentation errors. The MaxDist score gives a handle on local segmentation problems, such as individual surface points being moved away from the true surface. Such cases can result in interactive workload, even if the overall CA and Tc scores are low.

In addition, while the second segmentation stage does not necessarily deliver large improvement over registration-based label propagation in individual cases, we have shown that a two-stage approach improves the framework's sensitivity to the selected template image. While we have addressed this in the context of interactive segmentation, the results of this study can be applied in "automatic" atlas-based segmentation as well, where a single image is often used as a template. Clearly, as online segmentation proceeds, knowledge from increasing numbers of segmented images can be used to inform the interactive process. Ultimately, with sufficient segmented examples, a model can be built. The phase where several segmented images are available, but not sufficient to build a reliable model is the subject of further development of this work.

In this chapter, we also suggest a modification of the GC boundary term, which allows the method to couple with feature detectors. In our experiments, we assess the performance of GC when coupled with three well-known feature detectors against the original GC approach. Our experimental results suggest that the use of feature detectors may not provide any advantage over the original GC, when images demonstrate good object/background contrast. It may, however, improve the boundary identification ability of GC in challenging cases, where information from gradient is insufficient for the identification of the boundary of the anatomy of interest, such as in the prostate central gland. In this study, we coupled GC with feature detectors that respond to grey-level boundaries. However, detectors that identify textured edges may also be employed with our modified boundary term.

References

1. Allen PD, Graham J, Williamson DC, Hutchinson C (2006) Differential segmentation of the prostate in MR images using combined 3D shape modeling and voxel classification. In: Proceedings of the 3rd IEEE international symposium on biomedical imaging, vol 1–3, pp 410–413
2. Udupa JK, LeBlanc VR, Zhuge Y, Imielinska C, Schmidt H, Currie LM, Hirsch BE, Woodburn J (2006) A framework for evaluating image segmentation algorithms. Comput Med Imaging Graph 30(2):75–87
3. Moschidis E, Graham J (2010) Interactive differential segmentation of the prostate using graph-cuts with a feature detector-based boundary term. In: Proceedings of the 14th annual conference on medical image understanding and analysis, pp 191–195
4. Moschidis E, Graham J (2011) Propagating interactive segmentation of a single 3-D example to similar images: an evaluation study using MR images of the prostate. In: Proceedings of the 8th IEEE international symposium on biomedical imaging: from nano to macro, pp 1472–1475
5. Moschidis E, Graham J (2011) Evaluation of a framework for on-line interactive segmentation of similar 3-D images based on a single example. In: Proceedings of the 15th annual conference on medical image understanding and analysis, pp 287–291
6. Graaff VD (2001) Human anatomy, 6th edn. The McGraw-Hill Companies, Boston
7. Thorpe A, Neal D (2003) Benign prostatic hyperplasia. Lancet 361(9366):1359–1367
8. Tewari A, Shinohara K, Narayan P (1995) Transitional zone volume and transitional zone ratio: predictor of uroflow response to finasteride therapy in benign prostatic hyperplasia patients. Urology 45(2):258–265
9. Birkbeck N, Zhang J, Requardt M, Kiefer B, Gall P, Zhou SK (2012) Region-specific hierarchical segmentation of MR prostate using discriminative learning. In: MICCAI PROMISE12 Challenge
10. Gao Q, Rueckert D, Edwards P (2012) An automatic multi-atlas based prostate segmentation using local appearance-specific atlases and patch-based voxel weighting. In: MICCAI PROMISE12 Challenge
11. Vincent G, Guillard G, Bowes M (2012) Fully automatic segmentation of the prostate using active appearance models. In: MICCAI PROMISE12 Challenge
12. Kirschner M, Jung F, Wesarg S (2012) Automatic prostate segmentation in MR images with a probabilistic active shape model. In: MICCAI PROMISE12 Challenge

13. Maan B, van der Heijden F (2012) Prostate MR image segmentation using 3D active appearance models. In: MICCAI PROMISE12 Challenge
14. Ghose S, Mitra J, Oliver A, Martí R, Lladó X, Freixenet J, Vilanova JC, Sidibé D, Meriaudeau F (2012) A stochastic approach to prostate segmentation in MRI. In: MICCAI PROMISE12 Challenge
15. Malmberg F, Strand R, Kullberg J, Nordenskjöld R, Bengtsson E (2012) Smart paint—a new interactive segmentation method applied to MR prostate segmentation. In: MICCAI PROMISE12 Challenge
16. Toth R, Madabhushi A (2012) Deformable landmark-free active appearance models: application to segmentation of multi-institutional prostate MRI data. In: MICCAI PROMISE12 Challenge
17. Yuan J, Qiu W, Ukwatta E, Rajchl M, Sun Y, Fenster A (2012) An efficient convex optimization approach to 3D prostate MRI segmentation with generic star shape prior. In: MICCAI PROMISE12 Challenge
18. Litjens G, Karssemeijer N, Huisman H (2012) A multi-atlas approach for prostate segmentation in MR images. In: MICCAI PROMISE12 Challenge
19. Ou Y, Doshi J, Erus G, Davatzikos C (2012) Multi-atlas segmentation of the prostate: a zooming process with robust registration and atlas selection. In: MICCAI PROMISE12 Challenge
20. Makni N, Iancu A, Colot O, Puech P, Mordon S, Betrouni N (2011) Zonal segmentation of prostate using multispectral magnetic resonance images. Med Phys 38(11):6093–6105
21. Moschidis E, Graham J (2012) Automatic differential segmentation of the prostate in 3-D MRI using random forest classification and graph-cuts optimization. In: Proceedings of the 9th IEEE international symposium on biomedical imaging: from nano to macro, pp 1727–1730
22. Yin Y, Fotin SV, Periaswamy S, Kunz J, Haldankar H, Muradyan N, Turkbey B, Choyke P (2012) Fully automated 3D prostate central gland segmentation in MR images: a LOGISMOS based approach. In: Proceedings of SPIE medical imaging: image processing, vol 8314, pp 1–9
23. Litjens G, Debats O, van de Ven W, Karssemeijer N, Huisman H (2012) A pattern recognition approach to zonal segmentation of the prostate on MRI. In: Proceedings of the 15th international conference on medical image computing and computer-assisted intervention, vol 15, pp 413–420
24. Egger J, Penzkofer T, Kapur T, Tempany C (2012) Prostate central gland segmentation using a spherical template driven graph approach. In: Proceedings of the 5th image guided therapy workshop
25. Cootes TF, Taylor CJ (1995) Combining point distribution models with shape models based on finite element analysis. Image Vis Comput 13(5):403–410
26. Pentland A, Sclarrof S (1991) Closed-form solutions for physically based shape modeling and recognition. IEEE Trans Pattern Anal Mach Intell 13(7):715–729
27. Sclarrof S, Pentland A (1995) Modal matching for correspondence and recognition. IEEE Trans Pattern Anal Mach Intell 17(6):545–561
28. Cootes TF, Taylor CJ, Cooper DH, Graham J (1995) Active shape models—their training and application. Comput Vis Image Underst 61(1):38–59
29. Rother C, Kolmogorov V, Minka T, Blake A (2006) Cosegmentation of image pairs by histogram matching—incorporating a global constraint into MRFs, In: Proceedings of the 19th IEEE computer society conference on computer vision and pattern recognition, pp 1–8
30. Cheng DS, Figueiredo MAT (2007) Cosegmentation for image sequences. In: Proceedings of the 14th IEEE international conference on image analysis and processing, pp 635–640
31. Boiman O, Irani M (2006) Similarity by composition. In: Proceedings of the 20th annual conference on neural information processing systems, pp 177–184
32. Bagon S, Boiman O, Irani M (2008) What is a good image segment? A unified approach to segment extraction. In: Proceedings of the 10th European conference on computer vision, vol 4, pp 30–44

33. Čech J, Matas J, Perdoch M (2010) Efficient sequential correspondence selection by cosegmentation. IEEE Trans Pattern Anal Mach Intell 32(9):1568–1581

34. Batra D, Kowdle A, Parikh D, Luo J, Chen T (2010) iCoseg: interactive co-segmentation with intelligent scribble guidance. In: Proceedings of the 23rd IEEE computer society conference on computer vision and pattern recognition, pp 3169–3176

35. Vicente S, Rother C, Kolmogorov V (2011) Object cosegmentation. In: Proceedings of the 24th IEEE computer society conference on computer vision and pattern recognition, pp 2217–2224

36. Juan O, Boykov Y (2006) Active graph cuts. In: Proceedings of the 19th IEEE computer society conference on computer vision and pattern recognition, vol 1, pp 1023–1029

37. Rohlfing T, Brandt R, Menzel R, Russako DB, Maurer CR Jr (2005) Quo vadis, atlas-based segmentation? In: Suri J, Wilson DL, Laxminarayan S (eds) The handbook of medical image analysis-volume III: registration models. Kluwer Academic/Plenum Publishers, New York, NY, pp 435–486, Ch. 11

38. Fisher B, Modersitzki J (2008) Ill-posed medicine—an introduction to image registration. Inverse Problems 24:1–16

39. Boykov Y, Jolly M-P (2000) Interactive organ segmentation using graph cuts. In: Proceedings of the 3rd international conference on medical image computing and computer assisted intervention, no. 1935, pp 276–286

40. Boykov Y, Jolly M-P (2001) Interactive graph cuts for optimal boundary and region segmentation of objects in N-D images. In: Proceedings of the 8th IEEE international conference on computer vision, vol 1, pp 105–112.

41. Yoo TS (2004) Insight into images: principles and practice for segmentation, registration, and image analysis. A. K. Peters Ltd, Wellesley, MA

42. Zitová B, Flusser J (2003) Image registration methods: a survey. Image Vis Comput 21(11): 977–1000

43. Rueckert D, Sonoda LI, Hayes C, Hill DL, Leach MO, Hawkes DJ (1999) Nonrigid registration using free-form deformations: application to breast images. IEEE Trans Med Imaging 18(8):712–721

44. Thirion JP (1998) Image matching as a diffusion process. Med Image Anal 2(3):243–260

45. Glocker B, Komodakis N, Tziritas G, Navab N, Paragios N (2008) Dense image registration through MRFs and efficient linear programming. Med Image Anal 12(6):731–741

46. Komodakis N, Tziritas G, Paragios N (2007) Fast approximately optimal solutions for single and dynamic MRFs. In: Proceedings of the 20th IEEE computer society conference on computer vision and pattern recognition, pp 1–8

47. Cootes TF, Twining CJ, Petrović VS, Babalola KO, Taylor CJ (2010) Computing accurate correspondences across groups of images. IEEE Trans Pattern Anal Mach Intell 32(11): 1994–2005

48. Kroon DJ, Slump CH (2009) MRI modality transformation in demon registration. In: Proceedings of the 6th IEEE international symposium on biomedical imaging, pp 963–966

49. Nocedal J, Wright SJ (2006) Numerical optimization, 2nd edn. Springer, New York

50. Gu X, Pan H, Liang Y, Castillo R, Yang D, Choi D, Castillo E, Majumdar A, Guerrero T, Jiang SB (2010) Implementation and evaluation of various demons deformable image registration algorithms on GPU. Phys Med Biol 55:207–219

51. Vercauteren T, Pennec X, Perchant A, Ayache N (2007) Non-parametric diffeomorphic image registration with the demons algorithm. In: Proceedings of the 10th international conference on medical image computing and computer assisted intervention, vol 4792, pp 319–326

52. Komodakis N, Tziritas G (2007) Approximate labeling via graph-cuts based on linear programming. IEEE Trans Pattern Anal Mach Intell 29(8):1436–1453

53. Glocker B (2012) "mrf-registration.net," [Online]. Available: http://www.mrf-registration.net/

54. Zhang P, Cootes TF (2012) Automatic construction of parts+geometry models for initializing groupwise registration. IEEE Trans Med Imaging 31(2):341–358

55. Twining CJ, Marsland S, Taylor CJ (2004) A unified information-theoretic approach to the correspondence problem in image registration. In: Proceedings of the 17th international conference on pattern recognition, vol 3, pp 704–709
56. Goldberg A, Tarjan R (1988) A new approach to the maximum-flow problem. J ACM 35(4): 921–940
57. Moschidis E, Graham J (2010) A systematic performance evaluation of interactive image segmentation methods based on simulated user interaction. In: Proceedings of the 7th IEEE international symposium on biomedical imaging: from nano to macro, pp 928–931
58. Boykov Y, Kolmogorov V (2004) An experimental comparison of min-cut/max-flow algorithms for energy minimization in vision. IEEE Trans Pattern Anal Mach Intell 26(9): 1124–1137
59. Sonka M, Hlavac V, Boyle R (2008) Image processing analysis and machine vision, 3rd edn. Thomson, Toronto
60. Krčah M, Székely G, Blanc R (2011) Fully automatic and fast segmentation of the femur bone from 3D-CT images with no shape prior. In: Proceedings of the 8th IEEE international symposium on biomedical imaging: from nano to macro, pp 2087–2090
61. Canny J (1986) A computational approach to edge detection. IEEE Trans Pattern Anal Mach Intell 8(6):679–698
62. Kovesi P (1999) Image features from phase congruency. Videre 1(3):1–27
63. Smith S, Brady MJ (1997) SUSAN-A new approach to low level image processing. Int J Comput Vis 23(1):45–78
64. Morrone M, Ross J, Burr D, Owens R (1986) Mach bands are phase dependent. Nature 324(6094):250–253
65. Morrone M, Owens R (1987) Feature detection from local energy. Pattern Recogn Lett 6:303–313
66. Lee TS (1996) Image representation using 2D Gabor wavelets. IEEE Trans Pattern Anal Mach Intell 18(10):959–971
67. Kovesi P (2012) MATLAB and octave functions for computer vision and image processing. [Online]. Available: http://www.csse.uwa.edu.au/~pk/research/matlabfns/
68. Rajpoot K, Grau V, Noble J (2009) Local-phase based 3D boundary detection using monogenic signal and its application to real-time 3-D echocardiography images. In: Proceedings of the 6th IEEE international symposium on biomedical imaging: from nano to macro, pp 783–786
69. Bland M (2000) An introduction to medical statistics, 3rd edn. Oxford University Press, Oxford

Biography

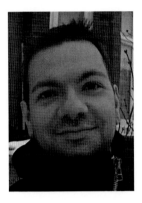

Dr. Emmanouil Moschidis received the B.Sc. degree in biomedical engineering from the Technological Educational Institute of Athens in 2005, the M.Sc. degree in biomedical engineering from the University of Lübeck in 2008, and the Ph.D. degree in medical image analysis from the University of Manchester in 2012. Since April 2012, he has worked as a research associate at the Institute of Population Health of the University of Manchester in the Centre for Imaging Sciences. His main research interests include image segmentation, image registration, and applications of pattern recognition, machine learning, and combinatorial optimization techniques in biomedical image analysis. Other interests include virtual and augmented reality in healthcare and medical decision support systems.

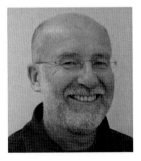

Dr. James Graham graduated in Physics from the University of Edinburgh in 1974. He obtained the Ph.D. in Structural Biology from the University of Cambridge in 1978. He has been active in Computer Vision and Biomedical Image Analysis for over 25 years. He is currently Reader in the Centre for Imaging Sciences at the University of Manchester.

3D Registration of Whole-Mount Prostate Histology Images to Ex Vivo Magnetic Resonance Images Using Strand-Shaped Fiducials

E. Gibson, M. Gaed, J.A. Gómez, M. Moussa, C. Romagnoli, S. Pautler, J.L. Chin, C. Crukley, G.S. Bauman, A. Fenster, and A.D. Ward

Abstract Determining the intra-prostatic spatial distribution and grade of prostate cancer before treatment may support improved diagnosis, therapy selection, or guidance of intra-prostatic lesion-focused therapies (e.g., radiation boosting or ablative focal therapy). Several in vivo imaging modalities are showing promise for imaging the intra-prostatic distribution of cancer. Evaluations of such imaging modalities ideally include comparisons to registered histological examinations of

E. Gibson (✉)
Biomedical Engineering Graduate Program, The University of Western Ontario,
London, ON, Canada

Robarts Research Institute, The University of Western Ontario, London, ON, Canada

M. Gaed • C. Crukley
Robarts Research Institute, The University of Western Ontario, London, ON, Canada

Lawson Health Research Institute, London, ON, Canada

J.A. Gómez • M. Moussa
Department of Pathology, The University of Western Ontario, London, ON, Canada

C. Romagnoli
Department of Medical Imaging, The University of Western Ontario, London, ON, Canada

S. Pautler
Lawson Health Research Institute, London, ON, Canada

Department of Surgery, The University of Western Ontario, London, ON, Canada

Department of Oncology, The University of Western Ontario, London, ON, Canada

J.L. Chin
Department of Surgery, The University of Western Ontario, London, ON, Canada

Department of Oncology, The University of Western Ontario, London, ON, Canada

G.S. Bauman
Lawson Health Research Institute, London, ON, Canada

Department of Oncology, The University of Western Ontario, London, ON, Canada

A.S. El-Baz et al. (eds.), *Abdomen and Thoracic Imaging: An Engineering
& Clinical Perspective*, DOI 10.1007/978-1-4614-8498-1_26,
© Springer Science+Business Media New York 2014

prostatectomy specimens, the clinically accepted "gold standard" for staging and grading prostate cancer. The registration of histology to ex vivo magnetic resonance (MR) images supports these challenging in vivo registrations by reconstructing 3D spatial information that is lost during the process of acquiring histology sections. In the work described in this chapter, ex vivo MR and histology images were acquired from nine formalin-fixed radical prostatectomy specimens which had been marked with extrinsic fiducials designed to be visible in these modalities. The histology images were registered retrospectively to the MR images using a novel algorithm based on the minimization of fiducial registration error between fiducial cross-sections on histology images and parametric fiducial curves on MR images. The 3D target registration error (TRE) was quantified based on the post-registration mis-alignment of manually identified homologous landmarks (3–7 per section, 184 in total), and was compared to two previously developed methods: (1) a method based on the guidance of the coarse slicing of specimens and (2) a method based on additional imaging of the images of the thick tissue slices. The proposed method yielded a mean $\pm$ standard deviation TRE of 0.71 ± 0.38 mm, 0.38–0.63 mm lower [95 % confidence interval (CI)] than the image-guided-slicing-based method, and within 0.13 mm (95 % CI) of the tissue-slice-imaging-based method. One component of the proposed method was able to refine the result from the image-guided-slicing-based method to within 0.13 mm (95 % CI) of the proposed method. The proposed method also resulted in a 70 % decrease in specimen processing time compared to the image-guided-slicing-based approach previously implemented at our center.

A. Fenster
Biomedical Engineering Graduate Program, The University of Western Ontario, London, ON, Canada

Robarts Research Institute, The University of Western Ontario, London, ON, Canada

Lawson Health Research Institute, London, ON, Canada

Department of Oncology, The University of Western Ontario, London, ON, Canada

Department of Medical Biophysics, The University of Western Ontario, London, ON, Canada

A.D. Ward
Biomedical Engineering Graduate Program, The University of Western Ontario, London, ON, Canada

Lawson Health Research Institute, London, ON, Canada

Department of Oncology, The University of Western Ontario, London, ON, Canada

Department of Medical Biophysics, The University of Western Ontario, London, ON, Canada

Introduction

The noninvasive determination of spatial distribution and grade of prostate cancer before treatment has the potential to support improved diagnosis, therapy selection, and focal therapy. For example, the accurate assessment of tumor grade and extent is required to support the decision to pursue active surveillance versus radical therapy. The current standard of systematic biopsies may fail to sample areas of cancer and/or the areas of highest cancer grade. Biopsies accurately targeted to the most suspicious lesions may increase the accuracy of diagnosis based on histological examination of biopsy tissue. Beyond biopsy, application of conformal treatments to intra-prostatic lesion (gross tumor) volumes with focused therapy (e.g., radiation boost or ablative focal therapy) requires precise tumor delineation before therapy. Monitoring of response to treatment or progression of cancer for men on active surveillance currently relies on prostate-specific antigen testing, an indirect assessment of tumor response. Noninvasive monitoring of intra-prostatic disease could augment decisions regarding treatment for these men. All of these clinical applications could be supported by imaging.

Many imaging modalities are showing promise for staging or grading prostate cancer in vivo, including single positron emission computed tomography using prostate-specific membrane antigen (PSMA) antibody-based tracers (Prostascint) [1, 2], positron emission tomography using choline-based tracers (e.g., ^{11}C-choline [3, 4] and ^{18}F-fluorocholine [5, 6]) and multi-parametric magnetic resonance (MR) imaging, comprising T2-weighted [7, 8], dynamic contrast enhanced [9, 10], diffusion-weighted [11, 12], and spectroscopic [13, 14] MR protocols. The evaluation of these imaging modalities ideally includes a comparison to tissue histopathology from prostatectomy specimens, the currently accepted clinical "gold standard." In the case of imaging of cancer distribution in the prostate, accurate registration of histopathology obtained from prostatectomy specimens with the in vivo imaging is required to assess the accuracy of the imaging in localizing and grading of intra-prostatic cancer foci.

Such imaging to histopathology registrations are challenging, in part, due to the processes involved in cutting histology sections from specimens for examination as part of current clinical protocols. For example, after radical prostatectomy, the prostate specimens are chemically fixed in formalin, causing tissue deformation and shrinkage. The fixed specimens are cut into 3–5-mm-thick slices, such that much of the spatial relationship between these pieces of tissue is lost. The slices are chemically treated to replace all water in the tissue with paraffin and are embedded in paraffin blocks, inducing further shrinkage. The paraffin blocks are mounted into a microtome cutting machine by hand, and oriented to align the front face of the tissue slice, seen through the translucent paraffin, with the microtome blade, introducing operator variability. Paraffin and tissue are sliced off the block until a full cross-section of tissue is visible (leaving as much tissue as possible in the paraffin block for medical records), and then a 4-μm-thick histology section is cut, resulting in a loss of 3D context and variability in the position and orientation within the tissue slice from which the histology section is taken. This section is unwrinkled and allowed to expand on a water bath before being mounted to a glass slide, potentially introducing further deformation. The deformation, loss of spatial information, and variability due to operators or processes, all present challenges to the registration of histology to in vivo images.

The techniques used to address these challenges fall into two major categories. *Prospective* techniques alter the processes involved in cutting histology sections from specimens to mitigate deformation, avoid loss of spatial information, or reduce variability. *Retrospective* techniques use assumptions about these processes and information (e.g., images or measurements) collected before, during, or after these processes to virtually undo the deformation, reconstruct lost spatial information, or account for variability. Many reconstruction methods use a combination of techniques from these two categories.

One common approach to the reconstruction of clinical specimens is to prospectively control the slicing of specimens into tissue slices [15–18], often using image guidance and specialized cutting devices to orient and position the cuts. These methods typically assume that histology sections are parallel and evenly spaced at a measured or pre-specified interval, an assumption usually supported by controlling the cutting of the initial tissue slices but undermined by the variability of the cutting process on the microtome [19]. An advantage of these approaches is that the position and orientation of the resulting histology can be pre-specified (to within the error of the image guidance and variability in the tissue slice and histology sectioning processes), allowing visual comparison of histological information from a single histology section with axis-aligned, rather than oblique, images. However, pre-specified tissue slice positions and orientations may not match those typically used in the standard pathology workflow and clinical reporting.

A second approach uses extrinsic fiducials and/or additional imaging to retrospectively reconstruct 3D spatial relationships of tissue sections lost during the histology acquisition, rather than prospectively constraining the spatial relationships. Extrinsic fiducials have been used to reorient histology images relative to one another [20, 21]. Additional imaging (typically photographs of tissue slices) has been used to account for tissue deformation [16, 22–25]. As in the guided-slicing approaches, these methods typically assume that histology sections are parallel and evenly spaced at a known interval, supported by prospectively controlling the cutting of tissue slices or retrospectively measuring them.

A third approach retrospectively reconstructs the spatial relationships between histology sections by registering histology images to 3D in vivo or ex vivo images of the intact prostate. Approaches that register directly to in vivo images hold the potential to reconstruct histology images with little disruption to the pathology workflow; however, they rely on the presence of intrinsic image information that may be disrupted by anatomic variability or even the disease processes of interest. Approaches that register to ex vivo images introduce some disruption to the pathology workflow due to additional imaging and have a similar reliance on intrinsic image information, but typically have more control over the imaging, allowing for images with a higher resolution and potentially more information in common with histology. Augmenting the intrinsic image information with extrinsic fiducials avoids the reliance on common image information (except for validation purposes), at the cost of additional disruption to the workflow to add the fiducials.

In the selection of appropriate methods for histology reconstruction, consideration of reconstruction accuracy is important. In the context of studies evaluating imaging modalities based on registration to 3D reconstructed histological information, reconstruction accuracy affects the studies' statistical power [26, 27] (i.e., the likelihood of the studies finding true statistically significant effects). Because of this effect, the use of a method with higher reconstruction error in a given study creates a requirement for a larger sample size, which can increase the effort needed for patient accrual, expose additional subjects to nonstandard-of-care tests and interventions and, given the high per-patient cost of imaging evaluation studies, substantially increase the cost of a study (see section "Comparison with Other Algorithms" in the discussion for an illustration). Thus, it is important to consider the comparison of registration accuracy amongst potential reconstruction methods for such studies.

Our institution has previously developed two approaches for histology registration. We first developed a prospective guided-slicing-based method [17] that used extrinsic strand-shaped fiducials internal to the prostate, ex vivo MR imaging, and time-consuming image guidance of a magnetically tracked stylus to mark the desired cutting plane with the goal of obtaining histology images along pre-specified planes corresponding to the in vivo imaging planes. To eliminate the need for magnetic tracking and image-guided slicing, we developed a second retrospective method [28] that used both internal and external fiducials, as well as additional ex vivo MR imaging of the tissue slices, yielding accurate registrations that accounted for the variability of microtome cutting and allowed the pathologist to slice specimens according to the standard pathology workflow.

The goal of the work described in this chapter was to evaluate a novel retrospective registration based on the optimization of correspondence errors of internal and external fiducials between histology and ex vivo imaging that did not use additional imaging of tissue slices (simplifying the process and reducing cost and processing time). We compared the accuracy of this method to our previously developed methods. In particular, the intent of the comparison to the image-guided-slicing-based method was to elucidate whether the image-guidance procedures were necessary for accurate registration, and the intent of the comparison to the tissue-slice-imaging-based approach was to elucidate whether the additional imaging contributed to increased registration accuracy. Because the use of internal fiducial markers may be prohibited in some centers, representing a barrier to translation, we also compared the proposed method to a variation that omitted internal fiducials. The intent of this comparison was to measure the loss of registration accuracy resulting from the elimination of internal fiducials from the registration workflow. Finally, in order to facilitate the acquisition of histology sections corresponding to pre-specified imaging planes (necessary to display corresponding histological information from an entire histology section alongside an imaging-axis-aligned in vivo image, and not possible with the proposed algorithm alone), we evaluated whether refining the results from our image-guided-slicing-based method using the optimization of fiducial correspondence errors in the proposed method would improve the accuracy of the image-guided-slicing-based method. This combination could potentially yield the accuracy of the registration-based method and the control of image-guided slicing. For these comparisons, we quantified the target registration error (TRE) of the registrations using homologous intrinsic landmarks identified on histology and MR images. These evaluations can be summarized by five questions answered by this work, enumerated as follows.

1. How accurate was the proposed method?
2. How did the accuracy of the proposed method compare to that of our previous image-guided-slicing-based method?
3. How did the accuracy of the proposed method compare to that of our previous tissue-slice-imaging-based method?
4. How did the use of internal fiducials impact registration accuracy?
5. Does applying fiducial correspondence error optimization to the image-guided-slicing-based method improve its accuracy?

This study was originally published in the Journal of Magnetic Resonance Imaging [29].

Materials and Imaging

As part of an ongoing prospective prostate imaging evaluation study, we obtained radical prostatectomy specimens from nine subjects. The inclusion criteria included: (1) aged 18 or older, (2) clinical stage T1 or T2 prostate cancer histologically confirmed on biopsy and (3) suitable for and consenting to radical prostatectomy. The exclusion criteria included: (1) prior therapy for prostate cancer, (2) use of 5-alpha reductase inhibitors within 6 months of the study start, (3) inability to comply with preoperative imaging, (4) allergy to contrast agents, (5) sickle cell or other anemias, (6) sources of artifact within the pelvis such as hip or penile prostheses, and (7) contraindications to MRI such as electronic implants, metal in the orbit or aneurysm clips. This study protocol was approved by the Human Subjects Research Ethics Board of our institution, and informed consent was given by all subjects.

Tissue Processing

An overview of the tissue processing for the study specimens is illustrated in Fig. 1. Prostate specimens were fixed in 10 % buffered formalin for 48 h immediately following surgery. Following fixation, extrinsic fiducials (described in detail in section "Fiducial Marking") were applied to the specimen, and the marked

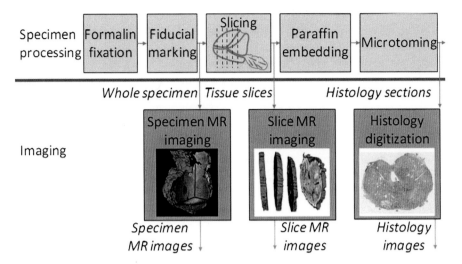

Fig. 1 An overview of the processing of the prostate specimens for histology and the imaging used in this study

specimen was imaged following the protocol described in section "Whole Specimen Ex Vivo MR Imaging." As in our hospital's standard prostate slicing protocol, the prostatic apex was removed and sliced parasagittally, the mid-gland was sliced into thick transverse slices, and the base was sliced parasagittally. Unlike our hospital's standard protocol, the orientation of the cut removing the apex was guided to coincide with in vivo imaging for another study [17], the mid-gland was embedded in agar prior to slicing, the mid-gland was sliced on a rotary cutter to yield parallel 4.4 ± 0.2-mm-thick slices, and in preparation for whole-mounting, the slices were not quartered. Only the mid-gland tissue slices were used for this study. The tissue slices were imaged following the protocol described in section "Tissue Slice MR Imaging." The tissue slices were decalcified and paraffin-processed following our hospital's large specimen processing schedule. Four-micrometer-thick whole-mount histology sections were cut from the resulting paraffin blocks and stained with hematoxylin and eosin (H&E). The resulting histology slides were digitized following the protocol described in section "Digital Histology Imaging."

Whole Specimen Ex Vivo MR Imaging

MR images of the intact prostate specimen (referred to as *specimen MR images* throughout this chapter) were acquired using a Discovery MR750 (GE Healthcare, Waukesha, WI, USA) at 3T using an endorectal coil (Prostate eCoil, Medrad, Inc., Warrendale, PA, USA). Specimens were positioned in approximately anatomical orientation in a sealed syringe, immersed in a fluorinated lubricant (Christo-Lube, Lubrication Technology Inc., Franklin Furnace, OH, USA) to reduce the proton signal surrounding the specimen and to eliminate artifacts. Specimens were imaged using two protocols: (1) a T1-weighted protocol used in the registration and accuracy evaluation that was sensitive to a gadolinium-based contrast agent in the extrinsic fiducials (3D SPGR, TR 6.5 ms, TE 2.5 ms, bandwidth ± 31.25 kHz, eight averages, field of view (FOV) 140 × 140 × 62 mm, slice thickness 0.4 mm, slice spacing 0.2 mm, 256 × 192 matrix, 312 slices, flip angle 15°, 25 min) and (2) a T2-weighted protocol used only in the accuracy evaluation that was sensitive to anatomical detail (3D FSE, TR 2,000 ms, TE 151.5 ms, bandwidth ± 125 kHz, three averages, FOV 140 × 140 × 62 mm, slice thickness 0.4 mm, slice spacing 0.2 mm, 320 × 192 matrix, 312 slices, 25 min).

Tissue Slice MR Imaging

MR images of the 4.4-mm-thick tissue slices (referred to as *tissue slice MR images* throughout this chapter) were also acquired. Tissue slices were immobilized with gauze in tissue-processing cassettes and immersed in Christo-Lube within a plastic bag. The tissue slices were imaged with the same MR scanner and coil as the specimen MR images, using the same MR protocols adjusted for a larger FOV to allow for spacing between slices and for the thickness of the cassettes.

Digital Histology Imaging

H&E-stained histology slides were digitized on a ScanScope GL (Aperio Technologies, Vista, CA, USA) bright field slide scanner at a 0.5 μm pixel size. These images were downsampled to yield images with a 0.03 mm pixel size (referred to as *histology images* throughout this chapter) for interactive fiducial and landmark localization (described in detail in sections "Fiducial Marking" and "Registration Accuracy").

Methods

Fiducial Marking

Prostate specimens were marked with two previously reported [17] types of strand-shaped fiducial markers designed to be visible on specimen MR and histology images: (1) external fiducial markers affixed to the surface of the specimen and (2) internal fiducials passed through the specimen. The strand shape of the markers

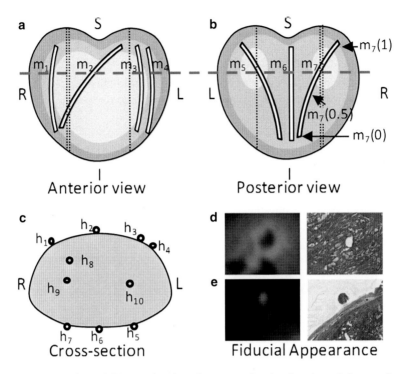

Fig. 2 An (**a**) anterior and (**b**) posterior view of a prostate showing the schematic layout of strand-shaped fiducials on the specimen, showing external fiducial curves m_1 through m_7, with internal fiducials m_8, m_9, and m_{10} shown as unlabeled *dotted lines*. (**c**) Cross-sectional view corresponding to *dashed line* in panels (**a**) and (**b**), showing fiducial cross-sections h_1 through h_{10}. (**d**) Internal and (**e**) external fiducials appearance on T1-weighted specimen MR and histology images

ensures the fiducials reliably intersect the thin histology planes. Fiducials were laid out as shown in Fig. 2. This layout was chosen such that the spatial configuration of fiducials intersecting with two different planes (i.e., two potential histology-specimen MR image alignments) could be distinguished under an affine transformation. Neighboring external fiducials, with the exception of fiducials 1 and 2 used to mark anterior left, were placed at approximately 45° angles relative to each other, so that the spatial configuration was sensitive to inferior–superior displacement and oblique orientation of the planes.

The external fiducials comprised cylinders of cortex tissue from lamb kidney ~30 mm in length and 1 mm in diameter (extracted using the cannula of a biopsy needle), soaked in a 1:40 solution of gadolinium-based contrast agent (Magnevist, Bayer AG, Germany) to 10 % buffered formalin. These fiducials were affixed to the surface of the specimen with a toughened, heat-resistant, ethyl cyanoacrylate glue (Loctite 411, Henkel Inc., Germany). The use of tissue as the fiducial material enabled the fiducials to adhere to the positively charged glass when the histology sections were mounted to slides, as tissue is typically negatively charged. Kidney cortex tissue in particular had material properties that were conducive to its use as a fiducial: (1) it was firm enough to stay intact through the physical and chemical processes of fiducial application and histology processing, (2) it was soft enough to avoid scoring the histology section when cut on a microtome, and (3) its appearance on histology images was distinct from that of prostate tissue, supporting fiducial localization. The gadolinium-based contrast agent enabled the fiducial to be visible on T1-weighted specimen MR images. The appearance of the external fiducials on T1-weighted specimen MR and histology images is shown in Fig. 2e.

The internal fiducials comprised cotton threads soaked in a 1:40 solution of gadolinium-based contrast agent to blue pathologist's ink (Tissue Marking Dye, Triangle Biomedical Sciences Inc., Durham, NC, USA). These threads were introduced through the specimen by passing a Quincke tip 18-gauge spinal cannula with stylet (BD Medical Inc., Franklin Lakes, NJ, USA) through the prostate, removing the stylet, passing the soaked cotton thread through the cannula, and removing the cannula, leaving the thread in place. The cotton thread was left in place during MR imaging and removed prior to tissue slicing. The gadolinium-based contrast agent and pathologist's tissue ink supported the visibility of the internal fiducials on the MR and histology images, respectively. The Quincke tip cannula has a bevel to one side that results in tissue being separated and moved laterally instead of being damaged. The appearance of the internal fiducials on T1-weighted specimen MR and histology images is shown in Fig. 2d.

The external and internal fiducials were interactively localized on the T1-weighted specimen MR images and histology images. On histology images, centers of the cross-sections of external and internal fiducials were manually selected in 3D Slicer (Surgical Planning Lab, Harvard Medical School, Boston, USA). On specimen MR images, the endpoints of the fiducials were manually selected in 3D Slicer, and the centerline of the entire fiducial strand was automatically computed using a fast-marching algorithm [30]. For some histology images, a subset of the fiducials were not visible, either due to an external fiducial being lost during processing or due to the histology section being taken from a plane past the endpoint of the fiducial. These histology sections were reconstructed using only the remaining visible fiducials.

Histology Registration

Each histology image was registered by minimizing the fiducial registration error (FRE) between the fiducial cross-sections on the histology image and the fiducial centerline on the corresponding specimen MR image over the space of affine transformations. Unlike minimizing the FRE of two sets of points over the affine transformations, minimizing the FRE between a set of points and a set of curves cannot be solved analytically. As this minimization may have local minima, and an exhaustive search of the nine-dimensional affine transformation space is computationally expensive, the minimization was instead performed using a three-step optimization: (1) identifying a plane in the specimen MR image for initialization using a discretized exhaustive search in a low-dimensional space, (2) computing a point-wise correspondence based on the identified plane between fiducial cross-sections on histology images and points along the fiducial strand on specimen MR images, and (3) optimizing the FRE iteratively in a high dimensional space. While steps 1 and 2 are closely linked, separating these two steps allows a more direct comparison to existing registration methods that can yield a slicing plane as an output. This algorithm is described formally in the following sections.

Reconstruction Algorithm Notation

The center point of the cross-section of the i-th fiducial on a histology image is denoted by the 2D point h_i (illustrated in Fig. 2c). The centerline of the i-th fiducial strand on a specimen MR image is denoted by the 3D parametric curve $m_i(s_i \in [0,1])$ (illustrated in Fig. 2a, b). Each point h_i corresponds to some point along $m_i(s_i \in [0,1])$, which can be uniquely defined by a particular value of s_i. Thus, we can describe all of the fiducial point correspondences as a correspondence vector $s = \langle s_1, s_2, \ldots, s_{10} \rangle$. For example, the correspondence vector $\langle 0.5, 0.5, 0.5, 0.5, 0.5, 0.5, 0.5, 0.5, 0.5, 0.6 \rangle$ would represent nine fiducials cross-sections on the histology image corresponding to the midpoints of the corresponding fiducial strands on the specimen MR image, and the tenth fiducial cross-section corresponding to a point 60 % along the length of the corresponding fiducial strand measured from the inferior-most endpoint.

The FRE after an affine transformation A was computed as

$$\text{FRE}(A) = \sum_{i=1}^{10} \|A h_i - C(A h_i, m_i)\|^2,$$

where $C(p,m)$ denotes the closest point on curve m to point p.

Correspondence vectors do not, in general, correspond to an affine transformation; however, each correspondence vector s defines a least squares best-fit affine transformation denoted A_s. In the iterative optimization, FRE is optimized over the space of correspondence vectors using the best-fit transformation

$$\text{FRE}(s) = \sum_{i=1}^{10} \|A_s h_i - C(A_s h_i, m_i)\|^2.$$

Reconstruction Algorithm Step 1: Plane Identification

An iterative minimization of FRE may converge to local minima. To mitigate this risk, we initialized the iterative minimization using the result of a discretized exhaustive search. Such a search in the nine-dimensional unbounded 2D–3D affine transformation space is not feasible. Instead, the search for an initialization was performed in a bounded three-dimensional space constrained to *reasonable* transformations, defined as the subspace of affine transformations that exactly align three fiducial cross-sections on a histology image to three points on the corresponding fiducial curves on the specimen MR image,

$$\widetilde{A} = \left\{ \left[\begin{matrix} m_{i_1}(s_{i_1}) & m_{i_2}(s_{i_2}) & m_{i_3}(s_{i_3}) \\ 1 & 1 & 1 \end{matrix} \right] \left[\begin{matrix} h_{i_1} & h_{i_2} & h_{i_3} \\ 1 & 1 & 1 \end{matrix} \right]^{+} \middle| \langle s_{i_1} s_{i_2} s_{i_3} \rangle \in [0,1]^3 \right\}$$

where i_1, i_2, and i_3 are the selected fiducial indices, and the operation M^+ denotes the matrix pseudoinverse. The minimization of FRE over this space was realized by exhaustively iterating over $\langle s_{i_1} s_{i_2} s_{i_3} \rangle$ at 0.01 intervals for the three curve parameters. The optimal curve parameters $\langle \check{s}_{i_1} \check{s}_{i_2} \check{s}_{i_3} \rangle$ define an initialization plane P through the points $m_{i_1}(\check{s}_{i_1})$, $m_{i_2}(\check{s}_{i_2})$, and $m_{i_3}(\check{s}_{i_3})$. This step is referred to as *plane identification* throughout this chapter.

The fiducial indices were selected to denote widely spaced fiducials including at least one diagonal fiducial. Fiducial indices 2, 4, and 7 (illustrated as m_2, m_4, and m_7 in Fig. 2a, b) were selected when all three were visible on the histology image; otherwise, fiducial indices were selected manually.

Reconstruction Algorithm Step 2: Correspondence Vector Identification

To initialize the iterative optimization, we computed the correspondence vector that represents the closest point to the initialization plane P for each fiducial curve. This step is referred to as *correspondence vector identification* throughout this chapter.

This approach was also used to compute correspondence vectors from planes generated by the alternative methods examined in this chapter, by computing the correspondence vector that represents the closest point to the plane from the alternative method for each fiducial curve. The generation of these planes is described in section "How Did the Accuracy of the Proposed Method Compare to That of Our Previous Image-Guided-Slicing-Based Method? (Question 2)" for the image-guided-slicing-based method and in section "How Did the Accuracy of the Proposed Method Compare to That of Our Previous Tissue-Slice-Imaging-Based Method? (Question 3)" for the tissue-slice-imaging-based method.

The initialization correspondence vector defines a least squares best-fit affine transformation that was used to assess the registration accuracy before iterative optimization.

Reconstruction Algorithm Step 3: Iterative Optimization

The iterative optimization of FRE was performed on the bounded ten-dimensional space of correspondence vectors, using a Nelder-Mead greedy simplex minimization, implemented as *fminsearch* in Matlab. The resulting correspondence vector defines a least squares best-fit affine transformation, taken as the result of the algorithm. This step is referred to as *iterative optimization* throughout this chapter.

Registration Accuracy

The registration error was measured using the post-registration 3D misalignment between pairs of homologous intrinsic point landmarks visible on histology and the specimen MR images. Landmarks were interactively localized in 2D on histology images and in 3D on the specimen MR image using 3D Slicer. Landmarks included corpora amylaceae, cysts, and atrophic ducts ~1 mm in diameter. The homology of the landmarks between histology and specimen MR images was determined based on spatial relationships with other salient image features close to the landmarks. Landmarks were identified by one observer (E.G.) under advisement from one radiologist (C.R.) and two genitourinary pathologists (M.M. and J.A.G.). An illustrative selection of landmarks is shown in Fig. 3.

The identification of homologous landmarks was supported by the use of tissue slice MR images. Because these images represent the same tissue as is imaged in specimen MR images, they could be virtually reassembled and aligned with the specimen MR image; this constrained the volume of the image to search for landmarks (after allowing for some tissue slice to specimen MR image misalignment) as histology sections were cut from a single tissue slice. Furthermore, because the Christo-Lube infiltrated cysts and ducts that were exposed on the cut faces of tissue slices and gave a signal void, many potential landmarks were emphasized on tissue slice MR images, supporting the identification of these same landmarks on specimen MR images.

The reconstruction error was measured based on the misalignment of homologous landmarks on histology and specimen MR images after registration. The misalignment vector for each landmark is denoted as TRE_j. Reconstruction error was quantified as the mean TRE, i.e., the mean magnitude of vectors TRE_j across 184 landmarks. The anisotropy of the reconstruction error was assessed by aggregating the vectors TRE_j under different reference frames and comparing the variances. First, the anisotropy with respect to the MR image coordinates was assessed by computing the variances along the principal components of the set of vectors $\{TRE_j | j \in 1..J\}$, which shared a common specimen MR-image-aligned reference frame; an isotropic error would be expected to yield three equal variances. Second, the anisotropy with respect to the histology image coordinates, which do not share a reference frame after registration, was assessed by decomposing each TRE_j into an out-of-plane component normal to the histology plane and an in-plane component parallel to the histology plane, computing the in-plane and out-of-plane variances. In this case, an isotropic error would yield an in-plane variance twice the out-of-plane variance because it can be considered as the sum of two 1-dimensional variances.

Because the measurement of TRE depends on the localization of landmarks which is subject to operator variability, the target localization error (TLE) was estimated for these landmarks on histology and specimen MR images. The TLE was quantified as an unbiased estimator of the standard deviation of repeated localizations of the same landmarks a day apart,

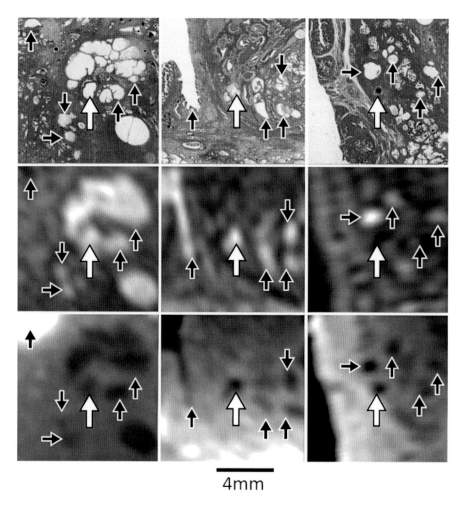

Fig. 3 Illustrative homologous landmarks (*white arrow*) used to measure the TRE. The homology of these landmarks was determined based on salient nearby features (*black arrows*), and were confirmed by a genitourinary pathologist (J.A.G.) and a radiologist specializing in prostate imaging (C.R.)

$$
\mathrm{TLE} = \sqrt{\frac{1}{J} \sum_{j=1}^{J} \frac{1}{K-1} \sum_{k=1}^{K} \left\| \mathbf{p}_{j,k} - \frac{1}{K} \sum_{k=1}^{K} \mathbf{p}_{j,k} \right\|^2},
$$

where $\mathbf{p}_{j,k}$ represents the k-th localization of the j-th landmark as a 2D (for histology images) or 3D (for specimen MR images) point, $K = 7$ repeated localizations and $J = 16$ landmarks.

Experiments

In this work, we characterized the registration accuracy of four approaches before and after iterative optimization. Based on these measurements, we addressed five key questions, as follows. (1) How accurate was the proposed method? (2) How did the accuracy of the proposed method compare to that of our previous image-guided-slicing-based method? (3) How did the accuracy of the proposed method compare to that of our previous tissue-slice-imaging-based method? (4) How did the use of internal fiducials impact registration accuracy? (5) Does applying fiducial correspondence error optimization to the image-guided-slicing-based method improve its accuracy?

How Accurate Was the Proposed Method? (Question 1)

To assess the reconstruction error of the proposed method, we computed the TRE after step 3 of the algorithm, and assessed the mean TRE and the anisotropy of the reconstruction error, as described in section "Registration Accuracy." Additionally, we assessed the robustness of the method by documenting the fiducial cross-sections that were absent on histology, and assessing the correlation of the number of remaining fiducials used in the registration with the TRE.

How Did the Accuracy of the Proposed Method Compare to That of Our Previous Image-Guided-Slicing-Based Method? (Question 2)

Our previously developed image-guided-slicing-based method yielded histology to MR image registrations, but involved complicated and time-consuming image guidance. To assess whether the image guidance was necessary for the registration, or whether the proposed method could achieve more accurate registrations using the same fiducials and imaging as our previous image-guided-slicing-based method, we compared the proposed method to the image-guided-slicing-based approach. Because the specimens in this study had been sliced using the image-guided-slicing-based approach [17], we were able to directly compare our retrospective reconstruction to this previous prospective approach. Although the previous approach selected the slicing planes to correspond to in vivo imaging planes, it also indirectly defined cutting planes on specimen MR images and assumed histology corresponded to these planes, yielding an output analogous to the plane identification step of the proposed algorithm (the first step in which a discretized exhaustive search for an initial plane was performed in a bounded three-dimensional space constrained to *reasonable* transformations). Applying the correspondence vector identification step of the proposed algorithm (the second step where the correspondence vector best fit to a given plane is calculated) to these planes yielded an affine registration based on image-guided slicing. We calculated the mean TRE of this registration and compared it to the proposed method.

How Did the Accuracy of the Proposed Method Compare to That of Our Previous Tissue-Slice-Imaging-Based Method? (Question 3)

While our previously developed tissue-slice-imaging-based method [28] yielded accurate registrations, it introduced an additional imaging step, increasing costs, processing time, and complexity. To assess whether this additional imaging was necessary for registration, we directly compared the proposed method to our tissue-slice-imaging-based method. In this previously developed method, the histology was first corresponded with the tissue slice MR image, ensuring that histology corresponded only to tissue within one tissue slice, and not across multiple slices (which is not possible, as each histology section is cut from a single tissue slice). The tissue slices were then virtually assembled using fiducial correspondences between tissue slices and the assembly was aligned to the specimen MR image using a least squares best-fit rigid transformation of fiducial markers. As in section "How Did the Accuracy of the Proposed Method Compare to That of Our Previous Image-Guided-Slicing-Based Method? (Question 2)," the correspondence vector identification step (the second step where the correspondence vector best fit to a given plane is calculated) of the proposed algorithm was applied to the resulting plane yielding a corresponding affine registration, and the iterative optimization step (the final step of the algorithm in which iterative optimization of FRE was performed on the bounded ten-dimensional space of correspondence vectors) was applied to refine the registration. Mean TRE was calculated after steps 2 and 3. Note that unlike many approaches that use tissue slice imaging [16, 22–25], the previous approach does not assume histology corresponds to the front face of the tissue slices, thus accounting for variability in microtome sectioning.

How Did the Use of Internal Fiducials Impact Registration Accuracy? (Question 4)

Although the application of our internal fiducials to the specimen is non-disruptive to clinical pathology assessment, it could be a barrier to translation of the proposed method to centers where such treatment of the tissue is prohibited, and additionally it adds complexity and time to the fiducial application process. In order to evaluate whether these internal fiducials were necessary for accurate registration, we performed the proposed registrations without using the internal fiducials, calculated the mean TRE, and compared it to that of the proposed algorithm.

Does Applying Fiducial Correspondence Error Optimization to the Image-Guided-Slicing-Based Method Improve its Accuracy? (Question 5)

The goals of the image-guided-slicing-based method (to obtain histology images along pre-specified planes) and the proposed method (to accurately determine the correspondence of histology to 3D imaging taking into account the variability in the process of acquiring histology) are not mutually exclusive. For example, if the application of the histology-imaging registration requires that histological information from a single section be displayed alongside axis-aligned imaging, image-guided slicing could be used to approximately constrain the position and orientation of the histology and the iterative refinement of FRE could be used to find the retrospective registration accurately. To assess the accuracy of this approach, the iterative optimization step of the proposed algorithm (the final step of the algorithm in which iterative optimization of FRE was performed on the bounded ten-dimensional space of correspondence vectors) was applied to the correspondence produced by the image-guided-slicing-based method, and the mean TRE was compared to that of image-guided-slicing-based method alone. This mean TRE was also compared to that of the proposed method.

Statistical Analyses

Statistical analyses were performed in Prism 5.04 (Graphpad Software, Inc., San Diego, USA). The TRE of each of the proposed algorithms were characterized using descriptive statistics [mean ± standard deviation (SD)] aggregated over all fiducials. Five key statistical comparisons were made for this study: one comparing the mean TRE of the image-guided-slicing-based method before and after iterative optimization, and four more comparing the mean TRE of the proposed method to each of the other methods. The mean TREs were first compared using a one-way repeated-measures analysis of variation (ANOVA) with five levels corresponding to the proposed algorithm, the proposed algorithm without internal fiducials, the image-guided-slicing-based method, the image-guided-slicing-based method with iterative optimization, and the tissue-slice-imaging-based method. Pairwise post hoc analyses using Bonferroni multiple comparison correction was used to assess the five key comparisons. To mitigate the impact of positive skew in the statistical comparisons, TRE measurements were transformed using a square-root function before statistical testing. After transformation, the D'Agostino and Pearson omnibus normality test detected deviation from normality only for the algorithm without internal fiducials, so post hoc analyses including this algorithm were confirmed with the nonparametric Wilcoxon matched-pairs signed rank test. Ninety-five percent confidence intervals (CI) on the differences were generated based on the post hoc analyses using the untransformed data, and should be interpreted in the context of their non-normality. To assess the robustness of the proposed method to the absence of some fiducial cross-sections on histology images, a Spearman correlation test was performed between the TRE for each landmark and the number of fiducials remaining on the corresponding histology image.

Results

The quantified registration accuracies and comparisons between them are given in Tables 1 and 2. A box plot of the five registration methods compared in this work is shown in Fig. 4. More in-depth results are given in the following sections.

Landmark Identification

Homologous landmark pairs were identifiable on all 34 histology–specimen MR image pairs, resulting in three to seven homologous landmarks on each of the three to five histology images per specimen (184 landmarks in total). Illustrative examples of the identified landmarks and the nearby salient features used to establish homology are shown in Fig. 3. The distribution of the landmarks is shown in Fig. 5, with 75 landmarks in the peripheral zone, 8 in the central zone, 66 in the transitional zone,

Table 1 TRE for four algorithms before and after iterative optimization. Algorithms compared in post hoc analyses are connected by lines, solid where a statistical difference was found, dashed when the analysis failed to detect a statistical difference

	Mean±SD TRE (mm) without iterative optimization	Mean±SD TRE (mm) with iterative optimization
Proposed method	0.76±0.43	0.71±0.38
No internal fiducials	0.95±0.84	0.92±0.82
Image-guided slicing	1.21±0.74	0.71±0.37
Tissue slice imaging	0.86±0.50	0.70±0.36

Table 2 Post hoc analyses comparing the five algorithms as 95 % CI (mm) on differences of mean TRE. For conciseness, algorithms after iterative optimization are marked "w/IO"

Method A	Method B	95 % CI (mm) $TRE_A - TRE_B$
Image-guided slicing	Proposed method w/IO	[0.38,0.63]
Image-guided slicing	Image-guided slicing w/IO	[0.38,0.62]
Image-guided slicing w/IO	Proposed method w/IO	[−0.12,0.13]
No internal fiducials w/IO	Proposed method w/IO	[0.09,0.34]
Tissue slice imaging w/IO	Proposed method w/IO	[−0.13,0.11]

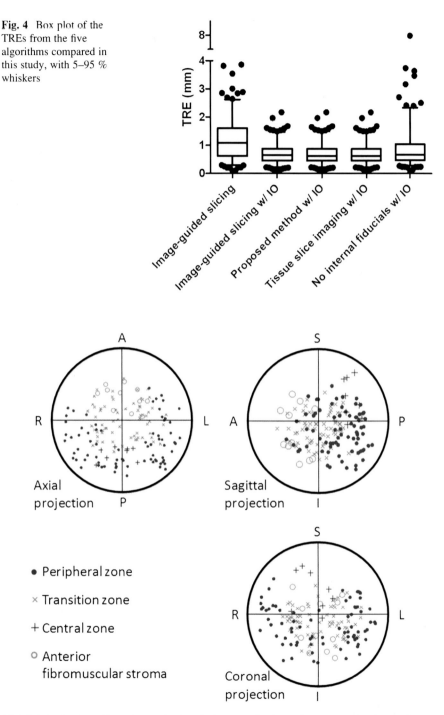

Fig. 4 Box plot of the TREs from the five algorithms compared in this study, with 5–95 % whiskers

Fig. 5 Distribution of homologous landmarks in normalized coordinates. Landmark coordinates were stretched such that the left/right, anterior/posterior, and inferior/superior extents matched for all specimens. Landmark *symbols* denote the zonal anatomy in which the landmark was identified

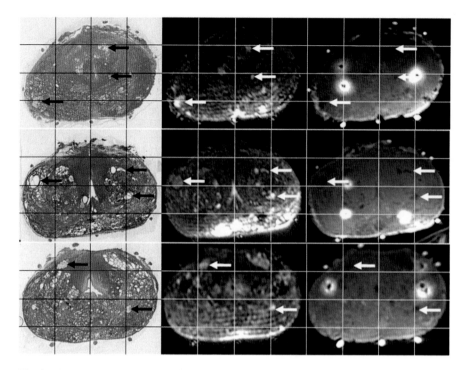

Fig. 6 Illustrative co-registered histology and specimen MR images. *White arrows* show example validation landmarks. Figure reproduced with permission from the Journal of Magnetic Resonance Imaging [29]

and 11 in the anterior fibromuscular stroma; the remaining 24 landmarks were not definitively categorized. Notably, no landmarks were identified near the apex and base because only mid-gland tissue slices were included in this study.

How Accurate Was the Proposed Method? (Question 1)

The key findings of this experiment were that the mean ± SD TRE was 0.71 ± 0.38 mm and that the specimen processing time, comprising fiducial marking, specimen MR imaging, localizing fiducials, and executing the reconstruction algorithm took 3 h; this was 8 h faster than the image-guided-slicing-based method and 2 h faster than the tissue-slice-imaging-based method.

Illustrative co-registered histology and specimen MR images are shown in Fig. 6. The mean ± SD TRE of 0.71 ± 0.38 mm was found to be anisotropic with variances of 0.33, 0.13, and 0.09 mm^2 in the principal directions of variation, measured in the MR image coordinate frame. However, the principal direction of variation was not aligned with an image axis. In the histology image coordinate frame the in-plane variance was 0.24 mm^2, and the out-of-plane variance was

0.39 mm (larger than the variances in the MR image coordinate frame). The TLE on histology images was 0.05 mm and the TLE on specimen MR images was 0.16 mm; these errors, combined in quadrature, are sufficiently small to interfere minimally with the measurement of TRE.

Of the 340 fiducial cross-sections expected on the histology images, 20 were not visible: 7 due to the sectioning plane being located past the endpoint of the fiducial and 13 due to the fiducial being lost during processing. The 95 % CI on the Spearman correlation coefficient for number of fiducials used in the registration [7 ($N = 1$), 8 ($N = 5$), 9 ($N = 7$) and 10 ($N = 21$)] with the TRE was -0.23 to 0.06.

The proposed method took 3 h per specimen, comprising 90 min for fiducial marking, 80 min for specimen MR imaging, 12 min for localizing fiducials, and 1 min for executing the reconstruction algorithm. In comparison, the image-guided-slicing-based method described in this work took ~11 h per specimen and the tissue-slice-imaging-based method took ~5 h per specimen.

How Did the Accuracy of the Proposed Method Compare to That of Our Previous Image-Guided-Slicing-Based Method? (Question 2)

The key finding of this experiment was that the image-guided-slicing-based approach yielded a mean ± SD TRE of 1.21 ± 0.74 mm, 0.38–0.63 mm higher (95 % CI) than the proposed algorithm.

How Did the Accuracy of the Proposed Method Compare to That of Our Previous Tissue-Slice-Imaging-Based Method? (Question 3)

The key finding of this experiment was that the mean ± SD TRE of the tissue slice imaging method was 0.70 ± 0.36 mm, within 0.13 mm (95 % CI) of the proposed algorithm. A Bland-Altman plot comparing the TRE of the tissue-slice-imaging-based method to the proposed method is shown in Fig. 7a.

How Did the Use of Internal Fiducials Impact Registration Accuracy? (Question 4)

The key finding of this experiment was that the proposed algorithm without internal fiducials yielded a mean ± SD TRE of 0.92 ± 0.82 mm, 0.09–0.34 mm higher (95 % CI) than the proposed algorithm with internal fiducials. Notably, all nine of

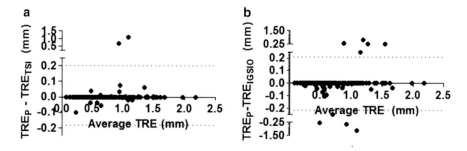

Fig. 7 Bland-Altman plots comparing (**a**) the mean TRE of the proposed algorithm (TRE_P) to that of the image-guided-slicing-based method after iterative optimization (TRE_{IGSIO}), and (**b**) the mean TRE of the proposed algorithm to that of the tissue-slice-imaging-based method (TRE_{TSI})

the outliers visible in Fig. 5 correspond to sections where one or more external fiducials were not visible on the histology image. When these sections were omitted, the difference remained significant but was less than 0.14 mm (95 % CI).

Does Applying Iterative Optimization to the Image-Guided-Slicing-Based Method Improve Its Accuracy? (Question 5)

The key finding of this experiment was that after iterative optimization, the image-guided-slicing-based approach yielded a mean ± SD TRE of 0.71 ± 0.37 mm, 0.38–0.62 mm lower than before iterative optimization and within 0.13 mm (95 % CI) of the proposed algorithm. A Bland-Altman plot comparing the TRE of the image-guided-slicing-based method to the proposed method is shown in Fig. 7b. The addition of iterative optimization to this method would require the localization of fiducials and execution of the software, adding approximately 15 min to the processing time.

Discussion

In this chapter, we presented a method for the accurate 2D–3D registration of whole-mount mid-gland prostate histology to ex vivo specimen MR images which yielded a submillimeter mean TRE, and reduced the time per specimen by 70 % relative to our previously implemented image-guided-slicing-based approach. These registrations, in conjunction with 3D–3D ex vivo–in vivo image registrations, can be used to support the evaluation of prostate imaging modalities.

Evaluation of the Proposed Algorithm

The accuracy of the registration algorithm was characterized and compared to four alternative registration approaches. The mean $\pm$ SD TRE of the proposed algorithm was 0.71 ± 0.38 mm with a higher component of error perpendicular to the identified histology image plane.

The method proved to be robust to the absence of one to three external fiducial cross-sections on histology images, an important result since this absence was observed for 5 % of cross-sections across 38 % of subjects. Although we failed to show a correlation between the number of fiducials visible on histology and the TRE, we speculate that missing higher numbers of fiducials than observed in this data set may result in an increase in registration error. The missing fiducials are due in part to the loss of fiducial cross-sections during tissue processing and in part due to tissue slicing not passing through the fiducials. The former could be mitigated by careful handling of the fiducial marked specimen during tissue processing, in particular when cutting tissue into thick slices. The latter problem could be mitigated by using longer fiducials covering a greater extent of the specimen.

Comparison with Other Algorithms

The mean TRE for the proposed algorithm without using tissue slice imaging was within 0.13 mm of the tissue-slice-imaging-based approach previously developed in our institute, suggesting the additional cost, complexity, and processing time of tissue slice MR imaging may not be warranted. The mean TRE was 0.38–0.63 mm lower than the image-guided-slicing-based method. The iterative optimization component of the algorithm (step 3) improved the mean TRE of the image-guided-slicing-based approach by 0.38–0.62 mm to be within 0.13 mm of the proposed method. Thus, if there is a need for controlling the histology section position and orientation, such as a need to display whole histology sections corresponding to whole imaging-axis-aligned in vivo images, then an image-guidance-based method could be combined with the proposed optimization of FRE to avoid sacrificing registration error.

Registration errors have resulted in researchers limiting the sizes of cancerous foci considered in studies [31, 32], and may have resulted in underestimations of the true underlying differences between cancerous and benign tissue [33]. The required accuracy for histology to in vivo imaging registrations depends on the research questions being answered. Furthermore, for a given study design, the TRE has an impact on the statistical power and the required sample size of the study. The reported mean TRE values can be considered in the context of a typical application of histology to in vivo imaging registrations: a prostate imaging validation study to detect signal differences between the cancer foci and normal tissue regions. A recent model of the statistical relationship between registration error and the statistical power for this type of imaging validation study [26, 27] can be used to quantify the impact of registration errors on the required sample size. Because the model also provides a mapping from mean TRE to the registration error metrics used in the model, this model can be used to compare the reported mean TRE values under the assumptions that the tumors are modeled as spherical regions, misalignment can be modeled as 3D Gaussian translational registration error and the reported TRE dominate the overall registration error from histology to in vivo images. In this scenario, using the proposed method with a mean TRE of 0.71 mm as a baseline, the image-guided-slicing-based method with a mean TRE of 1.21 mm would require 28 % more subjects to achieve the same statistical power. Considering the high cost per subject of imaging validation studies (e.g., $10,000 USD per subject in an ongoing prostate imaging study at our institution), this could have a substantial impact on the cost of the study. For example, in the aforementioned prostate imaging study, which plans to accrue 66 subjects, this 28 % increase in sample size would correspond to an additional cost of $190,000. Such sample size increases also increase the effort needed to accrue additional patients, time to complete studies, and expose additional subjects to nonstandard-of-care tests and interventions.

As we have demonstrated, the proposed method can be used without internal fiducials; however, this resulted in an increase in mean TRE. Using the previously described scenario, the proposed method without internal fiducials would require 11 % more subjects than with the internal fiducials, an increase that would correspond to an additional cost of $80,000 in the prostate imaging study at our institution. Some of this difference, however, was due to reduced robustness to missing fiducials on histology images. If all external fiducials were intact, the impact of absent internal fiducials was minimized, suggesting that the decrease in accuracy could be mitigated by careful handling and the use of longer extrinsic fiducial markers.

The proposed method requires some alteration of the pathology workflow, introducing fiducials and ex vivo MR imaging. However, this disruption is reduced compared to our previously implemented image-guided-slicing-based approach. The time required to collect data was reduced by 70 %. Furthermore, the retrospective registration allows the specimen to be cut following the standard slice orientations used in the pathologist workflow and in the resulting clinical reports.

Application

The proposed registration method has been applied in conjunction with precise contouring and grading of histology images and an interactive registration from ex vivo specimen MR images to in vivo multi-parametric MR images, enabling the mapping of information from histological examination to in vivo MR images for the evaluation of prostate cancer imaging. Oblique slices from two such cases containing Gleason score 7 peripheral zone cancer foci are shown in Fig. 8, illustrating the variability in the appearance of Gleason score 7 foci on T2-weighted MR imaging.

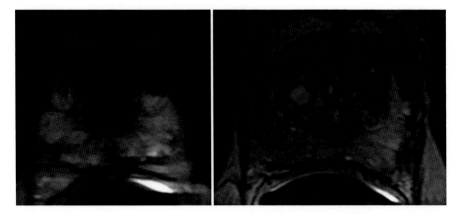

Fig. 8 Oblique slices from in vivo T2-weighted MR images from two subjects with contours of Gleason score 7 peripheral zone cancer foci mapped from histology images using the proposed method in conjunction with an interactive ex vivo to in vivo deformable registration. These cases illustrate the variable appearance of Gleason score 7 foci on T2-weighted MRI, and in particular the variability in the appearance of tumor boundaries

Limitations

The conclusions of this work should be considered in the context of two key limitations. First, only affine registrations were considered in our experiments. While previous work suggests that much of the deformation between whole-mount prostate histology and fixed ex vivo specimens can be accounted for by linear transformations, there is also evidence that some submillimeter nonlinear deformation is induced during the acquisition of histology [19]. Second, while the proposed method can theoretically be applied to specimens sliced without any guidance, it was tested on data from an existing study using image-guided slicing. This allowed for the direct comparison of image-guided-slicing-based and retrospective registrations; however, the variation in orientation of histology sections may underestimate what would be typically seen with less-controlled tissue handling.

Conclusion

In conclusion, the proposed fiducial-based 3D prostate whole-mount histology to ex vivo specimen MR image registration algorithm reduced our specimen processing time by 8 h per subject, a 70 % reduction, and yielded a mean ± SD TRE of 0.71 ± 0.38 mm. Our previous method based on the image-guided slicing of specimens into thick tissue slices yielded a mean TRE that was 0.38–0.63 mm higher (95 % confidence interval) and the proposed method executed without internal fiducials yielded a mean TRE that was 0.09–0.34 mm higher (95 % confidence interval). Under a statistical model relating TREs to the statistical power of an imaging study to detect mean signal differences between the smallest clinically significant [34] cancer foci and benign regions, the observed differences in registration error could result in 28 % and 11 % increases in sample size for the image-guided-slicing-based method and the proposed method without internal fiducials, respectively.

Acknowledgements This work was supported by the Natural Sciences and Engineering Research Council of Canada, Cancer Care Ontario, the Ontario Graduate Scholarship Program, the Ontario Institute for Cancer Research, and the Canadian Institutes of Health Research [CTP 87515]. A. Fenster holds a Canada Research Chair in Biomedical Engineering and acknowledges the support of the Canada Research Chair Program. A. D. Ward holds a Cancer Care Ontario Research Chair in Cancer Imaging.

References

1. Ellis RJ, Kaminsky DA (2006) Fused radioimmunoscintigraphy for treatment planning. Rev Urol 8(Suppl):S11–S19
2. Barrett JA, Coleman RE, Goldsmith SJ, Vallabhajosula S, Petry NA, Cho S, Armor T, Stubbs JB, Maresca KP, Stabin MG, Joyal JL, Eckelman WC, Babich JW (2013) First-in-man evaluation of 2 high-affinity PSMA-avid small molecules for imaging prostate cancer. J Nucl Med 54:380–387
3. Scher B, Seitz M, Albinger W, Tiling R, Scherr M, Becker H-C, Souvatzogluou M, Gildehaus F-J, Wester H-J, Dresel S (2007) Value of ^{11}C-choline PET and PET/CT in patients with suspected prostate cancer. Eur J Nucl Med Mol Imaging 34:45–53
4. Fei B, Wang H, Wu C, Chiu S-m (2007) Choline PET for monitoring early tumor response to photodynamic therapy. J Nucl Med 51:130–138
5. Beheshti M, Imamovic L, Broinger G, Vali R, Waldenberger P, Stoiber F, Nader M, Gruy B, Janetschek G, Langsteger W (2010) ^{18}F choline PET/CT in the preoperative staging of prostate cancer in patients with intermediate or high risk of extracapsular disease: a prospective study of 130 patients. Radiology 254:925–933
6. Kwee SA, Coel MN, Lim J, Ko JP (2005) Prostate cancer localization with ^{18}fluorine fluorocholine positron emission tomography. J Urol 173:252–255
7. Sciarra A, Barentsz J, Bjartell A, Eastham J, Hricak H, Panebianco V, Witjes JA (2011) Advances in magnetic resonance imaging: how they are changing the management of prostate cancer. Eur Urol 59:962–977
8. Barentsz JO, Richenberg J, Clements R, Choyke P, Verma S, Villeirs G, Rouvière O, Logager V, Fütterer JJ (2012) ESUR prostate MR guidelines 2012. Eur Radiol 22:746–757
9. Engelbrecht MR, Barentsz JO, Jager GJ, van der Graaf M, Heerschap A, Sedelaar JP, Aarnink RG, de la Rosette JJ (2000) Prostate cancer staging using imaging. BJU Int 86(Suppl 1):123–134
10. Ocak I, Bernardo M, Metzger G, Barrett T, Pinto P, Albert PS, Choyke PL (2007) Dynamic contrast-enhanced MRI of prostate cancer at 3T: a study of pharmacokinetic parameters. Am J Roentgenol 189:W192–W201
11. Vargas HA, Akin O, Franiel T, Mazaheri Y, Zheng J, Moskowitz C, Udo K, Eastham J, Hricak H (2011) Diffusion-weighted endorectal MR imaging at 3T for prostate cancer: tumor detection and assessment of aggressiveness. Radiology 259:775–784

12. Turkbey B, Shah VP, Pang Y, Bernardo M, Xu S, Kruecker J, Locklin J, Baccala AA, Rastinehad AR, Merino MJ, Shih JH, Wood BJ, Pinto PA, Choyke PL (2011) Is apparent diffusion coefficient associated with clinical risk scores for prostate cancers that are visible on 3-T MR images? Radiology 258:488–495

13. Vigneron DB, Males R, Noworolski S, Nelson SJ, Scheidler J, Sokolov D, Hricak H, Carroll P, Kurhanewic J (1998) 3D MRSI of prostate cancer: correlation with histologic grade. In: Proceedings of International Society for Magnetic Resonance in Medicine, pp 488

14. Zakian KL, Sircar K, Hricak H, Chen HN, Shukla-Dave A, Eberhardt S, Muruganandham M, Ebora L, Kattan MW, Reuter VE, Scardino PT, Koutcher JA (2005) Correlation of proton MR spectroscopic imaging with Gleason score based on step-section pathologic analysis after radical prostatectomy. Radiology 234:804–814

15. Chen LH, Ho H, Lazaro R, Thng CH, Yuen J, Ng WS, Cheng C (2010) Optimum slicing of radical prostatectomy specimens for correlation between histopathology and medical images. Int J Comput Assist Radiol Surg 5:471–487

16. Jackson AS, Reinsberg SA, Sohaib SA, Charles-Edwards EM, Jhavar S, Christmas TJ, Thompson AC, Bailey MJ, Corbishley CM, Fisher C, Leach MO, Dearnaley DP (2009) Dynamic contrast-enhanced MRI for prostate cancer localization. Br J Radiol 82:148–156

17. Ward AD, Crukley C, McKenzie CA, Montreuil J, Gibson E, Romagnoli C, Gómez JA, Moussa M, Chin J, Bauman G, Fenster A (2012) Prostate: registration of digital histopatho-logic images to in vivo MR images acquired by using endorectal receive coil. Radiology 263:856–864

18. Shah V, Pohida T, Turkbey B, Mani H, Merino M, Pinto PA, Choyke P, Bernardo M (2009) A method for correlating in vivo prostate magnetic resonance imaging and histopathology using individualized magnetic resonance-based molds. Rev Sci Instrum 80:104301–104306

19. Gibson E, Gómez JA, Moussa M, Crukley C, Bauman G, Fenster A, Ward AD (2012) 3D reconstruction of prostate histology based on quantified tissue cutting and deformation parameters. Proc SPIE Med Imaging 8317:83170N

20. Hughes C, Rouvière O, Mege-Lechevallier F, Souchon R, Prost R (2012) Robust alignment of prostate histology slices with quantified accuracy. IEEE Trans Biomed Eng 60:281–291

21. Bart S, Mozer P, Hemar P, Lenaour G, Comperat E, Renaud-Penna R, Chartier-Kastler E, Troccaz J (2005) MRI-histology registration in prostate cancer. In: Proceedings of Surgetica

22. Groenendaal G, Moman MR, Korporaal JG, van Diest PJ, van Vulpen M, Philippens ME, van der Heide UA (2010) Validation of functional imaging with pathology for tumor delineation in the prostate. Radiother Oncol 94:145–150

23. Taylor LS, Porter BC, Nadasdy G, di Sant'Agnese PA, Pasternack D, Wu Z, Baggs RB, Rubens DJ, Parker KJ (2004) Three-dimensional registration of prostate images from histology and ultrasound. Ultrasound Med Biol 30:161–168

24. Xu J, Humphrey PA, Kibel AS, Snyder AZ, Narra VR, Ackerman JJ, Song SK (2009) Magnetic resonance diffusion characteristics of histologically defined prostate cancer in humans. Magn Reson Med 61:842–850

25. Park H, Piert MR, Khan A, Shah R, Hussain H, Siddiqui J, Chenevert TL, Meyer CR (2008) Registration methodology for histological sections and in vivo imaging of human prostate. Acad Radiol 15:1027–1039

26. Gibson E, Fenster A, Ward AD (2012) Registration accuracy: how good is good enough? A statistical power calculation incorporating image registration uncertainty. In: Ayache N, Delingette H, Golland P, Mori K (eds) Proceedings of Medical Image Computing and Computer Assisted Intervention, vol 7511, pp 643–650

27. Gibson E, Fenster A, Ward AD (2013) The impact of registration accuracy on imaging validation study design: a novel statistical power calculation. Med Image Anal 17:805–815

28. Gibson E, Crukley C, Gómez JA, Moussa M, Bauman G, Fenster A, Ward AD (2011) Tissue block MRI for slice orientation-independent registration of digital histology images to ex vivo MRI of the prostate. In: Proceedings of International Symposium on Biomedical Imaging, pp 566–569

29. Gibson E, Crukley C, Gaed M, Gómez JA, Moussa M, Chin JL, Bauman GS, Fenster A, Ward AD (2012) Registration of prostate histology images to ex vivo MR images via strand-shaped fiducials. J Magn Reson Imaging 36:1402–1412

30. Sethian JA (1999) Level set methods and fast marching methods evolving interfaces in computational geometry, fluid mechanics, computer vision, and materials science. Cambridge University Press, Cambridge

31. Turnbull LW, Buckley DL, Turnbull LS, Liney GP, Knowles AJ (1999) Differentiation of prostatic carcinoma and benign prostatic hyperplasia: correlation between dynamic Gd-DTPA-enhanced MR imaging and histopathology. J Magn Reson Imaging 9:311–316

32. Engelbrecht MR, Huisman HJ, Laheij RJF, Jager GJ, van Leenders GJLH, Hulsbergen-Van De Kaa CA, de la Rosette JJMCH, Blickman JG, Barentsz JO (2003) Discrimination of prostate cancer from normal peripheral zone and central gland tissue by using dynamic contrast-enhanced MR imaging. Radiology 229:248–254

33. Rouvière O, Raudrant A, Ecochard R, Colin-Pangaud C, Pasquiou C, Bouvier R, Marechal JM, Lyonnet D (2003) Characterization of time-enhancement curves of benign and malignant prostate tissue at dynamic MR imaging. Eur Radiol 13:931–942

34. Epstein JI, Walsh PC, Carmichael M, Brendler CB (1994) Pathologic and clinical findings to predict tumor extent of nonpalpable (stage T1c) prostate cancer. JAMA 271:368–374

Biography

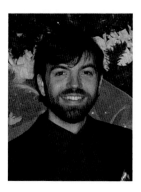

Eli Gibson received his B.A.Sc. in computer engineering from Simon Fraser University. He completed his Master's degree at Simon Fraser University in engineering under the supervision of Dr. Mirza Faisal Beg, pursuing research into the quantification and analysis of cortical thickness for early assessment of Alzheimer's and other forms of dementia. He is currently a Ph.D. Candidate under the supervision of Drs. Aaron Fenster and Aaron Ward at the Robarts Research Institute at The University of Western Ontario in London, Ontario, pursuing research into the evaluation of prostate cancer imaging via co-registration with histopathological reference standards.

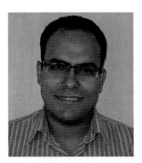

Dr. Mena Gaed completed his M.D. at Cairo University in Cairo, Egypt. He is currently pursuing a Master's degree in Pathology at the Schulich School of Medicine and Dentistry, The University of Western Ontario under the supervision of Dr. Aaron Fenster and Dr. Madeleine Moussa, focusing on the relationship between the appearance of prostate cancer on in vivo imaging modalities and the corresponding histopathological features on prostatectomy specimens.

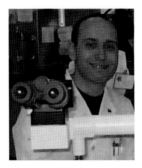

Dr. José A. Gómez is a Pathologist at London Health Sciences Centre in London, Ontario, specializing in Genitourinary Pathology. He is also an Associate Professor in the Department of Pathology at the Schulich School of Medicine and Dentistry, The University of Western Ontario in London, Ontario. Dr. Gómez's primary areas of interest are testicular neoplasms, the study of prognostic factors in prostatic adenocarcinoma, and the correlation of prostatectomy specimens with imaging modalities for the optimization of preoperative diagnosis, biopsy protocols and surgical planning.

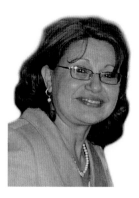

Dr. Madeleine Moussa is a Pathologist at London Health Sciences Centre in London, Ontario, specializing in Genitourinary Pathology and Nephropathology. She is also a Professor in the Department of Pathology at the Schulich School of Medicine and Dentistry, The University of Western Ontario in London, Ontario. Dr. Moussa's primary research areas are genitourinary cancers including prostate, bladder and kidney.

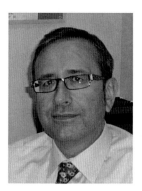

Dr. Cesare Romagnoli is a Radiologist at London Health Sciences Centre in London, Ontario, specializing in Abdominal and Musculoskeletal Imaging. He is also an Associate Professor in the Department of Medical Imaging at the Schulich School of Medicine and Dentistry, The University of Western Ontario in London, Ontario. Dr. Romagnoli's primary areas of research interest are in the application of 3D ultrasound imaging to prostate and rectal cancers.

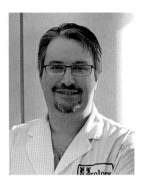

Dr. Stephen Pautler joined the staff at St. Joseph's Hospital (St. Joseph's Health Care, London) as an Assistant Professor with The University of Western Ontario, Department of Surgery in 2002, and was cross-appointed to the Department of Oncology in 2005. Dr. Pautler is a scientist with the Lawson Health Research Institute in London, Ontario. He has co-authored more than 90 peer-reviewed articles, several chapters, and has presented at numerous international urology meetings. His current interests include surgical robotics and urologic laparoscopy with the application of minimally invasive surgical techniques and image-guided ablative procedures for urologic cancers. Dr. Pautler is the co-director of the Endourology fellowship program and participates in the Society of Urologic Oncology fellowship program at The University of Western Ontario. Since 2012, he has been the Surgical Oncology Lead for the Southwest Regional Cancer Program, Cancer Care Ontario.

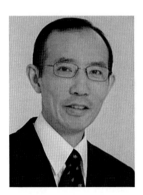

Dr. Joseph L. Chin is Professor of Urology and Oncology at the Schulich School of Medicine and Dentistry, The University of Western Ontario. He has been Chair of the Division of Urology at the University of Western Ontario, Head of the Provincial Surgical Oncology Program for the Southwestern Ontario Region, and Chair of the Royal College of Physicians and Surgeons of Canada Specialty Committee in Urology, responsible for the Training and Evaluation of Canadian

Urology Residents. Dr. Chin is currently Chair of the Division of Surgical Oncology at the University of Western Ontario. Dr. Chin has received many research grants from international and national granting agencies. His laboratory and clinical research interests are in prostate cancer management, including minimally invasive and alternative forms of management. His clinical practice at London Health Sciences Centre is concentrated in Urologic Oncology. He has been a Canadian leader in such procedures as robotic assisted laparoscopic prostatectomy, cryosurgery, and high intensity focused ultrasound for prostate cancer. Dr. Chin is an Editorial Board member of several major international Urology journals. He has published over 200 research papers and book chapters, mostly in the area of uro-oncology. Dr. Chin is President of the Canadian Urological Association for 2011–2013. He was appointed to the Order of Ontario in 2011 for his contributions to the field of prostate cancer, specifically in prevention and treatment, patient, and public education, and in fundraising for research.

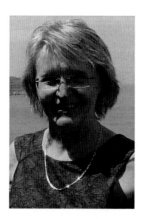

Cathie Crukley is a Research Assistant at the Lawson Health Research Institute in London, Ontario. Ms. Crukley is a Pathology Histotechnologist with a clinical career spanning 38 years, working as a bench technologist and later specializing in immunohistochemistry. Ms. Crukley has held several supervisory positions leading to Manager, Pathology Laboratories for the merged laboratory services of the three London, Ontario hospitals. In 2008, she moved into a research position with the CIHR Team in Image Guidance for Prostate Cancer. Ms. Crukley continues to grow in her research role as she supports 3D pathology processes for the Imaging Research Laboratories at Robarts Research Institute, The University of Western Ontario.

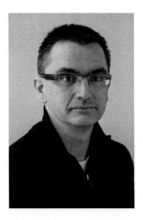

Dr. Glenn S. Bauman is a Radiation Oncologist specializing in genitourinary and central nervous system malignancies. He is also Professor and Chair/Chief of the Department of Oncology at the Schulich School of Medicine and Dentistry, The University of Western Ontario in London, Ontario and is an Associate Scientist at the Lawson Health Research Institute. Dr. Bauman's primary areas of research interest are in modeling of effects of uncertainty on radiation treatment delivery, multi-modality image guided radiotherapy, and cancer imaging.

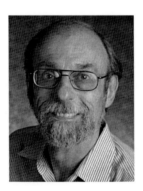

Dr. Aaron Fenster is the founding Director of the Imaging Research Laboratories (IRL) at the Robarts Research Institute and Professor in Radiology at the University of Western Ontario (UWO). In addition, he is the founder and Associate Director of the new interdisciplinary graduate program in Biomedical Engineering at UWO. He is also the Chair of the basic Science division of the Department of Medical Imaging and the Director for the Biomedical Imaging Research Centre at UWO. In 2010, he became the Centre Director and acting CEO of the newly formed Centre for Imaging Technology Commercialization—a federally funded Centre of Excellence in Commercialization and Research. Currently, he holds a Canada Research Chair-Tier 1 in Biomedical Engineering. He is the first recipient of the Premier's (Ontario) Discovery Award for Innovation and Leadership (2007), the Hellmuth

Prize for Achievement in Research at the UWO (2008), and the Canadian Organization of Medical Physicists (COMP) Gold Medal Award (2010). In 2011, he was inducted into the Canadian Academy of Health Sciences. Fenster's research has resulted in 250 papers in peer-reviewed journals, 37 patents (27 awarded and 10 pending), and the formation of four companies in London based on research in his laboratory. In addition, some of his patents have been licensed to 13 different companies, which have commercialized them for world-wide distribution.

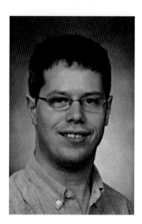

Dr. Aaron D. Ward is an Assistant Professor of Medical Biophysics, Biomedical Engineering, and Oncology at The University of Western Ontario, and a Scientist with the Lawson Health Research Institute in London, Ontario. At the London Regional Cancer Program, he co-leads the Imaging Research Laboratory within the Gerald C. Baines Centre for Translational Cancer Research and holds a Cancer Care Ontario Research Chair in Cancer Imaging. Dr. Ward's research program is in the area of development and evaluation of computational methods for medical image analysis, including image segmentation, registration, and computer-aided diagnosis and therapy guidance for cancer patients, with particular attention paid to the validation of algorithms using statistical measures appropriate to assessment of clinical utility and reliability. Current disease sites of interest include the prostate, lung, and brain.

Anatomical Landmark Detection

David Liu and S. Kevin Zhou

Abstract We present a landmark detection method that detects a large number of anatomical structures efficiently in a medical image. The method consists of two steps. The first step performs nearest neighbor matching, which exploits holistic image context to quickly obtain coarse estimates of landmark positions. The second step refines landmark positions while minimizing the overall computation time, by exploiting unary and pairwise context in a submodular optimization framework. The system is validated on a database of 2,500 CT volumes and shows significant speedup over traditional methods. Additionally, we present a method for training individual landmark detectors based on the Multiple Instance Learning framework. We introduce a spatial regularization term that encourages a concentrated detection response map, which is particularly suitable for medical images since landmarks are unique in a given image. This method gives better results than prior work when using few or even zero annotations.

Keywords Landmark detection • Multiple instance learning • Spatial regularization • Submodular optimization • Nearest neighbor

Introduction

An important area in medical image analysis is the development of methods for quickly finding the positions of certain anatomical structures, such as liver top, lung top, aortic arch, iliac artery bifurcation, femur head left and right, to name but a few. In multi-modality image registration (such as PET-CT) or in registration of follow-up scans, the fusion of multiple images can be initialized or guided by the positions of such anatomical structures [9, 25]. In vessel centerline tracing, vessel

D. Liu (✉) • S.K. Zhou
Imaging and Computer Vision, Siemens Corporate Technology, 755 College Road E,
Princeton, NJ 08540, USA
e-mail: David-liu@siemens.com; shaohua.zhou@siemens.com

A.S. El-Baz et al. (eds.), *Abdomen and Thoracic Imaging: An Engineering
& Clinical Perspective*, DOI 10.1007/978-1-4614-8498-1_27,
© Springer Science+Business Media New York 2014

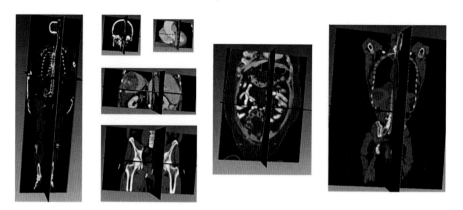

Fig. 1 The database used in this chapter has thousands of 3D CT scans with different body regions and severe pathologies

bifurcations can provide the start and end points of certain vessels to enable fully automated tracing [3]. In organ segmentation, the center position of an organ can provide the initial seed points to initiate segmentation algorithms [40]. In seminar reporting, automatically found anatomical structures can be helpful in configuring the optimal intensity window for display [38], or offer the text tooltips for structures in the scan [45].

We define an anatomical landmark (or landmark in brief) as a distinct and unique point position in an image that coincides with an anatomical structure. Some anatomical landmarks have little ambiguity, such as the apex of the left or right lung in a CT image. Other landmarks such as the liver center lack distinctiveness, because the center of mass of the liver often does not coincide with a unique anatomical structure and becomes ill-defined. In such a case, one can define a hypothetical bounding box that tightly bounds the liver, and define the liver center as the center of the bounding box.

We are interested in the problem of efficiently detecting a large number of landmarks from such scans, without reading DICOM tags or any textual information. This is challenging due the presence of imaging noise, artifacts, and body deformation. The field of view is also unknown. A practical landmark detection method must meet the following requirements. First, it must be robust to deal with pathological or anomalous anatomies such as fluid-filled lungs, air-filled colons, inhomogeneous livers caused by different metastasis, and resected livers after surgical interventions, different contrast agent phases, scans of full or partial body regions, and extremely narrow field of views. Figure 1 shows some examples of CT scans that illustrate the challenges. Second, since landmark detection is mostly a pre-processing step for computationally heavier tasks such as CAD and registration, it must run fast so that more time can be allocated for heavier tasks. Finally, the landmark detection accuracy depends on the subsequent applications. For example, for body region detection, exact 3D point positions are not needed; for registration, accurate landmarks are desired.

Landmark Detection Methods

State-of-the-art landmark detection methods are based on statistical learning [50]. In this paradigm, each landmark has a dedicated detector [32, 55]. In [37], volumes have consistent field of view, e.g., the database consists of only liver scans. In such a case, it is possible to predefine a region of interest (ROI) for each landmark detector. In general, however, the position of each landmark can vary significantly across different scans; in most cases, some landmarks such as the head or toe are not even present in a body scan. Under such cases, running multiple detectors independently of each other can result in false detections [32, 39]. To handle the problem of false detections, one can exploit the spatial relationship information between landmarks to reduce false detections. A model for describing the spatial relationship between landmarks is the Markov Random Field [4, 5].

Another important factor to consider when designing multiple landmark detectors is speed. Naively running each detector on the whole volume yields a time complexity proportional to the number of detectors and volume size. This poses significant computational resources when the number of landmarks of interest is large, or when the volumes are large. More efficient detection can be achieved with a sequential method [32]. This method assumes at least one of the landmark positions is known. Since the relative positions of landmarks in the human body are constrained (e.g., the kidney is below the heart in a typical CT scan), one can define a search range (sub-volume) for each unknown landmark relative to the known landmark positions. Detecting a landmark within a local search range instead of within the whole volume achieves faster speed.

In practice, however, none of the landmark positions is known a priori, and therefore the sequential method described above needs some pre-processing work to find the first landmark, also called the anchor landmark [32]. There are two major difficulties in finding the anchor landmark. First, as mentioned earlier, detectors are prone to false positives when used alone. This poses a chicken-and-egg problem: To find the anchor landmark robustly, we need to rely on the positions of other landmarks, which are, however, unknown. A second problem exists, even if the detectors had zero false positive rates: typical CT scans have small (partial) field-of-view, as opposed to imaging the whole body from head to toe. Since we do not know which landmarks are present in a partial field-of-view volume, it would require trying many detectors, each one running in the whole volume, until a landmark is found present. This process is a computational bottleneck of the sequential method. In other words, the key problem in the sequential method is to find the anchor landmark robustly and efficiently. This brings us to the topic of context exploitation in the next section.

Context Exploitation

Designing a useful landmark detection method should effectively exploit the rich contextual information manifested in the body scans, which can be generally categorized as *unary* (or *first-order*), *pairwise* (or *higher-order*), and *holistic* context.

The *unary context* refers to the local regularity surrounding a single landmark. The classical object detection approach in [49, 50] exploits the unary context to learn a series of supervised classifier to separate the positive object (herein landmark) from negative background. The complexity of this approach depends on the volume size.

The *pairwise or higher-order context* refers to the joint regularities between two landmarks or among multiple landmarks. Liu et al. [32] embed the pairwise spatial contexts among all landmarks into a submodular formulation that minimizes the combined search range for detecting multiple landmarks. Here the landmark detector is still learned by exploiting the unary context. In [55], the pairwise spatial context is used to compute the information gain that guides an active scheduling scheme for detecting multiple landmarks. Seifert et al. [44] encoded pairwise spatial contexts into a discriminative anatomical network.

The *holistic context* goes beyond the relationship among a cohort of landmarks and refers to the whole relationship between all voxels and the landmarks; in other words, regarding the image as a whole. In [58], shape regression machine is proposed to learn a boosting regression function to predict the object bounding box from the image appearance bounded in an arbitrarily located box and another regression function to predict the object shape. Pauly et al. [38] simultaneously regress out the locations and sizes of multiple organs with confidence scores using a learned Random Forest regressor. To some extent, image registration [22] can be regarded as using the holistic context.

In [32], no holistic context is used. Instead, the aforementioned "anchor landmark" is searched to trigger the whole detection process. There are two major problems of finding the anchor landmark. First, as mentioned earlier, detectors are prone to false positives when used alone. Detecting the "anchor landmark" utilizes only the unary context in exhaustive scanning. Since any false positive detection of the "anchor landmark" causes catastrophe in detecting the remaining ones, sometimes it requires trying many detectors, each one running in the whole volume, until a landmark is found present.

In this chapter we present an approach that leverages all three types of contexts. It consists of two steps:

- The first step uses nearest neighbor (NN) matching, which exploits holistic context to perform matching and transfers landmark annotations. This is significantly different from the regression approach as in [58] which scans through the image searching for landmarks. This is also different from the "anchor landmark" approach in [32]. Detecting the "anchor landmark" utilizes only the unary context in exhaustive scanning. Since any false positive detection of the "anchor landmark" causes catastrophe in detecting the remaining ones, sometimes it requires trying many detectors, each one running in the whole volume, until a landmark with very high confidence score is found. Finally we achieve a much faster algorithm for detecting landmarks.

- The second step uses submodular optimization to minimize overall computation time. The method exploits both unary and pairwise contexts and aims to minimize the overall computation. The approach was first introduced in [32] to minimize the total search range and later extended to minimize overall computation time in [31] by modifying the cost function in the submodular formulation.

Coarse Landmark Detection Using Nearest Neighbor Matching

Our method consists of two steps. The first step is coarse detection and involves finding a rough position estimate for all landmarks. After coarse detection, we refine the landmark positions through landmark detectors. This section focuses on the coarse detection step.

Assume that a volume is represented by a D-dimensional feature vector. Given a query (unseen input) vector $x \in R^D$, the problem is to find the element y^* in a finite set Y of vectors to minimize the distance to the query vector:

$$y^* = \arg \min_{y \in Y} d(x, y) \tag{1}$$

where $d(.,.)$ is the Euclidean distance function. Other choices can be used too. Once y^* is found, the coarse landmark position estimates are obtained through a "transfer" operation, to be detailed in section "Transferring Landmark Annotations".

Volume Features

To facilitate the matching, we represent each volume by a D-dimensional feature vector. In particular, we adopt a representation of the image using "global features" that provide a holistic description as in [47], where a 2D image is divided into 4×4 regions, eight oriented Gabor filters are applied over four different scales, and the average filter energy in each region is used as a feature, yielding in total 512 features. For 3D volumes, we compute such features from nine 2D images, consisting of the sagittal, axial, and coronal planes that pass through 25 %, 50 %, and 75 % of the respective volume dimension, resulting a 4,608-dimensional feature vector.

Efficient Nearest Neighbor Search

In practice, finding the closest (most similar) volume through evaluating the exact distances is too expensive when the database size is large and the data dimensionality is high. Two efficient approximations are used for speedup. Vector quantization [33] is used to address the database size issue and product quantization [24] for the data dimensionality issue.

A quantizer is a function $q(.)$ mapping a D-dimensional vector x to a vector $q(x) \in Q = \{q_i, i = 1, 2, \ldots, K\}$. The finite set Q is called the codebook, which consists of K centroids. The set of vectors mapped to the same centroid forms a Voronoi cell, defined as $V_i = \{x \in R^D | q(x) = q_i\}$. The K Voronoi cells partition the space of R^D. The quality of a quantizer is often measured by the mean squared error between an input vector and its representative centroid $q(x)$. We use the K-means algorithm [33] to find a near-optimal codebook. During the search stage, which has high speed requirement, distance evaluation between the query and a database vector consists of computing the distance between the query vector and the nearest centroid of the database vector.

These volume feature vectors are high dimensional (we use $D = 4{,}608$ dimensions), which poses difficulty for a straightforward implementation of the K-means quantization described above. A quantizer that uses only $1/3$ bits per dimension already has 2^{1536} centroids. Such a large number of centroids make it impossible to run the K-means algorithm in practice. Product quantization [24] addresses this issue by splitting the high-dimensional feature vector into m distinct sub-vectors as follows,

$$\underbrace{x_1, \ldots, x_{D^*}}_{u_1(x)}, \ldots, \underbrace{x_{D-D^*+1}, \ldots, x_D}_{u_m(x)} \qquad (2)$$

The quantization is subsequently performed on the m sub-vectors $q^1(u_1(x)), \ldots, q^m(u_m(x))$, where q^i, $i = 1, \ldots, m$ denote m different quantizers. In the special case where $m = D$, product quantization is equivalent to scalar quantization, which has the lowest memory requirement but does not capture any correlation across feature dimensions. In the extreme case where $m = 1$, product quantization is equivalent to traditional quantization, which fully captures the correlation among different features but has the highest (and practically impossible, as explained earlier) memory requirement. We use $m = 1{,}536$ and $K = 4$ (2 bits per quantizer).

A Note on Product Quantization and Related Work

The explosion of the amount of digital content has stimulated search methods for large-scale databases. An exhaustive comparison of a query with all items in a database can be prohibitive. Approximate nearest neighbors (ANN) search methods are invented to handle large databases, at the same time seeking a balance between efficiency and accuracy. Such methods aim at finding the nearest neighbor with high probability. Several multi-dimensional indexing methods, such as KD-tree [16], have been proposed to reduce the search time. However, for high-dimensional feature vectors, such approaches are not more efficient than the brute-force exhaustive distance calculation, whose complexity is linear with the database size and the data representation dimension [24].

One of the most popular ANN techniques is Locality-Sensitive Hashing [10]. However, most of these approaches are memory consuming. The method of [54] embeds the vector into a binary space and improves the memory constraint. However, it is outperformed in terms of the trade-off between accuracy and memory usage by the Product Quantization method [24].

Volume Size Clustering

The anisotropic resampling of volumes into the same size, as done in section "Volume Features", causes distortion in appearance. This could have negative impact on nearest neighbor search. For example, when a head scan and a whole body scan are resampled to the same number of voxels, their appearances could become more similar than they were in their original sizes, and hence negatively affecting the results in Eq. (1). We use the K-means algorithm [33] to cluster all database volumes into 30 categories based on the volume's physical dimensions. Given a query volume, it is first assigned to the category of volumes with similar physical sizes. Nearest neighbor search is then only performed within this category.

Transferring Landmark Annotations

Given a query, we use the aforementioned method to find the most similar database volume. Assume this database volume consists of N landmarks with positions $\{s_1,\ldots,s_N\}$. We simply "transfer" these landmark positions to the query, as illustrated in Fig. 2. In other words, the coarsely detected landmark positions are set as $\{s_1,\ldots,s_N\}$. In the next section, we discuss how to refine these positions.

Fine Landmark Detection with Submodular Optimization

After the step of NN matching, certain landmarks are located roughly. We now trigger the landmark detectors to search for a more precise position for each landmark only within local search ranges predicted from the first stage results. Running a landmark detector locally instead of over the whole volume reduces the

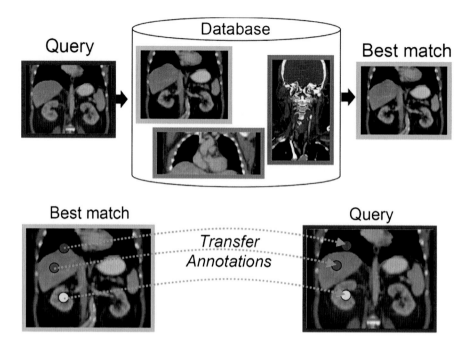

Fig. 2 Coarse landmark detection, a 2D illustration. Real system operates on 3D volumes. *Upper figure*: nearest neighbor search. *Lower figure*: annotated positions of database volume are transferred to query. The real system operates on 3D volumes

computation and also reduces false positive detections. The local search range of each detector is obtained off-line based on spatial statistics that capture the relative position of each pair of landmarks. Note that the two sets of landmarks in two stages can be different.

In order to speed up the detection, the order of triggering the landmark detectors needs to be considered. This is because, once a landmark position is refined by a detector, we can further reduce the local search ranges for the other landmarks by using the pairwise spatial statistics that embody the *pairwise context*.

The main goal in this section is to minimize the computational cost of multiple landmark detection. The computational cost is controlled by (1) the size of the image subspace (or *search space*) in which a detector is performing the search and (2) the unit cost of the landmark detector. We will first focus on item (1), and later extend the framework to item (2).

Having n landmarks detected, with $N - n$ landmarks remaining to detect, which detector should one use next, and where should it be applied, so that the overall computational cost is minimized? These two questions are tightly related, and the answer is simple: *determine the search space for each detector based on the already detected landmarks and pick the detector that has the smallest search space.* We will show theoretical guarantees of the algorithm in section "Greedy Algorithm",

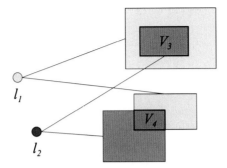

Fig. 3 Illustration of the search space definition in Eq. (4). Detected landmarks l_1 and l_2 provide search spaces for un-detected landmarks l_3 and l_4 (not shown). Final search spaces V_3 and V_4 for l_3 and l_4 are obtained by intersection. A greedy algorithm would prefer landmark l_4 over l_3 as the next landmark to detect since V_4 is smaller than V_3

and then in section "Another Search Space Criteria" extend the algorithm to take multiple factors into account, including the size of the search space and the unit cost of the detector (classifier).

Search Space

In sequential detection, landmarks already detected provide spatial constraints on the landmarks remaining to be detected. Consider an object consisted of N distinct landmarks. Denote by

$$\Lambda_{(1):(n)} = \{l_{(1)} \prec l_{(2)} \prec \ldots \prec l_{(n)}\}, n \leq N, \qquad (3)$$

the ordered set of detected landmarks. Denote by U the un-ordered set of landmarks that remains to be detected. For each landmark $l_i \in U$, its search space Ω_{l_i} is determined jointly by landmarks in $\Lambda_{(1):(n)}$, for example, by the intersection of the individual search spaces,

$$\Omega_{l_i}(\Lambda_{(1):(n)}) = \bigcap_{j, l_j \in \Lambda_{(1):(n)}} \Omega_{l_i}(\{l_j\}), \qquad (4)$$

where $\Omega_{l_i}(\{l_j\})$ denotes the search space for landmark l_i conditioned on the position of a detected landmark l_j. This is illustrated in Fig. 3. This definition could be restrictive, so we will discuss alternatives in sections "Another Search Space Criteria" and "Multiple Search Space Criteria".

Denote the search volume (or search area) of search space $\Omega_{l_i}(\Lambda)$ as $V(\Omega_{l_i}(\Lambda))$, which calculates the volume of $\Omega_{l_i}(\Lambda)$. Without loss of generality, assume the search volume is the cardinality of the set of voxels (pixels) that fall within the search space. Define the constant $\Omega_\phi \equiv \Omega_k(\phi), \forall k$, as the space of the whole image, which is a tight upper bound of the search space. The search volume has the following property:

Theorem 1 $\forall S \subseteq T$,

$$V(\Omega(S)) - V(\Omega(S \cup \{l\})) \geq V(\Omega(T)) - V(\Omega(T \cup \{l\})) \tag{5}$$

Set functions satisfying the above property are called *supermodular* [43].

Let us simplify the notation by omitting the subscript l_i from Ω_{l_i}. Define the complement $\overline{\Omega(S)} = \Omega_\phi \setminus \Omega(S), \forall S$, where Ω_ϕ has earlier been defined as the space of the whole volume.

Lemma 1 $\Omega(S \cup \{l\}) = \Omega(S) \cap \Omega(\{l\})$

This follows from the definition.

Lemma 2 *If* $S \subseteq T$, *then* $\Omega(S) \supseteq \Omega(T)$

Proof $T = S \cup (T \setminus S) \Rightarrow$ From Lemma 1, $\Omega(T) = \Omega(S \cup (T \setminus S)) = \Omega(S) \cap \Omega(T \setminus S) \subseteq \Omega(S)$.

Lemma 3 $\Omega(S) \setminus \Omega(S \cup \{l\}) = \Omega(S) \cap \overline{\Omega(\{l\})}$

Proof 　　 LHS $= \Omega(S) \setminus (\Omega(S) \cap \Omega(\{l\})) = \Omega(S) \cap \overline{(\Omega(S) \cap \Omega(\{l\}))} = \Omega(S) \cap (\overline{\Omega(S)} \cup \overline{\Omega(\{l\})}) = (\Omega(S) \cap \overline{\Omega(S)}) \cup (\Omega(S) \cap \overline{\Omega(\{l\})}) =$ RHS.

Lemma 4 *If* $\Omega(T) \subseteq \Omega(S)$, *then* $V(\Omega(S) \setminus \Omega(T)) = V(\Omega(S)) - V(\Omega(T))$

Lemma 5 *If* $\Omega(T) \subseteq \Omega(S)$, *then* $V(\Omega(T)) \leq V(\Omega(S))$

Finally we prove the supermodularity of $V(\Omega(.))$ in Theorem 1.

Proof of Theorem 1 From Lemma 2, $\Omega(S) \supseteq \Omega(T)$. Then $\Omega(S) \cap \overline{\Omega(\{l\})} \supseteq \Omega(T) \cap \overline{\Omega(\{l\})}$. From Lemma 3, we have $\Omega(S) \setminus \Omega(S \cup \{l\}) \supseteq \Omega(T) \setminus \Omega(T \cup \{l\})$. From Lemma 5, we have $V(\Omega(S) \setminus \Omega(S \cup \{l\})) \geq V(\Omega(T) \setminus \Omega(T \cup \{l\}))$. From Lemma 4, Q.E.D.

Lemma 6 $F(.)$ *in Eq.* (7) *is nondecreasing.*

Proof From Lemma 2 and Lemma 5, we have $\forall S \subseteq T$, we have $V(\Omega(T)) \leq V(\Omega(S))$, which shows $V(.)$ is nonincreasing. Consequently, $F(.)$ is nondecreasing.

Greedy Algorithm

The goal is to find the ordered set $\Lambda_{(2):(N)}$ that minimizes the cumulated search volume, i.e. ,

$$\Lambda'_{(2):(N)} = \underset{\Lambda_{(2):(N)}}{\operatorname{argmin}} \sum_{i=2}^{N} V(\Omega_{l_{(i)}}(\Lambda_{(1):(i-1)})). \tag{6}$$

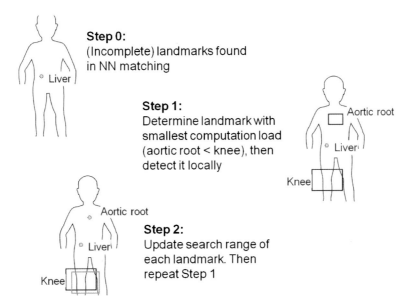

Fig. 4 Illustration of the greedy algorithm. Different box colors (*red* and *blue*) indicate search ranges provided by other landmarks (liver and aortic root)

Note that in Eq. (11) we do not include the first landmark l_1 as its search space is typically the whole image when no landmarks have been detected a priori. The first landmark can be detected using the method in section "Transferring Landmark Annotations", or by the method in section "Finding the Anchor Landmark". We will discuss these different methods in detail in section "Comparing Holistic-Anchoring and Sequential-Anchoring".

Define the cost function $C_k(\Lambda) = V(\Omega_k(\Lambda)), \forall k$. A greedy algorithm for finding the ordering $\{l_{(1)},\ldots,l_{(N)}\}$ that attempts to minimize the overall cost is to iteratively select the detector that yields the smallest cost. This is illustrated in Fig. 4 and proceeds as follows.

> Initialize $\Lambda = \{l_{(1)}\}$
> **for** $j=2,\ldots,N$ **do**
> $\quad\mid\quad l_{(j)} = \arg\min_k C_k(\Lambda_{(1):(j-1)})$
> $\quad\mid\quad$ Append $l_{(j)}$ to the ordered set $\Lambda_{(1):(j-1)}$
> **end**

This simple algorithm has nice theoretical properties. Define

$$F_k(\Lambda) = C_k(\phi) - C_k(\Lambda) \qquad (7)$$

Hence, $F_k(\phi) = 0$. From Lemma 6, $F_k(.)$ is a nondecreasing set function. From Eq. (1) and (7), $\forall S \subseteq T$,

$$F_k(S) - F_k(S \cup \{l\}) \leq F_k(T) - F_k(T \cup \{l\}) \qquad (8)$$

which means $F_k(.)$ is *submodular* [43]. Furthermore, since $C_k(\phi)$ is constant over k, Eq. (11) becomes

$$\Lambda'_{(2):(N)} = \underset{\Lambda_{(2):(N)}}{\operatorname{argmax}} \sum_{k=2}^{N} F_k \left(\Lambda_{(1):(k-1)} \right). \tag{9}$$

Lemma 7 $F(.) = \sum F_k(.)$ is submodular if $\forall k$, $F_k(.)$ is submodular [43].

Together, these properties bring us to the theorem that states the theoretical guarantee of the greedy algorithm.

Theorem 2 *If $F(.)$ is a submodular, nondecreasing set function, and $F(\phi) = 0$, then the greedy algorithm finds a set Λ', such that $F(\Lambda') \geq (1 - 1/e) \max F(\Lambda)$ [36].*

Optimizing submodular functions is in general NP-hard [34]. One must in principle calculate the values of $N!$ detector ordering patterns. Yet, the greedy algorithm is guaranteed to find an ordered set Λ such that $F(.)$ reaches at least 63 % of the optimal value.

Note that the ordering found by the algorithm is image-dependent, since the search space of the next detector is dependent on the position of the landmarks already detected. Therefore, the algorithm is not performing an "off-line" scheduling of detectors. For another example, when the search space of a landmark is outside the image or if its detection score is too low, then this landmark is claimed missing. This would influence the subsequent detectors through the definition of the search space and affect the final ordering.

Another Search Space Criteria

Another useful definition of search space can be defined as follows:

$$\Omega_{l_i}(\Lambda) = \min_{l \in \Lambda} \left\{ \Omega_{l_i}(l) \right\} \tag{10}$$

In each round of the greedy algorithm, each detected landmark provides a search space candidate for each un-detected landmark. Each un-detected landmark then selects the smallest one among the provided candidates. The greedy algorithm then selects the un-detected landmark that has the smallest search space. This is illustrated in Fig. 5. We call this search space criteria the *min-rule*, and the one in section "Search Space" the *intersection-rule*.

Denote $m_{l_i}(S) = argmin_{l \in S} \Omega_{l_i}(\{l\})$ as the landmark in the set of detected landmarks S that provides the smallest search range for detector l_i. Here we show that this definition also satisfies Theorem 1.

Lemma 8 $\forall S \subseteq T, V\ (\Omega(S)) \geq V\ (\Omega(T))$

Proof From definition, $\Omega(S) = \min_{l \in S} \Omega(\{l\})$, and $\Omega(T) = \min_{l \in T} \Omega(\{l\})$. Since $S \subseteq T$, we have $\Omega(S) \geq \Omega(T)$, and hence $V\ (\Omega(S)) \geq V\ (\Omega(T))$.

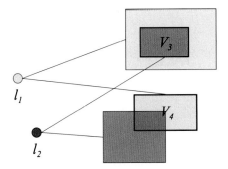

Fig. 5 Illustration of the search space definition in Eq. (10). Detected landmarks l_1 and l_2 provide search spaces for un-detected landmarks l_3 and l_4 (not shown). Final search spaces V_3 and V_4 for l_3 and l_4 are the minimum sets. This time, a greedy algorithm would prefer landmark l_3 over l_4 as the next landmark to detect since V_3 is smaller than V_4

Proof of Theorem 1

Case (i): $m_{l_i}(T) = m_{l_i}(T \cup \{l\})$. This means including l does not decrease the search space, and hence $V(\Omega(T)) = V(\Omega(T \cup \{l\}))$. But from Lemma 8, $V(\Omega(S)) \geq V(\Omega(S \cup \{l\}))$ always holds. Hence $V(\Omega(S)) - V(\Omega(S \cup \{l\})) \geq V(\Omega(T)) - V(\Omega(T \cup \{l\}))$.

Case (ii): $m_{l_i}(T) \neq m_{l_i}(T \cup \{l\})$. This means l provides a smaller search space than any other landmark in T, and hence $m_{l_i}(\{l\}) = m_{l_i}(T \cup \{l\})$. Since $S \subseteq T$, we also have $m_{l_i}(\{l\}) = m_{l_i}(S \cup \{l\})$. Hence, $V(\Omega(S \cup \{l\})) = V(\Omega(T \cup \{l\}))$. But from Lemma 8, $V(\Omega(S)) \geq V(\Omega(T))$ always holds. Hence $V(\Omega(S)) - V(\Omega(S \cup \{l\})) \geq V(\Omega(T)) - V(\Omega(T \cup \{l\}))$.

Multiple Search Space Criteria

Since submodularity is closed under linear combination with nonnegative scalars [43], multiple submodular functions can be optimized simultaneously. For example, one could combine the min-rule and intersection-rule. Note that the set of individual search spaces $\{\Omega_{l_i}(\{l_j\})\}_{i,j=1,\dots,N}$ need not be the same for the min- and intersection-rules. Under this combination, some detectors could obtain a search range from the min-rule, and some from the intersection-rule.[1, 2]

---

[1] If $\Omega_{l_i}(\{l_j\}), \forall i, j$, were the same for min- and intersection-rules, then the intersection-rule will always be selected, since the intersection operation yields non-larger spaces than individual ones.

[2] Linear combination is a common approach for finding Pareto-optimal solutions [6]. Since it can happen that $F_i(S) > F_i(T)$ while $F_j(T) > F_j(S)$, all we can hope for are Pareto-optimal solutions [6].

Cost of Detector

The algorithm introduced so far only considered the search space. In practice, different detectors have different costs and this should be taken into account during optimization. For example, if we have two detectors, then the algorithm above would select the next detector that has a smaller search space. However, this detector might have a much higher unit computational cost due to, for example, higher model complexity. One should multiply (and not linearly combine) search volume with the unit cost, since a detector is applied to *each* voxel within the search space and only the product reflects the cost correctly.

Fortunately, multiplication of a submodular function by a nonnegative scalar also maintains submodularity [43]. Denote q_i as the computational cost of detector i. The product $q_i C(\Omega_{l_i}(\Lambda))$ then considers the joint computational cost. Since $\forall i, q_i \geq 0, q_i C(\Omega_{l_i}(\Lambda))$ is submodular, the greedy algorithm can be applied and the same theoretical guarantees still hold.

The computational cost of a detector (classifier) can be estimated from, for example, the number of weak learners in boosting-based classifiers [50], the expected number of classifiers in a cascade of classifiers [50], or the empirical running time. Denote by $\alpha[l_j]$ the unit computation cost for evaluating the detector for landmark l_j. The goal is then to find the ordered set $\Lambda_{(1):(N)}$ that minimizes the *total computation*, i.e.,

$$\Lambda'_{(1):(N)} = \underset{\Lambda_{(1):(N)}}{argmin} \{\alpha[l_{(1)}] \, V(\Omega[l_{(1)}]) + \sum_{i=2}^{N} \alpha[l_{(i)}] V(\Omega[l_{(i)}|\Lambda_{(1):(i-1)}])\}. \quad (11)$$

When $\alpha[l_j] = 1$ for all j, this reduces to searching the minimum overall search range. We find that unit computation cost is roughly proportional to the physical disk size needed to store the detector model; hence, we set $\alpha[l(i)]$ as the model disk size.

The *greedy algorithm* for finding the ordering $\{l_{(1)}, \ldots, l_{(N)}\}$ that attempts to minimize the overall cost proceeds as follows:

> Initialize $\Lambda = \phi$.
>
> **for** $j=1, \ldots, N$ **do**
> $\quad$ $l_{(j)} = \arg\min_k \alpha[k] V(\Omega[k|\Lambda])$;
> $\quad$ Append $l_{(j)}$ to the ordered set Λ so that the new $\Lambda = l_{(1)}, \ldots, l_{(j)}$.
> **end**

In other words, in each round one triggers the detector that yields the smallest computation.

Again, *the greedy algorithm is guaranteed to find an ordered set Λ such that the invoked cost is at least 63 % of its optimal value* [32]! It is worth emphasizing that the ordering found by the algorithm is data-dependent and determined in run-time on the fly.

Finding the Anchor Landmark

The algorithm in the previous section finds an image-dependent ordering of detectors assuming at least one landmark $l_{(1)}$ has already been detected. We call $l_{(1)}$ the *anchor landmark*. Note that the anchor landmark can be a different landmark for different images. In section "Coarse Landmark Detection Using Nearest Neighbor Matching" we presented an approach for finding a coarse position estimate of certain landmarks based on NN matching. We call it the holistic-anchoring approach. An alternative approach was presented in [32], which finds the anchor landmark through running individual detectors. We call it the sequential-anchoring approach. Here we review this alternative approach and compare it with the holistic-anchoring approach in section "Comparing Holistic-Anchoring and Sequential-Anchoring"

Define $f(l)$ as the estimated frequency of appearance of landmark l in an image. Then, define the ordering of trials

$$m_1 = \arg\max_l\{f(l_1), \ldots, f(l_N)\} \tag{12a}$$

$$m_2 = \arg\max_l\{f(l_1), \ldots, f(l_N) | m_1 \text{not present}\} \tag{12b}$$

$$m_3 = \arg\max_l\{f(l_1), \ldots, f(l_N) | m_1, m_2 \text{not present}\} \tag{12c}$$

and so on. We can use this ordering of trials to detect the anchor landmark. Intuitively, since landmark m_1 appears most frequently, searching for it in the first trial would reduce most significantly the need for a subsequent trial (whole-image search). Landmark m_2 is the most frequent landmark under the condition that m_1 does not exist in the volume. This conditioning is to avoid m_2 being a landmark that is in the vicinity of m_1, in which case if m_1 is occluded, most likely m_2 is also occluded.

Since all of the detectors have similar accuracy and computational cost, such an ordering based on conditional frequency performs well. However, if some detectors have very different accuracy or cost than the others, those characteristics should also be taken into account.

The system starts with detecting the anchor landmark and initiates the greedy algorithm. If the greedy algorithm determines a search space but the corresponding detector fails to find the landmark, the greedy algorithm simply proceeds to the next round. If all subsequent landmarks are not found, the system is restarted with a different anchor landmark. The chance that the system produces more false positives than running the detectors independently is low. This is because, while the false positive rate of each detector could be high, the chance that multiple detectors produce false positives within their assigned search spaces is exponentially low. In fact there is a relationship between the overall false positive rate, detection rate, and the size of the individual search spaces. We have experiments and discussions on this topic in section "A Spatial Cascade of Classifiers".

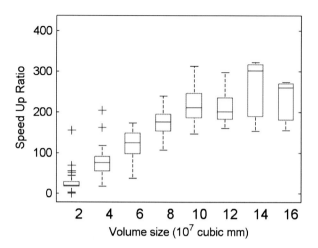

Fig. 6 Speedup ratio vs. volume size when comparing holistic-anchoring and sequential-anchoring for detecting body regions

Comparing Holistic-Anchoring and Sequential-Anchoring

In this experiment, we use the NN matching for detecting body regions that need rough landmark locations by utilizing the holistic context. This matching-based approach requires a database sufficiently large so that, given a query, the best match in the training database indeed covers the same body region(s) as the query. We collect 2,500 volumes annotated with 60 anatomical landmarks, including the left/right lung tops, aortic arch, femur heads, liver top, liver center, coccyx tip, etc. We use 500 volumes for constructing the training database and the remaining 2,000 volumes for testing. To ensure that each query finds a good match, we construct the database of 100,000 volumes in a near-exhaustive manner: In each iteration, we randomly pick one of the 500 volumes and then randomly crop and slightly rotate it into a new volume before adding it to the database. The annotated anatomical landmark positions in the original volume are transformed accordingly. The system runs on an Intel Xeon 2.33GHz CPU with 3GB RAM (Fig. 6).

Registration-based methods are not applicable since the test volumes cover a large variety of body regions. If each region is detected separately say using [49], the total detection time is proportional to the number of regions, as detecting each region requires a scan over the whole volume. The work in [8] reports a detection time around 2,000 ms for 9 landmarks, and median distance error around 22 mm on a GPU (parallelized) implementation. The work in [32] has the highest accuracy and fastest speed, so we compare against this work in better detail. As in Fig. 6 and Fig. 7, the implementation of [32], which is tuned to a similar detection accuracy as shown in Table 1, has a detection time of 450 ms for 6 landmarks that define the presence of right lung, skull, aorta, sternum, and liver; but the maximum time is 4.9 s, significantly larger than the median. This poses a problem for time critical subsequent tasks. The holistic-anchoring method has a nearly constant detection

	Median time(ms)	Average of Median errors (mm)
Sequential-anchoring	450	28.6
Holistic-anchoring	5	29.9

Fig. 7 The performance of detecting body regions using holistic-anchoring vs. sequential-anchoring

Table 1 Median detection errors (mm) for 6 different landmarks that define 5 body regions

	Sequential-anchoring	Holistic-anchoring
Lung apex right	24.1	27.1
Skull base	31.9	19.1
Aortic root	23.2	35.8
Lung center	20.6	24.5
Sternum bottom	37.3	35.1
Liver center	35.2	37.9

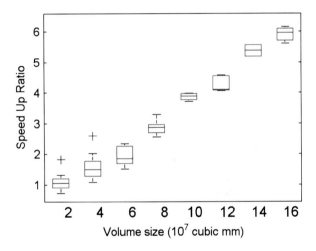

Fig. 8 Speedup ratio vs. volume size when comparing holistic-anchoring and sequential-anchoring for detecting the liver top

time of 5 ms, achieving a speedup of 90 times while maintaining similar detection accuracy. The speedup is even more significant if more regions are of interest as the detection does not depend on the number of regions. The NN matching code can be optimized and parallelized for faster speed. In general, a large detection error from NN matching, which is fine for body region detection purpose, is due to the large variability in the landmark appearance and its relative location to other landmarks.

When accurate positions are desired, we combine the holistic-matching with landmark detectors that exploit unary context. Now each landmark detector only needs to search in a local neighborhood around the rough position estimate given by the first stage, instead of searching in the whole volume. For detection of multiple landmarks, we further utilize pairwise spatial context for more improvements (Fig. 8).

Fig. 9 Performance
comparison of accurately
detecting the liver top

	Median time (ms)	Average of Median errors (mm)
Baseline [49]	340	1.3
Our method	**165**	1.3

Table 2 Errors (mm) in
accurately detecting
7 different landmarks
using NN matching and
submodular optimization

(mm)	Mean	Q95	Mean [32]
Trachea bifurcation	**2.5**	4.5	2.8
Left Lung Top	**2.6**	6.0	3.2
Right Lung Top	**3.2**	8.5	3.7
Liver Top	**2.5**	4.0	2.9
Liver Bottom	**6.4**	30.5	n.a.
Left Kidney Center	8.4	50.7	**6.3**
Right Kidney Center	**6.4**	39.2	7.0

Detecting One Landmark

We consider detecting the liver top. In Fig. 8 and Fig. 9, the baseline approach uses
a Probabilistic Boosting Tree (PBT) [49] to scan through the whole volume. Our
method uses the PBT only to search in a local neighborhood. Evidently our method
is much faster than the state-of-the-art due to the additional leverage of holistic
context. A bigger volume yields more pronounced speedup (as large as six-fold) as
the use of holistic context breaks down the dependency on volume size.

Detecting Multiple Landmarks

We further experiment accurately detecting 7 landmarks listed in Table 2 with three
example landmarks of trachea bifurcation, liver bottom, and left kidney center
shown in Fig. 10. Table 2 presents the mean detection error and the 95th percentile
error that exhibits the robustness of the combined approach. The results in [32] are
also included for comparison. We obtain better detection results except for the left
kidney center, whose annotations are quite ambiguous, while consuming less time
with a mean computation of 1.1s vs 1.3s for [32]. Due to space limitation, we omit
the results of other anatomical landmarks.

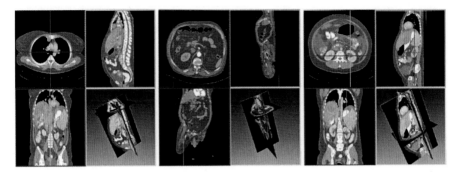

Fig. 10 Detected positions of trachea bifurcation, liver bottom, and left kidney center

Coarse-to-Fine Detection

In earlier discussions, we assumed each landmark is associated with a single detector. In implementation, a landmark has $R = 3$ detectors, each trained at different resolutions. Since training of landmark detectors is not the focus of this paper, we refer the reader to prior work in [49, 50]. In detection, we employ a coarse-to-fine strategy. Such multi-resolution techniques are frequently encountered when the solution to the original (high) resolution is either too complex to consider directly or subject to large numbers of local minima. The general idea is to construct approximate, coarser versions of the problem and to use the solution of the coarser problems to guide solutions at finer scales.

We run the algorithm in section "Finding the Anchor Landmark" using the coarsest-resolution detectors only. We then define a local (small) search space around each detected landmark and run higher resolution detectors within the local search space. The overall approach is efficient, because the coarse-resolution detectors have already rejected most of the voxels in the image.

At the end, the posterior probability of position x is taken from all resolutions using a log-linear model

$$p(x|I_{r_1}, \ldots, I_{r_R}) \propto \exp\left(\sum_{i=1}^{R} \alpha_{r_i} \phi_{r_i}(x)\right) \qquad (13)$$

where I_{r_i} is the volume at resolution r_i, $p(x|I_{r_i})$ is the posterior probability from the detector with resolution r_i, and the potential functions are given by $\phi_{r_i}(x) = \log p(x|I_{r_i})$. This can be shown equivalent to a products-of-experts model [21]. We also experimented with the mixture-of-experts model [23] of the form

$$p(x|I_{r_1}, \ldots, I_{r_R}) \propto \sum_{i=1}^{R} \alpha_{r_i} p(x|I_{r_i}). \qquad (14)$$

Table 3 Detection time (sec) per volume. N is the number of landmarks in the system

	Mean	Std	Q95	Max
Independent D_{8mm} $N = 63$	17.30	6.16	46.24	84.51
Greedy D_{8mm} $N = 63$	1.14	0.47	1.92	2.44
Independent D_{8mm} $N = 25$	6.72	6.40	17.73	35.00
Greedy D_{8mm} $N = 25$	0.65	0.43	1.26	5.08
Greedy D_{4mm} $N = 25$	1.30	0.87	3.30	6.11
Greedy D_{2mm} $N = 25$	2.70	1.74	7.15	9.05

While the products-of-experts tends to produce sharper classification boundaries, the mixture-of-experts tends to have a higher tolerance to poor probability estimates [27]. Our experiments suggest the use of the mixture-of-experts.

Notice that each position is associated with multiple subwindows at different resolutions, so a larger amount of local context is utilized. Using context in object detection is discussed in prior work [49, 50]. Our approach combines results from multiple resolutions and different subwindow sizes and hence is different from approaches where a single, optimal window size is determined [51].

In the following experiment, the database consists of 2046 volumes. We split the data into 70 % training, 10 % validation, and 20 % testing, while avoiding splitting a patient with multiple scans into both training and testing. The pairwise search spaces, $\Omega_{l_i}(\{l_j\})$, for each pair of landmarks l_i, l_j, are cuboids estimated from training and validation data. Using only training data to define a tight cuboid for one landmark given another could result in too confined search spaces if the detectors have large errors in testing. We obtain this error information from the validation set and enlarge the cuboids accordingly.

We have 63 landmarks including positions such as the center, top, and bottom of organs, bones, and bifurcations of vessels. In Table 3 we show the speed of landmark detection when all landmarks are detected independently versus the proposed method with the min-rule. Q95 is the 95th percentile. D_{8mm} denotes the system using detectors trained at 8 mm resolution running the greedy method (without coarse-to-fine), D_{4mm} uses the coarse-to-fine strategy with 8 and 4 mm resolution detectors, and D_{2mm} uses detectors at all three (8,4, and 2mm) resolutions.

Table 3 also includes experiments where only a subset of 25 landmarks are used in the system. We observe that the detection time of the greedy approach is not linearly proportional to the number of landmarks. In fact, when using "fewer" landmarks, the maximum time "increased" from 2.44 to 5.08 s. This can be understood because the search space of each detector is provided by the landmarks already detected, some of which are not present in the 25-detector system.

The detection speed versus volume size is shown in Fig. 11. The reason that smaller volumes do not consume much less time can be understood from Fig. 12, which shows that smaller volumes often require more number of trials to find the anchor landmark. Since each trial requires a whole image search, detection time increases.

The detection errors of the coarse-to-fine strategy are shown in Table 4.

Fig. 11 Detection time as a function of volume size. *Blue* (+): independent landmark detectors. *Red* (x): Greedy search

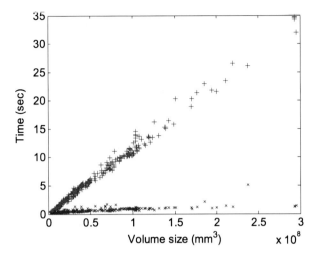

Fig. 12 Number of trials to find the anchor landmark as a function of volume size

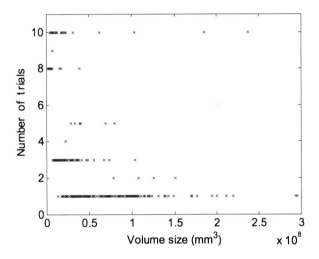

Table 4 Mean distance error in millimeters

	D_{8mm}	D_{4mm}	D_{2mm}
TracheaBif.	11.9	3.6	2.8
L.LungTop	22.2	3.5	3.2
R.LungTop	13.8	3.7	3.7
LiverDome	14.8	3.4	2.9
L.Kidney	13.6	6.7	6.3
R.Kidney	15.1	5.6	7.0

Two comparisons to recent literature can be made. First, the work in [8] reported a detection time around 2 s for 9 landmarks, and mean distance error around 28 mm. The system achieves lower distance errors in less time even on a standard

Table 5 Distance errors
in millimeters comparing
coarse-to-fine detection
using the product- and
mixture-of-experts

		Q25	Q50	Q95
Iliac Bifurcation	Baseline	6.76	13.96	22.72
	Product	4.67	8.43	**11.56**
	Mixture	**3.95**	**7.06**	13.99
Brachioc. Artery	Baseline	4.20	5.46	9.89
	Product	4.30	6.83	11.46
	Mixture	**3.63**	**5.19**	**8.77**

Intel Core2 Duo CPU 2.66GHz (whereas they used a GPU implementation for speedup). Second, the work in [55] reported larger distance errors (kidney error 9mm, versus 6 mm when using coarse-to-fine 8mm- and 4mm-resolution detectors) with detection time around 4 s for 6 landmarks, significantly slower than our system (1.3 s for 25 landmarks using coarse-to-fine 8mm- and 4mm-resolution detectors).

In Table 5 we compare the different coarse-to-fine approaches discussed in section "Coarse-to-Fine Detection". The baseline approach finds the top candidates at one resolution and initiates a finer-resolution detection around those top candidates. This has a shifting problem (much like in visual tracking) when only neighboring resolutions are considered and information from the earliest resolutions are lost. The mixture-of-experts often has the most accurate results and has reasonable tolerance to outliers.

Some detection results of vessels are shown in Fig. 13. Diseased vessels have high appearance variations, and yet we detect the carotid, iliac, renal, and brachiocephalic bifurcations with mean error 3.9, 7.2, 5.2, and 5.3 mm, respectively.

Table 6 shows confusion matrices of 8 mm detectors. This will be discussed further in section "A Spatial Cascade of Classifiers".

A Spatial Cascade of Classifiers

One might worry that a sequential detection approach could break down if the anchor landmark is incorrect or the first few detectors fail. Furthermore, the proposed search strategy was driven by computational cost considerations, and accuracy in terms of false positive rate and detection rate was not mentioned. Here we argue that the sequential "accept or reject" behavior of our method behaves similar to a Viola–Jones cascade of classifiers [50]. Intuitively, while the false positive rate of the first detector could be high, the rate that the first n detectors all fail is significantly lower.

More formally, if each detector has false positive rate f_i and detection rate d_i, the overall false positive rate and detection rate are $f = \prod f_i$ and $d = \prod d_i$ assuming independence. But f and d depend on the size of the search space, $\Omega_{l_i}(.)$. With a slight abuse of annotation, assume search space Ω_{l_i} is a cuboid, and $\lambda \Omega_{l_i}(.), \lambda > 0$, is

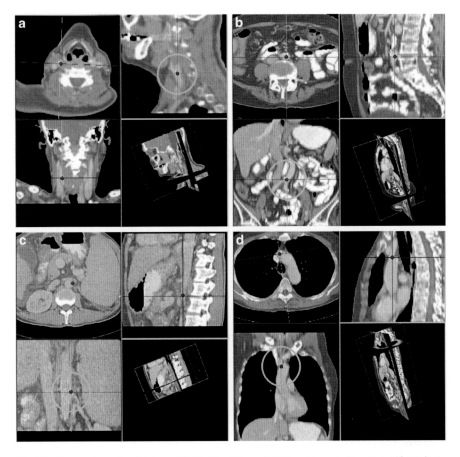

Fig. 13 Detected results of (**a**) carotid (**b**) iliac (**c**) renal (**d**) brachiocephalic artery bifurcations

an enlarged or shrunk cuboid with the same center. The operating point of the ROC curve can then be adjusted by tuning λ. As λ increases, the individual detectors behave more independently and there is less cascade-effect. As λ decreases, d_i and f_i decrease, and so do d and f. Tuning individual classifiers to adjust the overall f and d is also presented in the Viola–Jones cascade of classifiers.

On the other hand, in the Viola–Jones cascade, classifiers of the "same" landmark are chained together. Here, classifiers of "different" landmarks are chained and provide robustness through their joint spatial relationship. As shown in Table 6, this geometric cascade indeed reduces false positives without sacrificing the detection rate. Such a robustness property is desirable and is typically implemented by random fields [4, 5] or voting procedures [11]. If desired, one can still enforce a random field or perform voting on top of our method.

Table 6 Confusion matrices

	$F\,P_A$	$F\,N_A$	$F\,P_B$	$F\,N_B$
SkullBase	**0 (193)**	0 [50]	1 (192)	0 [50]
R.LungTop	**0 (84)**	1 [114]	1 (83)	1 [114]
LiverDome	0 (86)	2 [65]	0 [86]	2 [65]
R.HipTip	**0 (131)**	0 [94]	1 (130)	0 [94]
R.Knee	0 (265)	0 [12]	0 (265)	0 [12]
LiverBott.	2 (33)	1 [33]	2 (33)	1 [33]
TracheaBif.	0 (44)	0 [41]	0 (44)	0 [41]
LiverCent.	**0 (90)**	1 [136]	2 (88)	1 [136]
L.HumerusHead	0 (96)	1 [12]	0 (96)	1 [12]
R.HumerusHead	1 (80)	2 [7]	1 (80)	2 [7]
L.LungTop	**0 (61)**	1 [21]	1 (61)	1 [20]
L.HipTip	**0 (94)**	**1 [46]**	2 (92)	2 [45]
L.FemurHead	0 (124)	0 [16]	0 (124)	0 [16]
R.FemurHead	0 (120)	0 [16]	0 (120)	0 [16]
CoccyxTip	0 (118)	0 [16]	0 (118)	0 [16]
PubicSymph.Top	0 (133)	0 [23]	0 (133)	0 [23]
SternumTip	3 (51)	1 [22]	3 (51)	1 [22]
AortaBend	**0 (31)**	1 [53]	1 (30)	1 [53]
Brachioceph.	1 (35)	3 [132]	1 (35)	3 [132]
R.Kidney	2 (59)	5 [61]	2 (59)	5 [61]
L.Kidney	0 (71)	0 [76]	0 (71)	0 [76]

The first two columns (with subscript A) show the number of false positives and false negatives. Numbers in parentheses are the number of true negatives. Numbers in brackets are the number of true positives. The last two columns use detectors run independently. Detections with distance error larger than 5 voxels are false positives

Submodularity

The problem of maximizing a submodular function is of central importance, with special cases including Max Cut [19], maximum facility location [7]. While the graph Min Cut problem is a classical polynomial-time solvable problem, and more generally it has been shown that any submodular function can be "minimized" in polynomial time, maximization turns out to be an NP-hard problem [42]. The work of [32] is the first to apply the theory of submodularity to object detection. More specifically, we prove the submoduarity of the cost functions based on two search space criteria.

Information Gain and Entropy

Several works use maximization of information gain or entropy as objective function [28, 41, 55]. However, using information gain or entropy as objective could actually lead to arbitrary bad computation time!

Assume we have three landmarks, A, B, and C, with position x_A, x_B, x_C distributed along a 1-D line with position parameters $(\mu_A = 0, \Sigma_{AA} = 1), (\mu_B = 10, \Sigma_{BB} = 30),$ $(\mu_C = 10, \Sigma_{CC} = 110),$ and $\Sigma_{AB} = 5, \Sigma_{AC} = 110, \Sigma_{BC} = 50.$ This distribution could model the height of different people, with landmark A aligned with the CT scanner. Assume landmark A has already been detected. Which landmark should one detect next? The approach in [55] selects C since it yields a higher information gain than B. However, if the size of the search spaces of B and C are positively correlated with conditional covariance $\Sigma_{B|A}$ and $\Sigma_{C|A}$, the search space of B is actually smaller than the search space of C. Without considering other factors, this means the decision based on search space will be contrary to the one based on information gain. With different covariance matrices, the difference could be arbitrarily large. This can be understood when we realize that the objective of maximizing information gain does not have a direct relationship with saving computation time.

The advantages of information gain mentioned in those work, however, should not be neglected. Therefore, a framework that gracefully trades off between information gain and computation time would be useful.

Speedups

Other methods for reducing computational cost (from an algorithmic perspective, instead of hardware acceleration such as using GPU computing) in object detection include tree-structured search [20], coarse-to-fine detection [14], cascade of classifiers [50], branch-and-bound [29], reduction of classifier measurements [46], and searching in marginal space [57].

Multiple Objects of the Same Type in One Image

In medical imaging, most anatomical structures have distinct appearances. Real-world image datasets (such as those obtained from hand-held cameras and camcorders) including the PASCAL dataset often contain multiple objects of the same class (type). In that scenario, our algorithm can be embedded in a parts-based framework such as [12, 13] to speed up the search for object-parts.

Scaling Up to Many Landmarks

Our goal is to detect in the order of thousands of anatomical structures. With such a large number of detectors, the computational savings of our approach would be significant.

Multiple Instance Learning

In order to train a high-performing object detector, often a large amount of exact annotations is needed, which is tedious to obtain. In this chapter, we introduce Multiple Instance Learning (MIL) [26, 30, 52, 56] applied to anatomical landmark detection. The method aims to alleviate the manual annotation burden and to accommodate imprecise annotations. MIL uses instance bags as inputs for training. A positive instance bag contains at least one positive and a negative bag contains all negatives. In landmark detection, we construct a positive bag by placing a bounding box big enough to guarantee that a true positive exists inside the bounding box.

The above construction yields a positive bag with only one or very few positive instances. But traditional "Noisy-OR" rule [52] favors many high scores in a bag. To better cope with the bag construction, we use the soft max function in our formulation. This formulation not only generalizes the integrated segmentation and recognition (ISR) rule [52] but also degenerates to the famous AdaBoost algorithm when each positive bag has exactly one instance. This formulation is amenable to analytical derivation too.

Conventional MIL methods treat instances in a bag independently. This ignores the strong spatial context embedded in the bag construction, that is, neighboring instances are arranged in a grid and hence strongly correlated. For example, Fig. 14 shows two example landmarks of tracheal bifurcation and liver top in a computed tomography (CT) scan. These two landmarks are located at distinct positions with spatial context. We propose to exploit this strong spatial context for better detection. Another practical consideration in landmark detection is the post-processing to select the final results. Thus it is desirable to have a concentrated detection response

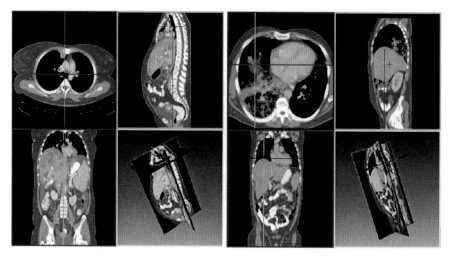

Fig. 14 The landmarks of tracheal bifurcation (*left*) and liver top (*right*) in a medical image featuring rich contextual information

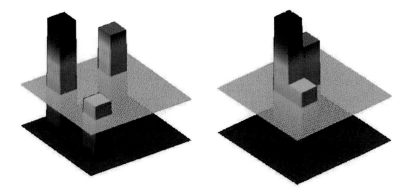

Fig. 15 A good response map should have a concentrated cluster as shown in the right map for better detection confidence. A measure of the tightness is the perimeter of two level sets from two maps, which is encouraged by our TV regularization framework

map, which is explicitly encouraged by our approach, so that the final detection results can be derived with more confidence.

Specifically we propose to use total variation (TV) to spatially regularize the MILBoost, resulting a Boosting algorithm incorporating spatial context and accommodating inexact annotations. Figure 15 illustrates the effect of the TV regularization that favors the output with a concentrated cluster or low perimeter. Finally, for faster detection we also derive empirical rules for pruning training instances.

Related Work on Multiple Instance Learning

The approach in [26] based on neural networks is one of the earliest MIL formulations though the term MIL was not yet used there. This is extended to a boosting context in [52], which proposes a cost function for the MIL problem in the setting of the AnyBoost framework [35]. Further in [52] MILBoost is shown to be superior to AdaBoost when given data with high incertitude. We use a smoothed max-based cost function, whose connection to existing formulations originally proposed in [26, 52] will be discussed later. Aside from these cost-based approaches there are also other attempts to solve the MIL problem, e.g., by modeling likelihood ratios as done in [30].

Spatial reasoning was applied to Boosting in [1], where the predicted label of a pixel (or patch) is influenced by the labels of neighboring pixels (or patches). Adding spatial regularization to Boosting in a non-MIL setting was done in [53]. In [53] the authors were the first to introduce a regularization kernel which is used to obtain base classifiers that output scores based on spatially clustered pixels. This regularization, however, is limited in several aspects. First, in many applications we do not expect discriminating pixels to be spatially clustered.

For example, in face detection the discriminating parts such as eyes, mouth, and nose are quite evenly distributed on the face and not clustered. Second, as [53] treats a non-MIL setting, the spatial regularization there does not exploit spatial relationships of instances in the same positive bag. Third, base classifiers could use features dependent on more than one pixel. We therefore propose a different regularization, which addresses all the above limitations.

Spatially Regularized MIL for Boosting

In MIL, instead of positive training instances we have positive bags. A positive bag with just one instance will be treated exactly like a positive instance in AdaBoost automatically by the formulas below. To make the notation more consistent and without loss of generality we can assume that all negative instances come also in bags with exactly one instance in it. We fix the notation as follows: Let n be the number of bags with corresponding labels $l_i \in \{+1, -1\}$, $i = 1, \ldots, n$. Bag i consists of n_i training instances: $\{x_i^1, \ldots, x_i^{n_i}\}$. The classifier assigns to each training instance a score $f(x_i^j) = y_i^j = \sum_{t=1}^{T} \lambda_t h_t(x_i^j)$, where h_t are the base classifiers, $\lambda_t \in \mathbb{R}$ denote their coefficients, and T is the number of base classifiers.

Formulation

We follow the AnyBoost framework [35] to minimize a cost function for our classifier. The total cost combines two components, the data term D and the regularization term R, into one:

$$C(f) = D(f) + \lambda R(f), \tag{15}$$

where $\lambda \geq 0$ is the weight parameter which denotes how much we want to regularize our results. According to the AnyBoost framework, Boosting may be seen as gradient descent in the space of functions generated by the base classifiers.

In AdaBoost (which is equivalent to all bags having exactly one instance) we assign scores y_i to each instance and then compute $D(f) = \sum_{i=1}^{n} \frac{1}{N_{l_i}} \exp(-l_i y_i)$, where $N_{-1} = \#\{i | 1 \leq i \leq n, \, l_i = -1\}$ and $N_{+1} = \#\{i | 1 \leq i \leq n, \, l_i = +1\}$ is the number of negative and positive bags, respectively. By the normalization, negative and positive bags contribute equally to the cost.

In MILBoost we must modify the cost function only for positive bags. The goal is to assign a score y_i to the whole positive bag and then penalize a low score by adding $\exp(-y_i)$ to the cost function. Ideally we would like to have $y_i = \max_{j=1,\ldots,n_i} y_i^j$. Unfortunately the max function is not differentiable. Therefore we use a smoothed max function with smoothing parameter k:

$$y_i = \frac{1}{k} \log \left(\sum_{j=1}^{n_i} \exp(ky_i^j) \right).$$

This function approaches the max function as the parameter k goes to infinity and is differentiable for all $k > 0$ (we used $k = 3$). Note that this function is the identity when we have exactly one instance in a bag, as is the case for negative bags. It also degenerates to AdaBoost when each positive bag has exactly one instance.

So the cost function for MILBoost is

$$D(f) = \sum_{i=1}^{n} \frac{1}{N_{l_i}} \exp \left(\frac{-l_i}{k} \log \left(\sum_{j=1}^{n_i} \exp(ky_i^j) \right) \right).$$

The gradient for sample x_i^j arising from the data term is then as follows:

$$\nabla D(f)(x_i^j) = \frac{-l_i \exp(-l_i y_i)}{N_{l_i}} \left(\frac{\exp(ky_i^j)}{\sum_{h=1}^{n_i} \exp(ky_i^h)} \right). \tag{16}$$

This formulation achieves two goals: A positive bag has high score exactly when at least one of its instances has high score and low score only when every instance has low score. If we set $k = 1$, the smoothed max function turns out to be equivalent to the integrated segmentation and recognition (ISR) rule [52] in the following sense. The probability for bag i according to the ISR rule is defined as $p_i = \frac{\sum_{j=1}^{n_i} \exp(y_i^j)}{1 + \sum_{j=1}^{n_i} \exp(y_i^j)}$, which is equal to $\sigma(y_i) = \frac{1}{1 + \exp(-y_i)}$, where y_i is the score of bag i computed with the smoothed max function with smoothing parameter $k = 1$ and $\sigma(\cdot)$ is the logistic function. Modeling probabilities as logistics of scores is common in the Boosting literature, see, for example, Eq. (9) in [17].

By using the smoothed max function with a high enough smoothing parameter k, the data term does not favor or penalize any specific distribution of scores inside a positive bag, except that it favors at least one high score. This is in contrast to the "Noisy Or" rule [52] which favors many high scores in a bag. Also the "Noisy Or" rule may be less suited for larger positive bags, which occur naturally when using inexactly annotated datasets in object detection, as then the "Noisy Or" rule will have high probability even when the positive bag has many instances to which the classifier assigns probabilities around 0.5 or a score of 0, respectively. Therefore the smoothed max function is better suited for object detection than the "Noisy Or" rule, as most positive bags only contain very few true positives.

Regularization Term

As was already mentioned, in object detection the classifier should assign high scores in a positive bag to a few clustered locations. To achieve this we propose to add the following Total Variation (TV) regularization: $R = \sum_{i=1}^{n} \frac{1}{n_i} \sum_{j=1}^{n_i} ||\nabla y_i^j||$, where $||\nabla y_i^j||$ is the norm of the discrete gradient. For 2D images or 3D volumes the positive bag most likely will have a grid structure. For 2D images the gradient can be written as $\nabla y_i^j = (y_i^{j_{\mathrm{right}}} - y_i^j, y_i^{j_{\mathrm{lower}}} - y_i^j)^{\mathsf{T}}$, where j_{right} is the index of the instance on the right-hand side of x_i^j and j_{lower} is the index of the instance just below of x_i^j. If the bag does not have a grid structure but consists of discrete points sampled from a manifold, then gradients can be defined as in section 2 of [18]. *Via the regularization, neighboring instances are not trained independently, in contrast to AdaBoost* [15].

The TV regularization allows for sharp peaks in the score map and favors spatially connected subsets of instances to which it assigns high scores. These subsets are favored to have low perimeter. This is also to be expected by the coarea formula: $\int_\Omega ||\nabla y|| dx = \int_{-\infty}^{\infty} P(\{y > t\}, \Omega) dt$, where $P(\{y > t\}, \Omega)$ is the perimeter of the level set $\{x \in \Omega | y(x) > t\}$ in the set Ω. A suitable version of the coarea formula of course also holds for our discrete setting. In other words, a regularized detector will output scores whose level sets have low perimeter. This is visualized in Fig. 15.

The regularization above is not differentiable, though convex. One may therefore either use sub-gradients or a smooth approximation to the above proposed regularization. The latter can be achieved by replacing the norm above by $\sqrt{\sum_{k=1}^{d} (\nabla y_i^j)_k^2 + \epsilon}$, where $\epsilon > 0$ is a constant and d is the dimension. Then the above regularization is smooth also for points with zero gradients. The gradient for sample x_i^j arising from the smoothed regularization term is, in the notation from [18], as follows:

$$\nabla R(f)(x_i^j) = -\operatorname{div}\left(\frac{\nabla y_i^j}{n_i \cdot \sqrt{\sum_{k=1}^{d}(\nabla y_i^j)_k^2 + \epsilon}}\right). \tag{17}$$

Other regularizations are possible. For example, we can use $R = \sum_{i=1}^{n} \sum_{j=1}^{n_i} ||\nabla y_i^j||^2$. This L_2 regularization will result in a classifier which does not vary strongly. This is desirable in case we have bags where neighboring probabilities should be similar.

Pruning in MIL

After training we obtain a series of T base classifiers. Evaluating all of them can be costly during detection, especially when we have trained many base classifiers. To lessen the computational load we propose to set rejection thresholds to reject false negatives early on. This is achieved as follows: Say we have a sample x which we want to classify and we have rejection thresholds $\theta(t)$ for $t \in R \subset \mathbb{N}$. If $t \in R$, $t < T$ and $\sum_{l=1}^{t} \lambda_l h_l(x) < \theta(t)$, then reject x without evaluating the remaining $T - t$ base classifiers. By setting the rejection thresholds we do not want to reject any true instances. In the context of MIL, however, we do not know which instances inside a positive bag have a positive label, so setting rejection thresholds based on them is not straightforward and therefore we cannot use formulas like the one in section 2 of [56], which is applicable only to a non-MIL setting. We generalize the approach in [56] and propose the following rejection thresholds which retain at least one instance in each positive bag:

$$\theta(t) = \min_{\{1 \leq i \leq n, l_i = 1\}} \left[\max_{\{1 \leq j \leq n_i\}} \sum_{s=1}^{t} \lambda_s h_s(x_i^j) \right]. \tag{18}$$

This is a good choice when we know that a bag contains usually one true positive, as is often the case in object detection, see also the discussion in the introduction. One can adapt the formula above in a straightforward manner for cases when we want to retain a certain number of instances from a positive bag. The complete algorithm is described in Fig. 16.

Comparing MILBoost with and Without Spatial Regularization

First, we detect the tracheal bifurcation as in Fig. 14 with 274 training datasets: 80 bags with one instance (which originate from exact annotations from an expert) and 194 bags with 1,000 instances each, of which one denotes the true (but unknown) position of our landmark. Our negative instances are sampled from the images at all positions different from the locations of instances in the positive bags. Our base classifiers are histograms over rectangle features as in [48]. The second experiment concerns the liver top, also shown in Fig. 14. Because the upper side of the liver is rather flat, it is difficult to annotate it precisely, rendering a difficult detection task. We used 300 training datasets: 100 annotations as accurate as possible and 200 positive bags with 1,000 examples inside each bag. For testing we consider an instance to be positive if it is not more than 2.5 mm away from the exact object location. Datasets cover different contrast phases and diseased livers. For comparison we consider MILBoost with no spatial regularization (this

Input

- Training bags $(l_1, x_1^1, \ldots x_1^{n_1}), \ldots, (l_n, x_n^1, \ldots, x_n^{n_n})$.

- T, the total number of base classifiers and λ, the weight for the spatial regularization in (15).

Initialization

- Take all positive bags and sample negative bags to form the subset Q for training.

- Define sampling intervals A, for example as $A = \{20, 40, 80, \ldots\}$.

Learning For $t = 1, \ldots, T$:

1. For all samples in Q set the gradients $\nabla C(f)(x_i^j) = \nabla D(f)(x_i^j) + \lambda \nabla R(f)(x_i^j)$ for $f = \sum_{k=1}^{t-1} \lambda_k h_k$ according to (16) and (17).

2. Select h_t as the base classifier with the lowest associated gradient $\sum_{i=1}^{n} \sum_{j=1}^{n_i} \nabla C(f)(x_i^j) h_t(x_i^j)$ and select λ_t, the weighting parameter for h_t, by line search to achieve a decrease in the cost function $C(f + \lambda_t h_t)$ from (15). Set $f = f + \lambda_t h_t$.

3. If $t \in A$:

   - Compute scores for all negative instances using the already trained classifiers

   - (Optional) Perform weight trimming [16] to trim off 10% of the negatives in Q.

   - Include in Q negative bags with high scores from all training instances to replace the negative instances which were trimmed off.

Output Series of base classifiers with rejection thresholds $\theta(t)$ as in (18).

Fig. 16 The algorithm of MILBoost with spatial regularization

corresponds to setting $\lambda = 0$ in Eq. (15)) and MILBoost with spatial regularization. Our specific choice of λ was chosen by cross-validation.

Figure 17 shows the ROC curves for MILBoost with and without spatial regularization for the two experiments. We tested the two methods on 100 test samples in the first experiment and on 300 test samples in the second experiment. A sample is counted as positive if it has a score higher than a certain threshold. The better ROC curve arising from the regularization is attributed to the fact that many high scores are penalized and therefore a lesser number of instances far from the true position of the object are assigned high scores. In Fig. 18 we show score maps to illustrate the influence of the regularization, which results in a more concentrated cluster of high scores and a final detection with more confidence.

Detection with Zero Annotations

In this experiment, we leverage the rich anatomical contextual information manifested in human body to test the idea whether we can use one landmark to provide "virtual" annotations for the learning and detection of another landmark. This way we learn the detector with zero annotation.

Fig. 17 The ROC curves for MILBoost with and without spatial regularization; top figure for the tracheal bifurcation; bottom figure for the liver top

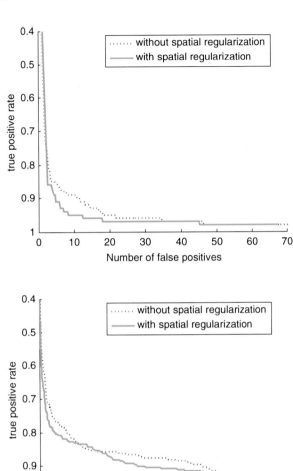

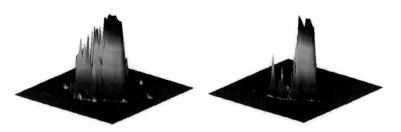

Fig. 18 The 2D slice of a score map for a classifier trained by MILBoost on the liver top dataset without spatial regularization (*left*) and MILBoost with spatial regularization (*right*). Note that the spatially regularized classifier will result in a lower false positive rate because it has fewer high scores and these are clustered tighter around the object's true position

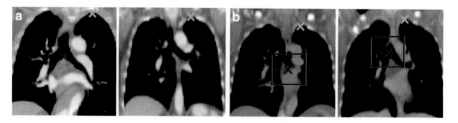

Fig. 19 The *crosses* indicate annotated positions with *blue* for left lung apex and *red* for tracheal bifurcation. Note that this is a 2D illustration; but the real system operates in 3D. (**a**) Exact annotations. (**b**) Virtual annotations

	Naive	PBT [48]	MILBoost [52]	**MILBoost with Spatial Reg.**
Q50	16.4	20.3	12.1	**6.6**
Q95	31.9	42.1	40.4	**21.4**
Mean	17.7	21.8	16.3	**8.4**
Max	100.9	42.8	49.6	**36.8**

Fig. 20 The error distance (in mm) in detecting the tracheal bifurcation landmark detection using virtual annotations

We experiment using the left lung apex and the tracheal bifurcation. From training data statistics, we know that the average translational shift from the left lung apex to the tracheal bifurcation is $[-48, -6, -88]$ mm. We simply shift the 200 lung apex annotations by such a constant amount to obtain "virtual" annotations for the tracheal bifurcation. The positive bag is formed as in Fig. 19. The same testing set is used as in the previous tracheal bifurcation detection task.

Figure 20 shows that the proposed MILBoost with spatial regularization consistently outperforms the other three methods: the naive method that evaluates the accuracy of the constant shift, the Probabilistic Boosting Tree (PBT) method [48], and the conventional MILBoost method [52]. To derive the final detected location, we used the mode of the response map. Figure 21 confirms the same finding both using plots and by visual inspection.

Summary

We first introduced a fast and accurate method to detect landmarks in 3D CT data. It is a state-of-the-art method in terms of detection speed and accuracy. The improvements to prior work arise from the leverage of holistic contextual information in the medical data via the use of an approximate nearest neighbor matching to quickly identify the most similar database volume and transfer its landmark positions, and the exploitation of unary and pairwise context via a submodular formulation that

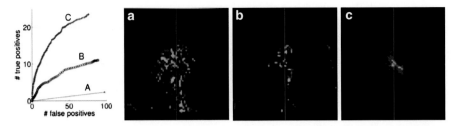

Fig. 21 The landmark detection performance and the instance score maps (2D cross-section) for the tracheal bifurcation detectors: (**a**) PBT [48], (**b**) conventional MILBoost [52], and (**c**) the proposed MILBoost with spatial regularization. The original test image is the left one in Fig. 19a. *Red* indicates highest detector response, followed by *green and blue*. In AdaBoost, many false positives are found far away from the ground truth position (center of image). The proposed method has the sharpest peak around the ground truth

aims to minimize the total computation for detecting landmark(s) and renders itself to a computationally efficiently greedy algorithm. The method has been successively validated on a database of 2,500 CT volumes. The method can be applied to different modalities such as MRI.

We then introduced a spatially regularized Multiple Instance Boosting algorithm which performs well on data which is annotated poorly. The proposed spatial regularization helps to incorporate the needed spatial context when dealing with inaccurately labeled data and gives better results than prior work when using few or even zero annotations.

Future directions include investigating the possibility to "convexify" the cost function [30]. This might result in an overall convex cost function, as our regularization is convex, too. In terms of application, one can incorporate the spatially regularized multiple instance learning algorithm in a tracking framework [2] for tracking medical devices such as catheters and guidewires in intervention procedures.

References

1. Avidan S (2006) Spatialboost: Adding spatial reasoning to adaboost. In: Proceedings of European conference on computer vision. Lecture notes in computer science, vol 3954. Springer, pp 386–396
2. Babenko B, Yang M-H, Belongie S (2009) Visual tracking with online multiple instance learning. In: IEEE conference on computer vision and pattern recognition, 2009 (CVPR 2009). IEEE
3. Beck T, Bernhardt D, Biermann C, Dillmann R (2010) Validation and detection of vessel landmarks by using anatomical knowledge. In: Proceedings of SPIE medical imaging. SPIE
4. Besag J (1986) On the statistical analysis of dirty pictures. J R Statist Soc B-48:259–302
5. Bishop CM (2006) Pattern recognition and machine learning, Springer, Berlin, p 383
6. Boyd S, Vandenberghe L (2004) Convex optimization. Cambridge University Press, Cambridge

7. Cornuejols G, Fischer M, Nemhauser G (1977) On the uncapacitated location problem. Ann Discrete Math 1:163–178
8. Criminisi A, Shotton J, Bucciarelli S (2009) Decision forests with long-range spatial context for organ localization in CT volumes. In: MICCAI workshop on Prob. Models for MIA. MICCAI
9. Crum WR, Phil D, Hartkens T, Hill D (2004) Non-rigid image registration: theory and practice. Br J Radiol 77:140–153
10. Datar PIM, Immorlica N, Mirrokni V (2004) Locality sensitive hashing scheme based on p-stable distributions. In: Proceedings of the symposium on computational geometry. ACM
11. Duda RO, Hart PE (1972) Use of the Hough transformation to detect lines and curves in pictures. Comm ACM 15:11–15
12. Felzenszwalb PF, Girshick RB, McAllester D, Ramanan D (2010) Object detection with discriminatively trained part-based models. IEEE Trans Pattern Anal Mach Intell 32(9):1627–1645
13. Felzenszwalb P, Huttenlocher D (2005) Pictorial structures for object recognition. Int J Comput Vision 61(1):55–79
14. Fleuret F, Geman D (2001) Coarse-to-fine face detection. Int J Comput Vision 41:85–107
15. Freund Y, Schapire R (1997) A decision-theoretic generalization of on-line learning and an application to boosting. J Comput Syst Sci 55:119–139
16. Friedman J, Bentley LJ, Finkel RA (1977) An algorithm for finding best matches in logarithmic expected time. ACM Trans Math Software 3(3):209–226
17. Friedman J, Hastie T, Tibshirani R (2000) Additive logistic regression: a statistical view of boosting. Ann Statist 38(2)
18. Gilboa G, Osher S (2008) Nonlocal operators with applications to image processing. Multiscale Model Simulat 7(3):1005–1028
19. Goemans MX, Williamson DP (1995) Improved approximation algorithms for maximum cut and satisfiability problems using semidefinite programming. J ACM 42:1115–1145
20. Grimson W (1990) Object recognition by computer: the role of geometric constraints. MIT Press, 1990.
21. Hinton G (1999) Products of experts. In: International conference on artificial neural networks (ICANN). ICANN
22. Izard C, Jedynak B, Stark CEL (2006) Spline-based probabilistic model for anatomical landmark detection. In: Proceedings of MICCAI. MICCAI
23. Jacobs R, Jordan MI, Hinton GE (1991) Mixtures of expert networks. Neural Comput 3:79–87
24. Jegou H, Douze M, Schmid C (2011) Product quantization for nearest neighbor search. IEEE Trans Pattern Anal Mach Intell 33:117–128
25. Johnson H, Christensen G (2002) Consistent landmark and intensity-based image registration. IEEE Trans Med Imag 21(5):450–461
26. Keeler JD, Rumelhart DE, Leow W (1990) In: NIPS, pp 557–563
27. Kittler J, Hatef M, Duin R, Matas J (1998) On combining classifiers. IEEE Trans Pattern Anal Mach Intell 20:226–239
28. Krause A, Guestrin C (2005) Near-optimal nonmyopic value of information in graphical models. In: Conference on uncertainty in artificial intelligence (UAI)
29. Lampert CH, Blaschko MB, Hofmann T (2008) Beyond sliding windows: Object localization by efficient subwindow search. In: IEEE conference on computer vision and pattern recognition
30. Li F, Sminchisescu C (2010) Convex multiple instance learning by estimating likelihood ratio. In: NIPS
31. Liu D, Zhou SK (2012) Anatomical landmark detection using nearest neighbor matching and submodular optimization. In: MICCAI
32. Liu D, Zhou SK, Bernhardt D, Comaniciu D (2010) Search strategies for multiple landmark detection by submodular maximization. In: Proc CVPR. IEEE
33. Lloyd S (1982) Least square quantization in pcm. IEEE Trans Inform Theory 28:129–137

34. Lovasz L (1983) Submodular functions and convexity, Springer, Berlin, pp 235–257
35. Mason L, Baxter J, Bartlett P, Frean M (2000) Boosting algorithms as gradient descent. In: NIPS, MIT, New York, pp 512–518
36. Nemhauser G, Wolsey L, Fisher M (1978) An analysis of the approximations for maximizing submodular set functions. Math Program 14:265–294
37. Okada T, Shimada R, Sato Y, Hori M, Yokota K, Nakamoto M, Chen Y, Nakamura H, Tamura S (2007) Automated segmentation of the liver from 3d ct images using probabilistic atlas and multilevel statistical shape model. In: Proceedings of MICCAI. MICCAI, pp 86–93
38. Pauly O et al (2011) Fast multiple organs detection and localization in whole-body mr dixon sequences. In: Proceedings of MICCAI. MICCAI
39. Peng Z, Zhan Y, Zhou XS, Krishnan A (2009) Robust anatomy detection from ct topograms. In: Proceedings of SPIE medical imaging. SPIE
40. Rangayyan R, Banik S, Rangayyan R, Boag G (2009) Landmarking and segmentation of 3D CT images. Morgan & Claypool Publishers, Los Altos
41. Roy N, Earnest C (2006) Dynamic action spaces for information gain maximization in search and exploration. In: American control conference. IEEE pp 6–11
42. Schrijver A (2000) A combinatorial algorithm minimizing submodular functions in strongly polynomial time. J Combinat Theory B(80):346–355
43. Schrijver A (2003) Combinatorial optimization, polyhedra and efficiency. Springer, Berlin
44. Seifert S et al (2009) Hierarchical parsing and semantic navigation of full body ct data. In: SPIE medical imaging. SPIE
45. Seifert S, Kelm M, Moeller M, Mukherjee S, Cavallaro A, Huber M, Comaniciu D (2010) Semantic annotation of medical images. In: SPIE medical imaging. SPIE
46. Sochman J, Matas J (2005) Waldboost - learning for time constrained sequential detection. In: IEEE conference on computer vision and pattern recognition. IEEE
47. Torralba A (2003) Contextual priming for object detection. Int J Comp Vis 53:169–191
48. Tu Z (2005) Probabilistic boosting-tree: Learning discriminative models for classification, recognition, and clustering. In: ICCV
49. Tu Z (2005) Probabilistic boosting-tree: Learning discriminative models for classification, recognition, and clustering. IEEE Int Conf Comput Vision 1589–1596
50. Viola P, Jones M (2004) Robust real-time face detection. Int J Comp Vis 57:137–154
51. Viola P, Platt J, Zhang C (2005) Multiple instance boosting for object detection. In: Proceedings of advances in neural information processing systems (NIPS). NIPS
52. Viola PA, Platt JC, Zhang C (2006) Multiple instance boosting for object detection. In: NIPS. MIT, Cambridge, pp 1417–1424
53. Xiang Z, Xi Y, Hasson U, Ramadge P (2009) Boosting with spatial regularization. In: NIPS, pp 2107–2115
54. Weiss A, Fergus TYR (2008) Spectral hashing. In: Advances in neural information processing systems
55. Zhan Y, Zhou X, Peng Z, Krishnan A (2008) Active scheduling of organ detection and segmentation in whole-body medical images. In: MICCAI
56. Zhang C, Viola PA (2008) Multiple-instance pruning for learning efficient cascade detectors. In: NIPS, Cambridge, pp 1681–1688
57. Zheng Y, Georgescu B, Ling H, Zhou S, Scheuering M, Comaniciu D (2009) Constrained marginal space learning for efficient 3D anatomical structure detection in medical images. In: IEEE conference on computer vision and pattern recognition. IEEE
58. Zhou SK (2010) Shape regression machine and efficient segmentation of left ventricle endocardium from 2d b-mode echocardiogram. Med Image Anal 14:563–81

Biography

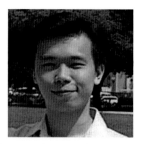

David Liu has been with Siemens Corporation, Corporate Technology, Princeton, New Jersey, since 2008, where he is a Technical Project Manager. He received the B.S. and M.S. degrees in electrical engineering from the National Taiwan University in 1999 and 2001, and Ph.D. in computer engineering from Carnegie Mellon University in 2008. He was a research intern at Microsoft Live Labs Research, Bellevue, Washington, in 2007. He is a recipient of the Outstanding Teaching Assistant Award from the ECE Department at Carnegie Mellon University in 2006, the Taiwan Merit Scholarship in 2005, the best paper award from the Chinese Automatic Control Society in 2001, the Garmin Scholarship in 2001 and 2000, and the Philips Semiconductors Scholarship in 1999.

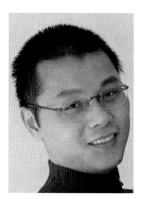

S. Kevin Zhou has been with Siemens Corporation, Corporate Technology, Princeton, New Jersey, since 2004, where he is Research Group Head. His main research interests include computer vision and image understanding, theoretic and applied machine learning, statistical computing and inference, and their applications to medical image analysis, biometrics, and multimedia. He received the Ph.D. degree in Electrical Engineering from University of Maryland College Park in 2004. He received the M.Eng. degree in Computer Engineering from National University of Singapore in 2000, and the B.Eng. degree in Electronic Engineering from University of Science and Technology of China in 1994. He has published two research monographs, one edited book, 25 journal papers and book chapters, over 100 peer-reviewed conference papers, 27 granted/published patents, and over 100 filled patent applications. He is a senior member of IEEE.

About the Editors

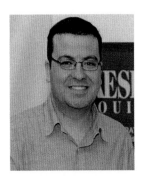

Ayman El-Baz, Ph.D., is Associate Professor in the Department of Bioengineering at the University of Louisville, KY. Dr. El-Baz has 14 years of hands-on experience in the fields of bioimaging modeling and computer-assisted diagnostic systems. He has developed new techniques for analyzing 3D medical images. His work has been reported at several prestigious international conferences (e.g., CVPR, ICCV, and MICCAI) and in journals (e.g., IEEE TIP, IEEE TBME, IEEE TITB, and Brain). His work related to novel image analysis techniques for lung cancer and autism diagnosis have earned him multiple awards, including first place at the annual Research Louisville 2002, 2005, 2006, 2007, 2008, 2010, 2011, and 2012 meetings, and the "Best Paper Award in Medical Image Processing" from the prestigious ICGST International Conference on Graphics, Vision and Image Processing (GVIP-2005). Dr. El-Baz has authored or coauthored more than 300 technical articles.

A.S. El-Baz et al. (eds.), *Abdomen and Thoracic Imaging: An Engineering & Clinical Perspective*, DOI 10.1007/978-1-4614-8498-1,
© Springer Science+Business Media New York 2014

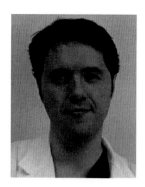

Luca Saba received the M.D. from the University of Cagliari, Italy, in 2002. Today he works in the A.O.U. of Cagliari. Dr. Saba research fields are focused on Multi-Detector-Row Computed Tomography, Magnetic Resonance, Ultrasound, Neuro-radiology, and Diagnostic in Vascular Sciences.

His works, as lead author, include more than 100 high impact factor, peer-reviewed, Journals as *American Journal of Neuroradiology, Atherosclerosis, European Radiology, European Journal of Radiology, Acta Radiologica, Cardiovascular and Interventional Radiology, Journal of Computer Assisted Tomography, American Journal of Roentgenology, Neuroradiology, Clinical Radiology, Journal of Cardiovascular Surgery, Cerebrovascular Diseases.* He is well-known speaker and has spoken over 45 times at national and international levels.

Dr. Saba has won 15 scientific and extracurricular awards during his career. Dr. Saba presented more than 450 papers and posters in National and International Congress (RSNA, ESGAR, ECR, ISR, AOCR, AINR, JRS, SIRM, AINR). He wrote nine book chapters and he is Editor of six books in the field of Computed Tomography, Cardiovascular, Plastic Surgery, Gynecological Imaging, and Neuro-degenerative imaging.

He is member of the Italian Society of Radiology (SIRM), European Society of Radiology (ESR), Radiological Society of North America (RSNA), American Roentgen Ray Society (ARRS), and European Society of Neuroradiology (ESNR) and serves as Reviewer of more than 30 scientific Journals.

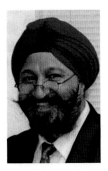

Dr. Jasjit S. Suri is an innovator, scientist, a visionary, an industrialist, and an internationally known world leader in Biomedical Engineering. Dr. Suri has spent over 20 years in the field of biomedical engineering/devices and its management. He received his Doctorate from University of Washington, Seattle and Business Management Sciences from Weatherhead, Case Western Reserve University, Cleveland, Ohio. Dr. Suri was crowned with Director Generals Gold medal in 1980 and the Fellow of American Institute of Medical and Biological Engineering for his outstanding contributions.

Index

A.S. El-Baz et al. (eds.), *Abdomen and Thoracic Imaging: An Engineering
& Clinical Perspective*, DOI 10.1007/978-1-4614-8498-1,
© Springer Science+Business Media New York 2014

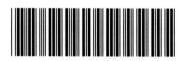